MICRONUTRIENT INTERACTIONS: VITAMINS, MINERALS, AND HAZARDOUS ELEMENTS

ANNALS OF THE NEW YORK ACADEMY OF SCIENCES

Volume 355

MICRONUTRIENT INTERACTIONS: VITAMINS, MINERALS, AND HAZARDOUS ELEMENTS

Edited by O. A. Levander and Lorraine Cheng

The New York Academy of Sciences
New York, New York
1980

Library of Congress Cataloging in Publication Data

Main entry under title:

Micronutrient interactions:

(Annals of the New York Academy of Sciences; v. 355)

Proceedings of a conference held Feb. 20–22, 1980 by the New York Academy of Sciences.

1. Vitamin metabolism—Congresses. 2. Trace element metabolism—Congresses. 3. Mineral metabolism—Congresses. 4. Metals—Toxicology—Congresses. I. Levander, O. A. II. Cheng, Lorraine. III. New York Academy of Sciences. IV. Series: New York Academy of Sciences. Annals; v. 355. Q11.N5 vol. 355 [QP771] 500s [612'.399] 80–25622
ISBN 0-89766-099-4
ISBN 0-89766-100-1 (pbk.)

CCP
Printed in the United States of America
ISBN 0–89766–099–4 (Cloth)
0–89766–100–1 (Paper)

ANNALS OF THE NEW YORK ACADEMY OF SCIENCES

VOLUME 355

December 1, 1980

MICRONUTRIENT INTERACTIONS: VITAMINS, MINERALS, AND HAZARDOUS ELEMENTS*

Editors and Conference Chairmen
O. A. LEVANDER and LORRAINE CHENG

CONTENTS

* This volume is the result of a conference entitled Micronutrient Interactions: Vitamins, Minerals, and Hazardous Elements, held on February 20–22, 1980 by The New York Academy of Sciences.

Financial assistance was received from:

- ABBOTT LABORATORIES
- HOFFMANN-LA ROCHE, INC.
- LEDERLE LABORATORIES
- MEAD JOHNSON NUTRITIONAL DIVISION
- NATIONAL INSTITUTES OF HEALTH
- NATIONAL SCIENCE FOUNDATION
- THE QUAKER OATS COMPANY
- SCIENCE AND EDUCATION ADMINISTRATION, USDA
- USV LABORATORIES

INTRODUCTORY REMARKS

Orville A. Levander

Vitamin and Mineral Nutrition Laboratory
Beltsville Human Nutrition Research Center
U.S. Department of Agriculture
Science and Education Administration
Beltsville, Maryland 20705

Nutrition and toxicology are attracting increasing attention from both health science professionals and the general public because of the relationship of these disciplines to the alleviation of certain human diseases and to the maintenance of good health. Unfortunately, the biological effects of most nutrients and toxicants are often studied only in isolation with little regard for interacting effects with other nutrients or hazardous elements. This reductionistic approach is probably due to the fact that most scientists are specialists who prefer to design and conduct unifactorial experiments. And yet people are constantly exposed to multiple nutritional and/or toxicological insults, so that the justification for multifactorial studies is apparent.

In the past, numerous conferences have discussed specific vitamins, minerals, or hazardous elements, but few meetings have considered the possible interactions among these substances. The purpose of the conference reported herein was to deal specifically with relationships among vitamins, minerals, and hazardous elements, and this was the first meeting organized especially to do so. Scientists who had done outstanding work with such interactions were assembled to allow for exchange and cross-fertilization of ideas and to encourage new investigators to initiate research in this field.

Historically, certain interactions—such as those of vitamin D and calcium, of copper, molybdenum, and sulfur, or of lead and calcium—have long been recognized and have generated considerable research. However, recent progress in the study of these interactions has greatly increased our understanding of their mechanisms at the biochemical level. Therefore, a discussion of these interactions seemed highly appropriate at this time.

The conference also seemed timely because of the growing realization among decision makers and standard setters of the need for a more general and integrative approach to nutritional and toxicological problems that takes into account relationships among several different factors. In the field of standard setting, for example, the requirement for a nutrient or the hazard of a poison cannot be determined without taking into account how these substances might interact with one another. Interactions of this type—which were discussed on the program and are of great current interest—include the effect of vitamin C on the nutritional availability of iron, the chemical reaction of nitrites with vitamins C and E, and the interaction of selenium and mercury.

The scope of the conference was limited to interactions of vitamins, minerals, and hazardous elements. Although a broader discussion of relationships among nutrients and toxicants would have been of interest, such an expanded conference would have been unwieldy at best. It is hoped that the conference, while admittedly limited in scope, will nonetheless promote thinking about interactions generally and help define, direct, and encourage research in an area on the threshold of rapid development. It is also anticipated that the published proceedings of this conference will serve as a valuable teaching tool, since no comparable compendium of information on interactions now exists.

THE CONTROL OF CALCIUM AND PHOSPHORUS METABOLISM BY THE VITAMIN D ENDOCRINE SYSTEM*

Hector F. DeLuca

Department of Biochemistry
College of Agricultural and Life Sciences
University of Wisconsin
Madison, Wisconsin 53706

Introduction

In 1919 Sir Edward Mellanby conclusively demonstrated the existence of a dietary factor responsible for the mineralization of bone.[1] McCollum and Steenbock carried out experiments showing the existence of a fat-soluble vitamin different from vitamin A that was responsible for mineralizing bone and the promotion of growth.[2,3] However, Huldshinsky and Chick provided clinical evidence that ultraviolet irradiation of rachitic children could result in the healing of the rachitic lesions.[4,5] Steenbock and Black then provided a clear demonstration that vitamin D could be generated not only in skin but also in food by ultraviolet irradiation of the sterol fractions.[6] This provided the necessary biochemical evidence for the fortification of food and the prevention of the widespread disease rickets. It also served as the groundwork for Askew *et al.* and Windaus and collaborators for the chemical isolation and identification of the mineralizing vitamin.[7,8]

Howland and Kramer investigated the necessity of vitamin D for the mineralization of bone and demonstrated quite clearly that a major reason for mineralization of bone in response to vitamin D is the elevation of plasma calcium and phosphorus concentrations.[9-11] More recent work by Neuman and collaborators revealed that plasma is normally supersaturated with calcium and phosphorus and the hydroxyapatite component of bone, whereas the serum of vitamin D–deficient animals is undersaturated.[12] Thus the major support of bone mineralization appeared to be the result of elevated plasma calcium and phosphorus concentrations.[13] On the other hand, there is clinical evidence to suggest that in addition to the elevation of plasma calcium and phosphorus concentrations, vitamin D may play a direct role in the mineralization process. Thus far, evidence for this concept is lacking, and it remains an open possibility. The current view is that vitamin D functions in mineralizing bone primarily by regulating calcium and phosphorus concentrations.

In addition to the regulation of plasma calcium and phosphorus levels, a role for vitamin D in the regulation of intestinal calcium absorption in response to needs for calcium has also been conclusively demonstrated.[14,15] Nicolaysen demonstrated that in animals or men deprived of calcium, the efficiency of absorption of calcium became markedly elevated, a process dependent upon the presence of vitamin D.[16] Inasmuch as the efficiency of calcium absorption remained elevated in animals as long as the skeleton required the calcium, Nicolaysen concluded that there must be some humoral factor elaborated that would inform the intestine of the skeletal needs

* This work was supported in part by Program Project Grant No. AM-14881 from the National Institutes of Health, Grant No. NAS9-15580 from the National Aeronautics and Space Administration, and the Harry Steenbock Fund of the Wisconsin Alumni Research Foundation.

0077-8923/80/0355-0001 $01.75/0 © 1980, NYAS

for calcium. He termed this "Nicolaysen's Endogenous Factor."[16] This endogenous factor has, at least in part, been demonstrated to be a vitamin D-dependent mechanism.[17,18]

During the past 15 years it has been conclusively demonstrated that to carry out these important regulations, vitamin D must be metabolically altered.[19,20] This alteration takes place first in the liver and subsequently in the kidney to produce a hormone, 1,25-dihydroxyvitamin D_3 [1,25-$(OH)_2D_3$]. The 1,25-$(OH)_2D_3$ functions to regulate plasma calcium, plasma phosphorus, and intestinal absorption of calcium. Pursuit of this investigation has led to the discovery of a major calcium- and phosphorus-regulating endocrine system, localized in the kidney, that elaborates a hormone derived from vitamin D to carry out these functions.

The Physiologic Sites of Action of Vitamin D in Regulating Calcium and Phosphorus Metabolism

To maintain the plasma calcium level at 10 mg/100 ml, calcium must be pumped from the intestinal lumen, the renal tubular fluid, and the bone fluid compartment to the extracellular fluid compartment.[19,20] In general, metabolic energy is required to drive these thermodynamically unfavorable reactions. This process has been clearly shown to be an active transport mechanism in the intestine.[21,22] It is almost certain that in the bone this is an active transport mechanism, although it has not been clearly demonstrated because of technical difficulties. Intestinal calcium transport or absorption is under direct control by the functional form of vitamin D.[19-21] Throughout the small intestine and even in segments of the large intestine, vitamin D stimulates the active transport of calcium against an electrochemical potential gradient.[21,22] When this system does not supply sufficient amounts of calcium, as for example under conditions of low calcium diets, calcium must be made available from other sources to meet the needs of the plasma. In the kidney, 99% of the filtered load of calcium is reabsorbed even in the absence of vitamin D and the parathyroid hormone (PTH).[23] The remaining 1% is under the control of these two humoral agents, although there is still some controversy regarding whether the active form of vitamin D is involved in the distal tubular conservation of the remaining 1% of the filtered load of calcium.[23-25] The major source of calcium available to support plasma calcium concentration in the absence of adequate amounts coming from the intestine is the bone fluid compartment.[26] The active form of vitamin D is believed to act together with PTH to mobilize calcium from the bone fluid compartment to the plasma compartment.[27] PTH is likely the major controlling factor in this process, although the presence of the active form of vitamin D is required for full expression of PTH in this system.[27]

In addition to its role in the calcium transport mechanisms, vitamin D is known to elevate plasma phosphate concentrations.[19,20] This is primarily carried out by stimulating intestinal transport of phosphate.[28-30] This system has been shown to be an active transport process involving the transfer of phosphate against an electrochemical potential gradient.[31] This system is quite independent of the calcium transport system activated by the same hormonal form of vitamin D. Although there has been a great deal of effort placed on determining whether vitamin D plays a role in renal tubular conservation of phosphate, this controversial question has not been resolved; but the current evidence suggests that vitamin D and its metabolites are not involved in the renal reabsorption of phosphate.[19,20] Phosphate is mobilized from bone together with calcium by the mechanism just discussed for calcium. These are the primary sites whereby vitamin D or its active form is involved in carrying out the regulation of calcium and phosphorus metabolism. FIGURE 1 illustrates diagrammatically the sites of action of vitamin D and PTH.

FUNCTIONAL METABOLISM OF VITAMIN D

Upon the administration of vitamin D to a vitamin D-deficient animal, some 20 hours are required before the intestine begins to transport calcium against an electrochemical potential gradient.[32] This inordinately long lag period was the chief clue that led to the discovery that vitamin D must be metabolized before function. With the synthesis of radioactive vitamin D of high specific activity, completed in the early 1960s, came the possibility of investigating the metabolism and transport of vitamin D.[33,34] Using this material and new methods of chromatography, it was demonstrated that vitamin D is metabolized to biologically active metabolites prior to the initiation of responses in the intestine and bone.[35] A crash program was then initiated, leading ultimately to the isolation in pure form of the first active form of vitamin D in 1968.[36] It was chemically identified as 25-hydroxyvitamin D_3 (25-OH-D_3) (see FIGURE 2).[36] It soon became evident that this compound must be metabolized further before function; and in 1970 and 1971, the major metabolite of 25-OH-D_3—found in the intestine of vitamin D-deficient animals given a single radioactive dose of vitamin D_3—was isolated in pure form.[37] By means of chemical and physical methods, it was unequivocally identified as 1,25-$(OH)_2D_3$.[37] Both of these metabolites were chemically synthesized to confirm their structures and to make quantities available for biological testing.[38,39]

25-OH-D_3 is formed primarily in the liver by a microsomal mixed-function monoxygenase that requires magnesium ions, molecular oxygen, and a cytosolic factor.[40-43] This microsomal system has been solubilized and its components isolated and reconstituted to reveal that this is a two-component mixed-function monooxygenase.[94] In addition to the microsomal 25-hydroxylase, apparently sterol mitochondrial 25-hydroxylase will also react to hydroxylate vitamin D to

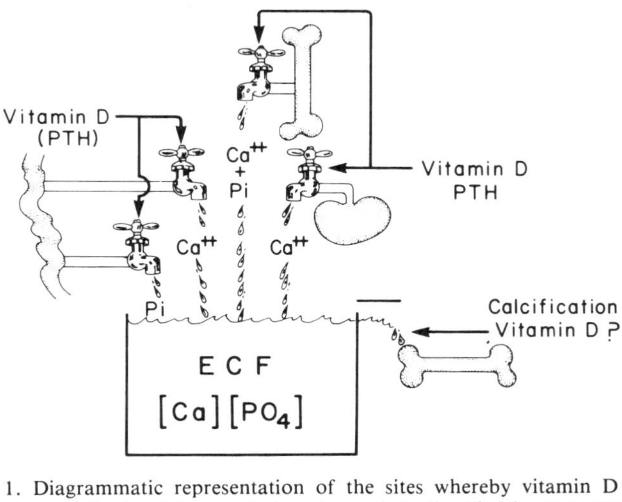

FIGURE 1. Diagrammatic representation of the sites whereby vitamin D functions to facilitate the transport of calcium and phosphorus into the blood compartment (ECF) in preparation for the calcification of bone.

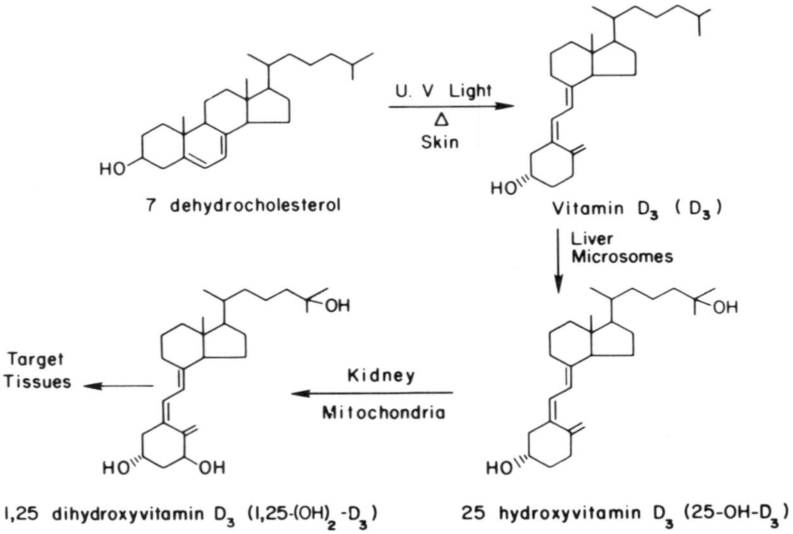

FIGURE 2. Biogenesis and functional metabolism of vitamin D_3.

25-OH-D.[43,44] However, this reaction has a very high Michaelis constant for vitamin D and likely functions only under conditions of high vitamin D dosage. In addition to these two 25-hydroxylase enzymes, some 25-hydroxylation of vitamin D has been demonstrated to occur in intestine and kidney.[45,46] Quantitatively these sites of 25-hydroxylation appear small, and furthermore, vitamin D accumulates markedly in the liver prior to appearance of 25-OH-D in the plasma.[47] Therefore it seems likely that the liver is the major site of 25-hydroxylation. 25-OH-D_3 is transported to the kidney where it undergoes its second obligatory modification.[37,48,49] This modification is carried out by mitochondrial three-component mixed-function monooxygenase.[50,51] The components of this system are shown in FIGURE 3. In this system, nicotinamide-adenine dinucleotide phosphate (NADPH) is generated internally in the mitochondria from operation of the tricarboxylic acid cycle and energy-dependent transhydrogenation. NADPH then brings about reduction of a flavoprotein called renal ferredoxin reductase. This in turn reduces an iron sulfur protein called renal ferredoxin. This component has been isolated in homogeneous form and shown to be a protein having a molecular weight (MW) of 11,800 and containing two-iron, two-sulfur clusters.[52] This iron sulfur protein in turn reduces a cytochrome P-450 that is specific for 25-OH-D_3. The P-450 utilizes molecular oxygen and incorporates one atom of oxygen into the 1α-position to form 1,25-$(OH)_2D_3$. This enzyme is found exclusively in the kidney and exclusively in the mitochondrial fraction in all higher animals except pregnant females.[48,49,53] The placenta, as well as the kidney, of pregnant females contains 25-OH-D_3-1α-hydroxylase.[54] Why the enzyme is found in the placenta is unknown at the present time.

In addition to noting these two obligatory hydroxylases for vitamin D, it is important to draw attention to an important reaction occurring in skin under normal physiologic circumstances. Unique among the vitamins is the fact that vitamin D is formed in skin under adequate exposure to ultraviolet light. 7-Dehydrocholesterol, found in abundant quantities in the epidermis, undergoes a chemical photolysis to form previtamin D_3 (not shown in FIGURE 2).[55,56] Previtamin D_3 is slowly converted

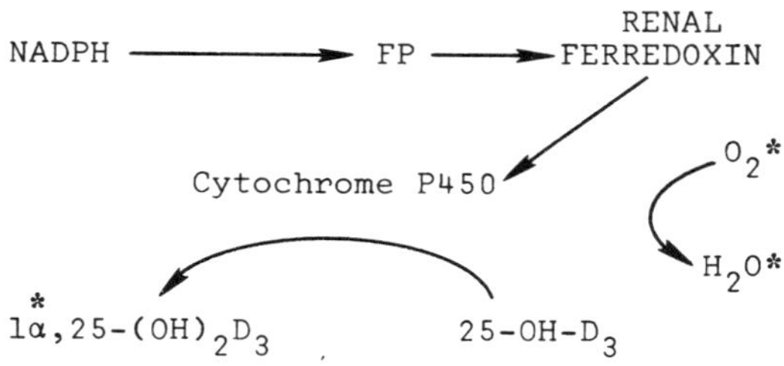

FIGURE 3. Components of the 25-OH-D_3-1α-hydroxylase of chicken kidney.

to vitamin D_3 in the skin.[55,57] Vitamin D_3 is then bound by the plasma transport protein and transported to the liver where it undergoes 25-hydroxylation. The transport protein for vitamin D has a molecular weight of 52,000 and is responsible for the transport of all of the vitamin D compounds known.[58-60] This protein is identical with the group specific protein isolated years before the metabolism of vitamin D was elucidated.[61] In any case, it is evident that under conditions of adequate amounts of sunlight or ultraviolet exposure, vitamin D is not required in the diet and hence cannot be considered as a dietary essential under these circumstances.

The essentiality of the conversions described in FIGURE 2 is illustrated by the fact that when they are anephric, vitamin D–deficient animals do not respond in terms of intestinal calcium transport or bone calcium mobilization to physiologic doses of vitamin D or 25-OH-D.[62,63] On the other hand, they respond equally well to 1,25-$(OH)_2D_3$ whether they have kidneys or not. Since 1,25-$(OH)_2D_3$ is not formed in the anephric nonpregnant animal, it can be concluded that 1,25-$(OH)_2D_3$ or a further metabolite thereof must be the metabolically active form in activating the calcium and phosphorus pump systems described in the earlier sections. Furthermore, since 1,25-$(OH)_2D_3$ is formed in the kidney and has its function in the intestine, it can most certainly be considered a hormone.[64] Finally, it must be noted that when given in small, frequent doses, 1,25-$(OH)_2D_3$ is the most potent form of vitamin D known. It is 10 times more active than vitamin D_3 and 2–5 times more active than 25-OH-D_3 in stimulating intestinal calcium transport, the mobilization of calcium from bone, the elevation of plasma phosphorus of rachitic rats, and the mineralization of bone.[65] At the present time, it appears that 1,25-$(OH)_2D_3$ is not metabolized further for function, although this has not been absolutely demonstrated. We can, therefore, consider for our discussion that 1,25-$(OH)_2D_3$ is the metabolically active form and that in true hormonal fashion, the synthesis of this compound is directly or indirectly strongly feedback regulated by plasma calcium and phosphorus concentrations.

THE REGULATION OF VITAMIN D METABOLISM

The Vitamin D Endocrine System

In 1971 Boyle *et al.* clearly demonstrated that the conversion of 25-OH-D_3 to 1,25-$(OH)_2D_3$ *in vivo* is intimately related to dietary and plasma calcium concentration as shown in FIGURE 4.[66,17] In a reciprocal fashion, the conversion of vitamin D to another metabolite, 24,25-dihydroxyvitamin D [24,25-$(OH)_2D_3$], is also regulated. The physiologic role of 24,25-$(OH)_2D_3$ is uncertain. However, current evidence suggests that this metabolite may well be an inactivation form of the vitamin. FIGURE 4 demonstrates that under conditions of normal plasma calcium

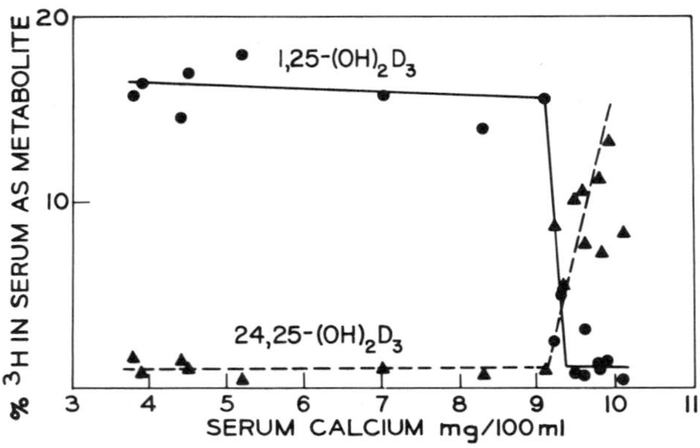

FIGURE 4. The relationship between serum calcium concentration and the conversion of radioactive 25-OH-D_3 to either 1,25-$(OH)_2D_3$ or 24,25-$(OH)_2D_3$. Rats were given a variety of diets with and without vitamin D to achieve the indicated serum calcium concentration. They were then injected intravenously with high specific activity radioactive 25-OH-D_3; and 6 hours later, radioactive metabolites accumulating in the plasma were determined following chromatography. Note that normal serum calcium concentration in our laboratory is 9.5 mg/100 ml.

concentration, the rats convert 25-OH-D to 1,25-$(OH)_2D_3$ or to 24,25-$(OH)_2D_3$. As the animals become hypocalcemic, the biogenesis of 1,25-$(OH)_2D_3$ is markedly increased and the conversion of 25-OH-D to 24,25-$(OH)_2D_3$ is markedly suppressed. Under conditions of hypercalcemia, 1,25-$(OH)_2D_3$ production is suppressed and 24,25-$(OH)_2D_3$ production is stimulated. Thus the need for calcium, as revealed by hypocalcemia, markedly stimulates production of this potent calcium-mobilizing hormone 1,25-$(OH)_2D_3$. Parathyroidectomy markedly suppresses the ability of hypocalcemia to stimulate production of 1,25-$(OH)_2D_3$.[67] Furthermore, the injection of PTH into such parathyroidectomized animals markedly stimulates production of 1,25-$(OH)_2D_3$. Since the parathyroid glands are believed to be the calcium-sensing organ of the body, it seems reasonable to postulate that the parathyroid glands secrete PTH in response to slight hypocalcemia. PTH, therefore, must have among its functions the stimulation of production of 1,25-$(OH)_2D_3$.[67,68] Since PTH stimulates conversion of 25-OH-D_3 to 1,25-$(OH)_2D_3$, it becomes crucial to understand which of the target organs of intestine and bone require additional PTH once the 1,25-$(OH)_2D_3$ is formed.[27] Experimental examination of this question revealed that the intestine responds to 1,25-$(OH)_2D_3$ equally well whether PTH is present or not. Furthermore, PTH does not stimulate intestinal calcium transport further. Thus the intestinal response to the hypocalcemic mechanism is clearly mediated by the PTH-stimulated conversion of 25-OH-D to 1,25-$(OH)_2D_3$.[18,69,70] On the other hand, the mobilization of calcium from bone does not take place in response to 1,25-$(OH)_2D_3$ in the parathyroidectomized animal. Similarly, PTH could not stimulate the mobilization of calcium in the vitamin D-deficient animal.[71] The presence of both hormones is required to mobilize calcium from bone to support plasma calcium concentration. This understanding made it possible to construct the calcium homeostatic mechanism as revealed in FIGURE 5. It is clear that in this system, the parathyroid glands monitor plasma calcium concentration and, in response to hypocalcemia, very rapidly secrete PTH. PTH is known to bind specifically to kidney and bone but not to intestine.[72] In the kidney, PTH blocks renal tubular reabsorption of phosphorus in a vitamin D-independent process,[73] enhances the renal tubular reabsorption of calcium,[74] and stimulates production of

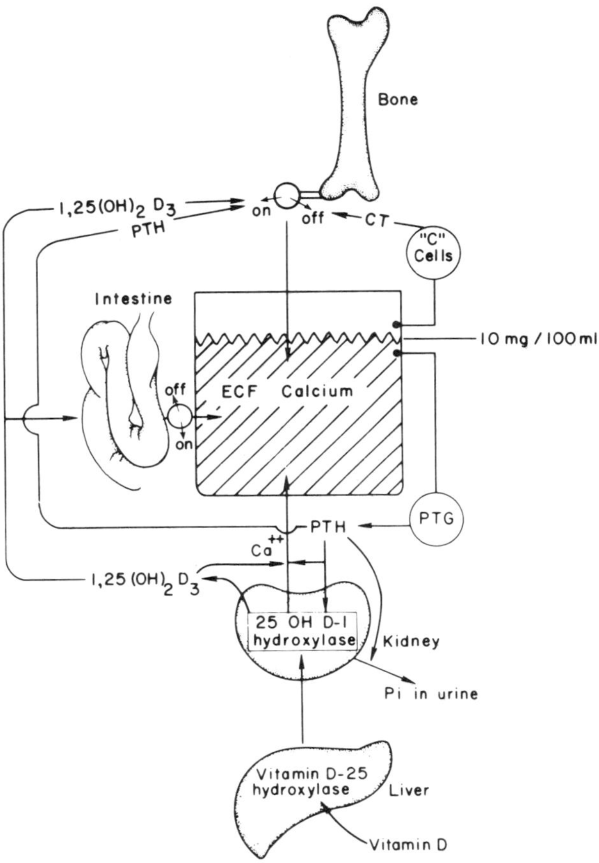

FIGURE 5. Diagrammatic representation of the mechanisms whereby serum calcium concentration is regulated by the parathyroid gland and the vitamin D endocrine system.

1,25-$(OH)_2D_3$ (see above). 1,25-$(OH)_2D_3$ then stimulates intestinal calcium absorption and, together with PTH, stimulates the mobilization of calcium from bone and renal tubular reabsorption of calcium. These sources of calcium drive the plasma calcium to normal levels, resulting in suppression of PTH secretion. It is evident that the regulation of plasma calcium concentration very heavily involves the vitamin D endocrine system working in conjunction with the parathyroid system.

NICOLAYSEN'S ENDOGENOUS FACTOR

The Regulation of Intestinal Calcium Absorption by the Vitamin D Endocrine System

From the above discussion, it is apparent that any condition that brings about even slight hypocalcemia will bring about increased PTH secretion, which in turn increases 1,25-$(OH)_2D_3$ production and thus results in the stimulation of intestinal

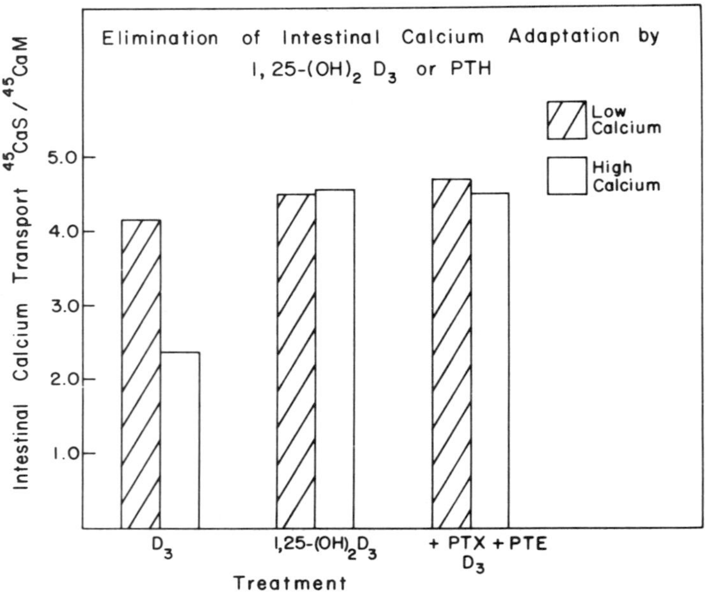

FIGURE 6. The efficiency of intestinal calcium transport in rats fed either a high calcium diet or low calcium diet and getting either vitamin D_3 or 1,25-$(OH)_2D_3$ as their sole source of vitamin D. Note also the effect of parathyroidectomy plus injected exogenous parathyroid hormone in animals given adequate amounts of vitamin D.

calcium transport. This explanation for Nicolaysen's endogenous factor was offered in 1971 when the vitamin D endocrine system was discovered by Boyle *et al.*[66,17] If this hypothesis were valid, it would be evident that an exogenous supply of 1,25-$(OH)_2D_3$ should eliminate the ability of the intestinal calcium absorption to adapt to dietary calcium levels. As shown in FIGURE 6, animals given a source of vitamin D but low levels of dietary calcium show a markedly elevated intestinal calcium absorption.[18] On the other hand, animals of the same age given a high calcium diet show low levels of intestinal calcium transport. If these animals are given an exogenous source of 1,25-$(OH)_2D_3$ instead, their intestinal calcium absorption becomes independent of dietary calcium. Similarly, if animals are parathyroidectomized and given an exogenous, but constant, source of PTH, they lose the ability to adjust their intestinal calcium absorption according to dietary calcium levels.[69,70] Thus it appears that the Nicolaysen endogenous factor is the parathyroid–vitamin D endocrine system.

The ability of the intestine to adapt to dietary calcium levels or to increase its efficiency of absorption to meet skeletal demands is of great importance in the protection of the skeleton. If there are increased demands for calcium that bring about hypocalcemia, the parathyroid system will react by secreting PTH. On a short-term basis in the presence of endogenous levels of 1,25-$(OH)_2D_3$, this will bring about increased mobilization of calcium from bone and increased conservation in the kidney. This results in a loss of bone. Normally, when the parathyroid system is stimulated, this stimulates production of 1,25-$(OH)_2D_3$, which results in an increase in intestinal calcium transport.[69,70] If this mechanism fails to occur, there will be increased reliance upon calcium from bone for support of plasma calcium concentration.

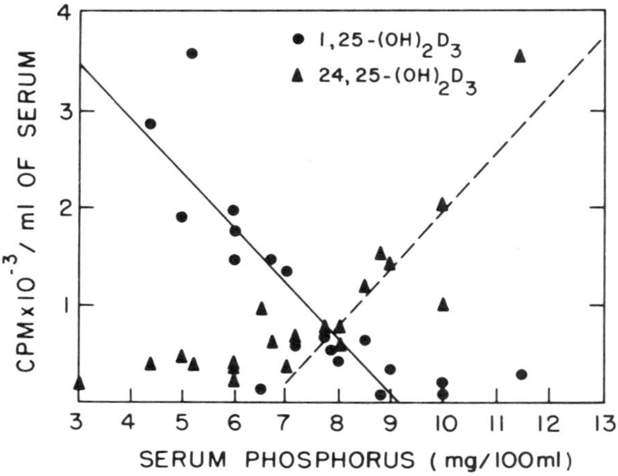

FIGURE 7. The relationship between serum phosphorus concentration in thyroparathyroidectomized rats fed a variety of dietary phosphorus levels and the ability of the animals to convert radioactive 25-OH-D_3 to 1,25-$(OH)_2D_3$ or 24,25-$(OH)_2D_3$. Rats were thyroparathyroidectomized and maintained on a diet containing a variety of levels of calcium and phosphorus to achieve the indicated phosphorus levels. After they had been on the diets for 2 weeks, they were injected with radioactive 25-OH-D_3; and 6 hours later, the metabolites accumulating in the blood were measured following chromatography. Normal serum phosphorus of rats in the intact state on these diets is 9–10 mg/100 ml.

Plasma calcium concentration is of critical importance to the function of nerve and muscle and the prevention of hypocalcemic tetany. Thus to prevent this circumstance, bone calcium will continue to be utilized. This chronic loss of skele' 'n over many years could lead to a thinning of bones and give rise to symptomatic osteoporosis. Thus the vitamin D endocrine system is of great importance in protecting the skeleton from loss and in protecting against an osteoporotic syndrome.

In addition to its function in the calcium systems, it has already been pointed out that 1,25-$(OH)_2D_3$ initiates the active transport of phosphate in the small intestine.[19,20] Furthermore, an important aspect of mineralization of bone is the elevation of plasma phosphorus concentration.[75,76] In fact, in rachitic children and rats, the primary problem in the failure of mineralization is the lack of phosphate in the plasma. Thus an important function of the vitamin D system is the elevation of plasma phosphorus concentration. Since 1,25-$(OH)_2D_3$ performs the activity of stimulating increased plasma phosphate concentrations, it is reasonable to suspect that phosphate is directly or indirectly involved in the regulation of 1,25-$(OH)_2D_3$ formation or metabolism. FIGURE 7 demonstrates that in the thyroparathyroidectomized animal, plasma phosphorus concentration plays an important role in the regulation of plasma 1,25-$(OH)_2D_3$ levels.[77] Thus under conditions of normal plasma phosphorus in the absence of parathyroid glands, no 1,25-$(OH)_2D_3$ is made and instead 24,25-$(OH)_2D_3$ is produced. Under conditions of marked hypophosphatemia, there is a marked stimulation of 1,25-$(OH)_2D_3$ production even in the absence of the parathyroid glands. Thus, hypophosphatemia brings about an accumulation of 1,25-$(OH)_2D_3$ in the plasma, presumably by stimulating production in the kidney; but this accumulation may also be the result of diminished destruction of 1,25-$(OH)_2D_3$. Whatever the cause, it is evident that the need for phosphate can also stimulate accumulation of the vitamin D hormone. The vitamin D hormone in turn

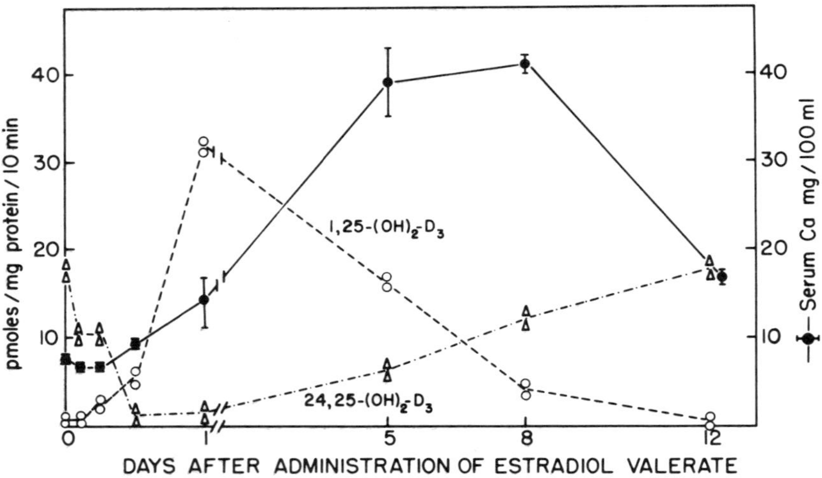

FIGURE 8. Changes in renal 25-OH-D_3-24-hydroxylase and renal 25-OH-D_3-1α-hydroxylase of adult male Japanese quail following an injection of 5 mg of estradiol valerate per kg body weight. (- - - - -) 1-hydroxylase; (- · · - · -) 24-hydroxylase; (———) serum calcium.

stimulates intestinal phosphate absorption and the mobilization of calcium and phosphate from bone.

In addition to calcium and phosphate, it is also evident that other endocrine systems may markedly affect the vitamin D endocrine system when there are increased demands for calcium. For example, in egg-laying birds when there are great demands for calcium, there is a marked stimulation of the 25-OH-D_3-1α-hydroxylase.[78,79] Thus it has been demonstrated that during the egg-laying cycle that follows ovulation, there is a marked stimulation of the 25-OH-D_3-1α-hydroxylase, resulting in markedly elevated plasma levels of 1,25-$(OH)_2D_3$.[78] Following completion of eggshell formation, plasma 1,25-$(OH)_2D_3$ levels subside, and upon the next ovulation cycle, the 1α-hydroxylase is again stimulated.

The stimulation of the 1α-hydroxylase in the egg-laying cycle is the result of the sex hormones. Thus, as shown in FIGURE 8, injection of estradiol into mature male birds brings about a suppression of the 24-hydroxylase and a marked elevation of the 1-hydroxylase.[80,81] This stimulation by estrogen requires the presence of testosterone and/or progesterone.[80-82] The three sex hormones together are responsible for stimulating 25-OH-D_3-1α-hydroxylase in the egg-laying bird. However, it is not clear whether this stimulation is direct or indirect. So far it has not been possible to demonstrate a stimulation of the 1α-hydroxylase by adding the sex hormones *in vitro* to cultures of kidney cells possessing the 1-hydroxylase.[83] Furthermore, parathyroidectomy of birds eliminates their ability to stimulate the 1-hydroxylase in response to an estrogen injection.[95] It is likely that this stimulation is mediated by the parathyroid glands or other, more direct regulatory mechanisms.

MECHANISM OF ACTION OF 1,25-$(OH)_2D_3$

A discussion of the vitamin D endocrine system would be incomplete without a discussion of how the vitamin D hormone might function in the target tissue. We have recently completed chemical synthesis of radioactive 1,25-$(OH)_2D_3$ of extremely high specific activity, permitting autoradiography studies to be carried out using frozen section methods.[84,85] Together with Walter Sumpf and Dr. Sar at the University of North Carolina, we have completed a number of these *in vivo* autoradiography studies.[86] Illustrated in FIGURE 9 is the subcellular localization of tritium-labeled 1,25-$(OH)_2D_3$ in the intestinal villus and crypt cells prior to the initiation of intestinal calcium transport. There is no question of nuclear localization, and a nuclear-mediated response of the intestine to 1,25-$(OH)_2D_3$ might be expected. It is, therefore, possible to visualize a steroid hormone mechanism for 1,25-$(OH)_2D_3$ as illustrated in FIGURE 10. As expected, receptors for 1,25-$(OH)_2D_3$ in the target tissues can easily be detected, using a sucrose density gradient and Scatchard analysis. The following receptors can be detected: in chick intestinal cytosol, a 3.7S (70,000 MW); in rat intestine, a 3.2S; in chick bone, a 3.7S; and in rat bone, a 3.2S.[87-91] Furthermore, the presence of receptors to 1,25-$(OH)_2D_3$ can be demonstrated in parathyroid glands, in skin epithelium, and in kidney preparations.[86,92,93,96]

SUMMARY

Vitamin D, which is normally produced in the skin under ultraviolet irradiation, is the building block for a new endocrine system that involves hydroxylation on the 25-position in the liver followed by 1α-hydroxylation in the kidney to produce the vitamin D hormone, 1α,25-$(OH)_2D_3$. This vitamin D hormone functions in the intestine, bone, and kidney to stimulate transport of calcium and phosphorus into the extracellular fluid compartment upon demand. The production of the vitamin D hormone is tightly feedback regulated directly or indirectly by calcium and phosphorus levels of the plasma. The vitamin D endocrine system is an important one in the regulation of calcium and phosphorus metabolism but is not solely respon-

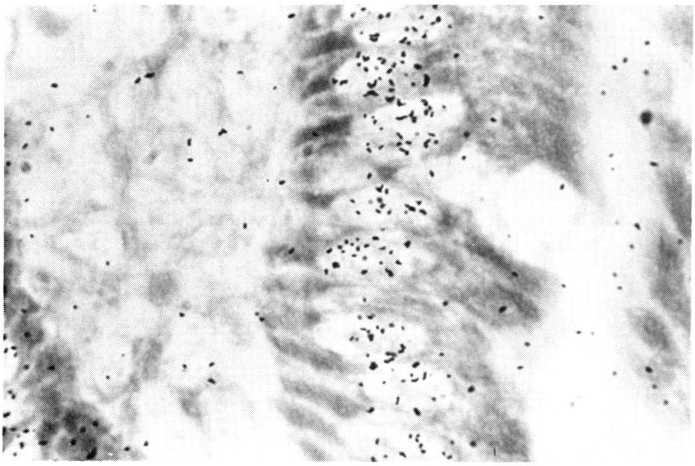

FIGURE 9. Frozen section autoradiography of intestine from a vitamin D-deficient rat 2 hours after receiving an intravenous injection of 1,25-$(OH)_2$-[26,27-^{3}H]D_3 (65 pmol). Note the exclusive nuclear localization of 1,25-$(OH)_2D_3$ in the intestinal villus cells, with no nuclear localization in the submucosa or in the goblet cells.

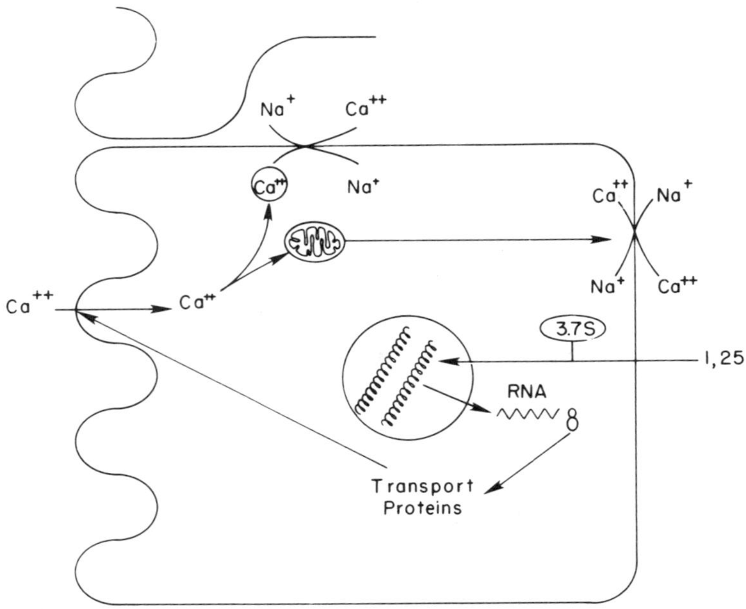

FIGURE 10. Diagrammatic representation of the expected mechanism whereby 1,25-$(OH)_2D_3$ initiates intestinal calcium transport. The 3.7S cytosol receptor in the chick has been clearly demonstrated, as has nuclear localization of the tritiated 1,25-$(OH)_2D_3$. Increased calcium permeability in the brush border membrane has also received experimental support, as has the need for sodium for calcium expulsion into the extracellular fluid compartment. The transfer of calcium across the absorptive cell by either vesicles or mitochondria has not been clearly established.

sible for the calcium and phosphorus transfer reactions occurring during reproduction. The vitamin D hormone functions in the target organs by a nuclear-mediated receptor-based mechanism probably involving the biogenesis of calcium and phosphorus transfer proteins. New target sites of 1,25-$(OH)_2D_3$ action in several tissues are suggested by this nuclear localization in those cells. Study of the vitamin D endocrine system has provided a new understanding of metabolic bone diseases and has provided new forms of vitamin D for their treatment. Thus a basic investigation of the regulation of calcium and phosphorus metabolism has rewarded medicine and science with new therapeutic approaches to disease problems.

REFERENCES

1. MELLANBY, E. 1919. Lancet **1:** 407–412.
2. MCCOLLUM, E. V., N. SIMMONDS, J. E. BECKER & P. G. SHIPLEY. 1922. J. Biol. Chem. **53:** 293–312.
3. STEENBOCK, H. & E. M. NELSON. 1923. J. Biol. Chem. **56:** 355–373.
4. HULDSHINSKY, K. 1919. Dtsch. Med. Wochenschr. **45:** 712–713.
5. CHICK, H., E. J. PALZELL & E. M. HUME. 1923. Med. Res. Coun. G.B. Spec. Rep. Ser. No. 77.
6. STEENBOCK, H. & A. BLACK. 1924. J. Biol. Chem. **61:** 405–422.

7. Askew, F. A., R. B. Bourdillon, H. M. Bruce, R. G. C. Jenkins & T. A. Webster. 1931. Proc. R. Soc. London Ser. B **107:** 76–90.
8. Windaus, A., O. Linsert, A. Luttringhaus & G. Weidlich. 1932. Ann. Chem. **492:** 226–241.
9. Howland, J. & B. Kramer. 1921. Am. J. Dis. Child. **22:** 105–119.
10. Shipley, P. G., B. Kramer & J. Howland. 1926. Biochem. J. **20:** 379–387.
11. Shipley, P. G., B. Kramer & J. Howland. 1925. Am. J. Dis. Child. **30:** 37–39.
12. Lamm, M. & W. F. Neuman. 1958. Arch. Pathol. **66:** 204–209.
13. DeLuca, H. F. 1967. Vitam. Horm. **25:** 315–367.
14. Templin, V. M. & H. Steenbock. 1933. J. Biol. Chem. **100:** 209–216.
15. Nicolaysen, R. 1943. Acta Physiol. Scand. **6:** 201–209.
16. Nicolaysen, R., N. Eeg-Larsen & O. J. Malm. 1953. Physiol. Rev. **33:** 424–444.
17. Boyle, I. T., R. W. Gray, J. L. Omdahl & H. F. DeLuca. 1972. Calcium control of the *in vivo* biosynthesis of 1,25-dihydroxyvitamin D_3: Nicolaysen's endogenous factor. *In* Endocrinology 1971. S. Taylor, Ed.: 468–476. Wm. Heineman Medical Books Ltd. London, England.
18. Ribovich, M. L. & H. F. DeLuca. 1975. Arch. Biochem. Biophys. **170:** 529–535.
19. DeLuca, H. F. 1978. Vitamin D. *In* The Fat-Soluble Vitamins. H. F. DeLuca, Ed. **2:** 69–132. Plenum Press. New York, N.Y.
20. DeLuca, H. F. & H. K. Schnoes. 1976. Ann. Rev. Biochem. **45:** 631–666.
21. DeLuca, H. F. 1978. Vitamin D and calcium transport. Ann. N.Y. Acad. Sci. **307:** 356–576.
22. Wasserman, R. H., Ed. 1963. The Transfer of Calcium and Strontium across Biological Membranes. Academic Press, Inc. New York, N.Y.
23. Steele, T. H., J. E. Engle, Y. Tanaka, R. S. Lorenc, K. L. Dudgeon & H. F. DeLuca. 1975. Am. J. Physiol. **229:** 489–495.
24. Sutton, R. A. L. & J. H. Dirks. 1978. Fed. Proc. Fed. Am. Soc. Exp. Biol. **37:** 2112–2119.
25. Sutton, R. A. L., C. A. Harris, N. L. M. Wong & J. Dirks. 1977. Effects of vitamin D on renal tubular calcium transport. *In* Vitamin D: Biochemical, Chemical, and Clinical Aspects Related to Calcium Metabolism. A. W. Norman *et al.*, Eds.: 451–453. Walter de Gruyter, Inc. Berlin, Federal Republic of Germany.
26. Talmage, R. V. 1969. Clin. Orthop. Relat. Res. **67:** 210–224.
27. Garabedian, M., Y. Tanaka, M. F. Holick & H. F. DeLuca. 1974. Endocrinology **94:** 1022–1027.
28. Harrison, H. E. & H. C. Harrison. 1961. Am. J. Physiol. **201:** 1007–1012.
29. Kowarski, S. & D. Schachter. 1969. J. Biol. Chem. **244:** 211–217.
30. Chen, T. C., L. Castillo, M. Korycka-Dahl & H. F. DeLuca. 1974. J. Nutr. **104:** 1056–1060.
31. Walling, M. W. 1977. Effects of 1α-dihydroxyvitamin D_3 on active intestinal inorganic phosphate absorption. *In* Vitamin D: Biochemical, Chemical, and Clinical Aspects Related to Calcium Metabolism. A. W. Norman *et al.*, Eds.: 321–330. Walter de Gruyter, Inc. Berlin, Federal Republic of Germany.
32. DeLuca, H. F. 1979. Nutr. Rev. **37:** 161–193.
33. Neville, P. F. & H. F. DeLuca. 1966. Biochemistry **5:** 2201–2207.
34. Norman, A. W. & H. F. DeLuca. 1963. Biochemistry **2:** 1160–1168.
35. Lund, J. & H. F. DeLuca. 1966. J. Lipid Res. **7:** 739–744.
36. Blunt, J. W., H. F. DeLuca & H. K. Schnoes. 1968. Biochemistry **7:** 3317–3322.
37. Holick, M. F., H. K. Schnoes, H. F. DeLuca, T. Suda & R. J. Cousins. 1971. Biochemistry **10:** 2799–2894.
38. Blunt, J. W. & H. F. DeLuca. 1969. Biochemistry **8:** 671–675.
39. Semmler, E. J., M. F. Holick, H. K. Schnoes & H. F. DeLuca. 1972. Tetrahedron Lett. **40:** 4147–4150.
40. Bhattacharyya, M. & H. F. DeLuca. 1974. Arch. Biochem. Biophys. **160:** 58–62.
41. Madhok, T. C., H. K. Schnoes & H. F. DeLuca. 1978. Biochem. J. **175:** 479–482.
42. Madhok, T. C. & H. F. DeLuca. 1979. Biochem. J. **184:** 491–499.
43. Pedersen, J. I., I. Holmberg & I. Bjorkhem. 1979. FEBS Lett. **98:** 394–398.
44. Bjorkhem, I. & I. Holmberg. 1978. J. Biol. Chem. **253:** 842–849.

45. TUCKER, G., III, R. E. GAGNON & M. R. HAUSSLER. 1973. Arch. Biochem. Biophys. **155:** 47–57.
46. BHATTACHARYYA, M. H. & H. F. DELUCA. 1974. Biochem. Biophys. Res. Commun. **59:** 734–741.
47. PONCHON, G. & H. F. DELUCA. 1969. J. Clin. Invest. **48:** 1273–1279.
48. FRASER, D. R. & E. KODICEK. 1970. Nature **228:** 764–766.
49. GRAY, R., I. BOYLE & H. F. DELUCA. 1971. Science **172:** 1232–1234.
50. GHAZARIAN, J. G., C. R. JEFCOATE, J. C. KNUTSON, W. H. ORME-JOHNSON & H. F. DELUCA. 1974. J. Biol. Chem. **249:** 3026–3033.
51. PEDERSEN, J. I., J. G. GHAZARIAN, N. R. ORME-JOHNSON & H. F. DELUCA. 1976. J. Biol. Chem. **251:** 3933–3941.
52. YOON, P. S. & H. F. DELUCA. 1980. Biochemistry **19:** 2165–2171.
53. GRAY, R. W., J. L. OMDAHL, J. G. GHAZARIAN & H. F. DELUCA. 1972. J. Biol. Chem. **247:** 7528–7532.
54. TANAKA, Y., B. HALLORAN, H. K. SCHNOES & H. F. DELUCA. 1979. Proc. Nat. Acad. Sci. USA **76:** 5033–5035.
55. ESVELT, R. P., H. K. SCHNOES & H. F. DELUCA. 1978. Arch. Biochem. Biophys. **188:** 282–286.
56. HOLICK, M. F., N. M. RICHTAND, S. C. MCNEILL, S. A. HOLICK, J. E. FROMMER, J. W. HENLEY & J. T. POTTS, JR. 1979. Biochemistry **18:** 1003–1008.
57. HOLICK, M. F. & M. B. CLARK. 1978. Fed. Proc. Fed. Am. Soc. Exp. Biol. **37:** 2567–2574.
58. BOTHAM, K. M., J. G. GHAZARIAN, B. E. KREAM & H. F. DELUCA. 1976. Biochemistry **15:** 2130–2135.
59. IMAWARI, M., K. KIDA & D. S. GOODMAN. 1976. J. Clin. Invest. **58:** 514–523.
60. HADDAD, J. G. & J. WALGATE. 1976. J. Biol. Chem. **251:** 4803–4809.
61. DAIGER, S. P., M. S. SCHANFIELD & L. L. CAVALLI-SFORZA. 1975. Proc. Nat. Acad. Sci. USA **72:** 2076–2080.
62. BOYLE, I. T., L. MIRAVET, R. W. GRAY, M. F. HOLICK & H. F. DELUCA. 1972. Endocrinology **90:** 605–608.
63. HOLICK, M. F., M. GARABEDIAN & H. F. DELUCA. 1972. Science **172:** 1146–1147.
64. DELUCA, H. F. 1974. Fed. Proc. Fed. Am. Soc. Exp. Biol. **33:** 2211–2219.
65. TANAKA, Y., H. FRANK & H. F. DELUCA. 1973. Endocrinology **92:** 417–422.
66. BOYLE, I. T., R. W. GRAY & H. F. DELUCA. 1971. Proc. Nat. Acad. Sci. USA **68:** 2131–2134.
67. GARABEDIAN, M., M. F. HOLICK, H. F. DELUCA & I. T. BOYLE. 1972. Proc. Nat. Acad. Sci. USA **69:** 1673–1676.
68. FRASER, D. R. & E. KODICEK. 1973. Nature London New Biol. **241:** 163–166.
69. RIBOVICH, M. L. & H. F. DELUCA. 1976. Arch. Biochem. Biophys. **175:** 256–261.
70. OMDAHL, J. L. & H. F. DELUCA. 1977. J. Nutr. **107:** 1975–1980.
71. RASMUSSEN, H., H. DELUCA, C. ARNAUD, C. HAWKER & M. VON STEDINGK. 1963. J. Clin. Invest. **42:** 1940–1946.
72. ZULL, J. E. & D. W. REPKE. 1972. J. Biol. Chem. **247:** 2195–2199.
73. FORTE, L. R., G. A. NICKOLS & C. S. ANAST. 1976. J. Clin. Invest. **57:** 559–568.
74. KLEEMAN, C. R., D. BERNSTEIN, R. ROCKNEY, J. T. DOWLING & M. H. MAXWELL. 1961. Studies on the renal clearance of diffusible calcium and the role of the parathyroid glands in its regulation. *In* The Parathyroids. R. O. Greep & R. V. Talmage, Eds.: 353–387. Charles C. Thomas. Springfield, Ill.
75. TANAKA, Y. & H. F. DELUCA. 1974. Proc. Nat. Acad. Sci. USA **71:** 1040–1044.
76. FRASER, D., S. W. KOOH & C. R. SCRIVER. 1967. Pediatr. Res. **1:** 425–435.
77. TANAKA, Y. & H. F. DELUCA. 1973. Arch. Biochem. Biophys. **154:** 566–574.
78. CASTILLO, L., Y. TANAKA, M. J. WINELAND, J. O. JOWSEY & H. F. DELUCA. 1979. Endocrinology **104:** 1598–1601.
79. KENNY, A. D. 1976. Am. J. Physiol. **230:** 1609–1615.
80. TANAKA, Y., L. CASTILLO & H. F. DELUCA. 1976. Proc. Nat. Acad. Sci. USA **73:** 2701–2705.
81. CASTILLO, L., Y. TANAKA, H. F. DELUCA & M. L. SUNDE. 1977. Arch. Biochem. Biophys. **179:** 211–217.
82. TANAKA, Y., L. CASTILLO, M. J. WINELAND & H. F. DELUCA. 1978. Endocrinology **103:** 2035–2039.

83. TRECHSEL, U., J. A. EISMAN, J. P. BONJOUR & H. FLEISCH. 1979. Evidence for a calcium-dependent, PTH-independent regulation of plasma 1,25-dihydroxyvitamin D in rats. *In* Vitamin D: Basic Research and Its Clinical Application. A. W. Norman *et al.*, Eds.: 511–513. Walter de Gruyter & Co. Berlin, Federal Republic of Germany.
84. NAPOLI, J. L., M. A. FIVIZZANI, A. J. HAMSTRA, H. K. SCHNOES & H. F. DELUCA. 1979. Anal. Biochem. **96:** 481–488.
85. NAPOLI, J. L., W. S. MELLON, M. A. FIVIZZANI, H. K. SCHNOES & H. F. DELUCA. 1980. Biochemistry. (In press.)
86. STUMPF, W. E., M. SAR, F. A. REID, Y. TANAKA & H. F. DELUCA. 1979. Science **206:** 1188–1190.
87. BRUMBAUGH, P. F. & M. R. HAUSSLER. 1973. Life Sci. **13:** 1737–1746.
88. KREAM, B. E., R. D. REYNOLDS, J. C. KNUTSON, J. A. EISMAN & H. F. DELUCA. 1976. Arch. Biochem. Biophys. **176:** 779–787.
89. KREAM, B. E., S. YAMADA, H. K. SCHNOES & H. F. DELUCA. 1977. J. Biol. Chem. **252:** 4501–4505.
90. KREAM, B. E., J. JOSE, S. YAMADA & H. F. DELUCA. 1977. Science **197:** 1086–1088.
91. MELLON, W. S. & H. F. DELUCA. 1980. J. Biol. Chem. **255:** 4081–4086.
92. COLSTON, K. W. & D. FELDMAN. 1979. J. Clin. Endocrinol. Metab. **49:** 798–800.
93. BRUMBAUGH, P. F., M. R. HUGHES & M. R. HAUSSLER. 1975. Proc. Nat. Acad. Sci. USA **72:** 4871–4875.
94. YOON, P. S. & H. F. DELUCA. 1980. Arch. Biochem. Biophys. (In press.)
95. CASTILLO, L., Y. TANAKA & H. F. DELUCA. 1979. (Unpublished results.)
96. SIMPSON, R. U. & H. F. DELUCA. 1980. Proc. Nat. Acad. Sci. (In press.)

DISCUSSION

A. B. EISENSTEIN (*Veterans Administration Medical Center, Brooklyn, N.Y.*): What happens to the l-hydroxylase in the kidney under circumstances of long-standing, but mild, hyperparathyroidism?

H. F. DELUCA: The only data that are available are in man. If this is primary hyperparathyroidism, then elevated levels of 1,25-dihydroxyvitamin D_3 [1,25-$(OH)_2D_3$] are found. However, the hydroxylase itself has not been measured, and the data could also have resulted from decreased destruction of 1,25-$(OH)_2D_3$.

L. HOWARD (*Albany Medical College, Albany, N.Y.*): Are there important differences that those of us who are using the compound should know about in regard to the D_3 and D_2 metabolites?

H. F. DELUCA: 1,25-$(OH)_2D_2$ and 1,25-$(OH)_2D_3$ are approximately equal in biological activity in mammals. In birds, of course, there is a very marked difference, and this is due to the conversion of vitamin D_2 metabolites to bile excretory products. In mammals, they're equivalently active.

J. G. BIERI (*National Institutes of Health, Bethesda, Md.*): Would you elaborate more on what's going on in the pregnant animals, since they don't need vitamin D?

H. F. DELUCA: Plasma levels of 1,25-$(OH)_2D_3$ during rigors of pregnancy and lactation are in fact high. Therefore, we thought that if we made the females totally vitamin D deficient, they would be unable to mobilize calcium and would be unable to support pregnancy and lactation.

That was not the case. The completely D-deficient mothers can mobilize calcium from their bone equivalently to D-replete mothers. Furthermore, their intestinal absorption of calcium increases. This means that there is some other humoral factor that is stimulating mobilization of calcium from bone and intestine at the time of pregnancy and lactation.

The fetus accumulates the same amount of calcium from the D-deficient mother as it does from the D-fed control; thus the transfer of calcium across the placenta apears normal. For the first few days of life, the pups also are able to absorb calcium from the intestine by a non-vitamin-D-dependent process as long as their calcium is provided in mother's milk. Since this milk cannot have vitamin D in any form, there is no support for the claim of a superactive water-soluble form of vitamin D in milk that we've heard so much about and for which there is no chemical evidence.

So it looks like there are certain calcium movements in the pregnant and lactating situation that are not vitamin D dependent. There's no question that the vitamin D system is a supplementary system that makes the animal better able to cope with recycling pregnancy; but at least on the first cycle, it is not essential and points to certain vitamin D–independent calcium transfer reactions.

J. G. Bieri: But do you think that this is applicable to the human situation after several pregnancies?

H. F. DeLuca: Well, I think a female who goes through pregnancy in a D-deficient state will have marked osteopenia and furthermore that she will stay that way after pregnancy unless she gets some form of vitamin D. It is my guess that she will not be able to support another pregnancy because there will not be a sufficient amount of calcium available in her bones to permit support of another fetus and lactation. Lactation is actually the biggest strain on calcium stores—much more so than the pregnancy itself. The rat is probably a reasonable model for man, but of course that's always a question anyone can ask. We don't know exactly the case in man. We can only extrapolate.

R. J. Dowling (*University of Pennsylvania Hospital, Philadelphia, Penn.*): Is it okay—in taking a patient receiving nothing by mouth—just to do urine calciums and phosphorus, or do you have to actually monitor the intake orally also? Can you expect that nothing of significance would be secreted into the intestine?

H. F. DeLuca: Well, undoubtedly some calcium will be excreted in intestine, but how much, I don't know.

R. J. Dowling: You mentioned that, normally speaking, there is very little calcium excreted in the urine.

H. F. DeLuca: No, there is a significant amount of calcium in the urine. When I said that 99% of the filtered load is reabsorbed, you have to bear in mind that man filters somewhere around 7 to 10 grams of calcium a day. Thus, 1% is a highly significant amount of calcium. Therefore, in man there is a significant urinary calcium.

R. J. Dowling: Is there any condition in which vitamin D may be implicated as actually demineralizing bone?

H. F. DeLuca: Under conditions of vitamin D intoxication, it is known that bone will demineralize. As a matter of fact, that is what led to the experiments in the first place—those that demonstrate that vitamin D does play a role in permitting parathyroid hormone to mobilize bone calcium when needed. But I think large amounts of vitamin D are required to demineralize bone. It does not occur under physiological circumstances because all the other systems are activated and the net effect is to mineralize bone rather than demineralize it.

R. J. Dowling: Is there any effect that you know of concerning vitamin A interacting along the pathway to cause demineralization?

H. F. DeLuca: I think Dr. Navia will talk about that. Maybe I shouldn't appropriate his talk.

C. S. Lieber (*Mount Sinai School of Medicine, New York, N.Y.*): What is our present concept of a mechanism of vitamin D abnormality in chronic users of microsomal inducers, such as antiepileptics?

H. F. DeLuca: This is a very interesting subject that has been controversial. There have been reports of osteomalacia associated with excessive or with chronic users of antiepileptic drugs. The idea, of course, is that microsomal P-450s are induced that destroy the active forms of vitamin D. Unfortunately, it hasn't gone beyond that, and we do know that the osteomalacia of this condition can be cured with the active forms of vitamin D. Also it can be done with larger amounts of vitamin D.

Now the problem is that there isn't uniform agreement as to what the incidence of osteomalacia is under conditions of antiepileptic treatment. Some clinicians say 30%, some say more; and I think it depends on the criteria that are used to evaluate the disease and where in the country it is examined. If it is in the South, they are getting lots of vitamin D from sunlight. In the North, they are not. So you will see the reports actually differ geographically.

VITAMIN E AND SELENIUM PROTECTION FROM *IN VIVO* LIPID PEROXIDATION*

Al L. Tappel

Department of Food Science
University of California
Davis, California 95616

In Vivo *Lipid Peroxidation*

There is a long history of experimentation on lipid peroxidation as it is influenced by interactions of oxidants, antioxidant nutrients, and nutrients that influence the stability of biological membranes. New evidence of these interactions and of the functions of the microsomal P-450 system has catalyzed a large investigational effort to unveil the extent to which lipid peroxidation is involved in pathological and normal biological reactions *in vivo*. TABLE 1 summarizes the important interactions of lipid peroxidation reactants, protective structures within the cell, the antioxidants vitamin E and selenium, antioxidant synergists, and initiators of the reaction. One particular area in which considerable growth in information has occurred in recent years has been that of selenium-glutathione peroxidase, where newer studies are beginning to quantitate the protection afforded by this enzyme relative to that afforded by vitamin E. The importance of studying nutrient interactions as well as oxidant interactions *in vivo* has received far more attention in recent research than in older research. Studies of less complicated, two-component systems have provided a good foundation of basic information, but *in vivo*, one cannot ignore the complexities of multiple interactions that are involved in lipid peroxidation. This reaction is of significance because it is among the major deteriorative reactions and is basic to understanding membrane and cellular aging processes and many disease processes.

Lipid peroxidation is the reaction of a polyunsaturated fat (LH) with an oxidant initiator to form a lipid free-radical intermediate (L·).[1-4] The lipid free radical reacts with oxygen to form a peroxy free radical (LOO·). The unpaired electrons of the peroxy free radical react to initiate relatively nonspecific hydrogen abstraction reactions as shown:

$$L\cdot + O_2 \rightarrow LOO\cdot$$

$$LOO\cdot + LH \rightarrow LOOH + L\cdot$$

Vitamin E serves as a chain-breaking antioxidant by the following reaction:

$$LOO\cdot + \text{vitamin E} \rightarrow LOOH + \text{vitamin E oxidized}$$

Metals in their lower oxidation state catalyze the homolytic decomposition of hydroperoxides, resulting in autocatalysis or branching reactions. Reactions that are damaging to biological membranes and tissues are caused by free radicals—including peroxy radicals, alkoxy radicals, and hydroxy radicals—and by other products, including hydroperoxides and carbonyls.

The membranes of subcellular organelles, especially mitochondria and microsomes, contain relatively large amounts of polyunsaturated fatty acids, and

* This research was supported by United States Public Health Service Research Grants AM 09933 and AM 06424 from the National Institutes of Arthritis and Metabolic Diseases, and by the National Live Stock and Meat Board.

0077-8923/80/0355-0018 $01.75/0 © 1980, NYAS

TABLE 1

INTERACTING COMPONENTS OF LIPID PEROXIDATION

Reactants:	Initiation by "Hazardous Elements":
Polyunsaturated lipids	1. Metabolic oxidants:
Vitamin A cooxidized	H_2O_2, O_2^-, HO·
Protective Structures:	2. Toxic metals:
Biological membranes, lipoproteins, etc.	Fe, Cu, Cd, Pb, Hg, Ag
Chain-Breaking Antioxidant:	3. Toxic oxidants of environment:
Vitamin E	ROOH, O_3, NO_2
Peroxide-Reducing Systems:	4. Some environmental toxicants:
Selenium-glutathione peroxidase	Some halogenated hydrocarbons, CCl_4 as an example
Glutathione-S-transferase	Cigarette smoke constituents
Antioxidant Synergists:	Alcoholic drinks
1. Reducing agents:	
Vitamin C, glutathione	
2. Metal chelation compounds:	
Specific proteins	

these membranes are the major sites of lipid peroxidation in the cells.[5-7] These two subcellular membranes contain fatty acids with 2, 4, 5, and 6 double bonds, for which the relative rates of *in vivo* and *in vitro* peroxidation are 1, 4, 6, and 8, respectively. Among the catalytic compounds that initiate lipid peroxidation in membranes are coordinated iron and heme proteins. Free radical lipid peroxidation reactions can be propagated through the polyunsaturated fatty acids of membrane phospholipids. These chain reactions are important, since a fatty acid hydroperoxide is produced for each completed peroxidation as the chain progresses. As mentioned above, branching reactions result from metal-catalyzed decomposition of peroxide. The chain of peroxidation can be relatively long before it is terminated by vitamin E or by a damaging reaction. The approximate molar ratio of polyunsaturated fatty acid to vitamin E in membranes is 1000:1.

Evidence for the occurrence of *in vivo* lipid peroxidation comes from several lines of investigation. This evidence comes from (a) the direct measurement in cells of accumulated products, such as fluorescent ceroid and lipofuscin pigments, and of thiobarbituric acid reactants; (b) the identification in animal breath of volatile scission products from lipid hydroperoxides; (c) the measurement *in vivo* of products of vitamin E that indicate that it has functioned to stop the chain reaction of lipid peroxidation; and (d) the successful replacement of vitamin E in the animal dietary by lipid antioxidants that are structurally dissimilar. Lipid peroxidation is one of the important concepts of experimental pathology and toxicology, in spite of the fact that some of the most convincing evidence for the role of lipid peroxidation *in vivo* is indirect.[5]

Selenium-Glutathione Peroxidase

The interrelationships and synergistic effects of vitamin E and selenium have been discussed in a number of reviews on selenium in nutrition.[8,9] As summarized below, recent experimental evidence shows that selenium is the active site of glutathione peroxidase. This enzyme is the subject of much current research, and it has been reviewed fairly extensively.[10-12] The interrelationships between selenium-glutathione peroxidase and lipid peroxidation are shown in FIGURE 1.

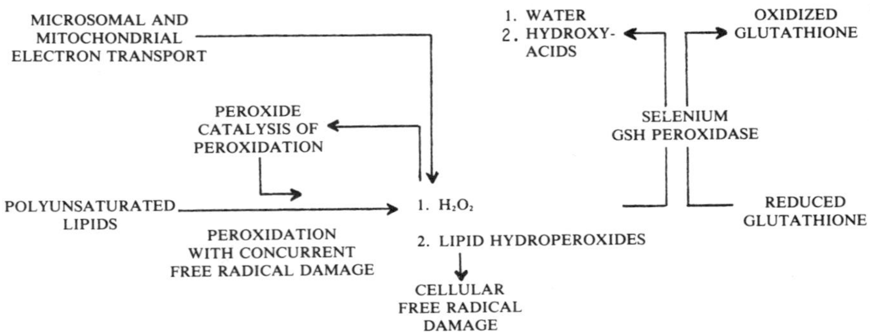

FIGURE 1. Relationships between selenium-glutathione peroxidase and *in vivo* lipid peroxidation.

Studies from this laboratory identified the catalytic site of rat liver glutathione peroxidase as selenocysteine.[13] ^{75}Se-labeled rat liver glutathione peroxidase was isolated at 30–50% purity with 20–30% yields in 4–5 days. Using these isolates, the selenium moiety in the enzyme was identified as selenocysteine by derivatizing the seleno group with either iodoacetate or ethylenimine in the intact protein, hydrolyzing the protein with 6 N HCl, and cochromatographing the ^{75}Se-labeled products with known standards. The enzyme was specifically labeled with [^{14}C]-iodoacetate on the ^{75}Se-labeled selenium atom and fractionated to yield the ^{14}C, ^{75}Se-labeled selenocysteine. It was concluded that the reduced form of glutathione peroxidase contains the selenocysteine selenol (-SeH) at the catalytic site.

To determine the mode of attachment of selenocysteine in the catalytic site of glutathione peroxidase, selenocysteine was stabilized by conversion to the carboxymethyl derivative. A selenium-containing tryptic fragment was partially purified by column chromatography through cellulose phosphate, Sephadex G-25 superfine, DEAE-agarose, and again through Sephadex G-25 superfine. Automated sequential Edman degradation yielded a residue of the phenylthiohydantoin of carboxymethylselenocysteine, indicating that the selenocysteine in the native enzyme is located within the polypeptide chain,[14] as shown:

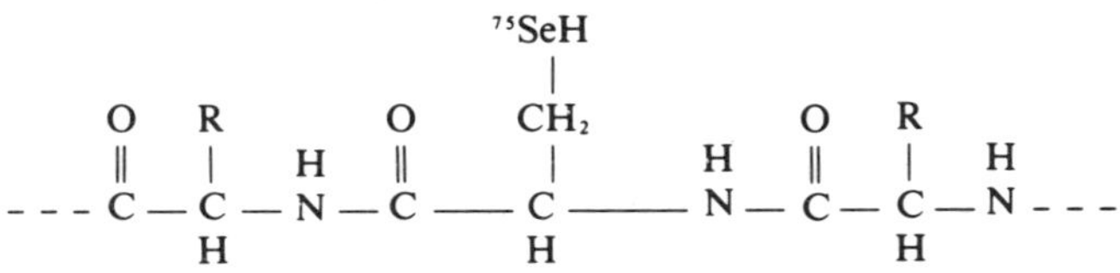

D. Lyons and C. Hawkes and coworkers found that rat liver *in vivo* and rat liver slices *in vitro* incorporated $^{75}SeO_3^{2-}$ into selenium-glutathione peroxidase and selenocysteine.[15] Incorporation of ^{75}Se into the enzyme was measured by SDS gel electrophoresis following partial purification by acetone precipitation and DEAE cellulose chromatography; incorporation into free selenocysteine was measured by purification of the carboxymethyl derivative on Dowex AG-50 X8 and DEAE cellulose. Added ^{3}H-labeled carboxymethyl-selenocysteine standard cochromatographed with the derivative in an amino acid analyzer system. Cycloheximide and puromycin strongly inhibited *in vitro* incorporation of ^{75}Se from $^{75}SeO_3^{2-}$. ^{75}Selenomethionine was 2.5 times more effective on a molar basis than was [^{75}Se]-selenocystine for *in vitro* synthesis of glutathione peroxidase. But, selenocystine is about 1.5

times as effective as selenomethionine at decreasing the incorporation of ^{75}Se from $^{75}SeO_3^{2-}$ into glutathione peroxidase. *In vivo* and *in vitro* isotope dilution studies indicated that selenocysteine and selenomethionine decreased the specific activity of ^{75}Se in glutathione peroxidase to about the same extent. Rat liver slices were incubated with [^{75}Se]-selenocysteine and [^{35}S]-cysteine before isolation and purification of aminoacyl-t-RNAs.[16] Isolated were three forms of [^{35}S]-cysteyl-t-RNA, all free of ^{75}Se, and one form of [^{75}Se]-selenocysteyl-t-RNA, which contained at least 99.8 mol % Se and less than 0.2 mol % S. Since the concentration of cysteine in the liver slices was about 10^2 times greater than that of selenocysteine, formation of selenocysteyl-t-RNA showed a 500-fold greater specificity for selenocysteine than for cysteine. This work supports our view that selenocysteine is incorporated during protein synthesis and implies that there is a unique codon for selenocysteine. Probable pathways for the incorporation of selenite into glutathione peroxidase are shown together with the metals that inhibit the enzyme:

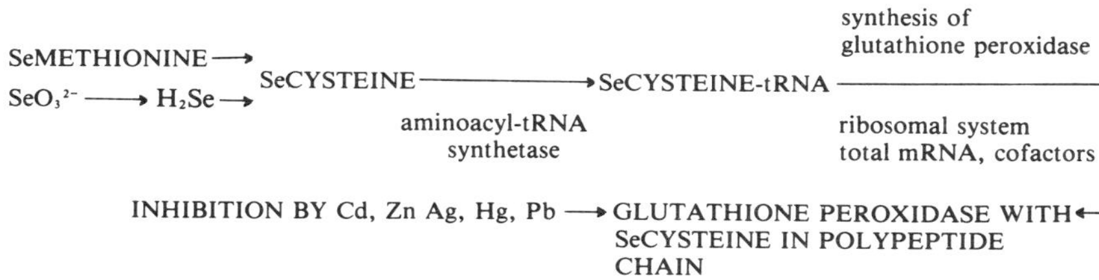

The inhibition of selenium-glutathione peroxidase by metal ions was studied by a direct spectrophotometric assay that monitors at 237 nm the decrease of GS^- concentration with time.[17] Cadmium(II) and zinc(II) ions were the most potent inhibitors, while silver(I), mercury(II), cobalt(II), and lead(II) inhibited to a lesser extent. Inhibition by these metals was competitive with respect to the donor substrate, glutathione (GSH). Competitive inhibition was verified for cadmium(II) ions by means of an assay employing Ellman's reagent. Inhibition by cadmium(II) ions was noncompetitive with respect to the acceptor substrate, *t*-butyl hydroperoxide. Correlation of inhibitor constants with chemical and physical properties showed a dependence on the softness of the metal ion as an acid and also a dependence on ionic size.

Production and Measurement of Hydrocarbon Gases from Lipid Peroxidation

Mechanisms have been postulated for the formation of the hydrocarbon gases ethane and pentane upon decomposition of ω3- and ω6-fatty acid hydroperoxides, respectively.[18-20] These mechanisms propose that alkoxy radicals undergoing β-scission are the most likely precursors for hydrocarbon gases. The following equations show that a pentane free radical is formed when an ω6-fatty acid hydroperoxide is cleaved from the chain on the side of the peroxy group that is closest to the methyl end:

$$\text{1 Mole } CH_3(CH_2)_4\underset{OOH}{C}-R + Fe^{2+} \rightarrow CH_3(CH_2)_4\underset{O\cdot}{C}-R + Fe^{3+} + OH\cdot$$

$$CH_3(CH_2)_4\underset{O\cdot}{C}-R \xrightarrow[\beta\text{-scission reaction}]{} CH_3(CH_2)_3\dot{C}H_2 + \underset{\underset{O}{\|}}{C}R$$

$$CH_3(CH_2)_3\dot{C}H_2 \xrightarrow[\text{H abstraction reaction}]{} CH_3(CH_2)_3CH_3 \text{ 0.01 Mole}$$

The free radical formed abstracts a hydrogen, forming pentane. Transition metals, iron and copper in particular, in their lower oxidation states are effective catalysts for the decomposition of hydroperoxides. Since the *in vivo* concentrations of iron, hematin, and copper are higher than those of other heavy metals, the assumption is that they catalyze decomposition of alkoxy radicals by β-scission, leading to the release of ethane and pentane.

Detection of lipid peroxidation *in vivo* has been limited because of limited methodology. Red cell hemolysis measurement to establish the state of vitamin E nutrition has been the principal method used to follow the course of vitamin E insufficiency or oxidant stress. As discussed below, recent studies with rats and mice have proven the hydrocarbon gas analysis measurements to be applicable to many different studies of lipid peroxidation *in vivo*.

The methods developed in this laboratory for measurement of hydrocarbon gas products of lipid peroxidation *in vivo* are summarized here.[21,22] Varian gas chromatographs with flame ionization detectors and fitted with six-way gas sample valves are used for analysis of hydrocarbon gases on 1/8 in. × 5–10 ft columns filled with activated alumina (60–80 or 80–100 mesh) and temperature programmed from 50 °C to 250 °C. Polar materials, such as aldehydes, ketones, and esters, are irreversibly adsorbed by the alumina. Alumina allows good separation of C_1 to C_8 paraffins. Individual rats are placed in a body chamber separated from the head chamber by rubber and Teflon® gaskets around the animal's neck. The two chambers are clamped together for an airtight seal. The rat is then exposed to commercial hydrocarbon-free air at a flow rate of 120 ml/minute for a minimum of 10 minutes prior to collection of a breath sample. The effluent side of the rat chamber is attached via a manifold to a stainless steel gas-sample loop partially filled with alumina. This trap is immersed in a semihard, ethanol–liquid nitrogen slurry during volumetric collection of a breath-air sample. After collection, the sample is injected into the column via the gas sample valve while the sample loop is heated. A comparison of peak areas—measured by peak height multiplied by the peak width at half-height— of a standard sample and the breath sample allows calculation of the molar amounts of individual hydrocarbon gases. The following computation for pentane, as an example, is applied:

$$\frac{\text{(pmoles pentane) (incoming flow rate of air)}}{\text{(100 g rat body wt) (sample volume)}} = \begin{array}{l}\text{total pentane produced/}\\ \text{100 g body wt/minute}\end{array}$$

Expression of hydrocarbon gases in these units is suggested as the most appropriate.

To date, only a few research groups have used evolved hydrocarbon gases to measure *in vivo* lipid peroxidation. Future use of the methodology should expand when one considers the large number of potential studies to be done. Systems for the collection of breath samples other than the one described above have been used. The use of whole-body chambers requires that respiratory gases be allowed to accumulate until a sufficient concentration is built up to be measured in a relatively small volume of head space. This type of chamber usually precludes making measurements within the first one-half hour after treatment of an individual animal with a toxicant, for example. For measurement of ethane produced by animals in whole-body chambers, Hafeman and Hoekstra have described a life-support apparatus, and Koster *et al.* have described the use of ethane-free pure oxygen.[18,23] Experience in our laboratory has shown that the use of individual animal chambers with only the animal's head exposed to the hydrocarbon-free air is most desirable.

TABLE 2

EVIDENCE THAT BREATH PENTANE COMES FROM *In Vivo* LIPID PEROXIDATION

1. *In vitro* decomposition of ω-6 polyunsaturated fatty acid hydroperoxides produces pentane.
2. *In vivo* pentane production is proportional to vitamin E deficiencies, selenium-glutathione peroxidase deficiencies, and dietary intake of ω-6 polyunsaturated fatty acids.
3. In vitamin E-deficient rats, pentane production is reversibly decreased when a nonbiological antioxidant (diphenyl phenylenediamine) is fed.
4. Halogenated hydrocarbon-induced *in vivo* lipid peroxidation, measured by conjugated diene formation, produces pentane in direct proportion to conjugated dienes.

Pentane Production as a Measure of Vitamin E Protection from In Vivo *Lipid Peroxidation*

A remarkable amount of evidence has now accumulated that pentane and ethane in the breath of animals derive from *in vivo* lipid peroxidation. This evidence is summarized in TABLE 2. To support the hypothesis that hydrocarbon gases produced *in vivo* come from decomposition of lipid hydroperoxides, *in vitro* studies were done.[19] Peroxidizing ω3- and ω6-fatty acids did not release hydrocarbon gases during a 20-hour iron-catalyzed peroxidation phase; but following the decomposition of hydroperoxides by addition of excess ascorbic acid, production of hydrocarbon gases was immediate. The major hydrocarbon gas products in iron-, copper-, or hematin-catalyzed peroxidation systems were ethane or ethylene from linolenic acid, and pentane from linoleic acid and arachidonic acid. Calculations of the ratios of hydrocarbon gases formed were based on fatty acid decrease and/or change in diene conjugation and peroxide values. Depending on the fatty acid, catalyst, and calculation basis used, pentane formation was as high as 1.3 mol %; ethane, 4.3 mol %; and ethylene, 10.6 mol %.

Two interesting studies of lipid peroxidation *in vivo* during vitamin E and selenium deficiency in the rat as measured by evolved ethane were reported by Hafeman and Hoekstra.[18,24] The relative amounts of ethane produced by rats fed various diets were, vitamin E- and selenium-supplemented:vitamin E-supplemented:selenium-supplemented:vitamin E- and selenium-deficient rats, 1:2.4:18.5:37. Through correlation of ethane production with pathological signs and death in the rats, evidence was provided that *in vivo* lipid peroxidation was linked to the gross deficiency syndromes.

In our laboratory, the expiration in rat breath of ethane and pentane was followed in rats fed a 10% corn oil diet with 0, 11, or 40 IU *dl*-α-tocopherol acetate/kg diet for seven weeks starting at age 21 days.[21] Pentane evolved by the rats not supplemented with vitamin E was significantly higher during the seven-week period than that evolved by either of the supplemented groups of rats. Ethane production by the nonsupplemented group was significantly higher than that of the group supplemented with 40 IU vitamin E/kg of diet by five weeks, and significantly higher than that of both supplemented groups by six weeks. By seven weeks, pentane production was tenfold greater in the nonsupplemented group than in either supplemented group, and ethane was about twofold greater. Ethane and pentane produced by the two supplemented groups were not significantly different from each other.

In another study, the effects of dietary vitamin E, selenium, and polyunsaturated fats on *in vivo* lipid peroxidation were studied.[22] Some of the results are shown in TABLE 3. Weanling rats were fed a basal torula yeast diet with varying amounts of vitamin E, selenium, and either 10% stripped corn oil, stripped lard, or coconut oil. By seven weeks, rats fed the doubly deficient lard or coconut oil diets had one-half the pentane production of rats fed the doubly deficient corn oil diet. Plasma linoleic plus arachidonic acid was 1.8 times greater on a wt % basis in rats fed corn oil than in rats fed lard or coconut oil. Pentane levels in rats fed 40 IU vitamin E/kg of the selenium-deficient diet with corn oil were one-sixth those of rats fed the same diet without vitamin E. The plasma level of vitamin E in the vitamin E-supplemented corn-oil-fed rats was about six times greater than that of rats fed the vitamin E-deficient corn oil diet. Selenium decreased pentane production to a level one-half that of the doubly deficient rats.

The above results agree with the concept that *in vivo* lipid peroxidation is inhibited by vitamin E and selenium-glutathione peroxidase, and that it is proportional to the polyunsaturated fatty acid content and inversely proportional to the chain-breaking antioxidant, vitamin E. Lipid peroxidation is initiated by reactions of the endoplasmic reticulum,[5,6] and probable major sources of lipid peroxidation are organs such as liver and testes. Hydroperoxides produced by lipid peroxidation *in vivo* at a steady state concentration should be reduced by selenium-glutathione peroxidase, and the amount of hydroperoxides reduced should be proportional to the enzyme present.

The hypothesis that pentane is an *in vivo* product of lipid peroxidation was confirmed further in a study of rats fed a diet deficient in vitamin E and supplemented with the nonbiological antioxidant *N,N′*-diphenyl-*p*-phenylene-diamine (DPPD).[25] Rats were fed a vitamin E-deficient diet starting at three weeks of age. After five weeks, 0.01% DPPD was added to the diets of one-half of the rats (group DPPD), while the diet of the other rats remained unchanged (group OE). Within two weeks of the diet change, rats fed DPPD exhaled 65% less pentane than did rats in group OE. After five weeks of being fed the DPPD-supplemented diet, the rats were again fed the basal vitamin E-deficient diet, and within three weeks, pentane levels were similar to those of rats in group OE.

These results strongly support the hypothesis that pentane is a product of *in vivo* lipid peroxidation and that it can be used as a reliable index. In the study just described, the DPPD apparently was incorporated into the body tissues and substituted for vitamin E in a protective antioxidant role.

The effects of vitamin E depletion and repletion were also studied. After eight, eight, and five weeks of being fed a vitamin E-deficient diet, three groups of rats were fed diets supplemented with 3.3, 11, and 200 IU *dl*-α-tocopherol acetate/kg of diet, respectively. There were significant decreases in pentane production by all of

TABLE 3

In Vivo LIPID PEROXIDATION PROPORTIONAL TO POLYUNSATURATED FATS AND PROTECTION BY DIETARY VITAMIN E AND SELENIUM

Vitamin E-Stripped Dietary Fat	Antioxidant Added/kg	Pentane (pmol/100 g/min)
Lard	0	3.9
Corn oil	0	9.7
Corn oil	0.1 mg Se	4.5
Corn oil	40 IU vitamin E	1.7
Corn oil	0.1 mg Se and 40 IU vitamin E	1.7

these rats within two weeks of the change to the vitamin E–supplemented diets. After five weeks, pentane breath levels stabilized in each group. Breath pentane levels were inversely proportional to the log of the dietary vitamin E concentration.

A small amount of pentane was produced by rats fed 200 IU vitamin E/kg of diet. This was probably representative of formation and decomposition of linoleic acid hydroperoxides that occurred before the free radical chain reaction was broken by vitamin E. The very low level of pentane production by these rats indicates that there is no other significant source of pentane *in vivo*. Tissue vitamin E levels vary with the logarithm of the dietary vitamin E level. According to one concept, a doubling in tissue vitamin E should halve the amount of pentane produced. Thus, the relationship obtained, which is significant at the 99% confidence level, is pentane $\propto$ 1/[tissue vitamin E] $\propto$ 1/log [dietary vitamin E]. The study described above supports the concept of a direct correlation between pentane production and *in vivo* lipid peroxidation.

When rats were treated with strong prooxidants, the time-response relationships showed that maximum pentane production occurred by 15–30 minutes following administration of carbon tetrachloride (CCl_4), bromotrichloromethane ($BrCCl_3$), and chloroform ($CHCl_3$).[26,27] The amount of pentane produced is correlated with the bond dissociation energies of these three compounds. This finding supports the concept that trichloromethyl radicals produced by homolytic cleavage of halomethanes induce lipid peroxidation. Conjugated dienes in various tissues were measured following administration of CCl_4 and $BrCCl_3$. The liver accounted for 85% and 94% of the total conjugated dienes measured after administration of CCl_4 and $BrCCl_3$, respectively. The amount of pentane produced during the 30-minute period following injection of these two compounds corresponded to about 0.2% of the lipid peroxides in the liver, measured as conjugated dienes at 30 minutes. Liver is probably the principal site of pentane production *in vivo*.

Effects of In Vivo *Toxicant Initiators Measured by Pentane Production*

A survey was recently done in this laboratory in which rats were treated with several compounds that are potential toxicants, in order to test the possibility that lipid peroxidation is involved in the acute toxicities of these compounds. Treatment of rats with a number of these compounds has shown essentially null results in that increased pentane production was not significant, as shown in TABLE 4.

Cadmium was previously found to decrease testicular glutathione peroxidase activity and to increase lipid peroxidation in this tissue.[28] While cadmium exhibits considerable toxicity in animals, zinc, a similar metal, does not. The effectiveness of

TABLE 4

TOXIC TREATMENTS WITHOUT SIGNIFICANT INVOLVEMENT OF *In Vivo* LIPID PEROXIDATION*

Cadmium, acute toxic dose injected, zinc injected as control.
Cholesterol or *Cholestanol*, fed as 1% of vitamin E–deficient diet during 1 year.
Vitamin D_3 up to 5×10^5 IU/kg $\pm$ 0.1 g cholesterol/kg orally for 5 days.
Vitamin A up to 5×10^5 IU/kg orally for 8 days.
Vitamin K_3 up to 0.3 g/kg orally for 10 days.

* Except as noted, rats were fed a standard laboratory chow diet.

cadmium as a lipid peroxidation-inducing agent, administered as an acute toxic dose to rats fed a standard laboratory chow diet, was tested by J. Downey, and zinc was similarly tested. Neither cadmium (2.2 mg/kg) nor zinc (100 mg/kg) administration resulted in increased pentane production when monitored for up to nine days after administration.

Dr. M. Bechtold followed the course of pentane production by groups of female rats fed a vitamin E-deficient diet over a one-year period. One group of rats was fed 1% cholesterol, and one group was fed 1% cholestanol, with the idea in mind that there might be differences in the stability of membranes and that these differences might show up as more peroxidizable membranes in the rats fed cholesterol. During the period of one year, there were no significant differences among the three groups of vitamin E-deficient rats as measured by pentane production.

It was reported by Russian workers that vitamin D toxicity in rats was decreased by administration of vitamin E.[29] Oral doses of vitamin D plus cholesterol were found to produce arterial lesions. R. Litov administered 5×10^5 IU vitamin D_3/kg with and without 0.1 g cholesterol/kg daily for five days with no evidence of lipid peroxidation as measured by pentane production, although physical symptoms indicated considerable toxicity to the rats.

Vitamin A, a known membrane destabilizer, is toxic in high dosages.[30] To test possible involvement of an acute toxic dose of vitamin A in induction of lipid peroxidation, R. Litov administered to rats as much as 5×10^5 IU of vitamin A ester concentrate/kg for eight days, and although gross physical evidence of toxicity was present in the animals, there was no increase in pentane production by these rats.

Vitamin K_3 (menadione of bacterial origin) is toxic in that it produces red blood cell hemolysis.[31] R. Litov also tested its potential as a peroxidizing agent by administering oral doses of 300 mg vitamin K_3/kg for 10 days to three rats. By the tenth day only one rat was surviving, but no increase in pentane production was seen by this time.

In other studies currently in progress, treatment of rats with oxidants or strong prooxidants has shown that lipid peroxidation is involved in the ensuing toxicity. TABLE 5 summarizes the results in terms of pentane production following treatment, with pentane production by vitamin E-deficient rats used as a point of comparison. By comparison with the relatively large amounts of pentane respired by oxidant-treated rats (10–1200 pmol/100 g/minute), vitamin E-supplemented rats produce very low levels of pentane (1–2 pmol/100 g/minute).

Dr. M. Bechtold and D. Gee are studying the possible relationship of the microsomal P-450 system to lipid peroxidation.[32] CCl_4 is metabolized by this system to the trichloromethyl free radical, and $CHCl_3$ is one product of metabolism. After intraperitoneal (ip) injection of 30 μl CCl_4/100 g, rats fed a standard laboratory chow diet produced three times less pentane than did rats fed a vitamin E-deficient diet. The relationship of pentane expired to $CHCl_3$ and acetone expired following injection of CCl_4 is being studied also.

Peroxides are generally strong oxidants. R. Litov has determined the effect of injecting rats with methyl ethyl ketone peroxide at 0.8 the LD_{50}. He has compared pentane production by vitamin E-supplemented and vitamin E-deficient rats (fed diets for six–nine weeks) following ip injection of 50 mg methyl ethyl ketone peroxide in mineral oil/kg at 20 minutes following injection. Rats fed a vitamin E-deficient diet produced 12 times more pentane than did vitamin E-supplemented rats following injection. Prior treatment of vitamin E-deficient rats by daily injection of 750 mg of vitamin C/kg/three days caused a doubling of pentane production over that by rats not treated with vitamin C, when lipid peroxidation was induced by methyl ethyl ketone peroxide injection.

TABLE 5

TOXIC CONDITIONS INVOLVING *In Vivo* LIPID PEROXIDATION

Condition or Treatment of Rat	Pentane Production (pmol/100 g body wt/min)	Time after Injection (min)
Vitamin E-deficient*	10	—
Carbon tetrachloride (30 μl/100 g)		
Laboratory chow-fed	10	30
Vitamin E-deficient	30	30
Methyl ethyl ketone peroxide (0.8 LD_{50})		
Vitamin E-supplemented	50†	20
Vitamin E-deficient	600†	20
Vitamin E-deficient, injected with vitamin C‡	1200†	20
Iron-injected§		
Vitamin E-deficient	50	—

* Rats were fed a 10% stripped corn oil diet for 7 weeks.

† Pentane production above basal levels.

‡ Rats were injected with 750 mg vitamin C/kg/day/3 days, and pentane was measured 24 hours later following injection with methyl ethyl ketone peroxide.

§ Rats were injected with 0.2 g iron as iron dextran/kg body wt three times over a 6-week period.

Iron has been reported to increase lipid peroxidation in vitamin E- and selenium-deficient rats as measured by ethane evolution, and a large amount of iron injected over a 28-day time period increased pentane production in rats fed a standard laboratory chow diet.[33,34] J. Downey is studying the effect of injecting iron, as iron dextran, in vitamin E-deficient rats. Three injections of 0.2 g/kg over a period of six weeks increased pentane production fivefold as compared with nontreated vitamin E-deficient rats.

This paper has brought out some of the many interactions that take place in lipid peroxidation reactions. The need for further studies of these interactions *in vivo* has been emphasized. Current research indicates that one of the best methods to study lipid peroxidation *in vivo* is the measurement of expired pentane. Recent studies using this technique show that vitamin E is the dominant antioxidant that provides protection and that selenium-glutathione peroxidase also provides significant defense against lipid peroxidation *in vivo.*

SUMMARY

Some of the vitamins and many of the metals that are being considered at this symposium interact in lipid peroxidation. Some of these interactions have been studied *in vivo*. Measurement of *in vivo* lipid peroxidation in the rat is accomplished by gas chromatographic analysis of pentane, a minor peroxidation product that is exhaled in the breath. In the rat, lipid peroxidation is proportional to dietary polyunsaturated lipids when the animal is deficient in antioxygenic agents. The chain-breaking antioxidant vitamin E is the main protector against *in vivo* lipid peroxidation. Dietary selenium, through its involvement in the biosynthesis of glutathione peroxidase, functions in a secondary antioxygenic role as a hydroperoxide reducer. In rats fed a vitamin E-deficient diet, injection of some hydroperoxides, iron, or vitamin C leads to initiation of *in vivo* lipid peroxidation, apparently by decomposing hydroperoxides to free radicals. Carbon tetrachloride, a toxic halogenated hydrocarbon, is metabolized by liver microsomes and initiates *in vivo* lipid peroxidation in the liver. These examples show that practical information on interactions involving *in vivo* lipid peroxidation can be obtained by studies that use the pentane method.

References

1. Pryor, W. A. 1976. *In* Free Radicals in Biology. W. A. Pryor, Ed. **1:** 1–49. Academic Press, Inc. New York, N.Y.
2. Mead, J. F. 1976. *In* Free Radicals in Biology. W. A. Pryor, Ed. **1:** 51–68. Academic Press, Inc. New York, N.Y.
3. Pryor, W. A. 1977. Med. Chem. N.Y. **5:** 331–359.
4. Tappel, A. L. 1978. Adv. Exp. Med. Biol. **97:** 111–131.
5. Plaa, G. L. & H. Witschi. 1976. Ann. Rev. Pharmacol. Toxicol. **16:** 125–141.
6. McCay, P. B. & J. L. Poyer. 1976. *In* Enzymes of Biological Membranes. A. Martonosi, Ed.: 239–256. Plenum Press. New York, N.Y.
7. Tappel, A. L. 1975. *In* Pathobiology of Cell Membranes. B. F. Trump & A. U. Arstila, Eds. **1:** 145–170. Academic Press, Inc. New York, N.Y.
8. Scott, M. L. 1973. *In* Organic Selenium Compounds: Their Chemistry and Biology. D. L. Klayman & W. H. H. Günther, Eds.: 629–661. Wiley-Interscience. New York, N.Y.
9. Ganther, H. E. 1974. *In* Selenium. R. A. Zingaro & W. C. Cooper, Eds.: 546–614. Van Nostrand Reinhold Co. New York, N.Y.
10. Flohé, L. 1976. *In* Proceedings of the Symposium on Selenium-Tellurium in the Environment, University of Notre Dame: 138–152. Industrial Health Foundation, Inc. Pittsburgh, Penn.
11. Flohé, L., W. A. Günzler & R. Ladenstein. 1976. *In* Glutathione: Metabolism and Function. I. M. Arias & W. B. Jakoby, Eds.: 115–138. Raven Press. New York, N.Y.
12. Ganther, H. E., D. G. Hafeman, R. A. Lawrence, R. E. Serfass & W. G. Hoekstra. 1976. *In* Trace Elements in Human Health and Disease. A. S. Prasad & D. Oberleas, Eds. **2:** 165–234. Academic Press, Inc. New York, N.Y.
13. Forstrom, J. W., J. J. Zakowski & A. L. Tappel. 1978. Biochemistry **17:** 2639–2644.
14. Zakowski, J. J., J. W. Forstrom, R. A. Condell & A. L. Tappel. 1978. Biochem. Biophys. Res. Commun. **84:** 248–253.
15. Lyons, D. W., C. W. Hawkes, J. W. Forstrom, J. J. Zakowski, C. J. Dillard, R. E. Litov & A. L. Tappel. 1978. Fed. Proc. Fed. Am. Soc. Exp. Biol. **37:** 1339.
16. Hawkes, W. C., D. E. Lyons & A. L. Tappel. 1979. Fed. Proc. Fed. Am. Soc. Exp. Biol. **38:** 820.
17. Splittgerber, A. G. & A. L. Tappel. 1979. Arch. Biochem. Biophys. **197:** 534–542.
18. Hafeman, D. G. & W. G. Hoekstra. 1977. J. Nutr. **107:** 656–665.
19. Dumelin, E. E. & A. L. Tappel. 1977. Lipids **12:** 894–900.
20. Donovan, D. H. & D. B. Menzel. 1978. Experientia **34:** 775–776.
21. Dillard, C. J., E. E. Dumelin & A. L. Tappel. 1977. Lipids **12:** 109–114.
22. Dillard, C. J., R. E. Litov & A. L. Tappel. 1978. Lipids **13:** 396–402.
23. Köster, U., D. Albrecht & H. Kappus. 1977. Toxicol. Appl. Pharmacol. **41:** 639–648.
24. Hafeman, D. G. & W. G. Hoekstra. 1977. J. Nutr. **107:** 666–672.
25. Downey, J. E., D. H. Irving & A. L. Tappel. 1978. Lipids **13:** 403–407.
26. Sagai, M. & A. L. Tappel. 1978. Toxicol. Lett. **2:** 149–155.
27. Sagai, M. & A. L. Tappel. 1979. Toxicol. Appl. Pharmacol. **49:** 283–291.
28. Omaye, S. T. & A. L. Tappel. 1975. Res. Commun. Chem. Pathol. Pharmacol. **12:** 695–711.
29. Spirichev, V. B., N. V. Blazheevich & I. M. Raskin. 1969. Vopr. Med. Khim. **15:** 123.
30. Rodahl, K. 1950. J. Nutr. **41:** 399–415.
31. Finkel, M. J. 1961. Clin. Pharmacol. Ther. **2:** 794–814.

32. GEE, D. L., M. M. BECHTOLD & A. L. TAPPEL. 1980. Fed. Proc. Fed. Am. Soc. Exp. Biol. **39:** 631.
33. DOUGHERTY, J. J. & W. G. HOEKSTRA. 1977. Fed. Proc. Fed. Am. Soc. Exp. Biol. **36:** 1151.
34. DILLARD, C. J. & A. L. TAPPEL. 1979. Lipids **14:** 989–995.

DISCUSSION

P. MARFEY (*State University of New York, Albany, N.Y.*): In your scheme, where you have implicated vitamin E as donating a hydrogen atom to the peroxy free radical, I assume that a carbon-based free radical can accept a hydrogen atom from vitamin E. For example, after β-scission you have a carbon-based free radical. Can that free radical abstract a hydrogen atom from vitamin E and become reduced?

A. L. TAPPEL: Yes, a carbon free radical can abstract hydrogen from vitamin E. What I show is the dominant quantitative situation wherein the free radical lipid usually reacts avidly with oxygen to give the hydroperoxy radical, and then that radical abstracts the hydrogen.

C. S. LIEBER (*Mount Sinai School of Medicine, New York, N.Y.*): With regard to the pentane measurements *in vivo,* how much of it can be derived from the gastrointestinal [GI] tract?

A. L. TAPPEL: We and the others who study this usually use animals that have been fasted for some period of time. In this way, we try to keep any gastrointestinal tract gases to a minimum.

C. S. LIEBER: How do you do it? Because even in starvation, you may have some GI production.

A. L. TAPPEL: Yes, the possibility hasn't been eliminated, but I think the amount has been reduced to a very low level.

C. S. LIEBER: Now the second question concerns pentane metabolism. How inert is it really?—because there has been some question concerning possible microsomal metabolism of pentane.

A. L. TAPPEL: We have not seen any absolute measurements of pentane metabolism. We believe that it is very low, and we have no evidence of its being metabolized.

W. R. HOLUB (*Life Systems Incorporated, Melville, N.Y.*): I have two short questions. One, did you try experiments with high or toxic levels of selenium and/or vitamin E? Second, have you looked at a physiological change that reflects peroxide production? I saw some work done on either measuring malonaldehyde or the sickling phenomenon, which is also related to antioxidant function.

A. L. TAPPEL: On topic one, we have used high levels of vitamin E and toxic levels of selenium, which produces glutathione peroxidase usually at a maximum level. Second, concerning physiological or pathological conditions that would generate lipid peroxidation, we have looked mainly at the effect of toxic compounds. Of course, animals that are partially vitamin E deficient might be considered to be in physiological or pathological conditions. They give off pentane in proportion to their vitamin E deficiency.

P. HOCHSTEIN (*University of Southern California School of Medicine, Los Angeles, Calif.*): Do you have any thoughts about the tissue source of pentane? You say the intestinal flora can be ruled out. How about plasma unsaturated fatty acids?

A. L. TAPPEL: Yes, Dr. Hochstein, the only case where we've done much about quantitating the source is in the injection of carbon tetrachloride, which is, of course, known to be a liver toxin. Therein, we measured the conjugated dienes formed from the peroxidizing lipid, and about 90% originated in the liver. So we assume, then, that 90% of the pentane came from that source. We don't have any other direct way of finding out what organs the pentane comes from.

E. M. GROSSMAN (*General Foods Research, Tarrytown, N.Y.*): As you know, there is quite a bit of push among many circles for the U.S. diet to change in the direction of increasing the polyunsaturated-saturated ratio to at least 1 from its current level of about ½. Could you speculate as to whether the normal vitamin E intake that is found in the average American diet would then be adequate to cover this increase in possible free radical generation.

A. L. TAPPEL: In a general way, any increase in consumption of vegetable oils would bring the requisite amount of vitamin E into the human body, and that probably would be a satisfactory balance.

Now I am concerned that people are exposed to mixed levels of toxicants, such as we enumerate; namely, oxidants in the air and also halogenated hydrocarbons. We don't know what level of protection these people are being afforded by their diets, but the pentane method does allow that measurement to be made. We have used it to monitor people, and so I think it will have more application.

L. M. KLEVAY (*Human Nutrition Laboratory, U.S. Department of Agriculture, Grand Forks, N. Dak.*): I have a comment related to Dr. Grossman's question. It seems that these data have important implications in the free radical theory of aging and experimental carcinogenesis. Then I have a question. Is superoxide dismutase involved in any of this?

A. L. TAPPEL: In that superoxide dismutase would catalyze superoxide to form hydrogen peroxide, which then could initiate lipid peroxidation, yes, it could well be involved.

K. C. BHUYAN (*Mount Sinai School of Medicine, New York, N.Y.*): Dr. Tappel, we have some evidence of lipid peroxidation in cataract in the human and also in experimental-animal-model cataract. I was trying to prevent this cataract by vitamin E and selenium; the results were not very encouraging, but we are continuing. Now, we find that high doses of selenium as selenite in rats produce cataract. These are selenium-injected rats, and cataract is produced within one to two weeks. Do you have any explanation for this toxic effect of selenium?

A. L. TAPPEL: We have no experience in that aspect of its toxicity.

K. C. BHUYAN: Now, what I have found is that there is a significant amount of superoxide dismutase in these lenses. There is no glutathione peroxidase, and there is insufficient catalase in the lenses. Do you have any comment on this?

A. L. TAPPEL: Sounds like a good example of interactions.

I. S. JAMALL (*University of Cincinnati Medical Center, Cincinnati, Ohio*): You alluded to the glutathione transferase system. Recent papers have been published on the glutathione peroxidase activity of the glutathione transferase, also called the selenium-independent glutathione peroxidase. What are your feelings on the relative importance of this selenium-independent glutathione peroxidase in various species?

A. L. TAPPEL: This is a very important topic; it hasn't been investigated much. Many of the conclusions relative to the human about selenium need have been drawn from the rat, an animal that is very dependent on selenium, whereas the human, for example, might be more dependent on the glutathione transferase system. So I think there need to be more comparative studies of these two enzymes.

H. SPRINCE (*Veterans Administration Medical Center, Coatesville, Penn.*): On this effect that you got with vitamin C, I think you infer that this was due to ascorbic acid reducing iron.

A. L. Tappel: Right.

H. Sprince: Also, iron doing the oxidizing. It must be remembered that ascorbic acid is in equilibrium with dehydroascorbic acid. Could dehydroascorbic acid have affected this? I think people are overlooking the fact that ascorbic acid can be a double-edged sword, and the effects of dehydroascorbic acid oxidations must be considered. What is your response?

A. L. Tappel: Yes, I don't want to make it sound too simple. If one did this in an *in vitro* system, then one could be sure of the mechanisms of the ascorbate reducing the iron and the iron catalyzing the peroxide decomposition. We think that's what's going on primarily *in vivo.* But, as you say, it could be more complicated.

INTERACTION OF VITAMIN C AND IRON*

Sean R. Lynch and James D. Cook

Division of Hematology
Department of Medicine
University of Kansas Medical Center
Kansas City, Kansas 66103

and

Veterans Administration Hospital
Kansas City, Missouri 64128

In early studies of food iron absorption, test meals consisted of single foods that had been biosynthetically labeled with radioiron.[1] Absorption varied considerably with individual food items, and in general, iron derived from animal tissue was more available than iron of vegetable origin.[1-3] More recently, it has been shown that the percentage absorption of iron from a given food item differs substantially when it is eaten in a meal containing two or more additional foods.[2-4] For example, soybean iron is much better absorbed than black bean iron if each is eaten separately, but a similar percentage of iron is absorbed from both bean sources when they are eaten together.[3] Absorption therefore appears to be a property of the overall composition of the meal rather than of the single food item. These studies led to a very important observation. If a small quantity of soluble inorganic iron is added to a biosynthetically labeled vegetable food just before it is eaten, percentage absorption of the two forms of iron is virtually identical.[5] The same is true of meals containing more than one vegetable food.[5-8] Therefore, it appears that when several foods are eaten together, nonheme iron destined for absorption behaves as though it were derived from a single common pool. Soluble inorganic iron salts used in fortification also enter this pool.[7,8] Iron absorption from it can be measured by determining the size of the pool and the percentage absorption of a soluble radioiron tracer added to the meal.[5-8]

Similar observations have been made for heme iron, which comes principally from hemoglobin and myoglobin of meat. Heme compounds enter a second common pool and share a set of properties different from those that govern nonheme iron absorption.[9] For example, heme is not degraded to any degree in the lumen of the gut but is taken up by the mucosal cells with iron still within the porphyrin ring.[10] Heme iron absorption is relatively independent of other components of the meal; ascorbic acid has no effect.[11,12] Absorption of heme iron can be measured by adding a small quantity of labeled hemoglobin to a meal just before it is eaten.[9] Virtually all dietary iron is absorbed from these two pools of heme and nonheme iron.[13]

In attempting to combat iron deficiency, most investigators have focused their attention on nonheme iron, which makes up over 90% of the iron in an average diet.[13] The percentage absorption of nonheme iron is only about one-tenth that of heme. Unlike heme iron, the availability of nonheme iron is critically dependent on several factors, some of which enhance and others of which inhibit its uptake.[14] Many chemical ligands present in food are known to have a powerful influence. For

* This work was supported by contract DSAN-C-0045 from the U.S. Agency for International Development and by Veterans Administration Interagency Agreement IGA V 589 (134)5-79033 from the U.S. Food and Drug Administration.

0077-8923/80/0355-0032 $01.75/0 © 1980, NYAS

example, carbonates, oxalates, phosphates, fiber components, and tannates impair absorption, while ascorbic acid, citric acid, tricarboxylic acids, amino acids, and sugars promote absorption. Of these, ascorbic acid has the greatest influence on iron assimilation.

Initial evidence suggesting that ascorbic acid can enhance iron absorption from certain foods was obtained in studies using meals eaten with and without citrus fruits.[1,15-20] For example, when 100 ml orange juice containing 40–50 mg ascorbic acid was added to a meal consisting of bread, butter, jam, tea or coffee, and an egg that had been biologically labeled with ^{59}Fe, absorption increased from 3.7 to 10.4%.[18] More recently, Rossander *et al.* studied a common Swedish "continental breakfast" and demonstrated that when orange juice containing 70 mg ascorbic acid is consumed with coffee and two wheat rolls, absorption is 2½ times higher than that from the same meal without orange juice.[20]

Moore and Dubach were the first to identify ascorbic acid as the cause of the increased absorption seen with meals containing fruit.[1] They demonstrated a similar increase in absorption with equivalent quantities of ascorbic acid. Their findings have subsequently been confirmed by others. Layrisse *et al.* demonstrated that nonheme iron absorption from a maize meal was increased severalfold when papaya was added to the meal.[19] The same degree of enhancement was achieved by adding ascorbic acid equivalent in amount to that contained in the papaya. Thus, although it is possible that there are factors other than ascorbic acid in fruit juices that enhance absorption, there is little doubt that ascorbic acid accounts for the major effect.

Ascorbic Acid as a Nonheme Common Pool Ligand

Early observations involving fruit juices led to a series of studies of the effect of ascorbic acid on the absorption of various forms of nonheme iron.[19,21-31] In two of the more recent investigations, ascorbic acid was added to meals prepared from maize, wheat, soya, and rice.[24,25] The cereal component of each meal had been labeled intrinsically with ^{55}Fe by hydroponic cultivation. $^{59}FeCl_3$, used as the extrinsic label for the nonheme pool, was added to the meal in trace quantities either immediately before the meal was eaten or to one of the ingredients before cooking. Supplemental iron in the form of a soluble iron salt, such as 2–5 mg ferric ammonium citrate or 4 mg ferrous sulfate, was incorporated into some of the meals. Ascorbic acid produced the same increase in absorption of both extrinsic and intrinsic radioiron labels over a wide range of absorption values and ascorbic acid concentrations (Figure 1). The composite mean absorption ratio of extrinsic to intrinsic radioiron was 1.13, a value very close to that of 1.10 reported by Cook *et al.* for meals containing no ascorbic acid.[5] These observations strongly support the conclusion that ascorbic acid acts as a ligand for the common nonheme iron pool and thus enhances absorption of all iron compounds in this pool to an equal extent. An important corollary is that extrinsic tagging allows valid comparisons to be made between meals eaten with and without supplementary ascorbic acid.

A number of ligands in food have a powerful inhibitory effect on absorption from the nonheme iron pool. The interaction of ascorbic acid with two of these, tannates and calcium/phosphate, has been studied.[32,31] Ascorbic acid reverses the strong inhibitory effect that tea exerts on nonheme iron absorption from cereal-based meals.[32] The degree of reversal of inhibition is directly proportional to the quantity of added ascorbic acid; absorption in the presence of ascorbic acid and tea may exceed absorption from the basal meal containing neither. The effect of ascorbic acid

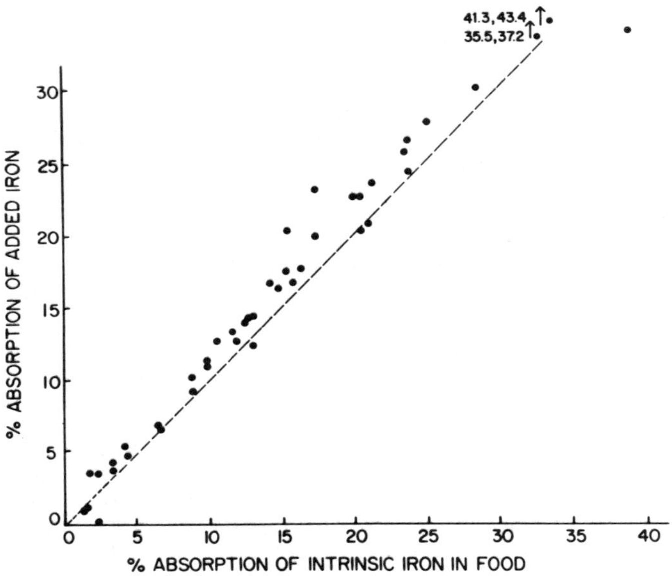

FIGURE 1. Nonheme iron absorption from test meals tagged simultaneously with intrinsic and extrinsic radioiron labels (see text for explanation).

on the inhibitory influence of calcium/phosphate on iron absorption was studied using a semisynthetic meal.[31] When inorganic calcium/phosphate was omitted from this meal, absorption increased about twofold, but the mean ratio of the meal with ascorbic acid to that without was similar whether or not calcium/phosphate was present. Apparently, ascorbic acid and known inhibitors of iron absorption have an opposite, but additive, effect on absorption from the nonheme common pool and can therefore be considered to act as competitive ligands.

The influence of ascorbic acid on iron absorption from meals containing other absorption promoters is less well defined. For example, meat and fish increase nonheme iron absorption when added to a vegetable meal. Cook and Monsen compared iron absorption from a standard meal containing beef, potatoes, cornmeal, peaches, ice milk, bread, and margarine with that of a semisynthetic meal of similar composition prepared with dextrimaltose, corn oil, and ovalbumin.[31] Nonheme iron absorption from the standard meal was much higher owing to its content of meat. Absorption from both these meals was enhanced by adding 100 mg of ascorbic acid. However, the mean absorption ratio of the meal with ascorbic acid to that without was 3.19 for the semisynthetic meal and only 1.67 for the standard meal, indicating that the enhancing effects of meat and ascorbic acid are not additive. A similar observation has been made with fish and ascorbic acid. Whereas 100 g fish increased the absorption of nonheme iron about threefold,[33] the percentage absorption of iron from a maize meal eaten with 100 g fish and fresh papayas containing approximately 70 mg ascorbic acid was the same as that from the meal eaten with the papayas alone.[19] Although it is not possible to draw definitive conclusions from this evidence, these two studies suggest that ascorbic acid and beef or fish are complementary rather than additive in their enhancing properties and that the addition of ascorbic acid to a meal containing meat or fish may have a relatively small influence on the quantity of nonheme iron absorbed.

Accumulating evidence indicates that the total intake of dietary iron is less important from a nutritional standpoint than the availability of that iron. A model has recently been proposed for estimating dietary iron absorption from any given meal based on the iron status of the individual, the content of heme and nonheme iron, and the content of enhancing constituents.[34] Of the many factors that have been said to influence iron absorption, only two were considered important enough for inclusion in the method for estimating available dietary iron. Meals were defined as having low, medium, or high iron availability based on the content of meat, poultry, or fish and of ascorbic acid. In this model, 1 g meat was considered roughly equivalent in its enhancing effect to 1 mg ascorbic acid. Estimates of nonheme iron absorption in subjects with 500 mg iron stores are shown in TABLE 1. The model defines the effect of these substances when added separately to a meal. It is less clear whether their effect is additive when both are contained in the meal. Presumably, the effect of 30–90 g meat, fish, or poultry *and* 25–75 mg ascorbic acid would be roughly additive and therefore would place the meal in the high iron availability category, but as previously discussed, this point is not clearly established.

INTERACTION OF ASCORBIC ACID AND CONTAMINANT IRON

Not all the iron in a meal is necessarily intrinsic to the food. Chemical assays of Indian diets have consistently revealed iron contents considerably in excess of those determined from food composition tables.[14] The disparity is believed to represent iron contamination either from the soil or from cooking utensils. The high prevalence of iron deficiency in these geographic areas of the world suggests that this iron is poorly absorbed. Therefore, the potential influence that ascorbic acid has on these less soluble forms of iron could be of considerable nutritional importance. Evaluation of ascorbic acid's effect is difficult because the chemical nature of the extraneous iron has not been identified and because suitable radiolabeled material is difficult to obtain. One study has addressed the problem indirectly.[30] Two likely food contaminants, ferric oxide, which is the major component of rust derived from cooking utensils, and ferric hydroxide, which forms much of the iron found in soil and unpurified water sources, were radiolabeled and added to a maize porridge meal; both were poorly absorbed, with mean values of 0.01% and 1.5%, respectively. The addition of 100 mg ascorbic acid increased absorption from ferric oxide to 0.5% and from ferric hydroxide to 6.7%. Although the relative increase was pronounced, absorption was still inappropriately low in the context of the meal and the iron-deficient population studied. This suggests that a significant proportion of each compound remains insoluble and unavailable to the common nonheme iron pool. Moreover, ferric hydroxide was absorbed only half as well as the intrinsic iron con-

TABLE 1

DIETARY IRON AVAILABILITY*

Meal Iron Availability	Meat, Fish, Poultry (g)		Ascorbic Acid (mg)	Nonheme Iron Absorption (%)
Low	< 30	and	< 25	3
Medium	30–90	or	25–75	5
High	> 90	or	> 75	8

* Based on data of Monsen *et al.*[34]

tained in maize porridge. Presumably most of the contaminating iron contained in food remains relatively unavailable for absorption despite the presence of ascorbic acid.

Quantitative Aspects

While many observers have noted that percentage nonheme food iron absorption rises with increasing ascorbic acid content of a meal, the quantitative effect of ascorbic acid has been examined rigorously in only two studies, which yielded similar results.[27,31] In one of them, ascorbic acid—ranging in amounts from 25 to 1,000 mg—was added to a semisynthetic meal containing 4.1 mg elemental iron. A linear relationship was observed between the absorption ratio of the meal with ascorbic acid to that without and the quantity of added ascorbic acid when both values were plotted on a logarithmic scale. A somewhat different relationship is seen when percentage absorption is plotted against the molar ratio of ascorbic acid to iron using linear scales (Figure 2). The response curve has two components. With the molar ratios below 7.5, which corresponds to approximately 100 mg ascorbic acid, there is a proportionately greater effect than with molar ratios above 7.5. It is interesting that when ascorbic acid is taken with pharmacologic doses of ferrous sulfate in the fasting state, a similar two-phase dose-response pattern occurs, although the degree of enhancement and the actual quantity of iron absorbed are very different in the two studies (Figure 3).[35]

The factors responsible for the two components of the dose-response curve are unknown, but it is tempting to speculate that the initial component may represent the effect that ascorbic acid has in rendering ferric iron soluble at the alkaline pH of the duodenum (see below). This would account for the relatively small increase in absorption seen when ascorbic acid was added to ferrous sulfate, since a large quantity

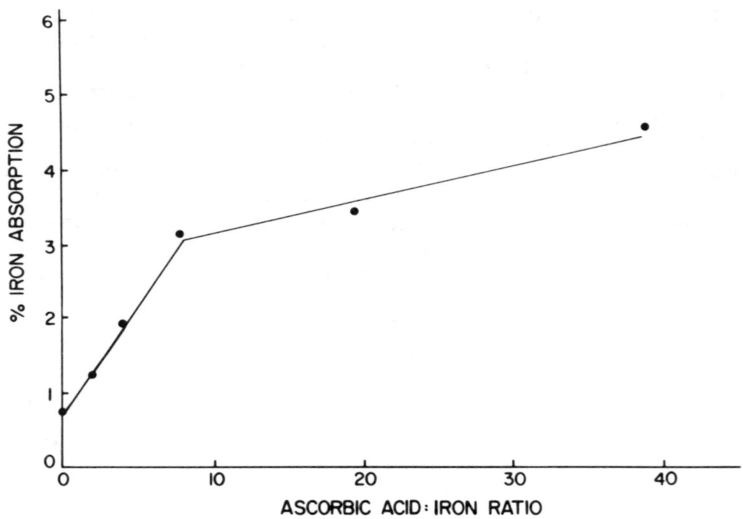

Figure 2. The effect of ascorbic acid on iron absorption from a semisynthetic meal. Geometric mean percentage iron absorption is plotted against the molar ratio of ascorbic acid to iron in the meal. (From the data of Cook and Monsen.)[31]

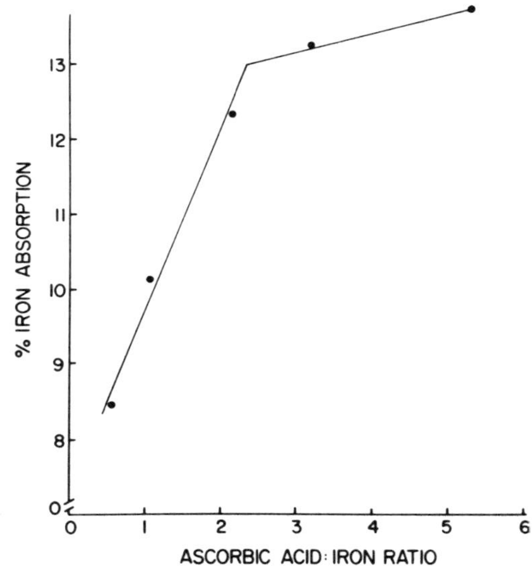

FIGURE 3. The effect of ascorbic acid on iron absorption from 30 mg elemental iron as ferrous sulfate. Percentage iron absorption is plotted against the molar ratio of ascorbic acid to iron. Since there were differences in basal absorption between groups of subjects receiving varying levels of ascorbic acid, the percentage absorption values plotted are those predicted from the absorption ratio with and without ascorbic acid for each group and the geometric mean basal absorption without ascorbic acid of the first group of subjects receiving 50 mg ascorbic acid. (Data from Brise and Hallberg.)[35]

of iron taken in this form would be expected to arrive at the absorptive surface of the duodenum as the soluble ferrous salt even in the absence of ascorbic acid.

Most of the published evidence dealing with the effect of ascorbic acid on vegetable iron absorption is derived from meals containing maize or rice. If the effect of varying iron status in these studies is removed by relating food iron absorption to a reference dose of ferrous sulfate and ascorbic acid, it is possible to compare the relative absorption of iron in different studies and in different population groups.[36] We have used the results obtained in a number of different investigations to construct a dose-response curve for iron absorption against molar ratio of ascorbic acid to iron in the meal (FIGURE 4).[19,24–26,29,30] All values have been adjusted to a reference absorption of 40%, a level that was considered indicative of iron deficiency. Although there is considerable variability between studies, the increase in percentage absorption is again directly proportional to the molar ratio of ascorbic acid to iron in the meal, emphasizing the singular importance of the quantity of ascorbic acid to nonheme iron absorption from vegetable meals.

MECHANISM OF ACTION

Ascorbic acid is effective only if it is present in the meal. In one study, 500 mg ascorbic acid taken with the meal increased absorption about sixfold, whereas the same quantity had little effect when taken four to eight hours prior to the meal.[31] In most investigations, ascorbic acid has been contained in an uncooked component of

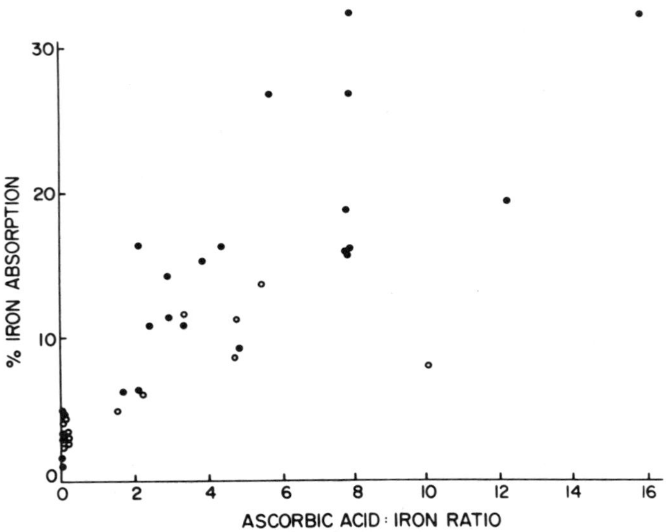

FIGURE 4. Enhancing influence of ascorbic acid on vegetable nonheme iron absorption. Mean percentage iron absorption, corrected for reference absorption, is plotted against the molar ratio of ascorbic acid to iron in the meals, Solid circles represent maize meals, and open circles represent rice meals (see text for explanation).

the meal or has been added just before consumption. Under certain circumstances, enhancement was also seen when it was incorporated into one of the ingredients prior to cooking. After boiling, approximately 70% of 50- and 100-mg supplements of ascorbic acid remained in the reduced form and significant enhancement of iron absorption was seen.[24] However, in baked foods, such as soy biscuits and wheat bread, very little ascorbic acid remained in the reduced state and no enhancement of iron absorption occurred.

A better understanding of the probable mode of action of ascorbic acid has been provided by the studies of Conrad and Schade.[37] When reducing agents are absent from food, iron in the common pool exists in ferric form. Ferric iron has a coordinating valence of 6, and in an aqueous solution, metal ions are bound to each other through water bridges. Since increases in pH make more hydroxyl ions available, metallic polymers or precipitated metallic hydroxides are formed, and the iron becomes inaccessible to the mucosal cell.[14] Conrad and Schade demonstrated that the addition of ascorbic acid to a ferric chloride solution at an acid pH causes displacement of hydrogen ions from ascorbate and the formation of a purple-colored complex that can be isolated by alcoholic precipitation. This iron chelate remains in solution over a wide pH range of 2–11. The reaction however must be initiated at acid pH (FIGURE 5). Both ferric chloride alone and ferric chloride plus ascorbate are insoluble at alkaline pH. Both become progressively more soluble as the pH is reduced by the addition of hydrochloric acid, and both are totally soluble at a pH of approximately 2. As pH is again raised with sodium hydroxide, ferric chloride is precipitated and very little remains soluble at a pH above 4. In contrast, the addition of ascorbic acid to ferric chloride yields a complex of iron that remains completely soluble at a higher pH. The importance of solubility to iron absorption was confirmed in gastrectomized rats. Radioiron absorption was measured from oral

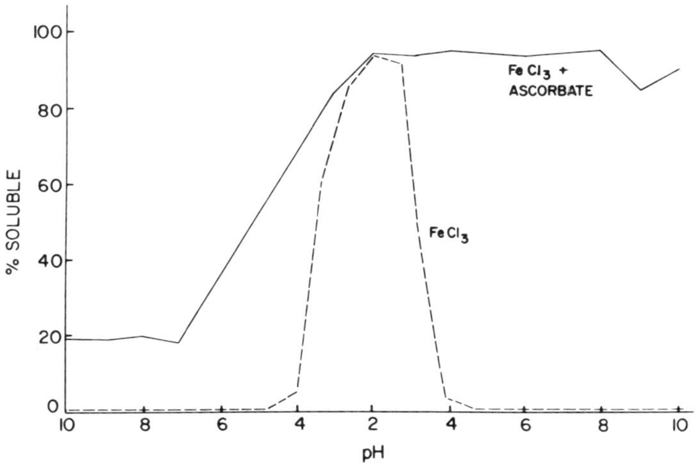

FIGURE 5. Effect of pH on the solubility of $FeCl_3$ with and without ascorbate. Both $FeCl_3$ (hatched line) and $FeCl_3$ to which an equimolar quantity of ascorbic acid had been added were relatively insoluble in NaOH. As the pH was reduced by the addition of HCl, both became soluble. $FeCl_3$ was again precipitated by realkalization with NaOH, while $FeCl_3$ with ascorbic acid remained soluble. (After Conrad and Schade.)[37]

test doses of ferric chloride to which ascorbic acid had been added. Mean percentage absorption for test doses containing ascorbic acid added before and after alkalization was 17 and 5.3, respectively. Similar results were obtained in experiments in which the test doses were instilled directly into the duodenum. When the two iron solutions were introduced into the stomach separately, approximately equal quantities of iron were absorbed.

Ascorbic Acid Fortification

In the past, attempts to improve iron nutrition in populations at risk for iron deficiency relied on iron fortification. The efficacy of this approach has been questioned, since added iron enters the nonheme pool of dietary iron and is affected by inhibitors of iron absorption prevalent in this type of diet. If the diet consists predominantly of cereals such as wheat, maize, and rice, which are poor sources of available iron, fortification iron is also poorly absorbed. Improvement in iron status may only be possible if fortification iron is added in a form less affected by dietary constituents or if a substance is added to the diet that renders both food iron and fortification iron more available. The former approach has led to the use of iron with ethylenediamine tetraacetic acid (EDTA) in pilot fortification studies. The latter might be made feasible by adding ascorbic acid to the diet.

Although theoretically attractive, a number of obstacles have been encountered in using ascorbic acid for dietary fortification. The initial investigations were based on the premise that optimal results would be obtained by adding both ascorbic acid and fortification iron to the diet to ensure a sufficiently large pool of nonheme iron on which ascorbic acid could act.[24] However, in selecting a suitable food vehicle for dual fortification, a number of practical problems were encountered. It is desirable for such a vehicle to be eaten in approximately the same quantities by all individuals. Ideally, the vehicle should not be added prior to cooking, since ascorbic acid is largely inactivated when subjected to the high temperatures used for baking. Common salt seemed to be the most suitable vehicle, but discoloration occurred when ascorbic acid and various iron compounds were added to it simultaneously.[25,26] The discoloration was particularly pronounced when cheaper grades of salt were used and after storage in hot, humid conditions. Nevertheless, it is possible to fortify common salt with 0.1% iron as ferric phosphate ($FePO_4$) and 1.25% ascorbic acid. This product can be stored under all but the most extreme tropical conditions provided that 2.5% starch is incorporated to retard the development of discoloration. However, $FePO_4$ is a relatively insoluble compound, and the influence of ascorbic acid on its absorption is variable. When added to rice and maize meals prior to cooking, it appears to enter the common pool completely, and the enhancement achieved by the addition of ascorbic acid is the same for $FePO_4$ as for intrinsic iron or added ferrous sulfate.[26] In contrast, when $FePO_4$ is added to a maize meal immediately before it is eaten, it remains relatively unavailable for absorption even when large quantities of ascorbic acid are present.[29] Cane sugar has been examined as a fortification vehicle,[29] but it is also unsatisfactory since it is commonly taken in tea and coffee and any soluble iron present produces a black discoloration due to the precipitation of tannins.[32] Finally, ascorbic acid fortification is expensive when compared with iron fortification, and this is an important consideration in developing countries.

Ascorbic Acid Supplementation

The recommended dietary allowance for ascorbic acid is currently set at 45 mg daily. However, it has been suggested that this quantity is not adequate for optimal health and that very large doses of ascorbic acid are desirable. Intakes as high as 2–3 g daily have been reported to be beneficial in reducing the frequency and severity of the common cold and possibly in reducing the risk of cancer.[31]

The long-term effects of such megadose quantities of ascorbic acid on iron balance in man are not known. In a limited survey among Americans living in the northwestern United States, Cook and Monsen found ascorbic acid intakes ranging between 0 and 2,000 mg with a mean of 280 mg.[31] Based on studies with a semisynthetic meal containing no meat, they concluded that 280 mg ascorbic acid would produce a twofold increase in iron absorption if taken with breakfast and a threefold increase if taken in divided doses during the day.

These estimates probably represent the maximum possible effect of ascorbic acid, and the actual increase in iron absorption may be considerably less for several reasons. Ascorbic acid is effective in promoting food iron absorption only if taken with the meal; some or all of the supplementary ascorbic acid may be taken separately from meals. Population groups eating large quantities of ascorbic acid are drawn more commonly from the affluent sections of society where the consumption of animal foods is relatively high. The estimates of the enhancing effect of ascorbic acid on iron absorption were based on a diet containing no meat or fish.[31] However, as indicated above, ascorbic acid may have a much smaller effect on percentage iron absorption from meals containing animal foods. The final consideration in estimating the potential hazards of megadose levels of ascorbic acid intake relates to the dose-response effect of ascorbic acid. From the relationship between iron absorption and the molar ratio of ascorbic acid to iron (Figure 2), 100 mg ascorbic acid may represent a near maximal effect. If this is so, the estimated increase in absorption produced by a daily intake of 280 mg ascorbic acid in a meat-containing diet would be approximately 20% if the supplement were eaten with breakfast and slightly less than 40% if taken in three divided doses with each meal of the day. Support for this argument has been obtained in pilot studies, which have shown remarkably little long-term effect on iron stores in volunteer subjects taking 2 g ascorbic acid over 24 months.[38]

Summary

Food iron is absorbed by the intestinal mucosa from two separate pools of heme and nonheme iron. Heme iron, derived from hemoglobin and myoglobin, is well absorbed and relatively little affected by other foods eaten in the same meal. On the other hand, the absorption of nonheme iron, the major dietary pool, is greatly influenced by meal composition. Ascorbic acid is a powerful enhancer of nonheme iron absorption and can reverse the inhibiting effect of such substances as tea and calcium/phosphate. Its influence may be less pronounced in meals of high iron availability—those containing meat, fish, or poultry. The enhancement of iron absorption from vegetable meals is directly proportional to the quantity of ascorbic acid present. The absorption of soluble inorganic iron added to a meal increases in parallel with the absorption of nonheme iron, but ascorbic acid has a much smaller effect on insoluble iron compounds, such as ferric oxide or ferric hydroxide, which are common food contaminants. Ascorbic acid facilitates iron absorption by forming a chelate with ferric iron at acid pH that remains soluble at the alkaline pH of the duodenum. High cost and instability during food storage are the major obstacles to using ascorbic acid in programs designed to combat nutritional iron deficiency anemia.

References

1. Moore, C. V. & R. Dubach. 1951. Observations on the absorption of iron from foods tagged with radioiron. Trans. Assoc. Am. Physicians **64:** 245–256.
2. Layrisse, M. & C. Martinez-Torres. 1971. Iron absorption from food. Iron supplementation of foods. *In* Progress in Hematology. E. B. Brown & C. V. Moore, Eds. **6:** 137–160. Grune & Stratton, Inc. New York, N.Y.
3. Martinez-Torres, C. & M. Layrisse. 1973. Nutritional factors in iron deficiency: food iron absorption. *In* Clinics in Haematology. S. T. Callender, Ed. **2:** 339–352. W. B. Saunders & Co. London, Philadelphia, Toronto.
4. Martinez-Torres, C., I. Leets, M. Renzi & M. Layrisse. 1974. Iron absorption by humans from veal liver. J. Nutr. **104:** 983–993.
5. Cook, J. D., M. Layrisse, C. Martinez-Torres, R. Walker, E. Monsen & C. A. Finch. 1972. Food iron absorption measured by an extrinsic tag. J. Clin. Invest. **51:** 805–815.
6. Björn-Rasmussen, E., L. Hallberg, B. Magnusson, L. Rossander, B. Svanberg & B. Arvidsson. 1976. Measurement of iron absorption from composite meals. Am. J. Clin. Nutr. **29:** 772–778.
7. Björn-Rasmussen, E., L. Hallberg & R. B. Walker. 1972. Food iron absorption in man. I. Isotopic exchange between food iron and inorganic iron salts added to food: studies on maize, wheat and eggs. Am. J. Clin. Nutr. **25:** 317–323.
8. Björn-Rasmussen, E., L. Hallberg & R. B. Walker. 1973. Food iron absorption in man. II. Isotopic exchange of iron between labelled foods and between a food and an iron salt. Am. J. Clin. Nutr. **26:** 1311–1319.
9. Martinez-Torres, C. & M. Layrisse. 1971. Iron absorption from veal muscle. Am. J. Clin. Nutr. **24:** 531–540.
10. Weintraub, L. R., M. B. Weinstein & H.-J. Huser. 1968. Absorption of hemoglobin

iron: the role of a heme-splitting substance in the intestinal mucosa. J. Clin. Invest. **47:** 531–539.
11. Callender, S. T., B. J. Mallett & M. D. Smith. 1957. Absorption of haemoglobin iron. Br. J. Haematol. **3:** 186–192.
12. Turnbull, A. L., F. Cleton & C. A. Finch. 1962. Iron absorption. IV. The absorption of hemoglobin iron. J. Clin. Invest. **41:** 1897–1907.
13. Björn-Rasmussen, E., L. Hallberg, B. Isaksson & B. Arvidsson. 1974. Food iron absorption in man. Applications of the two-pool extrinsic tag method to measure heme and nonheme iron absorption from the whole diet. J. Clin. Invest. **53:** 247–255.
14. Bothwell, T. H., R. W. Charlton, J. D. Cook & C. A. Finch. 1979. Iron Metabolism in Man. Blackwell Scientific Publications. Oxford, England.
15. Steinkamp, R., R. Dubach & C. V. Moore. 1955. Studies in iron transportation and metabolism. VIII. Absorption of radioiron from iron-enriched bread. Arch. Intern. Med. **95:** 181–193.
16. Callender, S. T. & G. T. Warner. 1968. Iron absorption from bread. Am. J. Clin. Nutr. **21:** 1170–1174.
17. Elwood, P. C., D. Newton, J. D. Eakins & D. A. Brown. 1968. Absorption of iron from bread. Am. J. Clin. Nutr. **21:** 1162–1169.
18. Callender, S. T., S. R. Marney, Jr. & G. T. Warner. 1970. Eggs and iron absorption. Br. J. Haematol. **19:** 657–665.
19. Layrisse, M., C. Martinez-Torres & M. Gonzalez. 1974. Measurement of the total daily dietary iron absorption by the extrinsic tag model. Am. J. Clin. Nutr. **27:** 152–162.
20. Rossander, L., L. Hallberg & E. Björn-Rasmussen. 1979. Absorption of iron from breakfast meals. Am. J. Clin. Nutr. **32:** 2484–2489.
21. Pirzio-Biroli, G., T. H. Bothwell & C. A. Finch. 1958. Iron absorption. II. The absorption of radioiron administered with a standard meal in man. J. Lab. Clin. Med. **51:** 37–48.
22. Apte, S. V. & P. S. Venkatachalam. 1965. The effect of ascorbic acid on the absorption of iron. Indian J. Med. Res. **53:** 1084–1086.
23. Kuhn, I. N., M. Layrisse, M. Roche, C. Martinez & R. B. Walker. 1968. Observations on the mechanism of iron absorption. Am. J. Clin. Nutr. **21:** 1184–1188.
24. Sayers, M. H., S. R. Lynch, P. Jacobs, R. W. Charlton, T. H. Bothwell, R. B. Walker & F. Mayet. 1973. The effects of ascorbic acid supplementation on the absorption of iron in maize, wheat and soya. Br. J. Haematol. **24:** 209–218.
25. Sayers, M. H., S. R. Lynch, R. W. Charlton, T. H. Bothwell, R. B. Walker & F. Mayet. 1974. Iron absorption from rice meals cooked with fortified salt containing ferrous sulphate and ascorbic acid. Br. J. Nutr. **31:** 367–375.
26. Sayers, M. H., S. R. Lynch, R. W. Charlton, T. H. Bothwell, R. B. Walker & F. Mayet. 1974. The fortification of common salt with ascorbic acid and iron. Br. J. Haematol. **28:** 483–495.
27. Björn-Rasmussen, E. & L. Hallberg. 1974. Iron absorption from maize. Effect of ascorbic acid on iron absorption from maize supplemented with ferrous sulphate. Nutr. Metab. **16:** 94–100.
28. Layrisse, M., C. Martinez-Torres, M. Renzy & I. Leets. 1975. Ferritin iron absorption in man. Blood **45:** 688–698.
29. Disler, P. B., S. R. Lynch, R. W. Charlton, T. H. Bothwell, R. B. Walker & F. Mayet. 1975. Studies on the fortification of cane sugar with iron and ascorbic acid. Br. J. Nutr. **34:** 141–151.
30. Derman, D., M. Sayers, S. R. Lynch, R. W. Charlton, T. H. Bothwell & F. Mayet. 1977. Iron absorption from a cereal-based meal containing cane sugar fortified with ascorbic acid. Br. J. Nutr. **38:** 261–269.
31. Cook, J. D. & E. R. Monsen. 1977. Vitamin C, the common cold, and iron absorption. Am. J. Clin. Nutr. **30:** 235–241.
32. Disler, P. B., S. R. Lynch, R. W. Charlton, J. D. Torrance, T. H. Bothwell, R. B. Walker & F. Mayet. 1975. The effect of tea on iron absorption. Gut **16:** 193–200.
33. Layrisse, M., C. Martinez-Torres & M. Roche. 1968. The effect of interaction of various foods on iron absorption. Am. J. Clin. Nutr. **21:** 1175–1183.

34. MONSEN, E. R., L. HALLBERG, M. LAYRISSE, D. M. HEGSTED, J. D. COOK, W. MERTZ & C. A. FINCH. 1978. Estimation of available dietary iron. Am. J. Clin. Nutr. **31:** 134–141.
35. BRISE, H. & L. HALLBERG. 1962. Effect of ascorbic acid on iron absorption. Acta Med. Scand. Suppl. **171**(376): 51–58.
36. COOK, J. D., M. LAYRISSE & C. A. FINCH. 1969. The measurement of iron absorption. Blood **33:** 421–429.
37. CONRAD, M. E. & S. G. SCHADE. 1968. Ascorbic acid chelates in iron absorption: a role for hydrochloric acid and bile. Gastroenterology **55:** 35–45.
38. COOK, J. D. 1980. Unpublished observations.

DISCUSSION

W. R. HOLUB (*Life Systems Incorporated, Melville, N.Y.*): Just some questions on protocol. Were your experiments on humans or in animals?

S. R. LYNCH: They were done on humans.

W. R. HOLUB: Oh, then two questions. One is on the biosynthetic sources of ^{59}Fe. Were the total assays of iron compared?—so that when you compared meat to vegetable sources, were you really giving equimolar ratios of total iron and not just radioactive iron? That is one question. The second question is, How were the different foods prepared?—because that would make a significant difference. For example, if the grains were cooked or simply ground up instead of sprouted, that would make the availability of iron quite different.

S. R. LYNCH: The amounts of iron naturally present in the meals were not changed in most studies. We fed what we thought were representative meals for the people being studied, so that in most instances, there was of course very much less heme iron than there was nonheme iron. The nonheme iron forms a very much bigger pool in the diet. No attempts were made to change this situation.

In some of the studies where iron supplements were being investigated, an iron salt was added in addition to the nonheme iron already present.

All of the meals were cooked, and this of course has important effects, particularly on the ascorbic acid. Experiments were done in which ascorbic acid was added prior to the cooking procedure. If the food was baked, virtually all the ascorbic acid was oxidized and its addition had no effect. If it was boiled, as is more common in most of the developing countries, not all of the ascorbic acid was lost—perhaps 30 or 40% was oxidized—and an enhancing effect was still seen. If you add enough, you can still see a very significant effect.

H. SPRINCE (*Veterans Administration Medical Center, Coatesville, Penn.*): I missed your point about the optimal pH for the solubility of ferric chloride salts in the presence of ascorbic acid. What is that roughly? Is it pH 4?

S. R. LYNCH: What I tried to show was that ferric chloride itself is really only soluble at acid pH. If you add ascorbic acid to a ferric chloride suspension at an alkaline pH, it makes very little difference to iron solubility; but if you first lower the pH to the acid range, you form a complex of iron and ascorbic acid that remains soluble as the pH is raised again. We think that as the pH falls in the stomach, the complex is formed; and it then remains soluble once the higher pH of the duodenum is reached.

H. SPRINCE: What was the optimal pH at which this effect first set in? Was it pH 4?

S. R. LYNCH: In the *in vitro* experiment I described, they actually took it down to 2. That probably isn't necessary, but I don't know exactly how low you would have to go.

H. SPRINCE: I'm just wondering too what would have happened if, instead of ascorbic acid, you had used the dehydro form. Has that been considered in this *in vitro* system?

S. R. LYNCH: I'm not aware of that if it has.

H. SPRINCE: What I'm really saying is, What is the effect of dehydroascorbic acid in solubilizing ferric salts?

S. R. LYNCH: The only evidence that I can really quote in relation to that question is the effect of baking a meal. Baking doesn't totally oxidize ascorbic acid but at least removes virtually all of the dehydro form. We don't see any improvement in absorption then.

UNIDENTIFIED SPEAKER: I guess we have seen two effects: one is reduction of iron, and the other is chelation. Probably the first thing that happened was reduction; and then after that, chelation and return to iron three. The ascorbic acid may also be oxidized to dehydroascorbic and diketogulonic acids. Could you discuss the possibility of iron chelation to the latter two compounds?

S. R. LYNCH: Our work does not provide an answer to this question, and I don't think it has been examined carefully. It has been stated, especially in the older literature, that iron must be in the reduced form to be absorbed. This may well not be true, and the observation may have reflected only the better solubility of ferrous compounds at the pH of the duodenum. Therefore, I think that all one can say is that iron and ascorbic acid form a soluble complex that makes iron available to the mucosal cell. This does not necessarily imply that the iron must be in the reduced form.

L. HOWARD (*Albany Medical College, Albany, N.Y.*): Dr. Lynch, just a small, practical question. You mentioned already that the absorption of the more water-soluble salts of iron is not greatly improved by ascorbic acid. Does that mean that therapeutic tablets that combine ferrous sulfate with vitamin C are nonsense?

S. R. LYNCH: Yes, I think it probably does mean almost that. There is some improvement in the absorption seen with ferrous sulfate. Brise and Hallberg have studied the effect of large doses of vitamin C on the absorption of a 30-mg dose of ferrous sulfate, and you do see an increase in absorption up to a little less than 1½ times. I think that this relatively small effect is unimportant because there is a large quantity of available iron already present. You don't need the small increase in percentage absorption, and the addition of ascorbic acid is, of course, expensive. Thus it is probably not appropriate to recommend the use of such combinations. Furthermore, as you increase absorption, you also increase side effects by the same degree. So I think, all in all, there really isn't any reason for adding ascorbic acid to soluble ferrous salts.

L. M. KLEVAY (*Human Nutrition Laboratory, U.S. Department of Agriculture, Grand Forks, N. Dak.*): It's interesting that the beneficial effect of ascorbic acid on iron absorption contrasts with the impairment of copper absorption that has been found in several species. I just bring this up now because I don't think any of the other speakers are going to get to it.

J. G. BIERI (*National Institutes of Health, Bethesda, Md.*): What's the relative effectiveness of animal protein vs. ascorbic acid in the absorption of the inorganic iron? Would it be more feasible to promote more animal protein intake than to go through the ascorbic acid route?

S. R. LYNCH: I think both are important. Dr. Monsen and her colleagues recently proposed a model in which they tried to look at this. The conclusion that they reached was that 1 mg of ascorbic acid was roughly equivalent in its effect to 1 g of animal protein.

VITAMIN A INFLUENCE ON CALCIUM METABOLISM AND CALCIFICATION*

Juan M. Navia and Suzanne S. Harris

Institute of Dental Research and
Department of Nutrition Sciences
University of Alabama
Birmingham, Alabama 35294

Background and General Overview

Vitamin A and Bone

Vitamin A represents a group of retinoid compounds that includes natural forms and synthetic analogs possessing different degrees of biologic activity. Retinol, retinal, and retinoic acid are three such compounds, with retinol being the most biologically important. Retinol has a major role in maintaining vision, reproduction, and the growth and development of epithelial tissues and skeletal tissues.[1-5] While these different functions can be fulfilled by retinol, such molecules as retinoic acid can maintain growth and the integrity of epithelial tissues, but not the reproductive process or vision. Therefore, animals provided with no source of vitamin A in the diet but supplemented with retinoic acid eventually become sterile and blind. β-Carotene in the intestine can also yield retinoic acid, after being cleaved at the central double bond by β-carotene-15,15-dioxygenase in the presence of molecular O_2 and a bile salt.[6,7] The resulting retinaldehyde is reduced to retinol by another soluble mucosal enzyme, retinaldehyde reductase, and a small portion can be oxidized to retinoic acid.[8]

The absorptions of retinol and retinoic acid are also quite different. Retinyl esters present in foods are hydrolized in the intestine to retinol, which is absorbed into the mucosal cells, reesterified with saturated long-chain fatty acids, and incorporated into lymph chylomicrons.[9] These chylomicrons enter the blood circulation via the lymphatic vessels. The retinyl esters remain in the "remnant" cholesterol-rich particles until they are entirely removed by the hepatic tissue.[10,11] Here the retinyl esters are stored after hydrolysis and reesterification predominantly to retinyl palmitate. Retinoic acid, however, has a different metabolic pattern. It is absorbed through the portal system and transported in plasma bound to serum albumin.[3,12,13] It is not stored in the liver but is rapidly excreted in urine and also in bile as a retinoyl-β-glucuronide.[14]

A major development in 1968 was the demonstration that retinol from the liver was actually transported to target tissues attached to a specific transport protein, the retinol-binding protein (RBP).[15] Human RBP is a single polypeptide chain [molecular weight (MW) 21,000] with a single binding site for one molecule of retinol. It circulates as retinol-RBP (holo-RBP) strongly associated with another protein, prealbumin.[16] Human prealbumin appears to have four binding sites for RBP.[17] This tetramer protein also contains a central channel, which is the site of thyroxine (T4) binding.[18] The holo-RBP–prealbumin complex represents an important system for retinol transport to target tissues and also for protection of RBP, an

* This work was supported by NIH-NIDR Grants No. DE-04862–03 and DE-02670-10 and by NIH-NIDR Training Grant No. DE-07020-05.

0077–8923/80/0355–0045 $01.75/0 © 1980, NYAS

important protein in the metabolism of retinol, from glomerular filtration and renal catabolism.[19] The major functions of RBP for retinol seem to be (a) regulation of the mobilization of vitamin A from liver stores; (b) protection of the labile retinol molecule from oxidative action; (c) solubilization of the fat-soluble molecule in an aqueous medium; and (d) delivery of retinol directly to the target tissue.

The latter is an especially important point, for it is known that vitamin A can have highly toxic effects on membranes when doses are not kept within the physiological limits.[20] A major contribution to the understanding of the metabolism of vitamin A came through the recognition that besides RBP, the serum transport protein, there were also specific receptor proteins, cellular retinol-binding proteins (CRBP), present within cells.[21] This discovery was followed by identification of a new protein receptor capable of binding retinoic acid in chicken embryos and rats.[22,23] The cellular retinoic acid–binding protein (CRABP) has been detected in several tissues, including skin and intestinal mucosa, but not in liver or lung.[24] Differences found in organ distribution of the cellular binding proteins of adult rats have suggested that these proteins are regulated differently during development,[25] implying that both retinol and retinoic acid have important metabolic roles as members of the retinoid (vitamin A) family of compounds.

One of the proposed biochemical functions of these compounds is similar to that of polyprenols in the biosynthesis of bacterial polysaccharides.[26] Retinol would serve as a carrier of specific mannosyl residues by means of a phosphorylated form of vitamin A. The synthesis of retinyl phosphate has been demonstrated in cultured hamster intestinal cells and in rat liver and intestine *in vivo*. The sugar nucleotide guanosine diphosphate (GDP)-mannose has been reported to be a donor of mannose to exogenous retinyl phosphate (RP), forming mannosyl retinyl phosphate (MRP). However, if exogenous RP is absent, the transfer results in formation of mannosylated polyisoprenoid dolichyl mannosyl phosphate (DMP). Similar reactions have been reported with galactosyl transfer reactions to form Gal-RP.[27] Both MRP and Gal-RP could be of great importance in the biosynthesis of glycoproteins for cell surfaces, which are essential to adhesion properties of cells, and other glycoproteins, such as serum alpha-macroglobulin (α-MG) in the rat.[28] This protein was found to be defective in vitamin A–deficient rats as a result of underglycosylation.

The detailed knowledge of the biochemistry of different vitamin A forms (retinol, retinal, retinoic acid) in the metabolism of various tissues contrasts with the dearth of information available on the biochemical role of retinoids in the development and maintenance of mineralized tissues, such as bones and teeth.

In 1938, Mellanby reported that dogs fed a diet high in cereals and deficient in vitamin A and carotenes exhibited signs of incoordination and extensive pathologic changes in the internal ear structures, with overgrowth of bone that pressured and altered the inner sensory tissues in the labyrinth.[29] Moore also described a particular type of blindness present at birth in calves of dams fed poor quality roughage diet.[30] Autopsy of these calves showed that the optic nerve was atrophied and the bony canal through which it passed was only one-half its normal diameter. Thus, Moore concluded that the atrophy was due to increased pressure of overgrown bone on the nerve.

After having established the bony defect, a search began to determine how these changes were brought about. Wolbach attributed the bone dysplasia to alterations in endochondral growth,[31] while Mellanby assigned the defect to alterations in the position and activity of osteoclasts and osteoblasts in developing bone.[32] In the deficient (A –) state, bone cells seemed to become more active but did not change in biochemical functions. Mellanby made reference to the fact that the amount of calcium in bone seemed to be roughly the same. The A + femurs had 0.131 g Ca/kg body weight, and the A− femurs had 0.134 Ca/kg body weight, in spite of the differences in morphologic appearance.

These investigators and others seemed to agree that there were definite changes in the long bones, characterized by a thick cancellous cortex in A− bones with no major change in total ash.[33-35] The increased bulkiness of the bone was due to excessive periosteal deposition of bone, and the enlarged marrow cavity was filled with fatty marrow. Remodeling of the cancellous fiber bone into compact lamellar plates of mature bone seemed to be decreased.[36]

Hayes and Cousins examined both endochondral and intramembranous bone growth in relation to the effect of vitamin A deficiency on actual size and histologic appearance in calves.[37] These authors concluded that since the increased apposition of bone was not observed in diaphysis of femurs, where osteoblastic activity is normally seen, vitamin A deficiency had interfered with differentiation of the periosteal progenitor cells into osteoclasts. Gallina *et al.*, using a similar experimental approach, measured mineral apposition in slow-growing bone using fluorescent tetracycline-fluorescein labels and concluded that lesions were due to increased appositional growth.[38] However, Brown and Hayes, also using tetracycline labeling to evaluate the effect of vitamin A deficiency on medullary bone in rats, found more unresorbed medullary bone than new bone in A− rats.[39] They concluded that resorption of medullary bone was reduced by vitamin A deficiency and that this was primarily responsible for the bone alterations.

This early work identified the lesion in bone, but did not resolve the question of whether the overgrowth of bone was due to increased osteoblastic activity or to decreased osteoclastic processes in osseous tissues.

Together with these histological studies of bone changes associated with vitamin A deficiency, several studies have been reported where biochemical changes were evaluated. Dziewiatkowski studied the metabolism of matrix components such as chondroitin sulfate *in vivo* in rats deficient in vitamin A, by administering $^{35}SO_4$ and measuring the uptake in various tissues.[40] The vitamin A-supplemented control rats had a larger amount of $^{35}SO_4$ [counts per minute (cpm)/mg bone] in the femur (24 hours after injections of the label) than did the deficient (A−) animals. The experiments were repeated with ^{32}P rather than $^{35}SO_4$, and vitamin A-treated rats were found to have more radioactive label in the femoral end than did the untreated A− samples. The conclusion of this investigation was that vitamin A deficiency decreased the uptake of $^{35}SO_4$ and ^{32}P into femurs and arrested the normal growth and development of the cartilage plate.

These results did not agree with investigations conducted by Frape *et al.*, who measured the uptake of $^{35}SO_4$ into vitamin A-deficient pigs.[41] They found a significant increase in ^{35}S activity in the costochondral junction of the A− pigs compared to controls. Havivi and Wolf also reported studies on bone growth and sulfation during vitamin A deficiency using a chick model, which is characterized by rapidly growing bones.[42] Control and experimental diets were fed from birth; and at two to three weeks, when the birds were starting to develop severe symptoms of deficiency, they were killed, and the calvaria and tibia dissected for analysis and *in vitro* culture studies. The uronic acid concentration in the epiphysis of A− tibia was found to be higher than in controls, and the $^{35}SO_4$ label was incorporated at higher concentrations into epiphyseal bone matrix of A− tibia slices incubated in Krebs-Ringer buffer for three hours. These observations led the authors to postulate that vitamin A deficiency caused an increase in bone matrix or bone cells.

These and other studies indicate that vitamin A deficiency does affect bone matrix formation and possibly cellular differentiation and function; however, the data are often conflicting.[43-46] Several different parameters have been measured:

histology, calcium content, sulfate uptake, uronic acid levels, and t-RNA methylase and alkaline phosphatase. Both increased and decreased calcium content of bone from vitamin A–deficient animals have been reported, as well as increased and decreased sulfate uptake. Different animal species and strains (i.e., calves, dogs, rats, chicks) have been used, and in all cases, bones analyzed or studied contained portions of tissues formed prior to the onset of the deficiency. Small, critical changes in response of some of these parameters could have been masked or confounded by the presence of bone formed under nutritionally adequate conditions.

Excess Doses of Vitamin A

Effects on Bone

The effects of overdoses of vitamin A have been evaluated in a number of animal species, i.e., dogs, rabbits and guinea pigs, ducks, chickens, and rats.[47–51] Doses ranging from 25,000 to 50,000 IU/day for a period of one to three weeks induce lack of appetite, reduced body weight gain, spontaneous fractures near the ends of long bones,[52] rarefaction and thinning of long bones, and ultimately death. Microscopic examination of long bones shows that the epiphyseal line becomes reduced in thickness due to continued erosion of the hypertrophic zone and a lack of compensatory increase in the number of cells in the proliferative zone.[51] There is excessive resorption in extensive areas of long bones, where remodeling activity is intense. In such areas, numerous osteoclasts can be observed on the periosteal aspect of the cortical bone. Capillary vessel engorgement is seen frequently, as well as evidence of blood extravasation and small hemorrhages even in the absence of fractures. During hypervitaminosis A, therefore, osteoid and poorly calcified matrix can be observed on the endosteal side, and osteoclasis on the periosteal surface, which leads to a weakening of the whole organ.

Acute vitamin A toxicity has been described in polar explorers as a result of eating the livers of polar bears and bearded seals, which are known to contain large amounts of vitamin A.[53] Consumption of eight ounces of liver may provide more than 3,000,000 IU of vitamin A. The symptoms include headache, vomiting, lassitude, and in some cases severe peeling of the skin within a day or two. Chronic hypervitaminosis A has been reported particularly in children, and the symptoms include anorexia, irritability, and tender swellings of the limbs, which limits mobility of the patient.[54]

In most of these cases, calcium and phosphorus in serum are normal or slightly elevated, and alkaline phosphatase and vitamin A concentrations are abnormally high. The effects of excess doses are not limited to skeletal tissue and seem to be widespread among other organs and glands. The biochemistry of such changes is not completely understood, but some studies suggest that they are mediated through an increased release of lysosomal enzymes.[55] This is especially true in osteoclastic activity of bone cultures treated with parathyroid hormone. Chertow *et al.* have recently reported studies on the effect of vitamin A on parathyroid hormone (PTH) secretion *in vitro*, using bovine parathyroid tissue, and also *in vivo* with humans.[56] They found a stimulation of PTH release by vitamin A that was dose and time dependent. Interestingly, retinoic acid did not stimulate PTH secretion. Vitamin A also increased the lysosomal cathepsin D activity of parathyroid tissue, and thus might lead to increased mobilization and secretion of PTH. This was confirmed in the human studies, where subjects given a 25,000-IU vitamin A palmitate intramuscular dose showed serum parathyroid hormone increase. These studies suggest that vitamin A, besides its direct osteoclastic-stimulating activity, increases PTH secretion *in vitro* through modification of the cells within the gland by stimulation of the secretion granule membrane or possibly through stimulation of lysosomal proteolytic activity. Even though there is a better understanding of the role of vitamin A excess on the lysosomal activity involved in resorption of both cartilage and bone, much remains to be understood about the specific biochemical role of the vitamin and its effects on normal differentiation and activity of bone cells.

Deficiency of Vitamin A

Glycosaminoglycans and Bone Calcification

Research conducted to study the effect of vitamin A deficiency on bone development indicates that (a) at a microscopic tissue level, there is a characteristic bone overgrowth that could be due to decreased osteoclastic activity or to increased osteoblastic activity; and (b) at a biochemical level, there seems to be a definite effect on matrix formation, but the magnitude and direction of effects on glycosaminoglycans are uncertain. Confusion arises from (a) use of a variety of animal species fed different, undefined diets; (b) the confounding effect of inanition characteristic of vitamin A-deficient animals; (c) methodology that does not allow for evaluation of truly deficient bone; and finally (d) estimation of effects of vitamin A in endochondral or intramembranous bones that have varying quantities of cartilage.

To minimize some of these limitations and allow for detection of biochemical changes in bones due to vitamin A deficiency, we used a standardized model system that allowed the collection of bone known to be formed after the animal is clinically deficient.[57] This animal model consisted of young guinea pigs fed a purified gel diet containing either no vitamin A (A –) or 57 mg retinyl acetate/kg diet (A +).[58] After the fifth week, the guinea pigs showed a sharp decrease in serum retinol levels, and their liver vitamin A stores were depleted. At that time, the right lower incisor was extracted from all guinea pigs (A + and A –), and a 1-cm nylon tube inserted into the alveolar cavity (Figure 1). The mucosal borders were then approximated, sutured, and normally healed within two or three days. Animals were kept on their dietary regimen, and the controls were pair fed to the A – group. Some of the A – guinea pigs were supplemented with either 1 or 10 μg retinoic acid daily (A – /A +) by gavage. Fourteen days after implantation, the guinea pigs were killed, and the nylon tube—now filled with newly formed bone (tissue implant, TI)—was removed from each mandible. The bone obtained came from the mandible, an intramembranous bone without cartilage, and cells were mostly osteoblasts. Thus, this model provided new bone formed under vitamin A deficiency or sufficiency conditions with little, if any, osteoclastic activity. The bone formed, TI, could then be used either for biochemical analysis or cultured in a medium adequate for bone for evaluation of its metabolism of radioactively labeled salts and compounds. Using this technique, it was determined that the total calcium content of the A – TI was significantly lower than that of the A + TI, and the uptake of ^{45}Ca seemed to be less in the A – TI compared to the other two groups.[59] The glycosaminoglycan (GAG) fraction from the A – and the A – /A + TI cultured with $^{35}SO_4$ contained significantly more $^{35}SO_4$ than did the same fraction from the A + TI (Table 1). Thus, the lack of dietary vitamin A increased the amount of sulfur present in the GAG fraction from bone samples formed during deficiency, suggesting an increase in the amount of sulfated GAG present in the bone.

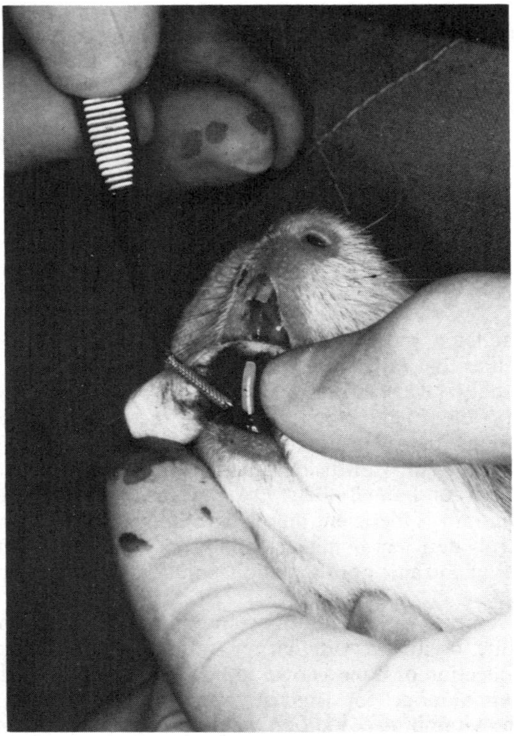

FIGURE 1. Insertion of a 1-cm nylon mesh tube into the alveolar cavity of an extracted incisor of a guinea pig. After suturing, bone is allowed to form, and the bone-filled implant is recovered for analysis and/or culture two weeks later.

Microscopic examination of histologic sections of these TI indicated the presence of highly cellular and loosely woven bone spicules.[60] Borders between areas of osteoid and stroma were not well defined. In contrast, bone tissue from guinea pigs supplemented with retinyl acetate (A+) or with retinoic acid (A−/A+) had a normal appearance of tightly organized bone spicules with normal osteoblastic rimming along the bone trabeculae. Retinoic acid, therefore, seemed to allow normal bone development when supplemented at a daily dose of 10 μg.

Several questions remain unanswered relative to the described effect of vitamin A deficiency on GAG metabolism, namely, whether the same effects take place in other types of bone, and whether the accumulation of sulfur is due to an increase in the amounts of GAG synthesized or to a defect in the degradation pathways of these compounds. To evaluate these questions, Harris and Navia used a neonatal rat calvarium model system, which, while being predominantly osteoblastic, did contain osteoclasts as well as some cartilage.[61] Two-day-old rat pup calvaria were cultured in BGJ media containing serum from A− rats or A+ rats dosed with 75,000 IU of retinyl acetate by gavage 2 hours prior to bleeding. The culture media were supplemented with either radiolabeled sulfate or glucosamine. As in the case of the guinea pig bone implant, the amount of ^{35}S sulfate in the GAG fraction from rat calvaria cultured with A− serum for 48 hours was significantly higher than the

TABLE 1

In Vitro INCORPORATION OF $^{35}SO_4$ INTO THE CPC-GAG PRECIPITATES OF TISSUE IMPLANTS FROM VITAMIN A-DEFICIENT GUINEA PIGS[59]

Experiment A: Tissue implants (TI) exposed to 5 μCi $^{35}SO_4$ for 48 hours

Groups*	Dry Weight TI† (mg)	CPC-GAG Ppt† (cpm ^{35}S/mg TI)
A+ (6)	6.83 ± 1.61	2405 ± 609
A− (6)	6.31 ± 1.93	4359 ± 1646‡
A−/A+ (5)	5.26 ± 0.64	4557 ± 1701‡

Experiment B: Tissue implants (TI) exposed to 0.5 μCi $^{35}SO_4$ for 48 hours

Groups*	Dry Weight TI† (mg)	Total Digest† (cpm ^{35}S/mg TI)	CPC-GAG Ppt‡ (cpm ^{35}S/mg TI)
A+ (9)	7.18 ± 1.93	7217 ± 1013	222 ± 67
A− (8)	6.91 ± 2.33	8001 ± 1670	353 ± 59‡
A−/A+ (10)	7.20 ± 1.55	7617 ± 1270	288 ± 65‡

* Number in parenthesis indicates the number of guinea pigs in each group.
† Data are expressed as mean ± standard deviation (SD).
‡ Significantly different compared to A+ at $P < 0.05$.

values obtained from calvaria cultured with A+ serum. The uptake of ^{35}S into GAG fraction of calvaria cultured with A− serum showed continuous increase over a 96-hour period, whereas ^{35}S uptake leveled off after 24 hours in the A+ group (FIGURE 2). When ^{14}C-glucosamine was added to the media, there was also a significant increase into GAG fractions in comparison to controls (TABLE 2).

The question of whether the alteration in sulfate uptake was due to an increased synthesis or decreased catabolism of the GAG was investigated in this same study, using a pulse-chase experiment.[61] Calvaria isolated in a similar manner to that in the previous experiment were incubated for 24 hours in media containing 0.5 μCi of ^{35}S and either A+ or A− serum, then transferred to media containing the same kind of serum but without labeled sulfate. The results, illustrated in FIGURE 3, confirmed that calvaria cultured in the presence of A− serum had significantly high incorporation of ^{35}S into GAG. What is more significant is that while there was a 65% loss of ^{35}S sulfate in the A+-incubated group, the values for the calvaria incubated under A− conditions maintained the initial concentrations of ^{35}S in the GAG. Thus, these studies suggest that bone cells under the influence of vitamin A deficiency lose their ability to regulate the metabolism of sulfated GAG, and that the defect is in the degradative pathway for these matrix molecules. Further studies are under way to characterize the molecular nature of these changes and the biochemical pathways affected, using an even simpler model of rat dentin/odontoblast cultures.

GENERAL COMMENTS AND CONCLUSIONS

Vitamin A is now known to be essential for the health and maintenance of the visual organ as well as the visual cycle, for the differentiation and maintenance of epithelial and skeletal tissues, for spermatogenesis, and for development and maintenance of the placenta. All these biologic functions of vitamin A can be fulfilled by retinol and to some extent by retinal, which can be formed from retinol in many of these tissues. Retinoid compounds, such as retinoic acid, are formed by

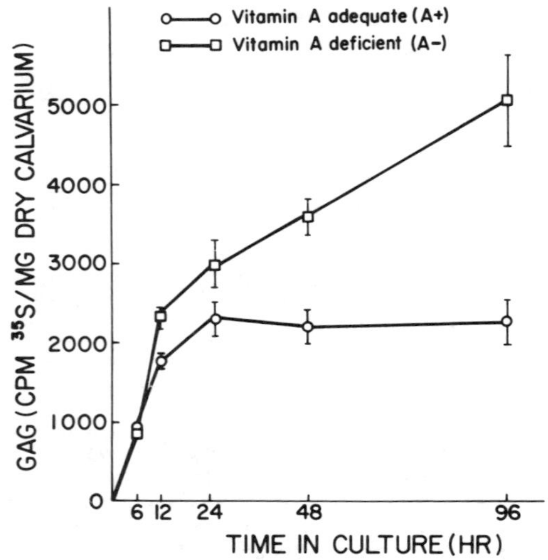

FIGURE 2. Mean rate of $^{35}SO_4$ uptake into the cetylpyridium chloride (CPC)-GAG precipitates of rat calvaria *in vitro*. These data were obtained using the same experimental conditions described in the text. The GAG fractions were precipitated with CPC, and aliquots counted for ^{35}S-sulfate. Each point represents the mean value for five observations, and the vertical bracket indicates plus and minus 1 standard error of the mean (SEM). (Reprinted from Reference 61 with permission of the American Institute of Nutrition.)

tissues through enzymatic oxidation of retinal and retinol and seem to be equally effective in fulfilling these biologic functions in some tissues (such as epithelia) but not in others (such as the eye, which, being unable to reduce retinoic acid, shows extensive degeneration of the rods and cones when only retinoic acid is available).

In the last 20 years, advances have been made in the biochemical understanding of retinoids, which has led to the identification of a specific transport protein for retinol as well as the identification of specific intracellular binding proteins for retinol and retinoic acid. Thus, the recognition has been made that retinol and retinoic acid are both metabolically active forms of vitamin A, with different specificities and metabolic pathways. This has led some researchers to postulate that there might be other forms of retinoids that could be physiologically synthesized in the tissues and that might be the potent, active metabolite responsible for specific biochemical roles within tissues.[62]

For skeletal tissues, the interactions between vitamin A and calcium metabolism have not been investigated extensively. After the initial morphologic studies—which described the profound effects of (a) vitamin A deficiency on bone development, characterized by a bulky overgrowth of tissue that suggested alteration of the remodeling process; and (b) vitamin A excess, which resulted in a marked loss of bone through activity of osteoclasts and increased action of PTH—there have been some efforts to ascertain the nature of the biochemical changes taking place under these conditions.

Development of standardized, controlled animal models to study the nature of the organic matrix of bone developed under vitamin A deficiency points to an alteration in the sulfated glycosaminoglycans, characterized by an accumulation of such molecules due to a defect in their degradation pathway. The exact molecular changes

TABLE 2

In Vitro INCORPORATION OF $^{35}SO_4$ OR [^{14}C]-GLUCOSAMINE INTO RAT CALVARIA[61]

Experiment 1*

Treatment†	Dry Weight‡ (mg)	cpm ^{35}S/mg Dry Calvarium	
		Total Digest‡	CPC-GAG Ppt‡
A+ (8)	10.6 ± 1.3	8817 ± 844	940 ± 177
A− (8)	11.3 ± 1.3	11318 ± 706§	1970 ± 300§

Experiment 2*

Treatment†	Dry Weight‡ (mg)	cpm [^{14}C]-Glucosamine/mg Dry Calvarium	
		Total Digest‡	CPC-GAG Ppt‡
A+ (18)	6.8 ± 0.7	7327 ± 894	1662 ± 244
A− (18)	7.3 ± 0.8	7752 ± 1185	1966 ± 537§

* Calvaria were incubated for 48 hours with 0.5 μCi $^{35}S\text{-}Na_2SO_4$ or [^{14}C]-glucosamine.
† Numbers in parenthesis indicate number of calvaria in each group.
‡ Data are expressed as mean ± SD.
§ Significantly different compared to A+ group at $P < 0.05$.

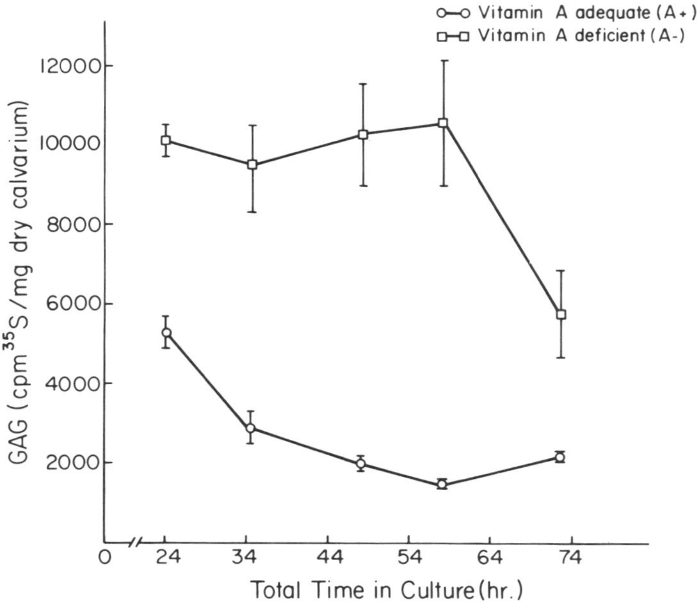

FIGURE 3. Mean loss of $^{35}SO_4$ from GAG fraction in rat calvaria. Two-day-old rat pup calvaria were incubated in a BGJ medium containing 0.5 μCi of $^{35}S\text{-}Na_2SO_4$ and serum from either A+ or A− rats. They were transferred to a nonradioactive medium after a 24-hour incubation, and calvaria were removed from this medium at various time intervals up to 48 hours (total incubation time: 72 hours). Total digests were precipitated with CPC, and the CPC-GAG fractions counted for radioactivity. Each point represents the mean of four replications, and the vertical bracket indicates plus and minus 1 SEM. (Reprinted from Reference 61 with permission of the American Institute of Nutrition.)

in the type and composition of GAG remain to be determinded, but the findings suggest that such changes can alter bone mineralization patterns and the structure of the resulting bone. One extremely interesting aspect is the ability of retinoic acid to substitute for retinol or retinal in these ossification mechanisms. The effect of vitamin A compounds on cell differentiation is still a factor of primary importance in these mineralization processes, but the biochemical consequence of such alterations in the type of cell formed seems to be changes in bone matrix glycosaminoglycans. Studies presently being conducted in simpler odontoblastic models might explain better the specific function and biochemical effects of the different retinoid metabolites.

Summary

Vitamin A deficiency has been shown to affect vision, reproduction, cellular differentiation, and maintenance of epithelial and skeletal tissues. Different vitamin A compounds, i.e., retinol and retinoic acid, vary in their ability to fulfill these biologic functions. Aside from vision, the exact molecular mechanisms of action for retinoids are largely unexplained. High doses of vitamin A are known to increase bone resorption through stimulation of lysosomal proteolytic activity, which also leads to increased secretion of PTH. Deficiency of retinol affects bone morphology by increasing bone thickness. Using a standardized guinea pig model, bone formed entirely during a retinol-deficient (A –) period contained less calcium and took up more ^{35}S into glycosaminoglycan (GAG) fractions *in vitro* than did control (A +) samples. Using rat calvaria, a pulse-chase experiment indicated that the rate of ^{35}S loss from calvaria cultured with A – serum was lower than in controls. Thus, retinol deficiency seems to increase the amount of sulfated GAG in bone through a defect in the degradation of GAG.

References

1. Wald, G. 1968. The molecular basis of visual excitation. Nature **219:** 800–807.
2. Mason, E. E. 1939. Relation of vitamins to the sex glands. *In* Sex and Internal Secretions. E. Allen, Ed. 2nd edit.: 1149. Williams & Wilkins Co. Baltimore, Md.
3. Bieri, J. G., E. G. McDaniel & W. E. Rogers, Jr. 1969. Survival of germ-free rats without vitamin A. Science **163:** 574–575.
4. Thompson, J. N. 1969. Vitamin A in development of the embryo. Am. J. Clin. Nutr. **22:** 1063–1069.
5. Barnicot, N. A. & S. P. Datta. 1972. Vitamin A and bone. *In* The Biochemistry and Physiology of Bone. G. H. Bourne, Ed. **8:** 197–279.
6. Goodman, D. S., H. S. Huang & T. Shiratori. 1966. Mechanism of the biosynthesis of vitamin A from b-carotene. J. Biol. Chem. **241:** 1929–1932.
7. Goodman, D. S. & J. A. Olson. 1969. The conversion of all-trans b-carotene into retinal. *In* Methods of Enzymology. Steroids and Terpinoids. R. B. Clayton, Ed. **15:** 462–475. Academic Press, Inc. New York, N.Y.
8. Fidge, N. H. & D. S. Goodman. 1968. The enzymatic reductions of retinol in rat intestine. J. Biol. Chem. **243:** 4372–4379.
9. Huang, H. S. & D. S. Goodman. 1965. Vitamin A and carotenoids. I. Intestinal absorption and metabolism of ^{14}C-labeled vitamin A alcohol and b-carotene in the rat. J. Biol. Chem. **240:** 2839–2844.
10. Goodman, D. S., H. S. Huang & T. Shiratori. 1965. Tissue distribution and metabolism of newly absorbed vitamin A in the rat. J. Lipid Res. **6:** 390–396.
11. Redgrave, T. G. 1970. Formation of cholesteryl ester-rich particulate lipid during metabolism of chylomicrons. J. Clin. Invest. **49:** 465–471.

12. Fidge, N. H., T. Shiratori, J. Ganguly & D. S. Goodman. 1968. Pathways of absorptions of retinal and retinoic acid in the rat. J. Lipid Res. **9:** 103–109.
13. Smith, J. E., O. O. Pomilch, Y. Muto & D. S. Goodman. 1973. The plasma transport and metabolism of retinoic acid in the rat. Biochem. J. **132:** 821–827.
14. Dunagin, P. E., Jr., E. H. Meadows, Jr. & J. A. Olson. 1965. Retinoyl beta-glucuronic acid: a major metabolite of vitamin A in rat bile. Science **148:** 86–87.
15. Kanai, M., A. Raz & D. S. Goodman. 1968. Retinol-binding protein: the transport protein for vitamin A in human plasma. J. Clin. Invest. **47:** 2025–2044.
16. Smith, J. E. & D. S. Goodman. 1979. Retinol-binding protein and the regulation of vitamin A transport. Fed. Proc. Fed. Am. Soc. Exp. Biol. **38:** 2504–2509.
17. Kopelman, M., U. Cogan, S. Mokady & M. Schinitzky. 1976. The interaction between retinol-binding proteins and prealbumins studied by fluorescence polarization. Biochim. Biophys. Acta **439:** 449–460.
18. Goodman, D. S. 1976. Retinol binding protein prealbumin and vitamin A transport. *In* Trace Components of Plasma: Isolation and Clinical Significance. G. A. Jamieson & T. J. Greenwalt, Eds.: 313–330. Liss. New York, N.Y.
19. Vahlquist, A., P. A. Peterson & L. Wibell. 1978. Metabolism of the vitamin A transport and visual dark adaptation in diseases of the intestine and liver. Scand. J. Clin. Lab. Invest. **38:** 301–308.
20. Dingle, J. T., H. B. Fell & D. S. Goodman. 1972. The effect of retinol and of retinol-binding protein on embryonic skeletal tissue in organ culture. J. Cell Sci. **11:** 393–402.
21. Bashor, M. M., D. O. Toft & F. Chytil. 1973. In vitro binding of retinol to rat tissue components. Proc. Nat. Acad. Sci. USA **70:** 3483–3487.
22. Ong, D. E. & F. Chytil. 1975. Retinoic acid binding protein in rat tissue. J. Biol. Chem. **250:** 6113–6117.
23. Sani, B. P. & D. L. Hill. 1974. Retinoic acid: a binding protein in chick embryo metatarsal skin. Biochem. Biophys. Res. Commun. **61:** 1276–1282.
24. Chytil, F. & D. E. Ong. 1979. Cellular retinol and retinoic acid–binding proteins in vitamin A action. Fed. Proc. Fed. Am. Soc. Exp. Biol. **38:** 2510–2514.
25. Ong, D. E. & F. Chytil. 1976. Changes in levels of cellular retinol and retinoic acid-binding proteins of liver and lung during perinatal development. Proc. Nat. Acad. Sci. USA **73:** 3976–3978.
26. DeLuca, L. M., G. C. Rosso & G. Wolf. 1970. The biosynthesis of a mannolipid that contains a polar metabolite of [15-^{14}C]-retinol. Biochem. Biophys. Res. Commun. **41:** 615–620.
27. Peterson, P. A., L. Rask, T. Helting, L. Ostberg & Y. Fernstedt. 1976. Formation and properties of retinyl phosphate galactose. J. Biol. Chem. **251:** 4986–4995.
28. Wolf, G., T. C. Kiorpes, S. Masushige, J. B. Schreiber, M. J. Smith & R. S. Anderson. 1979. Recent evidence for the participation of vitamin A in glycoprotein synthesis. Fed. Proc. Fed. Am. Soc. Exp. Biol. **38:** 2540–2543.
29. Mellanby, E. 1938. The experimental production of deafness in young animals by diet. J. Physiol. **94:** 380–398.
30. Moore, L. A. 1939. Relationship between carotene blindness due to constriction of the optic nerve, papillary edema and nyctalopia in calves. J. Nutr. **17:** 443–459.
31. Wolbach, S. B. 1947. Vitamin A deficiency and excess in relation to skeletal growth. J. Bone Jt. Surg. **29:** 171–192.
32. Mellanby, E. 1944. Nutrition in relation to bone growth and the nervous system. Proc. R. Soc. London Ser. B **132:** 28–45.
33. Irving, J. T. 1949. The effects of vitaminosis and hypervitaminosis A upon the incisor teeth and incisal alveolar bone of rats. J. Physiol. **108:** 92–101.
34. Frandsen, A. M. & H. Becks. 1962. The effect of hypovitaminosis A on bone healing and endochondral ossification in rats. Oral Surg. Oral Med. Oral Pathol. **15:** 474–487.
35. Howell, J. M. & S. N. Thompson. 1968. Observations on the lesions in vitamin A deficient adult fowls with particular reference to changes in bone and central nervous system. Br. J. Exp. Pathol. **48:** 450–454.
36. Hayes, K. C., S. W. Nielson & H. D. Eaton. 1968. Pathogenesis of the optic nerve lesion in vitamin A deficient calves. Arch. Ophthalmol. **80:** 777–787.
37. Hayes, K. C. & R. J. Cousins. 1970. Vitamin A deficiency and bone growth. I. Altered drift patterns. Calcif. Tissue Res. **6:** 120–132.

38. GALLINA, A. M., C. F. HELMBOLDT, H. E. FRIER, S. W. NIELSEN & H. D. EATON. 1970. Bone growth in the hypovitaminotic A calf. J. Nutr. **100:** 129–142.
39. BROWN, P. L. & K. C. HAYES. 1975. Effects of acute vitamin A deficiency on rat medullary bone. J. Dent. Res. **54:** 148.
40. DZIEWIATKOWSKI, D. D. 1954. Vitamin A and endochondral ossification in the rat as indicated by the use of ^{35}S and ^{32}P. J. Exp. Med. **100:** 10–24.
41. FRAPE, D. L., R. S. ALLEN, V. C. SPEER, V. W. HAYS & D. V. CATRON. 1959. Relationship of vitamin A to ^{35}S metabolism in the baby pig. J. Nutr. **68:** 189–201.
42. HAVIVI, E. & G. WOLF. 1967. Vitamin A sulfation and bone growth in the chick. J. Nutr. **92:** 467–473.
43. COUSINS, R. J., H. D. EATON, J. E. ROUSSEAU, JR. & R. C. HALL, JR. 1969. Biochemical constituents of the dura mater in vitamin A deficiency. J. Nutr. **97:** 409–418.
44. FIRSCHEIN, H. E. 1970. Collagen and mineral accretion rates in bone during vitamin A deficiency. Am. J. Physiol. **219**(5): 1183–1187.
45. HAVIVI, E. & R. TAL. 1974. Effect of vitamin A deficiency on several bone parameters in chicks. Int. J. Vitam. Nutr. Res. **44:** 8–13.
46. HAVIVI, E. & R. TAL. 1974. Vitamin A deficiency stimulated phosphatase activity in epiphyseal chick cartilage. Calcif. Tissue Res. **14:** 251–255.
47. MADDOCK, C. L., S. B. WOLBACH & S. MADDOCK. 1949. Hypervitaminosis A in the dog. J. Nutr. **39:** 117–137.
48. RODAHL, K. 1950. Hypervitaminosis A. Skrifter No. 95. Norsk Polarinstitutt. Oslo, Norway.
49. WOLBACH, S. B. & D. M. HEGSTED. 1953. Hypervitaminosis in young duck. AMA Arch. Pathol. **55:** 47–54.
50. WOLBACH, S. B. & D. M. HEGSTED. 1952. Hypervitaminosis and the skeleton of growing chicks. AMA Arch. Pathol. **54:** 30–38.
51. MOORE, T. & I. M. SHARMAN. 1979. Hypervitaminosis A combined calcium deficiency in rats. Int. J. Vitam. Nutr. Res. **49:** 14–20.
52. STEWART, R. J. C. 1975. Bone pathology in experimental malnutrition. World Rev. Nutr. Diet. **21:** 1–74.
53. RODAHL, K. & T. MOORE. 1943. The vitamin A content and toxicity of bear and seal liver. Biochem. J. **37:** 166–168.
54. CAFFEY, J. 1951. Chronic poisoning due to excess of vitamin A. Am. J. Roentgenol. Radium Ther. **65:** 12–26.
55. WANG, C. C., S. STRAIGHT & D. L. HILL. 1976. Destabilization of mouse liver lyposomes by vitamin A compounds and analogues. Biochem. Pharmacol. **25:** 471–475.
56. CHERTOW, B. S., G. A. WILLIAMS, R. M. NORRIS, G. R. BAKER & G. K. HARGIS. 1977. Vitamin A stimulation of parathyroid hormone: interactions with calcium, hydrocortisone and vitamin E in bovine parathyroid tissues and effects of vitamin A in man. Eur. J. Clin. Invest. **7:** 307–314.
57. KLOUDA, G. L. & J. M. NAVIA. 1974. An improved model system for the study of bone repair. Calcif. Tissue Res. **14:** 245–249.
58. NAVIA, J. M. & H. LOPEZ. 1973. A purified gel diet for guinea pigs. Lab. Anim. Sci. **23:** 111–114.
59. HARRIS, S. S. & J. M. NAVIA. 1977. Effect of vitamin A deficiency on calcium and glycosaminoglycan metabolism in guinea pig bone. J. Nutr. **107:** 2198–2205.
60. HARRIS, S. S., C. E. HUNT, C. J. ALVAREZ & J. M. NAVIA. 1978. Vitamin A deficiency and new bone growth: histologic changes. J. Oral Pathol. **7:** 85–90.
61. HARRIS, S. S. & J. M. NAVIA. 1978. Sulfate metabolism in rat calvaria cultured under vitamin A deficient conditions. J. Nutr. **108:** 1777–1782.
62. DE LUCA, H. A. 1979. Retinoic acid metabolism. Fed. Proc. Fed. Am. Soc. Exp. Biol. **38:** 2519–2523.

DISCUSSION

S. S. SHAPIRO (*Hoffmann-La Roche, Inc., Nutley, N. J.*): Several years ago, we showed in chondrocytes that *in vitro* in the presence of high levels of either retinoic acid or other synthetic retinoids, we altered the biosynthetic pathway of the GAGs [glycosaminoglycans] from the typical condroitin sulfates to heparin sulfates. Since these different GAGs will certainly be metabolized differently, might this be operative in bone, where you are now turning on heparin sulfate biosynthesis? This would result in apparent changes in degradation.

J. M. NAVIA: We are very much interested in knowing what types of cells are responsible for these biochemical changes. We are presently trying to identify the different types and amounts of glycosaminoglycans, and perhaps later we will identify the proteoglycans in bone and the metabolic pathways that lead to their synthesis under vitamin A-deficiency conditions. We do not know at this time whether the changes in GAG synthesis, such as the one you have seen in cartilage, are the same as the ones we detect in our bone system.

E. BARRETT (*Interesting Medicine, New York, N.Y.*): It may be a little premature to ask you, but would you discuss the possible implications of your studies on osteoporosis in humans.

J. M. NAVIA: We have not yet reached the stage in our research where we can address the question of osteoporosis. We are very interested in this problem and have just started some exploratory research efforts, so that within a year I hope I can answer your question better. This is a bone disorder that should be investigated, and we are doing just that at this time.

I. CLARK (*Rutgers Medical School, New Brunswick, N.J.*): Is there any difference in the ash content between your A-deficient and your A-supplemented calvaria?

J. M. NAVIA: We have checked the calcium concentration in guinea pig bone-containing implants, and we have seen a calcium decrease in bone formed under vitamin A deficiency. We have not done similar experiments in the rat calvaria experiments, where the bone is very immature and the model system is quite different. The rat calvaria are incubated for a very short period of time, 24 to 48 hours, and we do not get detectable changes in calcium concentration under these conditions.

I. CLARK: Because if there is a difference and you calculate per milligram calvaria, in the case where you have less mineral, you are bound to have more radioactive sulfur present.

J. M. NAVIA: Yes, I know; but we have checked on this, and there is an increase in sulfur uptake based on the glycosaminoglycan content of the bone.

J. G. BIERI (*National Institutes of Health, Bethesda, Md.*): Dr. Navia, did you say that 1 microgram retinoic acid daily is inadequate but 10 micrograms is sufficient?

J. M. NAVIA: Yes, I said this, because if you examine the data on sulfate incorporation, you will see that we could not obtain sufficiently high levels of sulfate uptake in vitamin A-deficient animals compared to controls when one microgram was used as a supplement. These were the first experiments we did, when we thought 1 microgram of retinoic acid was sufficient. In all other subsequent experiments, we increased the supplementation to 10 micrograms. As you could see in the histologic sections of bone, administration of 10 micrograms of retinoic acid gives a bone appearance that is indistinguishable from normal bone.

J. G. BIERI: Last year a group reported that in animals fed retinoic acid as their sole source of vitamin A, there was impairment in bone formation of the inner ear. Have you seen that before?

J. M. NAVIA: Yes, there are reports describing changes of the inner ear bones of animals deficient in vitamin A. Most of those studies were chronic studies, where disturbances of hearing and alterations in the integrity of the sensory tissue developed. Our studies involve short periods of time, so these deficiency syndromes are not seen in our model system.

VITAMIN A DEFICIENCY AND ABNORMAL METABOLISM OF IRON*

Robert E. Hodges,† Robert B. Rucker,‡ and Raymond H. Gardner‡

University of California
Davis, California 95616

Previous studies of experimental vitamin A deficiency in man by one of the authors (REH) led to the conclusion that anemia can result from lack of vitamin A.[1,2] This anemia was accompanied by low concentrations of iron in serum and by slightly decreased values for total iron-binding capacity. Administration of medicinal iron by mouth failed to elicit a hematologic response. Subsequent addition of vitamin A—in the form of either β-carotene or retinol—to the diet resulted in a prompt hematopoietic response.

The authors also have reviewed previous publications relating to the effects of vitamin A deficiency on hematopoiesis.[3] A number of these report an anemia associated with lack of this vitamin.[4-10] We have since conducted a series of studies designed to elucidate the mechanisms involved.[3,11-13] One of the most puzzling aspects of these studies is the occurrence *without* anemia of vitamin A deficiency in both man and experimental animals.[6,14-18] One explanation for this phenomenon is that an abrupt onset of vitamin A deficiency results in such severe illness that intakes of food and water fall to very low levels and the animals (or persons) become cachectic and hypovolemic. An acute onset of deficiency would result in hemoconcentration, which not only can mask an anemia but may give the impression of polycythemia. On the other hand, when deficiency develops slowly and is not very severe, the animals or persons presumably can maintain a normal circulating blood volume. Under these circumstances, the anemia that develops can be detected easily by routine hematologic tests.

Our studies of iron metabolism in vitamin A-deficient rats confirmed low concentrations of iron in their serum.[3,12,13] In addition, we found defective incorporation of radioactive iron (^{59}Fe) into erythrocytes. Next we investigated gastrointestinal absorption of ^{59}Fe. These studies disclosed that absorption of iron from the digestive tract of vitamin A-deficient rats was normal. Accordingly we studied the tissue distribution of iron and confirmed Wolbach's original observations that in the presence of vitamin A deficiency, excess iron is stored in the liver or spleen or both.[5,7] In addition, serum iron values were low.

One possible explanation for these findings could be a defect in the erythrocyte membrane as a result of inadequate vitamin A, since this vitamin is necessary for normal membrane synthesis. Indeed we had confirmed the earlier findings of Amine *et al.* that red blood cells are morphologically abnormal in vitamin A-deficient animals.[13,17] Presumably a defective cell membrane might result in abnormal fragility and a shortened half-life, resulting in a hemolytic anemia. This also could explain the excessive storage of iron and low serum iron, because intravascular hemolysis will result in accumulation of heme-iron in the liver or spleen or both.

* Supported by a grant from Hoffmann-La Roche, Inc., Nutley, N.J.

† Present affiliation: Department of Internal Medicine, University of Nebraska Medical Center, Omaha, Nebr. 68105.

‡ Department of Nutrition, College of Agricultural and Environmental Sciences.

0077-8923/80/0355-0058 $01.75/0 © 1980, NYAS

To test this hypothesis, we fed weanling rats a diet deficient in vitamin A until they had cessation of growth, rumpled fur, and other signs of deficiency, such as crusting of their eyelids. A control group was fed a normal diet. Samples of blood were collected from animals in both groups and labeled with ^{51}Cr, then reinjected into the original donor animals. This permitted estimates of erythrocyte survival over a period of 36 days.

Other studies included labeling of erythrocytes with ^{59}Fe. These studies will be reported elsewhere.

Results

The animals in this study were not anemic as judged by red blood cell counts, hemoglobin concentrations, and hematocrit values. There was a significant increase in splenic iron but not in hepatic iron. Erythrocyte survival curves were not significantly altered by vitamin A deficiency.

Discussion

A host of different nutrients have been suggested as essential for normal hematopoiesis. Most hematologists are understandably skeptical when another form of "deficiency anemia" is suggested. Certainly lack of iron, vitamin B_{12}, or folates will result in anemia. Other deficiency anemias have been suggested, including lack of vitamin B, niacin, vitamin E, ascorbic acid, zinc, and copper. Accordingly it is not surprising that the concept of "vitamin A-deficiency anemia" meets with little enthusiasm, especially when some investigators have been unable to confirm the observations of others.

The explanation must reflect certain differences in experimental design. Young, rapidly growing animals become deficient much more readily than do older animals. The diet of some animals may be absolutely devoid of vitamin A activity, whereas another group of animals may be fed a diet containing traces of this vitamin. The effect of vitamin A or lack of it on fluid distribution is well known. Deficiency of vitamin A results in a rise in cerebral spinal fluid pressure in most species studied, and in sheep it affects renal function.[18] There is very little information regarding the effects of vitamin A on circulating blood volume. Certainly severe cachexia from any cause may produce dehydration and hemoconcentration. Whether this explains the disparity between those studies demonstrating anemia as a result of vitamin A deficiency and studies failing to show anemia is conjectural. Certainly there is better agreement regarding abnormalities of iron metabolism in vitamin A-deficient animals and children. But the mechanisms involved are by no means clear. Increased hemolysis was an attractive theory, but the present study seems to indicate that this is not the mechanism.[19] Perhaps lack of vitamin A affects the binding of iron to carrier proteins or to intracellular proteins. Additional studies will be needed to elucidate this problem.

Conclusions

1. Vitamin A deficiency may be associated with an anemia, but this did not occur in the study reported here.

2. Alterations in iron metabolism occur in association with vitamin A deficiency. In the present study, excess iron was stored in the spleen.

3. Although erythrocyte morphology may be altered in vitamin A deficiency, the erythrocyte survival time, as estimated by ^{51}Cr tagging, was not significantly altered.

4. The cause of altered iron metabolism in vitamin A deficiency has not been determined, but it is not a result of increased hemolysis of erythrocytes.

References

1. Hodges, R. E. & J. E. Canham. 1970. Studies of experimental vitamin C deficiency and experimental vitamin A deficiency in man. *In* Proceedings of a Workshop on Problems of Assessment and Alleviation of Malnutrition in the United States. R. G. Hansen & H. N. Munro, Eds. GPO Publication No. 916.086. U.S. Government Printing Office. Washington, D.C.
2. Sauberlich, H. E., R. E. Hodges, D. L. Wallace, H. Kolder, J. E. Canham, J. Hood, N. Raica & L. K. Lowry. 1974. Vitamin A metabolism and requirements in the human studied with the use of labeled retinol. Vitam. Horm. **32:** 251–275.
3. Hodges, R. E., H. E. Sauberlich, J. E. Canham, D. L. Wallace, R. B. Rucker, L. A. Mejia & M. Mohanram. 1978. Hematopoietic studies in vitamin A deficiency. Am. J. Clin. Nutr. **31**(5): 876–885.
4. Findlay, G. M. & R. D. MacKenzie. 1922. The bone marrow in deficiency diseases. J. Pathol. **25:** 402–403.
5. Wolbach, S. B. & P. R. Howe. 1925. Tissue changes following deprivation of fat-soluble A vitamin. J. Exp. Med. **42:** 753–778.
6. Koessler, K. K., S. Mauer & R. Loughlin. 1926. The relation of anemia, primary and secondary, to vitamin A deficiency. J. Am. Med. Assoc. **87:** 476–482.
7. Blackfan, K. D. & S. B. Wolbach. 1933. Vitamin A deficiency in infants, a clinical and pathological study. J. Pediatr. **3:** 679–706.
8. Frank, M. 1934. Beitrag zur Hàmatologie der A-avitaminose. Monatsschr. Kinderheilkd. **60:** 350–355.
9. Wagner, K-H. 1940. Die experimentelle Avitaminose A beim Menschen. Hoppe Seyler's Z. Psysiol. Chem. **264:** 153–188.
10. O'Toole, B. A., R. Fradkin, J. Warkany, J. G. Wilson & G. V. Mann. 1974. Vitamin A deficiency and reproduction in rhesus monkeys. J. Nutr. **104**(11): 1513–1524.
11. Mejia, L. A., R. E. Hodges, G. Arroyave, F. Viteri & B. Torun. 1977. Vitamin A deficiency and anemia in Central American children. Am. J. Clin. Nutr. **30**(7): 1175–1184.
12. Mejia, L. A., R. E. Hodges & R. B. Rucker. 1979. Role of vitamin A in the absorption, retention and distribution of iron in the rat. J. Nutr. **109**(1): 129–137.
13. Mejia, L. A., R. E. Hodges & R. B. Rucker. 1979. Clinical signs of anemia in vitamin A-deficient rats. Am. J. Clin. Nutr. **32**(7): 1439–1444.
14. Sure, B., M. C. Kik & D. J. Walker. 1929. The effect of avitaminosis on hematopoietic function. I. Vitamin A deficiency. J. Biol. Chem. **83:** 375–385.
15. McLaren, D. S., M. Tchalian & Z. A. Ajans. 1965. Biochemical and hematologic changes in the vitamin A-deficient rat. Am. J. Clin. Nutr. **17**(9): 131–138.
16. Nockels, C. F. & E. W. Kienholz. 1967. Influence of vitamin A deficiency on testes, bursa of Fabricius, adrenal and hematocrit in cockerels. J. Nutr. **92:** 384–388.
17. Amine, E. K., J. Corey, D. M. Hegsted & K. C. Hayes. 1970. Comparative hematology during deficiencies of iron and vitamin A in the rat. J. Nutr. **100:** 1033–1040.
18. Corey, J. E. & K. C. Hayes. 1972. Cerebrospinal fluid pressure, growth, and hematology in relation to retinol status of the rat in acute vitamin A deficiency. J. Nutr. **102:** 1585–1593.
19. Gardner, R. H. 1979. The effect of vitamin A deficiency on hematopoiesis and iron metabolism. Master's Thesis. University of California. Davis, Calif.

Discussion

Unidentified Speaker: Have you done studies with rats maintained on retinoic acid? After you take retinoic acid away when they are retinol depleted, do you see any evidence for the anemia within a week or before they get too sick?

R. E. Hodges: We haven't studied deficiency of vitamin A and its effect on hematologic function with retinoic acid. This is another thing we would like to do. Vitamin A deficiency can be induced by feeding the animals retinoic acid for a long period of time, which keeps them alive and does not result in any significant storage of the vitamin. This permits the investigator to get a group of animals that become deficient almost immediately. With the techniques we used, it is necessary to follow the body weight each day and to follow the consumption of food. When they stop eating and stop gaining weight, then usually deficiency is imminent, and of course within a very short time they will develop rumpled fur and crusting of the eyelids and other evidence of deficiency. I think the suggestion about retinoic acid is a very good one, and it's one that we certainly intend to use.

H. F. DeLuca (*University of Wisconsin, Madison, Wis.*): Dr. Hodges, could you give us some additional information on the nature of the anemia. That is, is the number of red cells normal or abnormally low, or are they hypochromic, or is there any other information available on their nature?

R. E. Hodges: It is a normocytic normochromic anemia, but it's accompanied at least in men by low serum iron levels and total iron-binding capacity that's within the lower range of low normal.

H. F. DeLuca: The rate of formation of the red cells is normal also?

R. E. Hodges: We don't know this. This is another thing to study, and the fact that these rats do not incorporate iron-59 into their bone marrow at a normal rate suggests that perhaps it's not normal.

O. A. Levander (*Beltsville Human Nutrition Research Center, U.S. Department of Agriculture, Beltsville, Md.*): This is to confirm, more or less, your study on the red cell survival in the acutely deficient vitamin A rats. We've looked at the deformability of the red cells from such animals as measured by the filtration technique. We did not find any changes in filterability. If there is any relation between *in vitro* red cell deformability and *in vivo* red cell survivability, this would tend to lend support to your experiment.

R. E. Hodges: It is still tempting to think that there must be a defect and that perhaps these cells are destroyed a little more rapidly than normal, although certainly our evidence doesn't confirm that right now.

J. G. Bieri (*National Institutes of Health, Bethesda, Md.*): We've used a model of chronic A deficiency for some studies of possible keratomalacia in the rat, where we maintained rats on extremely low levels of retinoic acid after they were depleted of retinol. These levels run 50 to 100 micrograms per kilo of diet. The animals don't grow, they do have very serious eye lesions, and we keep these animals going for 6–8–10 weeks. We don't see any anemia in these animals.

R. E. Hodges: How old are the animals?

J. G. Bieri: We start them out as weanlings. We get them depleted of retinol in about five weeks and put them on retinoic acid, and then we keep dropping it down until they stop gaining weight. There might be a difference in experimental diets that might have to be looked at, such as the forms of iron in the diet and perhaps other factors.

R. E. Hodges: Yes I'm sure there are multiple variables. The fact that some people have reported anemia as routine and others have reported that it never occurs makes it even more challenging.

THE VITAMIN A–ZINC CONNECTION: A REVIEW

J. Cecil Smith, Jr.

Vitamin and Mineral Nutrition Laboratory
Beltsville Human Nutrition Research Center
U.S. Department of Agriculture
Science and Education Administration
Beltsville, Maryland 20705

Only within the last decade have data been obtained that support the concept of an interaction between zinc and vitamin A. However, nearly a quarter of a century ago, Stevenson and Earle casually noted low concentrations of serum vitamin A in swine with parakeratosis, a condition caused by dietary zinc deficiency. Massive doses of vitamin A acetate were of no apparent benefit in raising the serum vitamin A to normal.[1]

Soon afterwards, Vallee *et al.* suggested a possible metabolic relationship between zinc and vitamin A.[2,3] Their reasoning included the following: (1) Zinc is an integral part of the metalloenzyme alcohol dehydrogenase in yeast and horse liver.[4,5] Earlier it had been reported that alcohol dehydrogenase obtained from horse liver reversibly dehydrogenated vitamin A alcohol to vitamin A aldehyde in isolated retinal rods as well as in liver extracts.[6] (2) The eye (an active site of vitamin A metabolism) contains one of the highest concentrations of zinc in the body.[7] (3) Zinc-deficient swine showed low serum vitamin A, which was not reversed by vitamin A therapy.[1]

In addition, Vallee *et al.* noted the earlier work of Patek and Haig, who reported that 19 out of 24 patients with cirrhosis of the liver exhibited abnormal dark adaptation despite adequate dietary vitamin A.[2,3,8] Only massive doses of vitamin A improved the condition, and even then some patients appeared to be resistant to vitamin A therapy. Vallee *et al.* suggested that the poor response to vitamin A therapy in some of the cirrhotics was due to the altered zinc metabolism characteristic of that condition.[3]

Animal Studies

Saraswat and Arora and Arora *et al.* found that lambs fed a diet low in zinc but supplemented with vitamin A exhibited low levels of serum vitamin A when compared with the same lambs later fed the same diet supplemented with 50 ppm zinc.[9,10] Likewise, oral supplementation of zinc increased the efficacy of vitamin A therapy in lambs previously depleted of zinc and vitamin A.

Using both germ-free and conventional rats, Smith *et al.* demonstrated that animals fed a zinc-deficient vitamin A diet had plasma vitamin A concentrations that were nearly 50% lower than those of rats fed a zinc-adequate diet (Table 1).[11] Liver vitamin A concentrations were not altered. Vitamin A supplementation did not result in the plasma levels reverting to normal. However, zinc therapy alone for 14 days resulted in an elevation of plasma vitamin A levels to within normal range. All animals were fed *ad libitum*, and it was noted that growth may be involved in the zinc–vitamin A interaction. Nevertheless, it was hypothesized that zinc was necessary for the mobilization of vitamin A from the liver, as well as to maintain normal concentrations of plasma vitamin A.

0077-8923/80/0355-0062 $01.75/0

TABLE 1

LIVER AND PLASMA VITAMIN A CONCENTRATIONS IN ZINC-DEFICIENT RATS*

	Vitamin A	
	Liver† (μg/g)	Plasma† (μg/100 ml)
Zinc Adequate (*ad lib.*)	130 ± 14 (10)	39 ± 10 (8)
Zinc Deficient (*ad lib.*)	110 ± 47 (10)	20 ± 2.8 (8)
Level of Significance	NS	P < 0.001

* From Smith *et al.*, Reference 11.

† Mean ± standard deviation (SD); number of animals in each group is given in parenthesis.

A subsequent experiment compared parameters of vitamin A and zinc metabolism in three groups of animals fed (1) zinc-sufficient diet *ad libitum*; (2) zinc-deficient diet *ad libitum*; and (3) zinc-sufficient diet pair fed.[12] The intake of the pair-fed group was matched to that of the zinc-deficient, *ad libitum* animals in an effort to remove differences in food intake as a variable. This experiment showed low plasma vitamin A concentrations in the zinc-deficient rats (10 ± 2.0 μg/100 ml) compared to the zinc-adequate, *ad libitum* controls (40 ± 1.4 μg/100 ml). The pair-fed animals had intermediate levels of plasma vitamin A (27 ± 0.8 μg/100 ml), indicating an effect due to causes other than differences in food intake between the zinc-deficient and zinc-adequate pair-fed groups, since both groups received identical quantities of food daily. In addition, the specific vitamin A transport protein, retinol-binding protein (RBP), was shown to be significantly depressed in the plasma of the zinc-deficient animals compared to pair-fed controls. Indeed, the plasma RBP was decreased to a much greater extent than were total proteins (TABLE 2). This suggested that zinc deficiency results in depressing plasma RBP to a greater extent than many of the other plasma proteins. It has been suggested that RBP is more sensitive to protein and calorie intake than are other plasma proteins.[13] In contrast, the concentration of RBP in the liver was significantly decreased in only the zinc-deficient animals (FIGURE 1). The decreased food intake and the growth of the pair-fed animals did not alter the liver RBP concentration from the level found in the livers of the *ad libitum* controls. Only in the zinc-deficient group was liver RBP concentration significantly reduced, suggesting an effect of zinc per se on the synthesis of RBP.

TABLE 2

EFFECT OF ZINC DEFICIENCY ON PLASMA PROTEINS AND RETINOL-BINDING PROTEIN (RBP) IN RATS*

Treatment	Total Plasma Proteins† (mg/ml)	Plasma RBP† (ng/mg protein)
Zinc Adequate (*ad lib.*)	69.0 ± 1.1	49.7 ± 2.0
Zinc Adequate (pair fed)	68.1 ± 2.3	35.9 ± 1.2
Zinc Deficient	53.1 ± 1.8	13.9 ± 2.3
Difference (%)‡	22	61

* From J. E. Smith *et al.*, Reference 12.

† Mean ± standard error of the mean (SEM); seven animals in each group.

‡ Difference is a comparison of the zinc-adequate, pair-fed group with the zinc-deficient group.

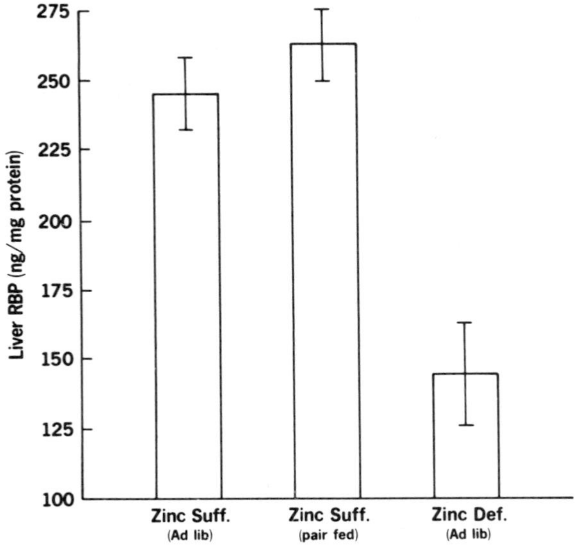

FIGURE 1. Effect of zinc deficiency on liver retinol-binding protein (RBP).

There was no evidence of increased rate of RBP turnover in the zinc-deficient animals.

Moderately reduced plasma vitamin A and RBP levels were evident in the pair-fed, zinc-sufficient rats compared to *ad libitum* controls (FIGURE 2). The reason for the depressions was not apparent. However, the growth rate of pair-fed animals was also depressed compared to the *ad libitum* controls because, although they were fed the identical diet, the quantity of food was restricted in the pair-fed group. Earlier studies by Rechcigl *et al.* demonstrated a positive linear correlation between vitamin A utilization and growth rate of rats.[14] Progressively increasing the level of dietary protein from zero to 18% increased the growth rate, food intakes, and vitamin A utilization. The liver vitamin A utilization was more closely correlated to growth rate than to food intake. Therefore, another set of experiments was carried out by Smith *et al.* that included four groups of animals: (1) animals restricted in growth to equal the growth of the zinc-deficient, *ad libitum* (weight-matched) group; (2) animals not allowed to grow by dietary restriction (zero growth); (3) animals fed the same quantity of food as the zinc-deficient (pair-fed) group; and (4) animals fed a zinc-supplemented diet *ad libitum*.[15] Three experiments were conducted at two different locations using different sources of animals. A total of 95 rats were used, including 24 that were germ free. Previous results showing lower plasma vitamin A levels in zinc-deficient animals were also confirmed. The results indicated that plasma vitamin A (and zinc) was depressed in animals severely restricted in food and growth, although they were fed a diet adequate in both vitamin A and zinc. In two out of three experiments, the restriction of food intake resulted in plasma vitamin A concentrations equal to the levels of the zinc-deficient animals (TABLE 3). Therefore the question was asked, "Is the effect of zinc on plasma vitamin A primary or secondary?"[15]

Smith *et al.* concluded that the normal mechanisms in animals for maintaining plasma vitamin A were altered either by zinc deficiency (which is accompanied by

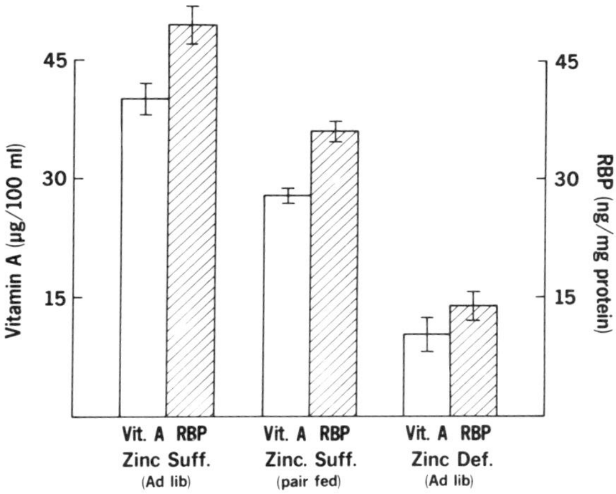

FIGURE 2. Effect of zinc deficiency on plasma vitamin A and retinol-binding protein.

decreased intake of food and decreased growth) or by growth depression resulting from intake restriction of a diet adequate in zinc and vitamin A.[15] In addition, zinc deficiency or food and growth restriction did not decrease liver vitamin A concentration, suggesting no impairment of vitamin A absorption and transport to the liver. However, an effect of zinc deficiency by impairing synthesis of liver RBP was proposed.[12,15]

Apgar, using a different approach, reasoned that since considerable vitamin A is deposited in the rat fetus during pregnancy, fetuses from zinc-deficient females who were fed no vitamin A during pregnancy should have reduced concentration of vitamin A if these females had an impaired ability to utilize (mobilize) the vitamin A stored in the liver.[16] Her results indicated that there was no difference in the concentration of vitamin A in the liver whether or not the dams received zinc with the vitamin A-deficient diet. In other experiments reported at the same time, Apgar fed a vitamin A-deficient diet throughout two pregnancies and lactations.[16] After the females were thus prepared, they were divided into two groups; one group continued to receive zinc supplementation, the other received no zinc. Both groups continued

TABLE 3

EFFECT OF ZINC DEFICIENCY AND GROWTH RESTRICTION ON PLASMA VITAMIN A IN RATS*

Group†	Number of Animals	Plasma Vitamin A‡ (µg/100 ml)
Zinc Adequate	63	34 ± 7.0[a]
Zinc Deficient	9	23 ± 5.7[b]
Zinc Adequate (zero growth)	9	23 ± 7.7[b]
Zinc Adequate (wt. matched to zinc deficient)	10	23 ± 4.7[b]

* From Smith *et al.*, Reference 15.

† All diets were adequate in vitamin A, 6900 µg/kg of retinyl acetate.

‡ Mean ± SD; values in the same column with different-lettered superscripts are significantly different at the $P < 0.001$ level.

to be fed a vitamin A–deficient diet. Cornification of the vagina, a sign associated with vitamin A deficiency, was not apparent in the zinc-deficient group after a period of up to seven months. The results were interpreted as indicating that the zinc-deficient females mobilized vitamin A. On the other hand, 30% or more of the vaginal smear cells were cornified in the zinc-supplemented group. Although unexplained, the more severe vitamin A deficiency in the zinc-supplemented group was apparently due to increased requirement, since those animals grew, whereas the zinc-deficient group did not grow and thus had a lower vitamin A requirement. From these and other data, Apgar concluded that "there is therefore no impairment in the ability of zinc-deficient rats to utilize their vitamin A stores and no evidence for a direct requirement for zinc in the utilization of vitamin A."[16]

A subsequent publication by Carney *et al.* concerned the effects of zinc deficiency on hepatic retinol mobilization and urinary excretion of vitamin A metabolites following an oral dose of radioactive retinyl acetate.[17] These authors concluded that zinc deficiency had no effect on mobilization of newly ingested vitamin A or urinary excretion of radioactive metabolites collected over a six-day interval. In addition, they suggested that the "low plasma vitamin A levels in zinc deficiency are probably the result of growth retardation rather than any role in vitamin A metabolism."[17]

In contrast, Duncan and Hurley came to a different conclusion using female rats who were depleted of vitamin A during growth, then mated and fed three (deficient, marginal deficient, or adequate) levels of zinc and three levels of vitamin A (also corresponding to deficient, marginal, or adequate intakes).[18] Parameters measured included weight change of dam during gestation, mean weight and malformation incidence of the full-term fetuses, and plasma and liver zinc and vitamin A levels in both the dams at term and in the 21-day-old fetuses. Low intake of zinc caused a reduction of the dams and fetuses' body weight. That is, the zinc-deficient dams lost an average of 15 g during gestation, and their fetuses weighed an average of 2.5 g per pup. The control dams gained 131 g, and their fetuses weighed an average of 5.3 g. As expected under these growth-restricted conditions, plasma vitamin A was markedly reduced in both the maternal and fetal animals. Statistically there was a significant interaction between plasma vitamin A and zinc. The authors concluded that the data indicated an interaction between zinc and vitamin A metabolism, possibly at the level of vitamin A mobilization from the liver. However, the experimental design did not attempt to control differences in growth or weight gain between the zinc-deficient animals and their controls. The effect of zinc on vitamin A metabolism may have been secondary due to the growth differences.

Thus, our laboratory and others now recognize that food and growth restrictions are complicating factors in the interpretation of any vitamin A–zinc interaction in the plasma and liver of immature rats or other growing experimental animals. Recently it has been suggested that the restriction of *protein* due either to the inanition that accompanies zinc deficiency or to food limitation of an adequate diet may be a factor in the inability to transport vitamin A into the plasma in sufficient quantity to maintain normal levels of the vitamin.[13]

In Vitro Studies

Several *in vitro* studies have concerned possible zinc–vitamin A interactions. Huber and Gershoff reported significant decreases in the alcohol dehydrogenase activity of zinc-deficient rats when either ethanol or retinol was the substrate.[19] Alcohol dehydrogenase from the retina appeared more sensitive to zinc deficiency than did liver alcohol dehydrogenase when adult males were used. However, in weanling rats born to females fed a zinc-deficient diet 1 to 3 days before parturition and throughout the 21-day suckling period, the activity of the alcohol dehydrogenase from both the liver and retina was significantly decreased regardless of whether ethanol or retinol was used as the substrate. Regrettably, growth and food intake were not controlled and might have affected the results, since the zinc-deficient animals grew significantly less than did the controls. Since this is the first report indicating decreased activity of alcohol dehydrogenase of the retina of zinc-deficient animals, it is imperative that these experiments be expanded to include pair-fed, food- and growth-restricted animals. Such experiments would also help clarify whether the alcohol dehydrogenase of the retina is similar to that in liver. An earlier study showed that vitamin A alcohol was dehydrogenated to vitamin A aldehyde in both isolated retinal rods and liver extracts, suggesting that the enzymes were similar.[6] However, the suggestion that the alcohol dehydrogenase of the retina is similar to the alcohol dehydrogenase of liver has been questioned recently.[20]

Other *in vitro* enzyme assay experiments included determining the activity of retinal reductase (an alcohol dehydrogenase) of the testes as well as the liver.[21] This experiment included a group of pair-fed animals as well as zinc-deficient and zinc-adequate animals fed *ad libitum*. The activity of retinal reductase was lower in the testes of the zinc-deficient animals compared to pair-fed controls. However, liver retinal reductase was not altered. From these experiments and those of Huber and Gershoff, it appears that retinal reductase activity of the eye (retina) and testis is more sensitive to zinc deficiency than is that of the liver.[19,21]

In a preliminary report, zinc enhanced the uptake of vitamin A by the seminiferous tubules of rat testes.[22] Other *in vitro* studies have concerned the effect of zinc on the rate of incorporation of radioactive retinol into bovine sperm.[23,24] There appeared to be an optimal concentration of zinc for maximal vitamin A *in vitro* uptake by sperm. However, various other factors—such as pH and concentration of carbohydrate, i.e., fructose—also influenced uptake, so any effect of zinc probably is nonspecific. That is, other trace elements might substitute for this function; only zinc was tested.

Ette *et al.* have administered 10 mg of $ZnSO_4$ intraperitoneally (ip) to normal weanling rats in order to study the short-term effect on plasma and liver concentrations of vitamins A and E.[25] Six hours after zinc administration, plasma vitamin A was increased, and liver concentrations decreased (TABLE 4). However, there was no effect on plasma and liver vitamin E concentrations, suggesting a specific effect on vitamin A and not on all fat-soluble vitamins. An *in vitro* study using liver homogenates indicated a marked increase in the release of vitamin A from the liver

TABLE 4

EFFECT OF A SINGLE INTRAPERITONEAL INJECTION OF ZINC ON PLASMA AND LIVER VITAMIN A IN NORMAL WEANLING RATS*†

	Liver Vitamin A‡ (μg/g)		Plasma Vitamin A‡ (μg/100 ml)	
Post Injection Time (hrs)	Saline	Zinc	Saline	Zinc
1	56 ± 2.5	49 ± 2.2	60 ± 2.7	81 ± 4.4
6	49 ± 2.1	15 ± 1.3	50 ± 4.2	160 ± 4.8
Significance	NS	P < 0.001	NS	P < 0.001

* 10 mg $ZnSO_4$.
† From Ette *et al.*, Reference 25.
‡ Mean ± SE; at least six animals per group.

tissue when incubated with 10 mg of $ZnSO_4$ per liver. The levels of $ZnSO_4$ used were extremely high in both the *in vivo* and *in vitro* studies. Indeed, our experience has been that ip injections of 1 mg of elemental zinc (~4 mg $ZnSO_4$) to weanling rats will result in one-half of the animals dying from the toxicity. The daily requirement for a growing weanling rat is in the area of 0.05–0.1 mg of zinc given ip. The results of Ette *et al.* must be confirmed using more physiologic levels.[25]

Human Studies

Our laboratory earlier reported a significant correlation between zinc and vitamin A in the plasma of children.[11] However, Hambidge *et al.* found no significant correlation of plasma zinc with serum vitamin A in 74 preschool (Head Start Program) children.[26] Nevertheless, plasma zinc was "low" in 34% of the children, and a near equal percentage (35%) had either "low" or "deficient" levels of serum vitamin A.[26] Earlier in 1972, Henkin and Smith studied serum zinc, vitamin A, and RBP in viral hepatitis patients.[27] All three parameters were depressed. However, there was no correlation between serum zinc and vitamin A. In contrast, serum zinc and RBP were significantly ($P < 0.03$) correlated, although the coefficient was only $r = 0.286$. Jacob *et al.* noted a positive correlation of plasma zinc with RBP in cystic fibrosis patients but not in controls.[28] In addition, they reported a significant correlation between plasma zinc and vitamin A—a finding similar to our earlier observation.[11]

Only within the last five years have zinc supplementation studies been designed to study a possible vitamin A-zinc interaction. In light of the earlier reports, [2,3,5,29] Halsted and Smith suggested an interaction among zinc, vitamin A, and impaired dark adaptation.[30] They further suggested that zinc supplementation may be helpful in vitamin A-resistant night blindness, a condition found in some alcoholic liver disease patients.[9]

We reported in a preliminary study that 6 consecutively selected alcoholic liver disease patients had low plasma levels of both zinc and vitamin A.[31] A larger study involving 119 alcoholic liver disease patients indicated that 52% exhibited both low plasma zinc (< 70 μg/100 ml) and vitamin A (< 30 μg/100 ml).[32] Thirty-three of the low zinc, low plasma vitamin A patients were randomly assigned to one of the following groups: (1) supplemented with zinc alone—oral $ZnSO_4 \cdot 7H_2O$, 220 mg BID* equivalent to 100 mg elemental zinc per day; (2) supplemented with vitamin A alone—50,000 IU of vitamin A acetate per day, orally; (3) supplemented with both zinc and vitamin A; and (4) placebo. With the exception of the zinc-alone group, which contained 9 subjects, all groups had 8 subjects for a total of 33. The results indicated that after 11 days of supplementing with either vitamin A, zinc, or a combination of both, plasma vitamin A was not significantly increased above the control group. The results must be considered tentative due to the short period of supplementation. However, there was no indication that zinc supplementation resulted in an alteration of plasma vitamin A in these patients.

Morrison *et al.* studied six stable alcoholic cirrhotics, who had low serum zinc concentrations and abnormal dark adaptation, compared to 21 age-matched controls (Table 5).[33] Two patients were treated first with oral vitamin A alone for two to four weeks. However, their dark adaptations returned to normal only after zinc was given for one to two weeks following the vitamin A treatment. Of three patients who were supplemented with zinc only, the dark adaptations returned to normal within

* BID means twice a day.

TABLE 5

EFFECT OF ZINC AND VITAMIN A THERAPY ON DARK ADAPTATION IN ALCOHOLIC CIRRHOTIC SUBJECTS*†

Patient	Initial	Vitamin A‡	Zinc§
1	3.2	2.6	2.1
2	3.0	3.2	2.2
3	3.1		2.2
4	2.5		2.1
5	4.3		3.1

* From Morrison *et al.*, Reference 33.
† Units log lux; age-matched controls 2.1 ± 0.2.
‡ 10,000 IU/day for 2–4 weeks.
§ 220 mg $ZnSO_4$/day for 1-2 weeks.

two weeks and were reduced in the third week. The sixth patient was treated with both vitamin A and zinc and attained a normal threshold within two weeks.

In another study from the same laboratory, Russell *et al.* reported that 14 out of 26 cirrhotic patients had abnormal dark adaptation.[34,35] Two of the 12 patients who were treated with oral vitamin A did not respond (dark adaptation did not improve). In these 2 patients, serum zinc concentrations were low (< 65 μg/100 ml). When zinc supplements (220 mg of zinc sulfate per day) were given, the dark adaptation became normal after one week. These data were supportive of the earlier suggestions of interactions between zinc, vitamin A, and impaired dark adaptation.[30]

A more recent study by Weismann *et al.* involved a double-blind clinical study in 30 patients with biopsy-proven alcoholic cirrhosis.[36] Zinc supplementation (134 mg daily) was given to 16 subjects, and a placebo to 14. The parameters included serum zinc, vitamin A, and carotene. Initial serum zinc concentrations were 86 μg/100 ml for the zinc-supplemented group and 81 μg/100 ml for the placebo group. After the six-week zinc supplementation period, serum zinc increased significantly but did not change for the placebo group. Serum vitamin A was not altered by either treatment. Inexplicably, serum carotene was decreased significantly in the zinc-treated group but did not change in the placebo group. Zinc supplementation was of no apparent benefit in improving dark adaptation. However, only one abnormal case was found in the zinc group prior to supplementation, and none in the placebo group. The subjects of this study were apparently not severely depleted of zinc, since their plasma zinc concentrations were 86 μg/100 ml prior to supplementation. This level would be considered within the normal range by most laboratories. In contrast, the subjects of the Morrison *et al.* study who responded to zinc supplementation all had serum zinc levels below 70 μg/100 ml.[33]

Earlier our laboratory had suggested that cystic fibrosis patients exhibited several of the abnormalities of vitamin A and zinc metabolism seen in zinc-deficient animals, including low blood vitamin A levels despite vitamin A supplementation and adequate liver vitamin A stores.[32] Smith *et al.* suggested an impaired liver vitamin A mobilization and transport system, since cystic fibrosis patients usually have adequate liver vitamin A stores.[37] Halsted and Smith reported low plasma levels of zinc in growth-retarded cystic fibrosis subjects.[38] In addition, Jacob *et al.* reported low hair zinc concentrations in cystic fibrosis patients, suggesting inadequate zinc nutriture.[28]

Recently, Palin *et al.* have reported the effect of oral zinc supplementation on plasma levels of vitamin A and retinol-binding protein in 53 subjects—36 cystic fibrosis patients and 17 siblings.[39] The patient and sibling groups were each divided into a zinc-supplemented and a placebo group and received their respective treatment for eight weeks. With the exception of an increased plasma zinc level for both groups receiving zinc, no significant changes occurred as a result of treatment, i.e., plasma vitamin A and RBP did not change. The authors noted that the cystic fibrosis patients were a "fairly healthy group" with a wide range of clinical statuses. In addition, the initial mean plasma zinc concentration for the cystic fibrosis patients prior to supplementation was 90 μg/100 ml, a level well within the normal range. However, the authors concluded that zinc supplementation was of no benefit in correcting the alterations in the vitamin A metabolism of the cystic fibrosis patients studied.

Brissot *et al.* used a correlative study to investigate the role of zinc, vitamin A, and RBP in 34 subjects with idiopathic hemochromatosis, 33 cases of alcoholic cirrhosis, 10 cases of nonalcoholic cirrhosis, and 34 normal controls.[40] Serum vitamin A and RBP were reduced in both alcoholic and nonalcoholic cirrhosis, whereas only the alcoholic cirrhosis group showed a reduced plasma zinc concentration. This is in contrast to earlier reports.[38,41] In the idiopathic hemochromatosis subjects, serum vitamin A was low despite normal RBP and zinc levels. The data were interpreted by the authors as giving little support to the hypothesis that low zinc levels are responsible for vitamin A and RBP abnormalities, because serum zinc was reduced only slightly (~25%) but RBP and vitamin A were reduced more severely (66 and 55%, respectively). The serum zinc levels for patients were within the normal levels reported by most other laboratories. Evidently, differences in analytic techniques accounted for the relatively higher values. However, as the authors acknowledged, there was a relative and significant decrease in serum zinc levels in the alcoholic cirrhosis patients. Nevertheless, the studies do "confirm a dramatic vitamin A deficiency" in alcoholic and nonalcoholic cirrhosis.[40] In addition, they confirm the low serum zinc concentrations in alcoholic cirrhotics, indicating an apparent deficiency of both vitamin A and zinc in cirrhotics. A review of alterations of zinc and vitamin A metabolism in alcoholic liver disease has been published by Cassidy *et al.*[42]

A recent report from India by Shingwekar *et al.* studied the effect of zinc supplementation on plasma levels of vitamin A and retinol-binding protein in vitamin A–deficient and protein-energy malnourished (PEM) children aged two to eight years.[43] The children were supplemented with 40 mg of zinc for 5 days for the PEM children and 10 days for the vitamin A–deficient children. Initial plasma zinc concentrations averaged 57 μg/100 ml for the severe PEM children and 71 μg/100 ml for the vitamin A-deficient children compared to 94 μg for the controls. Likewise, vitamin A and RBP were significantly reduced in both groups compared to controls. During the supplementation period, the children were maintained on their home diets without additional protein or vitamin A. After 10 days of zinc therapy,

TABLE 6

EFFECT OF ZINC SUPPLEMENTATION ON PLASMA RETINOL-BINDING PROTEIN (RBP) AND VITAMIN A IN PROTEIN-ENERGY MALNOURISHED CHILDREN*†

	Plasma‡ (μg/100 ml)		
	Zinc	RBP	Vitamin A
Day 0	57 ± 1.9	20 ± 0.9	13 ± 1.5
Day 5	126 ± 7.3	24 ± 0.9	18 ± 2.0
	P < 0.001	P < 0.01	P < 0.01

* 40 mg Zn/day; 19 subjects.
† From Shingwekar *et al.*, Reference 43.
‡ Mean ± SE.

the plasma vitamin A and RBP concentrations rose slightly, but not significantly, in the vitamin A-deficient children. However, there was a significant increase in both parameters of vitamin A metabolism (plasma vitamin A and RBP) in the PEM children after 5 days of zinc therapy (TABLE 6). The authors recognized that the degree of zinc deficiency, based on the plasma zinc concentration, was more severe in the PEM children than in the vitamin A-deficient children. The response during the short duration of 5 days is remarkable, especially since the children continued to be fed the inadequate diet and apparently received no additional vitamin A.

SUMMARY AND CONCLUSIONS

A general summary of typical results involving animal studies is shown in TABLE 7. A consistent and established finding is a reduction of plasma vitamin A concentration in zinc-deficient animals despite diets adequate in vitamin A. However, it appears that the depressed plasma vitamin A is not a result of zinc deficiency per se but rather is nonspecific, resulting from food- and growth-restriction factors associated with zinc deficiency.

Food restriction apparently is the critical factor, since both immature and mature nongrowing zinc-deficient animals have exhibited the decreased plasma vitamin A concentration. However, this point needs clarification. Liver vitamin A concentration is usually unaltered by the zinc deficiency, suggesting no defect in absorption or transport to the liver.

In regard to retinol-binding protein, it appears from the animal studies that zinc deficiency per se has an effect on both the plasma and liver RBP concentrations. We have hypothesized that zinc deficiency impairs RBP synthesis. It is speculated that only severe zinc deficiency results in a deficit of a sufficient magnitude for impairment of vitamin A metabolism at the cellular level. For example, retinene reductase, an apparent zinc-metallo alcohol dehydrogenase of the retina, appears to be sensitive to a severe zinc deficiency in animal studies. In humans, impaired dark adaptation

TABLE 7

SUMMARY OF RESULTS OF STUDIES CONCERNING VITAMIN A-ZINC INTERACTION

Animal Studies	Reference	Comparison to Normal
Zinc deficient or growth restricted:		
Plasma vitamin A	1, 11, 17, 18	lower
Liver vitamin A	11, 16, 18	no difference
Plasma RBP	12	lower
Zinc deficient only:		
Liver RBP	12	lower
Human Studies		**Vitamin A Status***
Zinc supplementation studies:		
Cirrhosis (alcoholic)	32	no change
	36	no change
	33	improved
	34	improved
Cystic fibrosis	39	no change
Vitamin A-deficient children	43	no change
Protein-energy malnourished children	43	improved

* Alteration in vitamin A status after zinc supplementation, i.e., change in plasma vitamin A, retinol-binding protein, and/or improvement in dark adaptation.

may be a result of inadequate supplies of the metabolizable zinc necessary to maintain the activity of the enzyme system. Thus, the conversion (dehydrogenation) of vitamin A alcohol to vitamin A aldehyde is impaired, with a resulting abnormality in dark adaptation, i.e., night blindness.

Indeed, the limited number of human studies suggest that zinc supplementation may be beneficial to vitamin A metabolism only in conditions where zinc deficiency is prevalent as indicated by low (< 70 μg/100 ml) plasma zinc. Conversely, zinc supplementation is of little benefit in conditions where vitamin A metabolism is altered but zinc status is normal. Therefore, definitive clinical studies involving primary zinc deficiency must be conducted before final conclusions can be made regarding the interrelationships of zinc and vitamin A in health and disease.

References

1. Stevenson, J. W. & I. P. Earle. 1956. Studies on parakeratosis in swine. J. Anim. Sci. **15:** 1036–1045.
2. Vallee, B. L., W. E. C. Wacker, A. F. Bartholomay & F. L. Hoch. 1957. Zinc metabolism in hepatic dysfunction. II. Correlation of metabolic patterns with biochemical findings. N. Engl. J. Med. **257:** 1055–1065.
3. Vallee, B. L., W. E. C. Wacker, A. F. Bartholomay & F. L. Hoch. 1959. Zinc metabolism in hepatic dysfunction. Ann. Intern. Med. **50:** 1077–1091.
4. Vallee, B. L. & F. L. Hoch. 1957. Zinc component of yeast alcohol dehydrogenase. Proc. Nat. Acad. Sci. **41:** 327–338.
5. Vallee, B. L. & F. L. Hoch. 1957. Zinc in horse liver alcohol dehydrogenase. J. Biol. Chem. **225:** 185–195.
6. Bliss, A. F. 1951. The equilibrium between vitamin A alcohol and aldehyde in the presence of alcohol dehydrogenase. Arch. Biochem. **31**: 197–204.
7. Underwood, E. L. 1977. Trace Elements in Human and Animal Nutrition. 4th edit. Academic Press, Inc. New York, N.Y.
8. Patek, A. J., Jr. & C. Haig. 1939. The occurrence of abnormal dark adaptation and its relation to vitamin A metabolism in patients with cirrhosis of the liver. J. Clin. Invest. **18**: 609–616.
9. Saraswat, R. C. & S. P. Arora. 1972. Effect of dietary zinc on the vitamin A level and alkaline phosphatase activity in blood sera of lambs. Indian J. Anim. Sci. **42:** 358–362.
10. Arora, S. P., E. E. Hatfield, F. C. Hinds & U. S. Garrigus. 1973. Influence of dietary zinc on the activity of blood vitamin A, alcohol dehydrogenase and carbonic anhydrase in lambs. Indian J. Anim. Sci. **43:** 140–144.
11. Smith, J. C., Jr., E. G. McDaniel, F. F. Fan & J. A. Halsted. 1973. Zinc: a trace element essential in vitamin A metabolism. Science **181:** 954–955.
12. Smith, J. E., E. D. Brown & J. C. Smith, Jr. 1974. The effect of zinc deficiency on the metabolism of retinol-binding protein in the rat. J. Lab. Clin. Med. **84:** 692–697.
13. 1977. Liver vitamin A mobilization during zinc deficiency and restricted food intake. Nutr. Rev. **35:** 213–215.
14. Rechcigl, M., Jr., S. Berger, J. K. Loosli & H. H. Williams. 1962. Dietary protein and utilization of vitamin A. J. Nutr. **76:** 435–440.
15. Smith, J. C., Jr., E. D. Brown, E. G. McDaniel & W. Chan. 1976. Alterations in vitamin A metabolism during zinc deficiency and food and growth restriction. J. Nutr. **106:** 569–574.
16. Apgar, J. 1977. Mobilization of vitamin A by the zinc deficient female rat. Nutr. Rep. Int. **15:** 553–559.
17. Carney, S. M., B. A. Underwood & J. D. Loerch. 1976. Effects of zinc and vitamin A deficient diets on the hepatic mobilization and urinary excretion of vitamin A in rats. J. Nutr. **106:** 1773–1781.
18. Duncan, J. R. & L. S. Hurley. 1978. An interaction between zinc and vitamin A in pregnant and fetal rats. J. Nutr. **108:** 1431–1438.

19. HUBER, A. M. & S. N. GERSHOFF. 1975. Effects of zinc deficiency on the oxidation of retinol and ethanol in rats. J. Nutr. **105:** 1486–1490.
20. VALLEE, B. L. 1977. Discussion of papers by Vallee and Falchuk. *In* Alcohol and Nutrition, T. K. Li, S. Schenkar & L. Lumeng, Eds.: 152–153. Proceedings of a Workshop, Indianapolis, Ind., September 26–27. Research Monograph No. 2. National Institute on Alcohol Abuse and Alcoholism.
21. SUNDARESAN, P. R., F. O. COPE & J. C. SMITH, JR. 1977. Influence of zinc deficiency on retinal reductase and oxidase activities in rat liver and testes. J. Nutr. **107:** 2189–2197.
22. AHLUWALIA, B., A. DEVI & J. F. J. CLARK. 1973. Enhancement with zinc in the incorporation of labelled vitamin A acetate in the seminiferous tubules of rat testes. (abst.). Fed. Proc. Fed. Am. Soc. Exp. Biol. **34:** 947.
23. SWARUP, D. & N. P. JOHNSON. 1974. Incorporation of labeled retinol and retinoic acid in bovine spermatozoa: effect of zinc on the rate of incorporation. Int. J. Vitam. Nutr. Res. **44:** 370–374.
24. SWARUP, D. & H. SEKHON. 1975. Incorporation of labelled retinol in bovine spermatozoa. III. Effect of zinc, fructose and pH on the incorporation. Nutr. Rep. Int. **12:** 255–259.
25. ETTE, S. I., T. K. BASU & J. W. T. DICKERSON. 1979. Short-term effect of zinc sulphate on plasma and hepatic concentrations of vitamin A and E in normal weanling rats. Nutr. Metab. **23:** 11–16.
26. HAMBIDGE, K. M., P. A. WALRAVENS, R. M. BROWN, J. WEBSTER, S. WHITE, M. ANTHONY & M. L. ROTH. 1976. Zinc nutrition of preschool children in the Denver Head Start Program. Am. J. Clin. Nutr. **29:** 734–738.
27. HENKIN, R. I. & F. R. SMITH. 1972. Zinc and copper metabolism in acute viral hepatitis. Am. J. Med. Sci. **264:** 401–409.
28. JACOB, R. A., H. H. SANDSTEAD, N. W. SOLOMONS, C. RIEGER & R. ROTHBERG. 1978. Zinc status and vitamin A transport in cystic fibrosis. Am. J. Clin. Nutr. **31:** 638–644.
29. KLEIN, S. 1972. Defects in twilight vision and in sensitivity to dazzle in patients with chronic liver disease: implications for driver safety. Dtsch. Gesundheitswes. **27:** 1235–1238.
30. HALSTED, J. A. & J. C. SMITH, JR. 1974. Night blindness and chronic liver disease. Gastroenterology **67:** 193–194.
31. SMITH, J. C., JR., E. D. BROWN, S. C. WHITE & J. D. FINKELSTEIN. 1975. Plasma vitamin A and zinc concentrations in patients with alcoholic cirrhosis. Lancet **1:** 1251–1252.
32. SMITH, J. C., JR., E. D. BROWN & W. A. CASSIDY. 1977. Zinc and vitamin A: interrelationships. *In* Zinc Metabolism, Current Aspects in Health and Disease. M. Hambidge, Ed.: 29–44. A. R. Liss. New York, N.Y.
33. MORRISON, S. A., R. M. RUSSELL, E. A. CARNEY & E. V. OAKS. 1978. Zinc deficiency: a cause of abnormal dark adaptation in cirrhotics. Am. J. Clin. Nutr. **31:** 276–281.
34. RUSSELL, R. M., S. A. MORRISON, F. R. SMITH, E. V. OAKS & E. A. CARNEY. 1978. Vitamin A reversal of abnormal dark adaptation in cirrhosis. Ann. Int. Med. **88:** 622–626.
35. 1979. Cirrhosis, abnormal dark adaptation and vitamin A. Nutr. Rev. **37:** 73–75.
36. WEISMANN, K., E. CHRISTENSEN & V. DREYER. 1979. Zinc supplementation in alcoholic cirrhosis. Acta Med. Scand. **205:** 361–366.
37. SMITH, F. R., B. A. UNDERWOOD, C. R. DENNING, A. VARMA & D. S. GOODMAN. 1972. Depressed plasma retinol-binding protein levels in cystic fibrosis. J. Lab. Clin. Med. **80:** 423–433.
38. HALSTED, J. A. & J. C. SMITH, JR. 1970. Plasma zinc in health and disease. Lancet **1:** 322–324.
39. PALIN, D., B. A. UNDERWOOD & C. R. DENNING. 1979. The effect of oral zinc supplementation on plasma levels of vitamin A and retinol-binding protein in cystic fibrosis. Am. J. Clin. Nutr. **32:** 1253–1259.
40. BRISSOT, P., A. LE TREUT, G. DIEN, M. COTTENCIN, M. SIMON & M. BOUREL. 1978. Hypovitaminemia A in idiopathic hemochromatosis and hepatic cirrhosis. Digestion **17:** 469–478.
41. HALSTED, J. A., B. HACKLEY, C. RUDZKI & J. C. SMITH, JR. 1968. Plasma zinc concentrations in liver diseases. Gastroenterology **54:** 1098–1105.
42. CASSIDY, W. A., E. D. BROWN & J. C. SMITH, JR. 1978. Alterations in zinc and vitamin A metabolism in alcoholic liver disease: a review. *In* Zinc and Copper in Clinical

Medicine. K. M. Hambidge & B. L. Nichols, Jr., Eds.: 59–79. SP Medical and Scientific Books. New York, N.Y.

43. Shingwekar, A. G., M. Mohanram & V. Reddy. 1979. Effect of zinc supplementation on plasma levels of vitamin A and retinol-binding protein in malnourished children. Clin. Chim. Acta **93:** 97–100.

Discussion

Unidentified Speaker: Is there any danger of an excess of intake of zinc in these patients?

J. C. Smith, Jr.: There is a danger with large amounts of zinc. However, we have given 150 mg of zinc per day for 10 weeks to patients with decubitus ulcers. There is nausea in a small percentage of subjects, especially with zinc sulfate. Some side effects have been reported, i.e., impairment of copper metabolism.

G. K. Davis (*University of Florida, Gainesville, Fla.*): Have you looked at the intestinal mucosa of your animals? With zinc deficiency or vitamin A deficiency, this is a major site of change. I would expect that if you saw interactions at all, this would be one place you ought to look.

J. C. Smith, Jr.: Thank you, Dr. Davis, we have not. The first thing we suspected when we noted the low plasma A in zinc-deficient animals was an impaired absorption of the vitamin A across the gut. However, we do not think this is the case. We have found that absorption of vitamin A is apparently normal in zinc-deficient animals. In fact, the vitamin A concentration is frequently higher in the liver of zinc-deficient animals. We have not examined the turnover rate of the liver vitamin A.

L. J. Machlin (*Hoffmann-La Roche, Inc., Nutley, N.J.*): Does vitamin A deficiency affect the zinc absorption?

J. C. Smith, Jr.: I cannot state specifically that zinc absorption is affected by vitamin A deficiency. However, vitamin A–deficient animals exhibit normal plasma and liver zinc concentrations, suggesting no impairment of zinc absorption.

J. G. Bieri (*National Institutes of Health, Bethesda, Md.*): I think that this particular nutrient interaction is a good example of how difficult, if not almost impossible, it is to set up the ideal experimental conditions. I commend Dr. Smith for presenting such a clear evaluation of the different results obtained by different investigators. If you don't actually work in this field, you might read somewhat more prominent publications and get one viewpoint, whereas there certainly are other viewpoints.

M. D. Schneider (*University of Tennessee, Knoxville, Tenn.*): In looking for the zinc, why did you just concentrate on the plasma and not take a look at the red cell membrane zinc concentrations? Might that be a better marker for changes in the zinc levels in the body?

J. C. Smith, Jr.: Well, in general, red cell zinc has not been responsive to acute zinc deficiency. Animals become zinc deficient within 14 days. However, the turnover time for the red cell is approximately 120 days. So in acute zinc deficiency, we do not see any change in the red blood cell zinc level. We examined the whole red blood cells, not the membrane only. In sum, red blood cell zinc concentration has not been a sensitive indicator of zinc status in either animals or humans.

H. Sprince (*Veterans Administration Medical Center, Coatesville, Penn.*): Alcoholics, of course, are known to lose a great deal of zinc. Is there any evidence of vitamin A deficiency in alcoholics?

J. C. SMITH, JR.: We examined 119 alcoholic liver disease patients and found that 52% exhibited both low plasma zinc and vitamin A. An additional 5% exhibited low plasma vitamin A concentration only.

L. J. MACHLIN: Some recent work would indicate that there is a fairly rapid exchange of plasma zinc with the red blood cell membrane zinc. So if you measured the membrane, this would probably just be a reflection of the plasma. As you indicated, the whole cell is not very responsive.

J. C. SMITH, JR.: That is a good point.

UNIDENTIFIED SPEAKER: Have you had a chance to look at sickle-cell patients? They are supposed to have a low zinc status.

J. C. SMITH, JR.: No, we have not.

[**Note added in proof:** Since the preparation of the manuscript, the author has received a paper confirming that alcoholic cirrhotics frequently have low serum concentrations of vitamin A and zinc as well as impaired dark adaptation. Vitamin A supplementation alone did not correct the impaired dark adaptation in 6 out of 28 subjects. However, zinc therapy was reported to normalize their dark adaptation. (McClain, C. J., D. H. Van Theil, S. Parker, L. K. Badzin & H. Gilbert. 1979. Alterations in zinc, vitamin A, and retinol-binding protein in chronic alcoholics: a possible mechanism for night blindness and hypogonadism. *Alcoholism: Clin. Exp. Res.* **3:** 135–141.)]

INTERACTIONS OF VITAMINS WITH ESSENTIAL MINERALS: GENERAL DISCUSSION

Moderator: J. G. Bieri

Nutritional Biochemistry Section
National Institute of Arthritis, Metabolism, and Digestive Diseases
National Institutes of Health
Bethesda, Maryland 20205

P. MARFEY (*State University of New York, Albany, N.Y.*): I would like to come back to Dr. Lynch's talk, where he discussed the absorption of iron.

I was wondering if one can say something about which oxidation state of iron is being absorbed. Is it the ferric or the ferrous form? Are there any studies done along these lines? I would guess that the iron that was present in heme probably would not survive in the ferrous form. I would imagine that it is absorbed in the ferric state. But what about the other class?

S. R. LYNCH (*University of Kansas Medical Center, Kansas City, Kans.*): I can say something about heme. It appears that heme is absorbed as such—as the intact heme protoporphyrin ring. The oxidation state probably isn't material to the absorption of the heme iron, and it is governed by a set of luminal parameters different from those for nonheme.

A lot of work has been done in experimental animals, attempting to define the effect of oxidation state on the absorption of nonheme iron. However, the studies that we've done do not address that question in man.

H. E. GANTHER (*University of Wisconsin, Madison, Wis.*): I'd like to ask Dr. Tappel a question about the identification of selenocysteine in glutathione peroxidase. I believe the evidence that has been published from your laboratory is based mainly upon the cochromatography of the unknown derivative of selenium from the enzyme with carboxymethyl derivatives of selenocysteine standards.

Now you have done mass spectroscopy of the selenocysteine standards. I have not seen this done on the unknown. Do you have any evidence from mass spectra on the unknown form from the enzyme?; and if not, why is that evidence not available?

A. L. TAPPEL (*University of California, Davis, Calif.*): Yes, that certainly is a good point. We started to try to identify the prosthetic group by mass spectroscopy, but, as you know from your experience, that's very difficult.

The first problem is to get enough prosthetic group from this enzyme, and then there is the problem of selenocysteine decomposition. So we solved the problem, as Dr. Ganther indicated, by preparing standards of the selenocysteine, derivatized to protect it, and then identified by cochromatography both on ion-exchange and amino acid analysis, and also two-dimensional thin-layer chromatography. We found these methods to be sufficient for identification. Since all of that took much effort, we did not go back and do what I think would be fairly laborious, that is, preparing enough prosthetic group for mass spectroscopy.

UNIDENTIFIED SPEAKER: Dr. Tappel, you mentioned use of chlorinated hydrocarbons, such as carbon tetrachloride, in forming oxidative products. How about other halogenated organic molecules, such as mono- or disubstituted chlorinated organic molecules?

A. L. TAPPEL: You are implying that there are many halogenated compounds that are very important to assay. There have been a few assays of some of these

0077-8923/80/0355-0076 $01.75/0 © 1980, NYAS

relative to lipid peroxidation. I think the big problem heretofore has been to have a good method of detection. For example, chloroform has very low activity as an initiator of lipid peroxidation, and it's only with a test like the pentane method that one can really tell whether or not it does initiate *in vivo*. So all these other compounds are on the list to be tested later.

W. G. HOEKSTRA (*University of Wisconsin, Madison, Wis.*): I have two comments relative to Dr. Tappel's presentation, and particularly in relation to an earlier comment about causing cataracts with selenite.*

We've been doing experiments like those of Dr. Tappel's but monitoring ethane instead of pentane. We've been feeding omega-3 fatty acids in order to get enough of those in the body tissue so that there is a substantial production of ethane. Other than that, our results are quite comparable to those of Dr. Tappel.

We've been using selenium and vitamin E-deficient rats and are measuring ethane to identify some antagonists or agents that stimulate peroxidation. The doubly deficient animals are very sensitive to agents like carbon tetrachloride, which are potent stimulators of peroxidation.

My group has looked at effects of selenite and selenate in rather large dosages. Selenite is a very potent prooxidant; it's a stimulator of lipid peroxidation in these deficient rats if administered in high quantities in a rather sudden dosage. Selenate, however, did not stimulate peroxidation, which is a bit confusing because the story is that selenate goes through selenite in its metabolism. Perhaps the cataracts that are induced by selenite result from this prooxidant effect of selenite.

Secondly, we've recently done some work with the isolated perfused rat liver, looking at glutathione peroxidase biosynthesis with the idea of trying to determine if selenocysteine is a closer precursor than are selenide and selenite. We've been adding radioactive forms of selenium to the perfusion medium and also adding large quantities of carrier selenium compounds to see if they dilute out the radioselenium incorporation. Our results imply that selenide and selenite are closer precursors to glutathione peroxidase than is selenocysteine. This is an indirect approach, but the implications are that the selenium from selenocysteine has to be removed from that molecule and put into another precursor that can also arise from selenite to get incorporated into glutathione peroxidase.

It seems questionable whether there is a separate transfer RNA for selenocysteine and whether free selenocysteine is really the molecule that is incorporated directly into the enzyme.

A. L. TAPPEL: I'd like to respond to the last concern that you have, Dr. Hoekstra, which is a good one. With isotope dilution studies of the type you mentioned, we have also done similar studies both in the intact animal and in liver slices. It's true that with results like you got—and we get very similar ones in some cases—one cannot strongly defend the concept of selenocysteine being close to the glutathione peroxidase just from isotope dilution studies.

But on the other hand, from tracer studies where the selenium incorporation is followed through the selenocysteine and into the glutathione peroxidase, we find that the isotope is moving from the selenocysteine to the glutathione peroxidase.

And then you are concerned about the transfer RNA, and I'm sure that you will want confirmation. We have very strong evidence of a selenocysteine-specific transfer RNA. This is by isolation in experiments where there is radioactive labeling of sulfur transfer RNA and selenium transfer RNA at the same time to show the differentiation. This is yet to be published in detail.

A more critical experiment is to transfer radioactive selenium from the

* See the discussion of Dr. Tappel's paper, page 30.

selenocysteyl transfer RNA to the protein glutathione peroxidase. We've done that also, and the labeling is consistent with the transfer.

W. G. Hoekstra: I'll be interested to see the evidence, because we can't rationalize our data with the direct incorporation of free selenocysteine into glutathione peroxidase in a perfused liver. The selenium certainly gets there, but you can dilute that out very effectively with selenite and selenide; and on the other hand, you can't dilute out the incorporation of radioselenite very well with selenocysteine.

A. L. Tappel: Right. Yes, I agree. We too thought that isotope dilution studies would be very straightforward, as Professor Hoekstra has indicated, and they weren't, so we were as surprised as you are.

Unidentified Speaker: Coming back to Dr. Lynch's paper and his implications about the absorbability of metallic micronutrients and vitamin C, I think consideration ought to be given also to the possible effects of dehydroascorbic acid as well as ascorbic acid, because dehydroascorbic is more lipophilic or is a lipophilic derivative of ascorbic acid and ascorbic acid per se is not lipophilic. If chelation does take place, the metallic micronutrients on a dehydro form might be a quicker way of getting these substances into the body.

S. R. Lynch: I don't have any direct answer, but I could perhaps comment on another compound—the palmitate derivative of ascorbic acid that we've tested recently. It is more lipophilic and appears to have about the same effect as ascorbic acid. Incidentally, the reason for examining this compound is that you can bake it into bread without destroying it, so that it is effective in bread even after it has been baked.

J. G. Bieri: Does isoascorbic acid have this effect on iron?

S. R. Lynch: I'm not sure of the answer to that question.

N. F. Suttle *(Moredun Research Institute, Edinburgh, Scotland)*: Dr. Lynch, in his presentation, mentioned very briefly the mucosal effects on iron absorption. I believe I'm right in saying that the test meal system that he is using largely bypasses any opportunity for mucosal effects.

What is the situation when there is an opportunity for mucosal reaction, such as a continued dietary vitamin C supplementation, for example? Does the individual eventually react by lowering its efficiency of absorption and countering the effects of vitamin C?

S. R. Lynch: That's a very important question that I really don't have time to deal with fully. I think there is no doubt that the body iron stores, presumably through the mucosa, do have an effect on iron absorption from this sort of meal. You can show an inverse correlation between the serum ferritin concentration, which is a measure of body iron stores, and percentage iron absorption from our meals.

The question of particularly large doses of ascorbic acid is very pertinent, since there are a lot of people taking this sort of dose and potentially this might lead to very large quantities of iron being absorbed.

I don't have any direct answer. One might suspect that the effect may not be that great for a number of reasons. First of all, I think that people often take these doses of ascorbic acid apart from meals, and the effect really is only seen if you take them together with meals. Secondly, many people who are taking this sort of dose eat a western diet that already makes iron fairly available for absorption. Therefore, the effect might be less. Thirdly, the sort of dose response that we see shows a much smaller increment above amounts of ascorbic acid of about 100 mg, so the effect might not be as great as you might expect from such a large dose.

There is one pilot study that Dr. Cook has done that perhaps has a bearing on this. What he did was measure serum ferritin levels in I think it was five normal volunteers over a period of two years. These people were taking doses of vitamin C up to about 2 g a day, and in fact there was very little effect on the serum ferritin levels, suggesting that in some way adaptation did occur.

INTERACTIONS OF THIAMIN, RIBOFLAVIN, AND OTHER B-VITAMINS

H. E. Sauberlich

Division of Nutrition Technology
Letterman Army Institute of Research
Presidio of San Francisco, California 94129

The biosynthesis and metabolism of nutrients in the body frequently require the concerted action of several of the B-complex vitamins. In many instances, these interactions are exceedingly critical and any alterations lead to biochemical and clinical abnormalities. Disease conditions may often represent the net result of deviations in several B-complex interactions. Angular stomatitis and glossitis have been shown in some instances to respond clinically to the administration of riboflavin or pyridoxine. The burning feet syndrome is probably likewise the result of multiple vitamin deficiencies, including that of pantothenic acid. Fatty livers may result from a deficiency of a number of the B-complex vitamins, including pantothenic acid, biotin, vitamin B_6, nicotinic acid, and vitamin B_{12}. Deficiencies of folic acid, vitamin B_{12}, and other B-complex vitamins have been reported to be associated with several neurological disorders and skin defects. The disorders are probably not the result of a single vitamin deficiency but the cumulative manifestation of several vitamin inadequacies of the diet. Interrelationships between several fat-soluble vitamins and B-complex vitamins have been reported. Although numerous vitamin interactions exist, only a few can be considered in this report.

NIACIN (NICOTINIC ACID)

The major role of niacin is in the formation of nicotinamide adenine dinucleotide (NAD) and nicotinamide adenine dinucleotide phosphate (NADP). However, niacin-deficient animals do not appear to have any serious impairment of oxidative reactions. Deficiency signs cannot be correlated with known metabolic functions of niacin coenzymes. Thus, niacin may have an essential role in unidentified nonoxidative reactions. The nicotinamide-containing coenzymes are involved in tissue respiration, glycolysis, and fat synthesis. Consequently, nicotinic acid participates in diverse metabolic pathways in concert with other vitamins. Undoubtedly, because of the extensive roles of nicotinic acid, the clinical features of pellagra are complex and involve the skin, digestive tract, and nervous system. McLester and Darby stated in 1952 that "while lack of nicotinic acid dominates the picture, pellagra is in truth a disease of multiple deficiencies—nicotinic acid, protein, riboflavin, and perhaps haemopoietic factors."[1] Tryptophan and vitamin B_6 are now recognized as specific factors involved. Subjects with pellagra may have a vitamin B_6 deficiency, as evidenced by low plasma pyridoxal phosphate levels that can be returned to normal levels with oral pyridoxine supplementation.[13]

Excess leucine in the diet may antagonize the functions of vitamin B_6 and impair the conversion of tryptophan to nicotinic acid.[2,3,10] Thus, the administration of leucine to human subjects resulted in an increase in the urinary excretion of quinolinic acid;[2,4] and for the rat, leucine administration resulted in a decrease in hepatic quinolinate phosphoribosyltransferase.[5] Vitamin B_6 supplementation nor-

0077-8923/80/0355-0080 $01.75/0 © 1980, NYAS

malized both the tryptophan-niacin metabolism and the tolerance to leucine.[3] The explanation for these observations is not certain, but may be related to an increased requirement for vitamin B_6 to metabolize the excess leucine by the pyridoxal phosphate-dependent leucine aminotransferase. An individual marginally deficient in vitamin B_6 would then be prone to the effects of excess leucine. Nicotinic acid formation from tryptophan is impaired in vitamin B_6-deficient subjects.[6] In such deficient subjects, urinary excretion of quinolinic acid and other metabolites is markedly increased following a tryptophan load. FIGURE 1 depicts the interactions of vitamin B_6 in the formation of nicotinic acid from tryptophan.

The formation of nicotinic acid from tryptophan requires not only the participation of pyridoxal phosphate but of niacin and riboflavin as well. Riboflavin deficiency caused a reduction in the activity of kynurenine hydrolase.[9] Kynurenine hydrolase is an NADPH- and flavin adenine dinucleotide (FAD)-dependent enzyme and is an enzyme that is relatively low in the hamster. Thus, Yeh and Brown have stated that "if the conversion of tryptophan to NAD was disturbed by the depression of 3-hydroxykynureninase in vitamin B_6 deficient hamsters, and the activity of the kynurenine hydroxylase was low in this species, the level of pyridine nucleotides would be reduced and the activity of kynurenine hydrolase would be further depressed during vitamin B_6 deficiency. No direct evidence for this theory was available at the

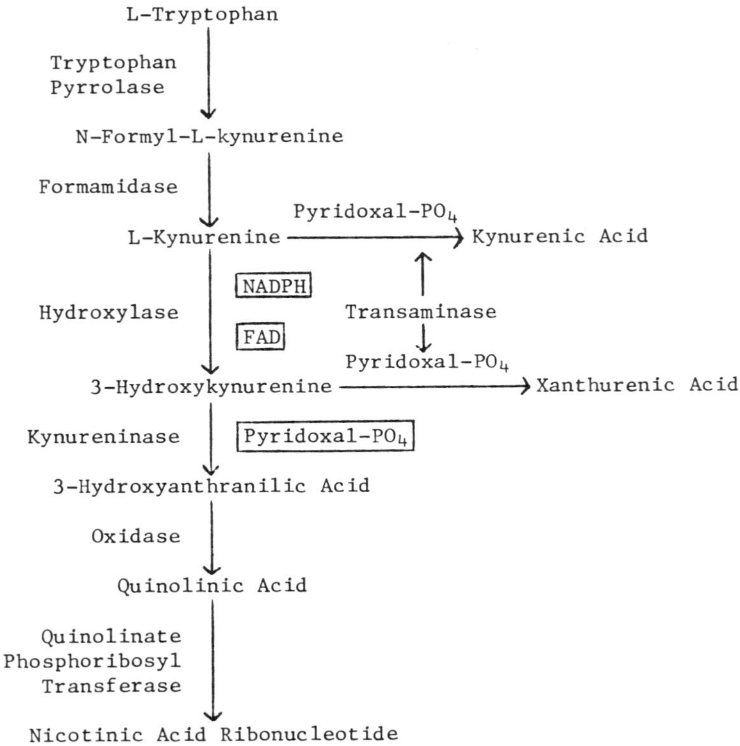

FIGURE 1. Involvement of vitamin B_6, riboflavin, and niacin in the conversion of tryptophan to nicotinic acid.

present time, but the urinary data are consistent with it."[7] In earlier studies, however, Snyderman *et al.* observed that infants deprived of vitamin B_6 for 60 days lost their ability to convert tryptophan to nicotinic acid.[8] The elevation in the amount of quinolinic acid excreted during vitamin B_6 deficiency has suggested that vitamin B_6 might be necessary for the further metabolism of quinolinic acid (FIGURE 2).[6] Quinolinic acid decarboxylase has been indicated to be a pyridoxal phosphate-dependent enzyme.

Yeh and Brown have studied extensively the effects of vitamin B_6 and tryptophan loading on the urinary excretion of tryptophan metabolites in mammals.[7] TABLE 1 represents a few of their observations. The urinary excretions of xanthurenic acid, kynurenine, and 3-hydroxykynurenine were significantly increased in the vitamin B_6-deficient hamster. The excretions of quinolinic acid, kynurenic acid, and acetylkynurenine were not significantly increased.

In vitamin B_6-deficient women, the percentages of the tryptophan load excreted as kynurenic acid, xanthurenic acid, acetylkynurenine, kynurenine, 3-hydroxykynurenine, and quinolinic acid were all significantly increased (TABLE 1).[7] Since 3-hydroxykynureninase is a pyridoxal phosphate-dependent enzyme, the increased excretions of kynurenic acid, xanthurenic acid, acetylkynurenine, kynurenine, and 3-hydroxykynurenine are explainable as a result of depressed enzyme activity during vitamin B_6 deficiency. However, the elevation in the amount of qui-

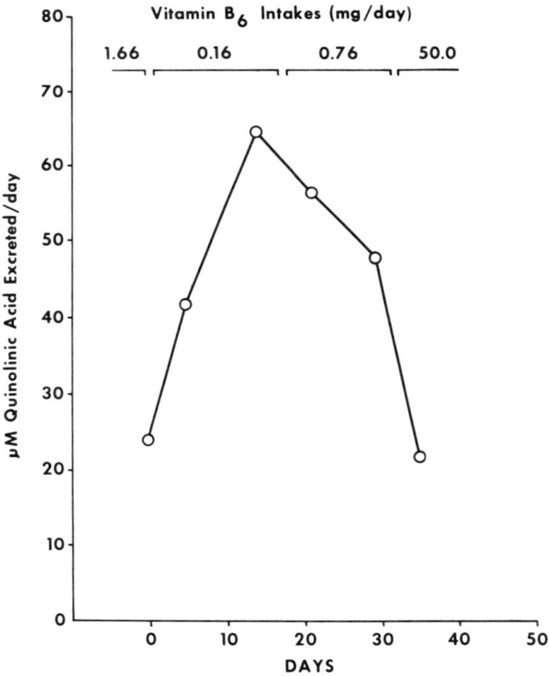

FIGURE 2. Effect of vitamin B_6 intake on the urinary excretion of quinolinic acid following a 2-gram load of L-tryptophan. Average excretion for six adult male subjects fed a diet providing 150 grams of protein per day. (Adapted from Kelsay *et al.*)[6]

TABLE 1

EFFECT OF VITAMIN B_6 DEFICIENCY ON THE URINARY EXCRETION OF METABOLITES FOLLOWING A TRYPTOPHAN LOAD*†

	Hamsters		Women	
Metabolite	Normal (%)	B_6 Deficient (%)	Normal (%)	B_6 Deficient (%)
Kynurenic Acid	0.33	0.55	0.49	1.68
Xanthurenic Acid	0.18	1.08	0.20	7.80
Acetylkynurenine	8.47	10.00	0.02	2.26
Kynurenine	10.30	23.00	0.13	8.23
3-Hydroxykynurenine	1.01	4.60	0.07	14.40
Quinolinic Acid	0.51	0.21	0.33	0.97

* Adapted from Yeh and Brown.[7]

† Percentage was calculated as: μmoles of metabolite in 24-hour urine after tryptophan load minus μmoles of metabolite in 24-hour urine before tryptophan load, divided by μmoles of tryptophan administered. Six hamsters and six women used in the studies.

nolinic acid as well as of 3-hydroxyanthranilic acid excreted during vitamin B_6 deficiency (FIGURE 1) cannot be accounted for by an inhibitory effect of vitamin B_6 deficiency on 3-hydroxykynureninase. As noted above, it has been suggested that vitamin B_6 might be necessary for the further metabolism of quinolinic acid.[6,11] Of note, the level of NAD in the body is regulated by a feedback inhibition on the activity of tryptophan pyrrolase (dioxygenase) by the tissue levels of pyridine nucleotides.[12] Thus, the formation of niacin from tryptophan is under the control of the vitamin itself.

RIBOFLAVIN

Flavoproteins are ubiquitous and may contain various numbers of molecules of FAD or of flavin mononucleotide (FMN) or both per molecule of enzyme. Riboflavin in association with NAD may function in oxidoreductase systems:

$$\text{NAD(P)H} + \text{H}^+ + \text{Acceptor}$$

$$\xrightarrow[\text{FAD;FMN}]{\text{flavoprotein}} \text{NAD(P)}^+ + \text{Reduced Acceptor}$$

For example, ferriductase, known also as NADH-FMN oxidoreductase, has been proposed for the mobilization of iron from ferritin. Riboflavin deficiency was reported to decrease hepatic iron mobilization and probably impaired the absorption of dietary iron, but it did not appear to interfere with iron-induced biosynthesis of ferritin.[24] The mechanism involved remains unclear.

The ultrastructural changes in the myelinated peripheral nerves in riboflavin deprivation resemble those classically noted in vitamin B_{12} deficiency.[15-17] Evidence exists that riboflavin-dependent oxidoreductase systems are involved in the synthesis of 5′-deoxyadenosylcobalamin coenzyme and in the activation of the vitamin B_{12} prosthetic group of the 5-methyltetrahydrofolate-homocysteine methyltransferase (FIGURE 3).[18-20]

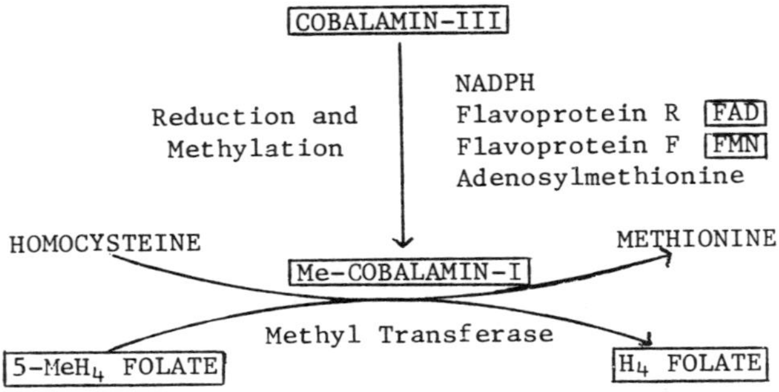

FIGURE 3. Interaction of vitamin B_{12} and folic acid.[20]

However, the neurological sequelae of a riboflavin deficiency are not mediated by a defective vitamin B_{12} function due to a requirement for a riboflavin-dependent oxidoreductase system in vitamin B_{12} coenzyme synthesis and function.[14] Riboflavin deficiency did not produce an increase in the odd-chain fatty acids of neural lipids, a characteristic of vitamin B_{12} deficiency.[21-23] Moreover, the vitamin B_{12}-dependent reactions, methylmalonyl coenzyme A mutase and 5-methyltetrahydrofolate-homocysteine methyltransferase, were not impaired by riboflavin deficiency (FIGURE 4).[19] A specific mechanism for the neural injury associated with a riboflavin deficiency remains to be established.

RIBOFLAVIN AND VITAMIN B_6

Riboflavin deficiency has often been associated with oral lesions, like cheilosis, angular stomatitis, and glossitis. Patients with these lesions sometimes fail to respond to riboflavin treatment alone and require supplementation with vitamin B_6 or other B-complex vitamins.[25] In some instances, erythrocyte glutamic oxaloacetic transaminase (EGOT) activity was very low, which was corrected largely by vitamin

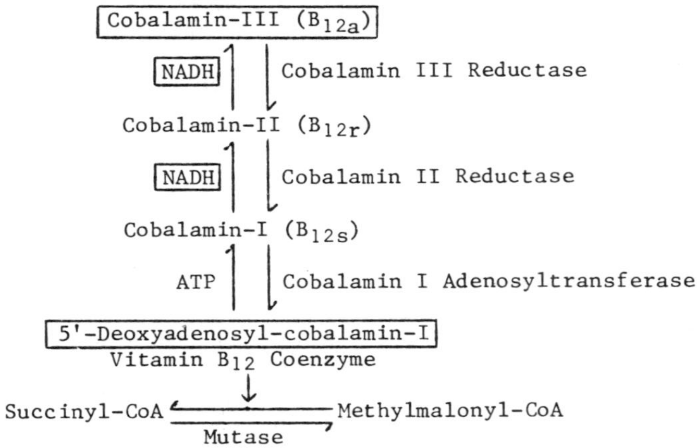

FIGURE 4. Activation of vitamin B_{12}.[19]

TABLE 2

EFFECT OF VITAMIN SUPPLEMENTS ON ERYTHROCYTE TRANSAMINASE ACTIVITY IN PATIENTS WITH ORAL LESIONS*

	Erythrocyte GOT Activity‡					
	Initial		Riboflavin Supplemented		Vitamin B_6 Supplemented	
Patient Group†	Activity	% S	Activity	% S	Activity	% S
Riboflavin Responsive (7)	2.07	26	1.68	19	2.45	15
Vitamin B_6 Responsive (6)	0.87	79	0.96	68	1.40	19

* Adapted from Krishnaswamy.[25]

† Patients were given daily 10 mg of riboflavin parenterally for 8–10 days followed by 5 or 10 mg of pyridoxine daily parenterally for 8–10 days. Values in parentheses indicate number of subjects studied.

‡ Erythrocyte glutamate-oxaloacetate transaminase activity expressed as μmoles of pyruvate formed/hour/10^8 cells. The *in vitro* stimulation response (% S) was determined by the addition of 50 μg of pyridoxal phosphate to the assay tube.

B_6 treatment and responded only minimally to riboflavin (TABLE 2). In other subjects, however, the erythrocyte transaminase activity was normal or elevated, but riboflavin supplementation was required to cure the oral lesions. These observations suggested that in riboflavin deficiency, pyridoxine may not be properly utilized, and as a result, a conditioned deficiency of vitamin B_6 may exist. Vitamin B_6 deficiency may also occur in pellagrins, which is reflected in low EGOT activity.[26]

Riboflavin deficiency in the rat slowed the uptake of labeled pyridoxine into the liver and decreased the conversion of pyridoxine to its metabolites.[27-29] Pyridoxine phosphate oxidase in the livers of riboflavin-deficient rats was only 15% of that of control animals (FIGURE 5).[28] Riboflavin deficiency also lowered pyridoxal kinase activity but did not influence pyridoxal phosphate phosphatase activity. The results

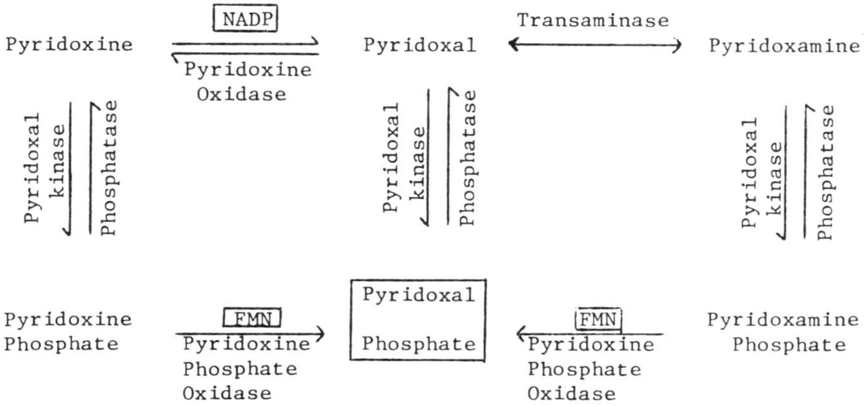

FIGURE 5. Participation of riboflavin and nicotinic acid in pyridoxal phosphate formation.

TABLE 3

EFFECT OF RIBOFLAVIN SUPPLEMENTATION ON THE FORMATION OF PYRIDOXAL PHOSPHATE BY RIBOFLAVIN-DEFICIENT SUBJECTS*

Subjects†	Riboflavin Deficiency Signs: Biochemical	Riboflavin Deficiency Signs: Clinical	PLP Ratio‡
Riboflavin Deficient	+	+	3.61 ± 0.76 (10)
After Riboflavin Treatment	−	−	5.60 ± 1.01 (7)
Normal Controls	−	−	8.25 ± 0.72 (4)

* Adapted from Lakshmi and Bamji.[29]

† Deficient subjects had abnormal erythrocyte glutathione reductase tests and oral lesions. Treatment consisted of the administration of 5 mg of riboflavin for 10 days.

‡ Pyridoxal phosphate ratio = (Blood PLP level 15 min after 5 mg IM pyridoxine)/(Initial blood PLP level). Mean ± standard error (SE) with number of subjects indicated within parentheses.

suggest that the slower rate of pyridoxal phosphate synthesis in riboflavin deficiency may be due to an impairment in the pyridoxine phosphate oxidase reaction as well as to a reduction in the pyridoxal kinase activity.

Lakshmi and Bamji studied further vitamin B_6 metabolism in human subjects who showed both biochemical and clinical signs of a riboflavin deficiency.[29] Normal and deficient subjects were administered pyridoxine, and their blood pyridoxal phosphate levels followed. Subjects with riboflavin deficiency signs had significantly lower blood levels of pyridoxal phosphate when compared to the control subjects. Clinical and biochemical deficiency signs as well as the ability to convert pyridoxine to pyridoxal phosphate were all improved by riboflavin treatment (TABLE 3).

In vitro studies demonstrated also an impaired ability of erythrocytes obtained from the riboflavin-deficient subjects to synthesize pyridoxal phosphate from pyridoxine (TABLE 4). Erythrocyte pyridoxal phosphatase activity was also depressed in the riboflavin-deficient subjects. The *in vitro* synthesis of pyridoxal phosphate from pyridoxine or pyridoxamine phosphate was markedly improved in the deficient subjects by riboflavin treatment. Phosphatase activity was also increased. In the case of the human, these data suggest that riboflavin deficiency imposes a constraint on

TABLE 4

ERYTHROCYTE PYRIDOXAL PHOSPHATE PHOSPHATASE ACTIVITY AND *In Vitro* ERYTHROCYTE SYNTHESIS OF PYRIDOXAL PHOSPHATE FROM PYRIDOXINE*

Subjects†	PLP Synthesis from Pyridoxine (ng/ml cells)	Phosphatase Activity‡
Riboflavin Deficient	0.19 ± 0.03 (7)	370 ± 25 (8)
After Riboflavin Treatment	0.55 ± 0.04 (3)	562 ± 55 (8)
Normal Controls	0.76 ± 0.11 (6)	678 ± 27 (6)

* Adapted from Lakshmi and Bamji.[29]

† Deficient subjects had abnormal erythrocyte glutathione reductase tests and oral lesions. Treatment consisted of the administration of 5 mg of riboflavin for 10 days.

‡ Pyridoxal phosphate phosphatase activity = ng PLP hydrolyzed/ml cells/30 minutes. Mean ± SE with number of subjects indicated within parentheses.

pyridoxal phosphate synthesis, but the effect may be diminished due to the lower pyridoxal phosphatase activity. This is in contrast to the decreased pyridoxal kinase activity reported for riboflavin-deficient rats.[27] Thus, discrepancies appear to exist in the observations on riboflavin interactions in vitamin B_6 metabolism.

Although the erythrocyte is normally an active site for the conversion of pyridoxine into active forms of vitamin B_6, erythrocytes from patients with homozygous or heterozygous β-thalassemia have a reduced *in vitro* rate of conversion of pyridoxine to pyridoxal and pyridoxal phosphate.[30] The rate of *in vitro* conversion of pyridoxine was increased by incubation of the blood from such patients with riboflavin. Presumably the effect was mediated through the synthesis in the erythrocyte of FMN from riboflavin, which in turn stimulated the flavoprotein, pyridoxine phosphate oxidase (FIGURE 5). *In vivo* studies supported this concept.[30] When a β-thalassemia patient was given oral supplements of riboflavin, the rate of pyridoxine conversion increased to normal within three weeks (TABLE 5). After stopping riboflavin supplementations, the rate decreased considerably during the first three weeks, and continued to decrease steadily. The duration of the increased conversion rate appeared to correspond approximately to the normal life span of erythrocytes. This would suggest that the pyridoxine phosphate oxidase enzyme is defective in the thalassemia patient. The significance of the ability of erythrocytes to convert pyridoxine to physiological forms of vitamin B_6 remains to be established. Nevertheless, the data available suggest that the erythrocytes are capable of metabolizing a significant proportion of the pyridoxine ingested.

VITAMIN B_6 AND VITAMIN C

Interrelationships between vitamin B_6 and vitamin C have been observed. Selivanova and associates reported that the urinary excretion of 4-pyridoxic acid, the major metabolite of vitamin B_6, was elevated with an increased intake of ascorbic acid.[31,32] Baker *et al.* followed whole blood ascorbic acid levels in normal adult men subjected to depletion and repletion of vitamin B_6 (FIGURE 6).[33] Whole blood level of ascorbic acid progressively fell during the vitamin B_6-depletion phase and returned

TABLE 5

EFFECT OF RIBOFLAVIN SUPPLEMENTS ON ERYTHROCYTE METABOLISM OF VITAMIN B_6 IN A β-THALASSEMIA PATIENT*

Weeks on Study	Riboflavin Supplement (mg/day)	*In Vitro* Conversion of Pyridoxine to Pyridoxal† (%)
0	0	33
1	20	53
3	20	87
8	20	100
9	0	87
11	0	70
17	0	45
25	0	33
Controls	0	95

* Adapted from Anderson *et al.*[30]

† *In vitro* conversion of 500 ng pyridoxine per ml of blood 37 °C in 1 hour. Sum of pyridoxal phosphate and pyridoxal formed, and measured by *L. casei* assay.

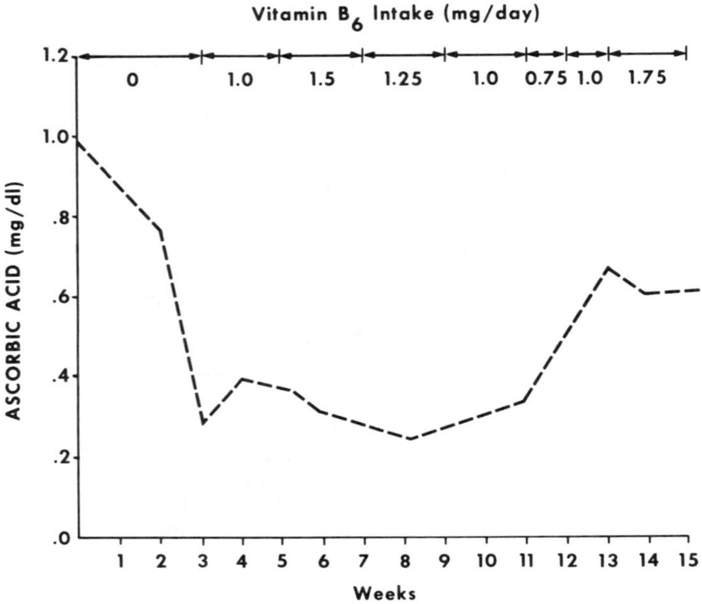

FIGURE 6. Effect of vitamin B_6 depletion and repletion on whole blood ascorbic acid levels in adult men. The formula diet fed provided 100 grams of protein per day. (Adapted from Baker *et al.*)[33]

to normal levels upon repletion with pyridoxine. In a subsequent study on vitamin C deficiency in adult men, the urinary excretion of free pyridoxine was measured.[34] During the vitamin C–depletion period, a 3½-fold increase occurred in the free urinary pyridoxine, even though the subjects were receiving a constant daily intake of 2.5 mg of pyridoxine. Upon repletion with ascorbic acid, urinary free pyridoxine levels progressively fell until they returned to the levels observed during the control period. During the repletion period, the intake of pyridoxine also remained constant. The above observations suggest that an interaction exists between vitamin B_6 and vitamin C, but the precise interrelationship remains to be clarified.

VITAMIN B_6 AND VITAMIN B_{12}

Vitamin B_6 deficiency has been reported to cause an impairment in vitamin B_{12} absorption in the rat that results in a lowering of vitamin B_{12} levels in the serum and in reduced vitamin B_{12} stores in the liver.[35,36] These observations are summarized in TABLE 6. In contrast, vitamin B_{12}-deficient rats were observed to have elevated serum glutamic-oxaloacetic transaminase activity (SGOT), which was considered due to some damage in organs rich in transaminase, such as the liver.[36] The mechanism and significance of the interaction between these two vitamins remain unclear.

Subsequently, Cheny *et al.* reported that the lowering of erythrocyte glutamic-oxaloacetic (EGOT) and erythrocyte glutamic-pyruvic (EGPT) transaminase activities in the rat was specific to vitamin B_6 deprivation.[37] Deficiencies in riboflavin,

TABLE 6

INTERRELATIONSHIP BETWEEN VITAMIN B_6 AND VITAMIN B_{12} IN THE RAT*

Group No.†	Treatment‡ Vitamin B_6	Vitamin B_{12}	Serum Vitamin B_{12} (pg/ml)	Liver Vitamin B_{12} (ng/g)	SGOT§ (units/ml)
A (10)	−	+	656 ± 51	335 ± 11	32 ± 4
B (10)	+	+	1020 ± 68	464 ± 30	77 ± 3
C (13)	+	−	115 ± 10	24 ± 6	117 ± 8

* Adapted from Ranke *et al.*[36]
† Numbers in parentheses denote number of rats used.
‡ Where indicated, diet contained 5 mg/kg of pyridoxine and 50 μg/kg of vitamin B_{12}.
§ Serum glutamate-oxaloacetate transaminase activity.

thiamin, pantothenic acid, niacin, or biotin did not produce any significant alterations in either EGOT or EGPT activities.

BIOTIN

Human tissues contain four major biotin-dependent carboxylases: (a) pyruvate carboxylase, a gluconeogenic enzyme (FIGURE 7); (b) propionyl-CoA carboxylase, associated with the catabolism of valine, isoleucine, and fatty acids with odd-numbered chain lengths (FIGURE 8); (c) β-methylcrotonyl-CoA carboxylase, associated with the degradation of leucine (FIGURE 9); and (d) acetyl-CoA carboxylase, which participates in the formation of malonyl-CoA for the initiation of fatty acid synthesis.[38]

Patients with defects in the activities of pyruvate carboxylase, propionyl-CoA carboxylase, or β-methylcrotonyl-CoA carboxylase have been reported.[38-43] In some patients, the organic aciduria responds to treatment with high levels of biotin, consistent with a reduced affinity for biotin in a transport protein or in the biotin-linking enzyme, holocarboxylase synthetase. In the overall metabolic reactions involving biotin, participation of pantothenic acid in the form of coenzyme A is required. In the metabolism of leucine, valine, and isoleucine, in addition to biotin, pyridoxal phosphate, NAD, and FAD are required (FIGURES 8 and 9).

Leucine, valine, and isoleucine, following an initial transamination reaction with pyridoxal phosphate to form the corresponding α-keto acids, are oxidatively decarboxylated to form acetyl-CoA derivatives. The subsequent reactions are similar to the metabolism of fatty acids. The propionyl-CoA formed from valine and

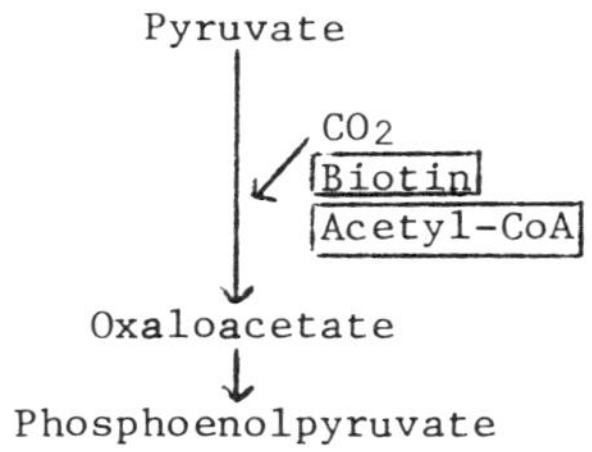

FIGURE 7. Metabolism of pyruvic acid to oxaloacetic acid.

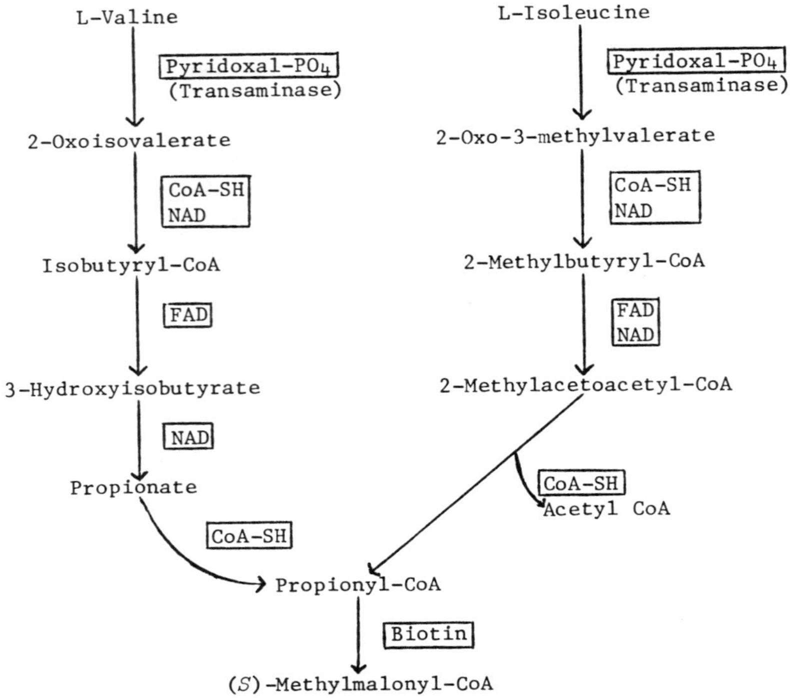

FIGURE 8. Interactions of vitamins in the metabolism of valine and isoleucine.

isoleucine requires biotin for its conversion to methylmalonyl-CoA. In the metabolism of leucine, the conversion of β-methylcrotonyl-CoA to β-methylglutaryl-CoA is a biotin-requiring reaction.

The hereditary condition maple syrup urine disease is associated with an aberrant metabolism of valine, leucine, and isoleucine as a result of defective biotin action. Transamination is unaffected, but normal oxidative decarboxylation with acetyl-CoA formation does not occur in children afflicted with this disorder. A similar defect has been reported in a patient with a dietary deficiency of biotin.[40]

Isovaleriacidemia represents a defect in the metabolism of leucine and is associated with high levels of isovaleric acid in the plasma. The metabolic defect appears to be due to an inadequate functioning of the riboflavin-dependent dehydrogenase catalyzing the conversion of isovaleryl-CoA to β-methylcrotonyl-CoA (FIGURE 9).

BIOTIN AND PANTOTHENIC ACID

Propionate metabolism in man requires pantothenic acid and biotin in its conversion to methylmalonic acid.[44-46] As noted above, valine and isoleucine may serve as a source of propionate (FIGURE 10). Outward signs of an interaction between biotin and pantothenic acid appear to exist. Both biotin deficiency and pantothenic

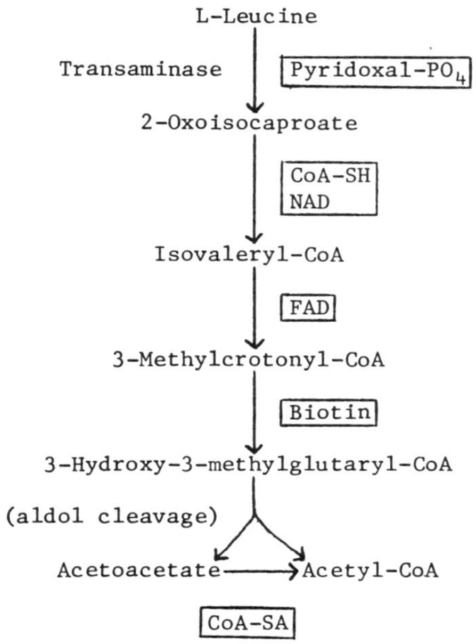

FIGURE 9. Vitamins required for the metabolism of leucine.

acid deficiency result in the depigmentation of the fur of black mice. Biotin deficiency may be aggravated by a simultaneous pantothenic acid deficiency. The addition of biotin to the diet not only protects the animals from a biotin deficiency, but also reduces the severity of the symptoms of a pantothenic acid deficiency. Biotin deficiency is associated with extensive fatty infiltration of the liver and kidney, which emphasizes its importance in the metabolism of fat.[47]

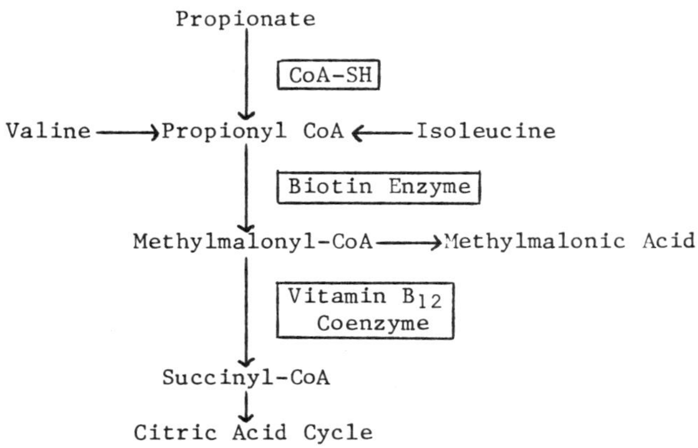

FIGURE 10. Interactions of vitamin B_{12}, biotin, and pantothenic acid in propionic acid metabolism.

VITAMIN B_{12}

In mammals, vitamin B_{12} is required in the following reactions: (a) methylation of homocysteine and (b) the conversion of methylmalonyl-CoA to succinyl-CoA (FIGURES 3 and 4). The former also requires folic acid to complete the methylation reaction. Vitamin B_{12} deficiency gives rise to an increase in tissue levels of methylmalonyl-CoA and propionyl-CoA.[48] Thus, the human subject deficient in vitamin B_{12} is often observed to excrete excess amounts of methylmalonic acid in the urine. Since this reaction requires vitamin B_{12} but not folic acid, increased urinary excretion of methylmalonic acid does not occur with a folate deficiency.[49]

The elevated levels of propionyl-CoA and methylmalonyl-CoA that occur in a vitamin B_{12} deficiency may inhibit the biosynthesis of malonyl-CoA, which is required for elongation processes, such as the conversion of linoleate to arachidonate.[50] Vitamin B_{12} deficiency promotes a greater synthesis and accumulation of odd-number and branched-chain, 15- and 17-carbon, fatty acids. Elevated levels of these fatty acids were observed in the spinal cord phosphatidyl choline of a child with deranged vitamin B_{12} metabolism.[51] Reports have suggested that the development of neurological lesions of pernicious anemia may be due in part to the progressive accumulation of branched-chain and odd-numbered saturated fatty acids into neural cerebrosides and phospholipids. Methylmalonic aciduria occurs as a rare genetic disease. Patients with this disease have a low level of vitamin B_{12} coenzyme (FIGURE 4).

VITAMIN INTERACTIONS IN SERINE AND GLYCINE METABOLISM

Serine biosynthesis and metabolism represent an example of interactions of several B-complex vitamins. Serine can originate from 3-phosphoglycerate through the participation of NAD and pyridoxal phosphate (FIGURE 11). Serine gives rise to many other substances in the body and serves as a source of the single-carbon units needed for the synthesis of methyl and formyl groups. The amino acid serves as a major source of glycine through cleavage by the tetrahydrofolic acid–dependent serine transhydroxymethylase. Serine is generally catabolized by deamination to pyruvate.

Glycine may be metabolized for energy, serve as one-carbon units, or be utilized in the formation of other biological compounds. Glycine, through the interaction of pyridoxal phosphate and succinyl-CoA, forms δ-aminolevulinic acid, which is converted to porphobilinogen, the precursor of porphyrins. Glycine may be metabolized via several pathways. One pathway, important in both plants and animals, involves four proteins and the interaction of pyridoxal phosphate, NAD, FAD, and tetrahydrofolic acid.

FOLIC ACID AND VITAMIN C

Anemia is often observed in vitamin C–deficient patients. A normochromic, normocytic, or macrocytic type of anemia is generally observed, although megaloblastic anemia has been reported for some patients.[52–57] The presence of megaloblastic anemia in some scorbutic patients has given rise to the consideration that either a dietary deficiency of folic acid existed or that folate metabolism was impaired in vitamin C deficiency.[58,59] In some instances, the megaloblastic anemia was effectively treated with ascorbic acid alone, while in other reports, supplements of

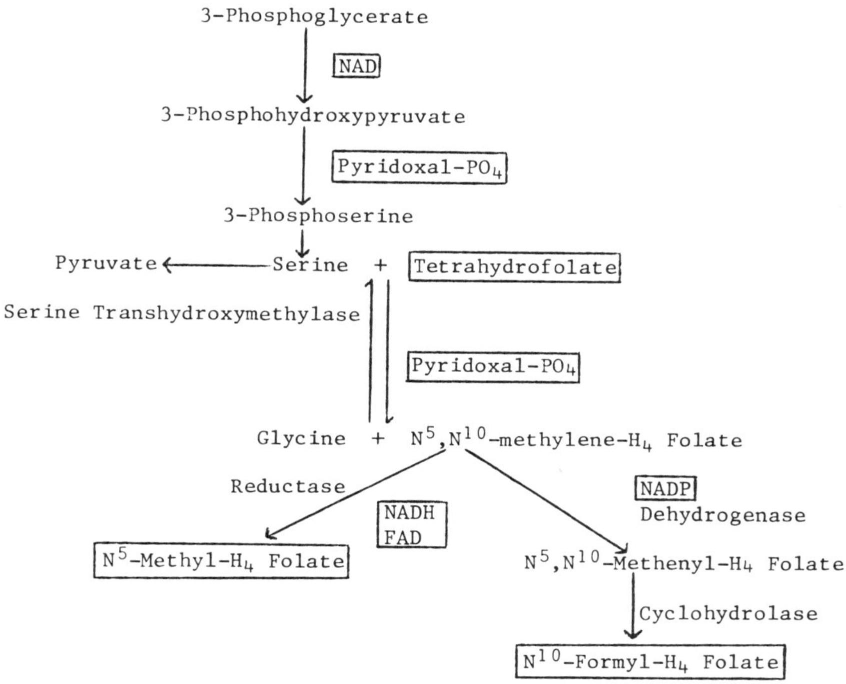

FIGURE 11. Interactions of vitamins in the metabolism of serine.

folic acid were required.[53,56] Stokes *et al.* more recently studied megaloblastic anemia in a patient with scurvy.[58] Based on hematological response and the urinary excretion of folate metabolites following the treatment with 5-formyl tetrahydrofolic acid, the investigators suggested that the anemia of scurvy is caused in part by the removal of tetrahydrofolates from the metabolic pool. They considered ascorbic acid to play an important role in the prevention of the oxidation of tetrahydrofolates to 10-formylfolic acid. It should be noted that only a small amount of the administered folate was recovered in the urine. The majority of the folate catabolized apparently results in other metabolites not measured in this study.[60] Therefore, ascorbic acid may have a greater effect on these other metabolic pathways of folic acid.

VITAMIN B_1 (THIAMIN)

Pyruvate metabolism involves the essential paticipation of thiamin pyrophosphate in concert with the actions of lipoic acid, coenzyme A, NAD, and FAD (FIGURE 12). Although a vitamin B_1 deficiency can be produced readily in the human experimentally, the clinical signs and symptoms observed cannot be fully explained by known functions of the vitamin. Erythocyte transketolase activity falls early in a thiamin deficiency. A deficiency of vitamin B_6 or riboflavin had no effect on erythrocyte transketolase activity in the rat.[61] However, thiamin deficiency has been reported to influence liver aminotransferase activities in the rat.[62] Liver alanine

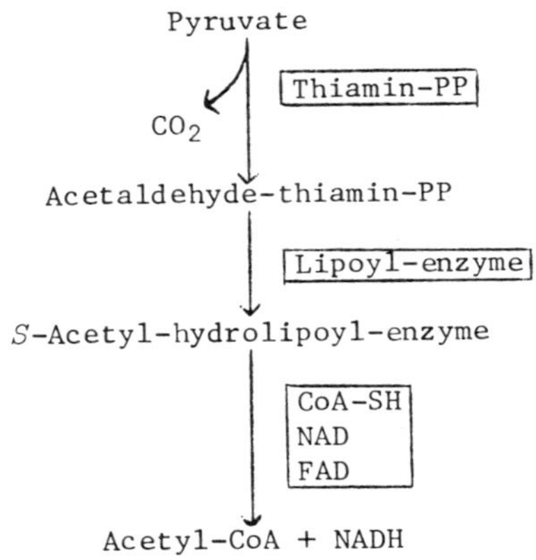

FIGURE 12. Interactions of thiamin with other vitamins in pyruvate metabolism.

aminotransferase activity was increased and liver aspartate aminotransferase activity decreased in thiamin-deficient rats. Although not established, the accumulation of metabolites, such as pyruvic acid, in thiamin-deficient animals may affect aminotransferase activity.

SUMMARY

Interactions of the B-complex vitamins are essential in the performance of metabolic and catabolic reactions in the body. Even vitamin C and the fat-soluble vitamins may be involved in these interactions. Clinical and biochemical aberrations associated with various disease states can often be explained on the basis of these vitamin interrelationships. Health and nutritional well-being are dependent upon the maintenance and proper functioning of these vitamin-dependent metabolic pathways.

REFERENCES

1. McLESTER, J. S. & W. J. DARBY. 1952. Nutrition and Diet in Health and Disease: 263. W. B. Saunders Co. Philadelphia, Penn.
2. KRISHNASWAMY, K., S. BAPURAO, T. C. RAGHURAM & S. G. SRIKANTIA. 1976. Effect of vitamin B_6 on leucine induced changes in human subjects. Am. J. Clin. Nutr. **29:** 177–181.
3. BAPURAO, S. & K. KRISHNASWAMY. 1978. Vitamin B_6 nutritional status of pellagrins and their leucine tolerance. Am. J. Clin. Nutr. **31:** 819–824.
4. BELAVADY, B., S. G. SRIKANTIA & C. GOPALAN. 1963. The effect of oral administration of leucine on the metabolism of tryptophan. Biochem. J. **87:** 652–655.
5. GHAFOORUNISSA & B. S. NARASINGA RAO. 1973. Effect of leucine on enzymes of the tryptophan-niacin metabolic pathway in rat liver and kidney. Biochem. J. **134:** 425–430.
6. KELSAY, J., L. T. MILLER & H. LINKSWILER. 1968. Effect of protein intake on the excretion of quinolinic acid and niacin metabolites by men during vitamin B_6 depletion. J. Nutr. **94:** 27–31.
7. YEH, J. K. & R. R. BROWN. 1977. Effects of vitamin B_6 deficiency and tryptophan loading on urinary excretion of tryptophan metabolites in mammals. J. Nutr. **107:** 261–271.

8. Snyderman, S. E., L. E. Holt, Jr., R. Carretero & K. Jacobs. 1953. Pyridoxine deficiency in the human infant. J. Clin. Nutr. **1:** 200–207.
9. Hayaishi, O. & H. Okamoto. 1971. Localization and some properties of kynurenine-3-hydroxylase and kynurenine aminotransferase. Am. J. Clin. Nutr. **24:** 805–806.
10. Gopalan, C. & K. S. Jaya Rao. 1975. Pellagra and amino acid imbalance. Vitam. Horm. N.Y. **33:** 505–528.
11. Rose, D. P. & P. A. Toseland. 1973. Urinary excretion of quinolinic acid and other tryptophan metabolites after deoxypyridoxine or oral contraceptive administration. Metabolism **22:** 165–171.
12. Dietrich, L. S. 1971. Regulation of nicotinamide metabolism. Am. J. Clin. Nutr. **24:** 800–804.
13. National Institute of Nutrition. 1978. Annual Report: 55–56. Hyderabad, India.
14. Frenkel, E. P., R. L. Kitchens, H. E. Savage, R. A. Seibert & M. Lane. 1979. Lack of effect of riboflavin deficiency on vitamin B_{12}-related metabolic pathways and fatty acid synthesis. Am. J. Clin. Nutr. **32:** 10–15.
15. Norton, W. N., I. Daskel, H. E. Savage, R. A. Seibert & M. Lane. 1976. Effects of riboflavin deficiency on the ultrastructure of rat sciatic nerve fibers. Am. J. Pathol. **85:** 651.
16. Frenkel, E. P. 1973. Abnormal fatty acid metabolism in peripheral nerves of patients with pernicious anemia. J. Clin. Invest. **52:** 1237.
17. Pant, S. S., A. K. Asbury & E. P. Richardson, Jr. 1968. The myelopathy of pernicious anemia. A neuropathological reappraisal. Acta Neurol. Scand. Suppl. **44**(35): 7.
18. Weissbach, H. 1971. Studies on vitamin B_{12} metabolism in HeLa cells. Arch. Biochem. Biophys. **142:** 231.
19. Mahoney, M. J., A. C. Hart, V. D. Steen & L. E. Rosenberg. 1975. Methylmalonicacidemia: biochemical heterogeneity in defects of 5′-deoxyadenosylcobalamin synthesis. Proc. Nat. Acad. Sci. **72:** 2799.
20. Fujii, K., J. H. Golivan & F. M. Huennekens. 1977. Activation of methionine synthetase: further characterization of the flavoprotein system. Arch. Biochem. Biophys. **178:** 662–670.
21. Frenkel, E. P., R. L. Kitchens & J. M. Johnston. 1973. The effect of vitamin B_{12} deprivation on the enzymes of fatty acid synthesis. J. Biol. Chem. **248:** 7540–7546.
22. Frenkel, E. P., R. L. Kitchens, L. B. Hersch & R. Frenkel. 1974. Effect of vitamin B_{12} deprivation on the *in vivo* levels of coenzyme A intermediates associated with propionate metabolism. J. Biol. Chem. **249:** 6984–6991.
23. Mukherjee, A., P. A. Srere & E. P. Frenkel. 1976. Studies on the mechanism by which hepatic citrate synthase activity increases in vitamin B_{12} deprivation. J. Biol. Chem. **251:** 2155–2160.
24. Zaman, Z. & R. L. Verwilghen. 1977. Effect of riboflavin deficiency on activity of NADH-FMN oxidoreductase (ferriductase) and iron content of rat liver. Biochem. Soc. Trans. **5**(1): 306–308.
25. Krishnaswamy, K. 1971. Erythrocyte glutamic oxaloacetic transaminase activity in patients with oral lesions. Int. J. Vitam. Nutr. Res. **41:** 247–252.
26. Krishnaswamy, K. 1971. Erythrocyte transaminase activity in human vitamin B_6 deficiency. Int. J. Vitam. Nutr. Res. **41:** 240–246.
27. National Institute of Nutrition. 1978. Annual Report: 46–51. Hyderabad, India.
28. Lakshmi, A. V. & M. S. Bamji. 1974. Tissue pyridoxal phosphate concentration and pyridoxaminephosphate oxidase activity in riboflavin deficiency in rats and man. Br. J. Nutr. **32:** 249–255.
29. Lakshmi, A. V. & M. S. Bamji. 1976. Regulation of blood pyridoxal phosphate in riboflavin deficiency in man. Nutr. Metab. **20:** 228–233.
30. Anderson, B. B., M. Saary, A. D. Stephens, G. M. Perry, I. C. Lersundi & J. E. Horn. 1976. Effect of riboflavin on red-cell metabolism of vitamin B_6. Nature **264:** 574–575.
31. Selivanova, V. M. 1960. Excretion of vitamin B_6 in the urine of a healthy individual. Bull. Exp. Biol. Med. **50:** 37.
32. Selivanova, V. M., V. K. Agashin & I. N. Polyakova. 1963. The effect produced by

ascorbic acid on the 4-pyridoxic passage with urine in healthy humans. Vopr. Pitan. **22:** 55.
33. BAKER, E. M., J. E. CANHAM, W. T. NUNES, H. E. SAUBERLICH & M. E. MCDOWELL. 1964. Vitamin B_6 requirement for adult men. Am. J. Clin. Nutr. **15:** 59–66.
34. BAKER, E. M., R. E. HODGES, J. HOOD, H. E. SAUBERLICH, S. C. MARCH & J. E. CANHAM. 1971. Metabolism of ^{14}C- and ^{3}H-labeled L-ascorbic acid in human scurvy. Am. J. Clin. Nutr. **24:** 444–454.
35. YEH, S. D. & B. F. CHOW. 1959. Vitamin B_{12} absorption in pyridoxine-deficient rats: further studies. Am. J. Clin. Nutr. **7:** 426.
36. RANKE, B., E. RANKE & B. F. CHOW. 1960. The interrelationship between vitamin B_6 and B_{12} deficiencies in rats. J. Nutr. **71:** 411–415.
37. CHENEY, M. C., D. M. CURRY & G. H. BEATON. 1965. Blood transaminase activities in vitamin B_6 deficiency: specificity and sensitivity. Can. J. Physiol. Pharmacol. **43:** 579–589.
38. SAUNDERS, M., L. SWEETMAN, B. ROBINSON, K. ROTH, R. COHN & R. A. GRAVEL. 1979. Multiple carboxylase defects and complementation studies with propionicacidemia in cultured fibroblasts. J. Clin. Invest. **64:** 1695–1702.
39. NYHAN, W. L. 1974. Heritable Disorders of Amino Acid Metabolism: Patterns of Clinical Expression and Genetic Variation. John Wiley and Sons, Inc. New York, N.Y.
40. SWEETMAN, L., L. SUHR & W. L. NYHAN. 1979. Deficiencies of propionyl-CoA and 3-methylcrotonyl CoA carboxylases in a patient with a dietary deficiency of biotin. (abst.). Clin. Res. **27:** 118.
41. BARNES, N. D., D. HULL, L. BALGOBIN & D. GOMPERTZ. 1970. Biotin-responsive propionicacidaemia. Lancet **2:** 244–245.
42. GOMPERTZ, D., G. H. DRAFFAN, J. WATTS & D. HULL. 1971. Biotin-responsive β-methylcrotonylglycinemia. Lancet **2:** 22–24.
43. WEYLER, W., L. SWEETMAN, D. MAGGIO & W. L. NYHAN. 1971. Deficiency of propionyl-CoA carboxylase and methylcrotonyl-CoA carboxylase in a patient with methylcrotonylglycinuria. Clin. Chim. Acta **76:** 321–328.
44. ABIKO, Y. 1975. Metabolism of coenzyme A. *In* Metabolism of Sulfur Compounds (Metabolic Pathways) **7:** 1. Academic Press, Inc. New York, N.Y.
45. BONJOUR, J. P. 1977. Biotin in man's nutrition and therapy—a review. Int. J. Vitam. Nutr. Res. **47:** 107–118.
46. MCCORMICK, D. B. 1975. Biotin. Nutr. Rev. **33:** 97–102.
47. BANNISTER, D. W. 1976. The biochemistry of fatty liver and kidney syndrome. Biochem. J. **156:** 167–173.
48. FRENKEL, E. P., R. L. KITCHENS, L. B. HERSH & R. FRENKEL. 1974. Effect of vitamin B_{12} deprivation on the *in vivo* levels of coenzyme A intermediates associated with propionate metabolism. J. Biol. Chem. **249:** 6984–6991.
49. SAUBERLICH, H. E., R. P. DOWDY & J. H. SKALA. 1974. Laboratory Tests for the Assessment of Nutritional Status. CRC Press, Inc. Boca Raton, Fla.
50. PEIFER, J. J. & R. D. LEWIS. 1979. Effects of vitamin B_{12} deprivation on phospholipid fatty acid patterns in liver and brain of rats fed high and low levels of linoleate in low methionine diets. J. Nutr. **109:** 2160–2172.
51. KISHIMOTO, Y., M. WILLIAMS, H. W. MOSER, C. HIGNITE & K. BIEMANN. 1973. Branched chain and odd-numbered fatty acids and aldehydes in nervous system of a patient with deranged vitamin B_{12} metabolism. J. Lipid Res. **14:** 69–77.
52. COX, E. V., M. J. MEYNELL, B. E. NORTHAM & W. T. COOKS. 1966. The anaemia of scurvy. Am. J. Med. **42:** 220–227.
53. ASQUITH, P., M. H. OELBAUM & D. W. DAWSON. 1967. Scorbutic megaloblastic anaemia responding to ascorbic acid alone. Br. Med. J. **4:** 402.
54. GOLDBERG, A. 1963. The anaemia of scurvy. Q. J. Med. **32:** 51–64.
55. COX, E. V., M. J. MEYNELL & W. T. COOKE. 1962. Scurvy and anaemia. Am. J. Med. **32:** 240–250.
56. ZALUSKY, R. & V. HERBERT. 1961. Megaloblastic anaemia in scurvy with response to 50 micrograms of folic acid daily. New Engl. J. Med. **265:** 1033–1038.
57. CHAZAN, J. A. & S. P. MISTILIS. 1963. The pathophysiology of scurvy. Am. J. Med. **34:** 350–358.

58. STOKES, P. L., V. MELIKIAN, R. L. LEEMING, H. PORTMAN-GRAHAM, J. A. BLAIR & W. T. COOKE. 1975. Folate metabolism in scurvy. Am. J. Clin. Nutr. **28:** 126–129.
59. MAY, C. D., E. N. NELSON & C. V. LOWE. 1950. Pathogenesis of megaloblastic anaemia in infancy: interrelationship between pteroylglutamic acid and ascorbic acid. Am. J. Dis. Child. **80:** 191–206.
60. MURPHY, M., M. KEATING, P. BOYLE, D. G. WEIR & J. M. SCOTT. 1976. The elucidation of the mechanism of folate catabolism in the rat. Biochem. Biophys. Res. Commun. **71:** 1017–1024.
61. BRIN, M. 1962. Erythrocyte transketolase in early thiamine deficiency. Ann. N.Y. Acad. Sci. **98:** 528–541.
62. STIELAU, W. J., R. A. FREEDLAND & J. H. MEYER. 1965. Effects of B-vitamin deficiencies and of starvation on liver enzyme activities of growing rats. J. Nutr. **87:** 109–116.

DISCUSSION

H. SPRINCE (*Veterans Administration Medical Center, Coatesville, Penn.*): If I have followed you correctly, pyridoxine is transformed to pyridoxic acid, and ascorbic acid hastens this reaction.

H. E. SAUBERLICH: Yes, ascorbic acid has been reported to increase the amount of pyridoxic acid formed and excreted.

H. SPRINCE: Is taking huge doses of ascorbic acid apt to increase the requirement for vitamin B_6?

H. E. SAUBERLICH: That was the suggestion of the report published by the Russian investigators, although I'm not sure that anyone has repeated these findings. I understand that a group at Oregon State has been looking into this possibility.

INTERACTIONS OF VITAMIN E WITH VITAMIN C, VITAMIN B_{12}, AND ZINC

Lawrence J. Machlin and Edda Gabriel

Department of Clinical Nutrition
Hoffmann-La Roche, Inc.
Nutley, New Jersey 07110

In the past, clarification of the interaction of vitamin E with selenium, polyunsaturated fatty acids, vitamin A, and iron has led to an understanding of many previously perplexing observations concerning vitamin E status in man and animals. The interactions of vitamin E with vitamin C, vitamin B_{12}, and zinc are less well explored. Greater knowledge of these interactions will, undoubtedly, lead to a better understanding of both the biochemical function of vitamin E and the clinical manifestations of a deficiency of this vitamin.

Interaction with Vitamin C

Effect of Vitamin E on Vitamin C Synthesis

In vivo synthesis of ascorbic acid (AA) is reduced in livers of vitamin E–deficient rats.[1,2,3] A number of signs of a vitamin E deficiency resemble those of scurvy. For example, in the pig, hemorrhages are often observed.[4] In the rat, skin ulcerations, suggesting defective collagen synthesis, are seen after a prolonged deficiency of vitamin E.[5] These scorbutic-like symptoms might be explained by a defect in AA synthesis in vitamin E–deficient animals *in vivo.* Chen and Barnes have reported that plasma levels of both total and reduced AA are lower in vitamin E–deficient rats or guinea pigs than in controls.[6,7] However, there was no effect of dietary vitamin E on total urinary excretion of AA in the guinea pig, and there was no evidence that vitamin E influenced the time of onset of scurvy in AA-deficient animals. Furthermore, no relationship of dietary vitamin E level to plasma AA has been observed in the dog, pig, lamb, or chicken.[8,4,9,10] In addition, neither liver AA in the rat and chicken nor urinary AA in the rat is influenced by vitamin E status.[5,10] Finally, tyrosine metabolism, an indicator of AA function, is not altered by a vitamin E deficiency.[5,11] Thus, except for the report of lowered plasma AA in vitamin E–deficient rats and guinea pigs, there are few data to support the hypothesis that AA synthesis is decreased in a vitamin E deficiency.[6,7] The *in vitro* observation of lowered AA synthesis in livers from vitamin E–deficient animals could be explained by the susceptibility of gulonolactone oxidase to the effects of lipid peroxidation.[1-3,12-14] Gulonolactone oxidase is a key enzyme in the synthesis of AA.[15]

Effect of Vitamin C on E Status

Dietary supplements of AA had inconsistent effects in reducing the incidence of encephalomalacia (ENC) in chickens but did reduce the incidence of exudative diathesis (ED) (Figure 1).[16-18] ED is caused by a simultaneous deficiency of selenium and vitamin E. Selenium has little or no effect on the incidence of ENC. This would suggest that AA might "spare" selenium but not vitamin E in the chicken. Indeed,

0077-8923/80/0355-0098 $01.75/0 © 1980, NYAS

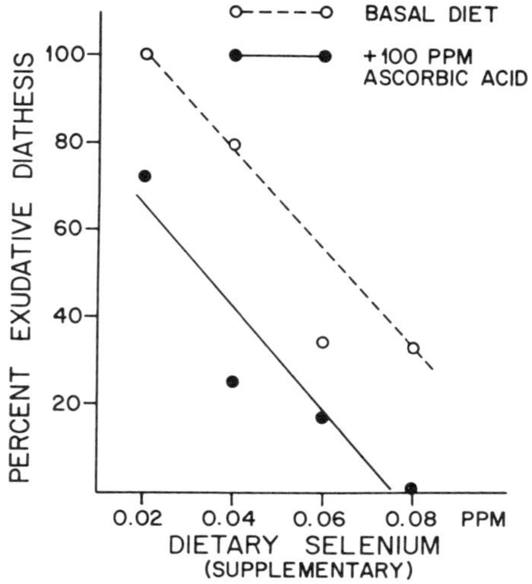

FIGURE 1. Effect of dietary ascorbic acid on exudative diathesis in chickens. (Based on Combs and Pesti.)[18]

Combs and Pesti have shown that dietary AA increases plasma glutathione peroxidase (FIGURE 2) and reduces the requirement for selenium.[18] AA apparently produces these effects by increasing the absorption of selenium.[18] This is probably a consequence of the reducing activity of AA. In these same studies, dietary AA did not affect absorption of vitamin E.

In livers of vitamin E-deficient guinea pigs, dietary AA maintained normal respiration and swelling rates of liver mitochondria.[19] Moreover, at several levels of

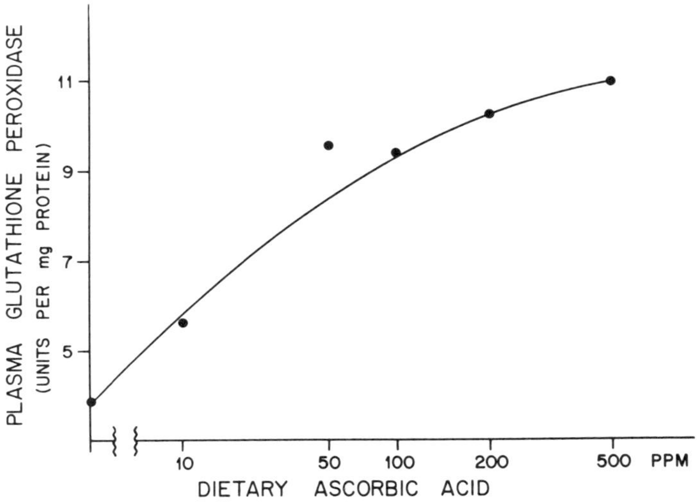

FIGURE 2. Effect of dietary ascorbic acid on plasma glutathione peroxidase in the chicken. (Based on Combs and Pesti.)[18]

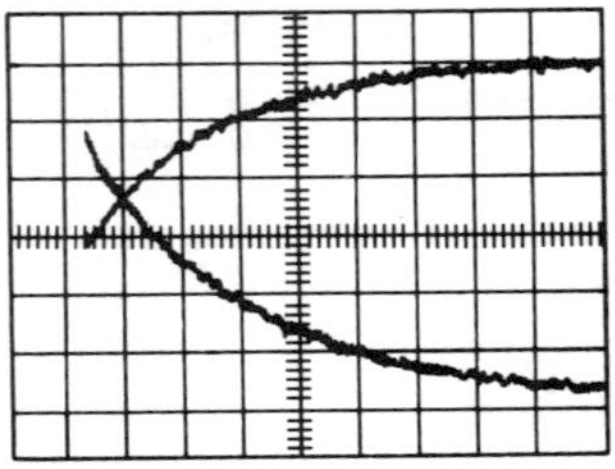

FIGURE 3. Oscillograms for the reaction between the vitamin E radical and vitamin C. (From Packer *et al.*[25] Reproduced with permission from *Nature*.)

vitamin E intake, addition of AA resulted in slightly increased levels of plasma vitamin E. These observations suggest that dietary AA had a vitamin E–like effect or "spared" vitamin E or both. Unfortunately, AA had no effect on erythrocyte hemolysis, and no other effects of AA on classical vitamin E–deficiency signs (e.g., myopathy, testis degeneration) were reported.

In summary, AA clearly spares selenium in the chicken by increasing selenium absorption. However, a sparing effect on vitamin E has not been consistently demonstrated, and more definitive studies on this subject are needed.

Free Radical Reaction between Vitamin E and Vitamin C

According to the "antioxidant hypothesis," vitamin E–deficiency diseases are a consequence of *in vivo* peroxidation of unsaturated fatty acids.[20] A chief criticism of this theory is that *in vivo* peroxidation should result in tocopherol destruction.[21,22] However, no clear evidence for either the disappearance of tocopherol from tissues or the appearance of oxidized metabolites has been presented. One possible explanation for the absence of detectable destruction of tocopherol is that tocopherol is converted to a free radical, which then reacts with either glutathione or AA to regenerate tocopherol.[23-25] Packer *et al.* have shown that following pulse radiolysis of an aerated solution of tocopherol, there is formation of a phenoxy radical, which subsequently disappears with the simultaneous appearance of an ascorbate radical (FIGURE 3).[25] Thus, there is chemical evidence that AA might participate in the regeneration of a tocopherol radical. The ascorbate radical can be enzymatically reduced back to AA by a nicotinamide adenenine dinucleotide hydride (NADH)-

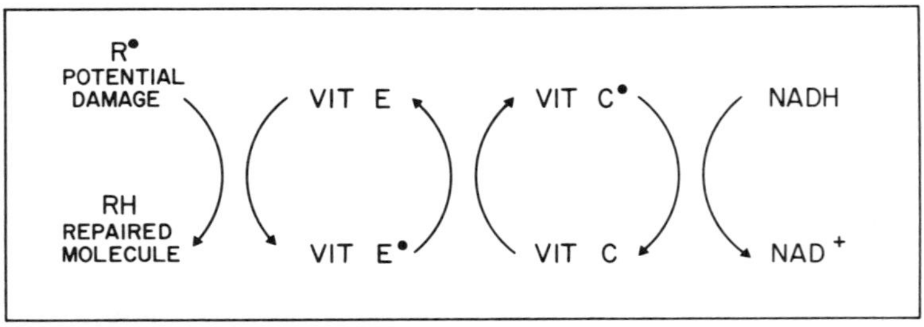

FIGURE 4. Proposed scheme for *in vivo* regeneration of vitamin E from vitamin E radical (probably phenoxy radical) by vitamin C (R•, VIT E•, VIT C• are radicals). (From Packer *et al.*[25] Reproduced with permission from *Nature*.)

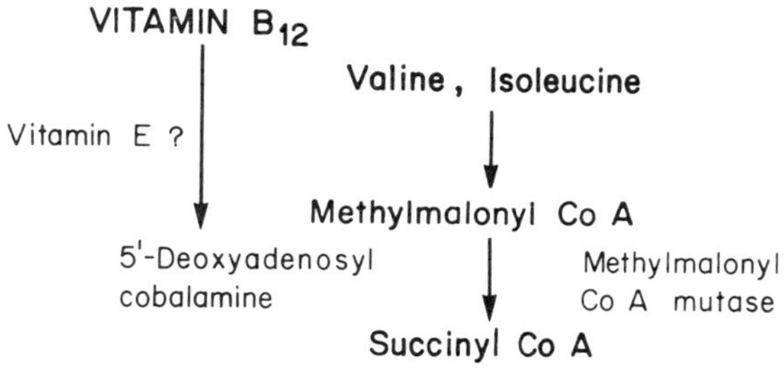

FIGURE 5. Proposed roles of vitamins E and B_{12} in metabolism of methylmalonic acid.

dependent system.[26] Thus, there exists a possible mechanism for continuously regenerating tocopherol, which could continue to function as an antioxidant (FIGURE 4). Evidence for the existence of such a mechanism operating *in vivo* is needed before the true physiological significance of such a hypothesis can be assessed.

INTERACTIONS WITH VITAMIN B_{12}

Methylmalonyl–coenzyme A mutase requires 5′-deoxyadenosylcobalamin as a cofactor (FIGURE 5). Since this enzyme is necessary for the metabolism of methylmalonate, a deficiency of vitamin B_{12} results in a methylmalonicacidemia. Barness found that urinary excretion of methylmalonic acid, observed in some premature infants, disappeared or decreased when vitamin E was administered.[27] In addition, in two patients with cystic fibrosis, administration of vitamin E was followed by disappearance of urinary methylmalonate. Oski *et al.* found an inverse relationship between serum tocopherol and vitamin B_{12} levels (TABLE 1).[28] A possible biochemical explanation for these findings, suggested by Pappu *et al.*, is that a vitamin E deficiency may interfere with the conversion of vitamin B_{12} to its coenzyme, 5′-deoxyadenosylcobalamin.[29] They found that excretion of urinary methylmalonate was 41 ± 5 μM/24 hours in vitamin E–deficient rats compared with 11 ± 4 μM/24 hours in control animals. None of the animals were deficient in vitamin B_{12}, and the concentration of cyanocobalamin in serum and liver of vitamin E–deficient rats was the same as the controls. This suggests that the vitamin E deficiency did not interfere with absorption, storage, or transport of cyanocobalamin. Other *in vitro* experiments demonstrated that the activity of methylmalonyl-CoA mutase was lower in liver preparations from vitamin E–deficient rats. Furthermore, addition of 5′-deoxyadenosylcobalamin, the cofactor for the mutase, restored the enzymatic conversion *in vitro*. This suggests that vitamin E may be required for the

TABLE 1

INFLUENCE OF TOCOPHEROL ON SERUM VITAMIN B_{12}*

Tocopherol Status	Number of Patients	Serum: Tocopherol (mg/dl)	Serum: Vitamin B_{12} (pg/ml)
Low†	12	0.29	1,570
Normal‡	14	0.87	410

* Oski *et al.*[28] † Less than 0.5 mg/dl. ‡ More than 0.5 mg/dl.

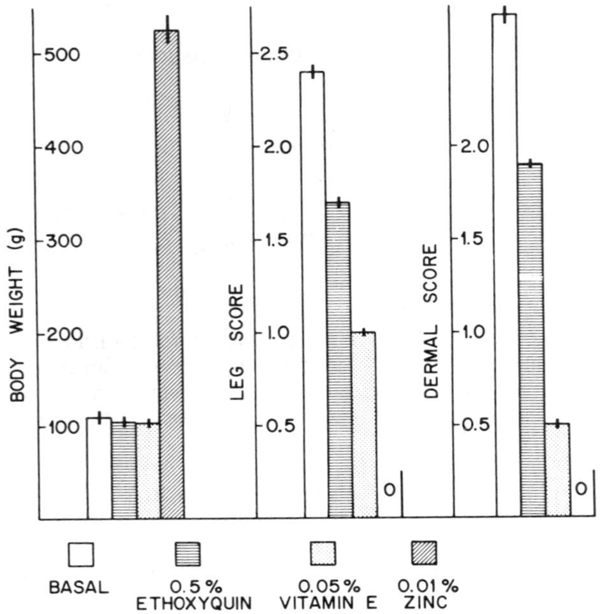

FIGURE 6. Effect of vitamin E on symptoms of zinc deficiency in the chicken. Basal diet contained 30 IU vitamin E per kg. (Based on Bettger *et al.*)[39]

conversion of vitamin B_{12} to its coenzyme 5′-deoxyadenosylcobalamin. Pappu *et al.* have suggested that accumulation of methylmalonate in the liver might explain the inhibition of succinic acid oxidation in vitamin E deficiency.[29] In addition, they point out that there is impaired DNA synthesis in the anemia observed in vitamin E-deficient monkeys similar to that resulting from a vitamin B_{12} deficiency.[30] Exactly how a decrease in the 5′-deoxyadenosylcobalamin could lead to such an anemia remains to be investigated.

INTERACTION WITH ZINC

Chvapil *et al.* have proposed that zinc can function as a stabilizer of biomembranes.[31] This is based on the observation that zinc can stabilize lysosomes *in vitro,* inhibit lipid peroxidation in livers of CCl_4-treated rats,[31] and inhibit spontaneous or osmotic hemolysis of erythrocytes.[32,33] Vitamin E also has the ability to stabilize membranes.[34,35] Formation of irreversibly sickled cells (ISC) in patients with sickle-cell anemia is thought to be related to abnormal membrane function. It is of interest that administration of either zinc or vitamin E to sickle-cell anemia patients results in a decreased number of ISC.[36,37] A deficiency of either zinc or vitamin E results in testis degeneration and an elevation of arachidonic acid in testes lipid.[38] Although vitamin E and zinc show some common biochemical and nutritional effects, there have been few studies concerned with their interaction.

Bettger *et al.* found that chicks fed a low-zinc diet developed severe skin lesions on the toes and foot pads, as well as gross joint abnormalities.[39] Supplementation of the zinc-deficient diet with vitamin E significantly reduced the severity of the skin

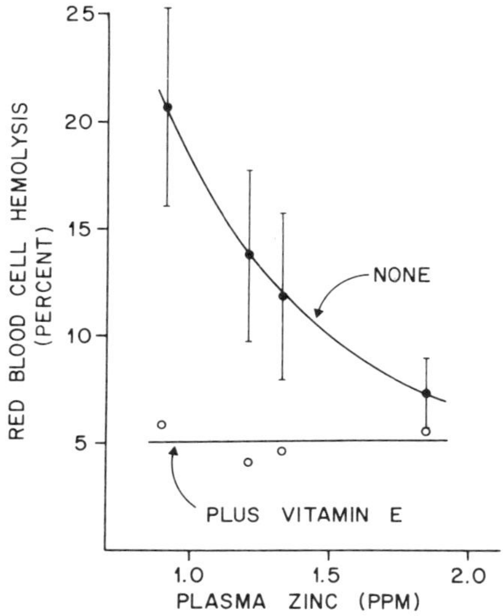

FIGURE 7. Influence of zinc on peroxidative hemolysis. Four-week-old rats were fed diets containing 7, 14, 36, or 520 ppm zinc with or without 200 ppm vitamin E for five weeks. Plasma zinc was determined. Washed red blood cells from these animals were incubated with H_2O_2 for 1 hour at 24 °C, and percent hemolysis determined.

and joint pathology but had no effect on the decreased rate of growth in the zinc-deficient chicks (FIGURE 6). Incubation of skin in a buffer containing copper resulted in the release of thiobarbituric acid–reactive substances. Production of this indicator of peroxidation was reduced when diets were supplemented with either zinc or vitamin E. These observations support the hypothesis that zinc plays an analogous

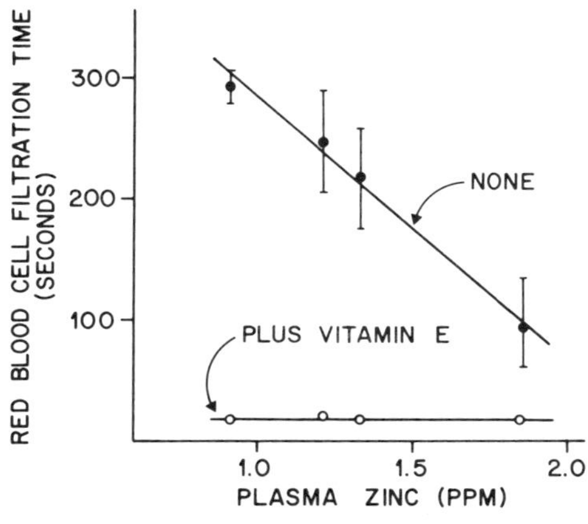

FIGURE 8. Influence of zinc on red blood cell (RBC) filtration time. See FIGURE 7 for animal treatment. Filtration time was that required for 2 ml of a 2% RBC suspension to pass through a 3.0 μ Nuclepore filter using a vacuum of 10 cm of water. Cell suspensions were incubated at 37 °C for three hours prior to measurement of filtration time.

TABLE 2

LACK OF AN EFFECT OF ZINC ON TESTICULAR DEGENERATION AND PLASMA PYRUVATE KINASE (PK) AND GLUTAMIC OXALACETIC TRANSAMINASE (GOT) IN VITAMIN E-DEFICIENT RATS (EXPERIMENT 1)

Dietary		Testis	Plasma	
Zinc (ppm)	Vitamin E (ppm)	Weight* (g)	PK† (units/ml)	GOT† (units/l)
7	2	2.1 ± 0.2	5.4 ± 0.8	284 ± 32
14	2	1.9 ± 0.2	5.8 ± 0.6	282 ± 28
36	2	1.9 ± 0.2	5.9 ± 0.5	295 ± 58
520	2	2.0 ± 0.1	5.6 ± 0.5	332 ± 82
7	200	3.8 ± 0.2	0.2 ± 0.02	60 ± 3
14	200	3.6 ± 0.1	0.2 ± 0.06	72 ± 11
36	200	3.6 ± 0.1	0.2 ± 0.04	70 ± 5
520	200	3.6 ± 0.2	0.2 ± 0.03	70 ± 8

* Rats were fed experimental "zinc" diets for 16 weeks after a 4-week period on a vitamin E-deficient diet. Eight animals per group. Numbers are mean ± standard error.

† Rats were fed experimental "zinc" diets for 5 weeks after a 4-week period on purified diets with or without vitamin E. Eight animals per group.

biochemical role to that of vitamin E, by stabilizing membrane structure and thus reducing peroxidative damage to the cell.

We have recently addressed ourselves to the question of whether dietary zinc would influence vitamin E-deficiency signs.

Male rats fed either vitamin E-deficient or replete diets for four weeks post-weaning were transferred to diets containing (by analysis) 7, 14, 36, or 520 parts per million (ppm) zinc. After five weeks on these diets, plasma zinc levels were 0.9, 1.2, 1.3, and 1.8 ppm, respectively. The growth rate of rats fed the lowest level of zinc was not significantly different from those fed the higher levels. In red blood cells (RBC) from rats deficient in vitamin E, the percent hemolysis after 1 hour exposure to H_2O_2 at 24 °C was inversely related to the plasma zinc level (FIGURE 7). Hemolysis was less than 6% in RBC from rats fed vitamin E, regardless of the zinc level. The filtration time for 2 ml of a 2% RBC suspension to pass through a 3.0 μ Nuclepore filter after a 3-hour incubation at 37 °C was also reduced by zinc in cells from vitamin E-deficient animals (FIGURE 8). Filtration times were very rapid in RBC from rats

TABLE 3

EFFECT OF DIETARY ZINC ON GROWTH OF VITAMIN E-DEFICIENT AND REPLETE RATS (EXPERIMENT 2)*

	Body Weight Gain† (g)	
Zinc (ppm)	No Vitamin E‡	200 ppm Vitamin E
6	51 ± 6	105 ± 7
18	56 ± 5	113 ± 5
500	49 ± 6	120 ± 8

* Weanling rats were fed purified diets containing 16 ppm Zn, with or without vitamin E, for five weeks and then transferred to diets with the levels of Zn indicated for eight weeks.

† Mean ± standard error of 10 animals per group for eight-week period on experimental Zn diets.

‡ Plasma tocopherol levels of rats on these diets were less than 0.1 mg/dl.

TABLE 4

EFFECT OF DIETARY ZINC ON RED BLOOD CELL ZINC (EXPERIMENT 2)*

Dietary Zinc (ppm)	Red Blood Cell Zinc (ppm)
6	7.11 ± 0.34
18	7.32 ± 0.34
500	7.53 ± 0.35

* Red blood cells were obtained from 10 animals per group after three weeks on experimental diets. Values are mean ± standard error.

fed vitamin E. Zinc status did not affect myopathy [as indicated by plasma pyruvate kinase (PK) or glutamic oxalacetic transaminase (GOT) levels] or testes degeneration in vitamin E-deficient animals (TABLE 2). Thus, zinc appears to increase the stability of the RBC to oxidative stress during *in vitro* incubation but has no effect on vitamin E-deficiency signs in other tissues.

In a second experiment, rats were transferred to diets containing 6, 18, or 500 ppm zinc at six weeks postweaning and maintained on these diets for eight weeks. The zinc level did not significantly affect weight gain during this period in either vitamin E-deficient or replete rats (TABLE 3). When RBC from the vitamin E-deficient animals were incubated in air at 28 °C, malondialdehyde (MDA) formation was detectable after 1½ hours and increased linearly thereafter (FIGURE 9). The zinc level had no significant effect on MDA formation, indicating that zinc was not

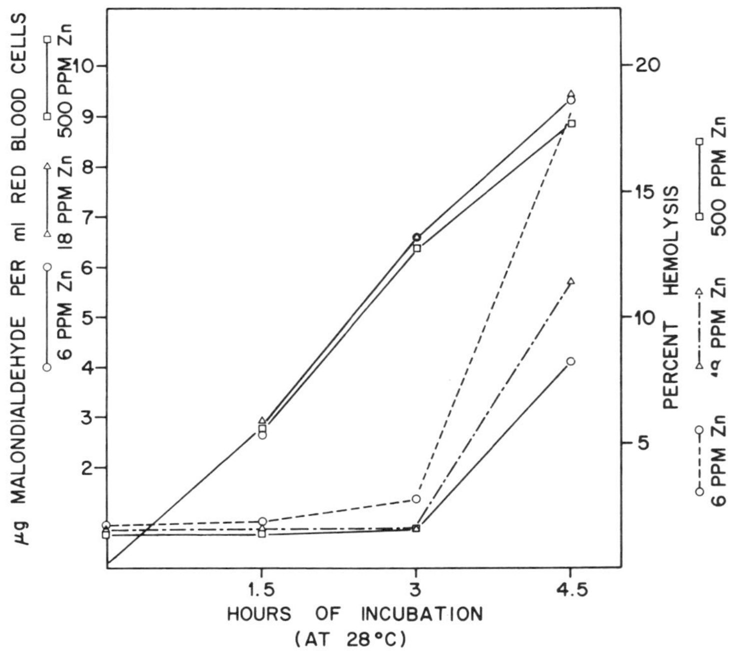

FIGURE 9. Effect of dietary zinc on hemolysis and malondialdehyde formation in red blood cells (RBC) from vitamin E-deficient rats fed diets containing 6, 18, or 500 ppm zinc for eight weeks. A 4% suspension of RBC in phosphate-buffered saline was incubated in air at 28 °C. No H_2O_2 or any other oxidant was added.

acting as an antioxidant. Hemolysis was detectable after 4½ hours incubation and was significantly reduced in RBC from zinc-supplemented animals. This is clear evidence that peroxidation precedes hemolysis in vitamin E–deficient red cells and would indicate that zinc stabilizes the RBC membrane against events that occur following peroxidation. In this study, dietary zinc levels did not significantly affect the zinc content of the RBC (TABLE 4). Zinc, however, is known to be incorporated into the RBC membrane.[40] It is possible that an increase in the dietary zinc levels did result in an increase in zinc in the RBC membrane. However, since the membrane accounts for less than 2% of the mass of the RBC, the large quantity of zinc in the nonmembrane portion of the cell probably would obscure any changes that occur in the membrane.

Zinc is a component of over 70 metalloenzymes, and undoubtedly many deficiency signs, such as growth depression, result from a reduced level of one or more of these enzymes. In addition to its structural role in enzymes, zinc, as well as vitamin E, may function as a membrane stabilizer. This role might account for the pathology observed in such tissue as the RBC, skin, and joints when either of these nutrients is absent and would explain why either nutrient might prevent such pathology.

Our results suggest that in the red blood cell, zinc is not functioning as an antioxidant but apparently stabilizes the membrane against damaging events that occur following peroxidation. Further investigation is required to fully explain the biochemical basis for the interaction between these nutrients and to obtain quantitative data concerning the effect of zinc status on the dietary requirement for vitamin E and vice versa.

REFERENCES

1. CAPUTTO, R., P. B. MCCAY & M. P. CARPENTER. 1958. Requirements of Mn^{++} and Co^{++} for the synthesis of ascorbic acid by liver extract of animals deprived of tocopherol. J. Biol. Chem. **233:** 1025.
2. CARPENTER, M. P., A. E. KITABCHI, P. B. MCCAY & R. CAPUTTO. 1959. The activation by tocopherol and other agents of ascorbic acid synthesis by liver homogenates from vitamin E deficient rats. J. Biol. Chem. **234:** 2814.
3. MCCAY, P. B., M. P. CARPENTER, A. E. KITABCHI & R. CAPUTTO. 1959. In vitro activation of the synthesis of ascorbic acid in liver extracts of tocopherol-deficient rats. Arch. Biochem. **82:** 472.
4. BROWN, R. G., B. A. SHARP, L. G. YOUNG & A. VAN DREUMAL. 1971. Serum ascorbate levels in swine with cardiac muscular dystrophy (Mulberry Heart Disease) and hepatosis dietetica. Can. J. Anim. Sci. **51:** 537.
5. MACHLIN, L. J., R. FILIPSKI, J. NELSON, L. R. HORN & M. BRIN. 1977. Effects of a prolonged vitamin E deficiency in the rat. J. Nutr. **107:** 1200.
6. CHEN, L. H. & K. J. BARNES. 1976. Nutritional relationship of vitamin E and vitamin C in rats. Nutr. Rep. Int. **14:** 699.
7. CHEN, L. H. & K. J. BARNES. 1976. Nutritional relationship of vitamin E and vitamin C in guinea pigs. Nutr. Rep. Int. **14:** 89.
8. HAYES, K. C., S. W. NIELSEN & J. E. ROUSSEAU, JR. 1969. Vitamin E deficiency and fat stress in the dog. J. Nutr. **99:** 196.
9. DE MILLE, F., R. G. BROWN & J. G. BUCHANAN-SMITH. 1972. Ascorbic acid metabolism in lambs and the effect of vitamin E or ethoxyquin and rumen development. Can. J. Anim. Sci. **52:** 411.
10. BIERI, J. G. & A. A. ANDERSON. 1960. Peroxidation of lipids in tissue homogenates as related to vitamin E. Arch. Biochem. Biophys. **90:** 105.
11. EL-KHATIB, S., U. A. CHENAU, M. P. CARPENTER, R. E. TRUCCO & R. CAPUTTO. 1964.

Possible presence of lipid peroxides in tissues of tocopherol deficient animals. Nature **201:** 188.
12. Caputto, R., R. E. Trucco & A. E. Kitabchi. 1961. The interrelationship between gulonolactone oxidase and the process of lipid peroxidation. Ann. N.Y. Acad. Sci. **92:** 79.
13. Chatterjee, I. B. & R. W. McKee. 1965. Lipid peroxidation and biosynthesis of L ascorbic acid in rat liver microsomes. Arch. Biochem. Biophys. **110:** 254.
14. Kitabchi, A. E., P. B. McCay, M. P. Carpenter, R. E. Trucco & R. Caputto. 1960. Formation of malondialdehyde in vitamin E deficiency and its relation to the inhibition of gulanolactone oxidase. J. Biol. Chem. **235:** 1591.
15. Chatterjee, I. B., M. C. Kar, M. C. Ghosh & B. C. Guha. 1961. Aspects of ascorbic acid biosynthesis in animals. Ann. N.Y. Acad. Sci. **92:** 36.
16. Dam, H., I. Kruse, I. Prange & E. Sondergaard. 1948. Influence of dietary ascorbic acid, nordehydroguaiaretic acid and cystine on vitamin E deficiency symptoms in chicks. Biochim. Biophys. Acta **2:** 32.
17. Combs, G. F., Jr. & M. L. Scott. 1974. Antioxidant effects on selenium and vitamin E function in the chick. J. Nutr. **104:** 1297.
18. Combs, G. F., Jr. & G. M. Pesti. 1976. Influence of ascorbic acid on selenium nutrition in the chick. J. Nutr. **196:** 958.
19. Chen., L. & M. L. Chang. 1978. Effect of dietary vitamin E and vitamin C on respiration and swelling of guinea pig liver mitochondria. J. Nutr. **108:** 1616.
20. Tappel, A. L. 1962. Vitamin E as the biological lipid antioxidant. Vitam. Horm. N.Y. **20:** 493.
21. Green, J. & J. Bunyan. 1969. Vitamin E and the biological antioxidant theory. Nutr. Abstr. Rev. **39:** 321.
22. Diplock, A. T. 1978. The biological function of vitamin E and the nature of the interaction of the vitamin with selenium. World Rev. Nutr. Diet. **31:** 178.
23. Pryor, W. A. 1976. The role of free radical reactions in biological systems. *In* Free Radicals in Biology **1:** 1–47. Academic Press, Inc. New York, N.Y.
24. Tappel, A. L. 1968. Will antioxidant nutrients slow aging processes? Geriatrics **23:** 97.
25. Packer, J. E., T. F. Slater & R. L. Wilson. 1979. Direct observation of a free radical interaction between vitamin E and vitamin C. Nature **278:** 737.
26. Schneider, W. & H. Staudinger. 1965. Reduced nicotinamide-adenine dinucleotide-dependent reduction of semidehydroascorbic acid. Biochim. Biophys. Acta **96:** 157.
27. Barness, L. A. 1967. Vitamin B_{12} deficiency with emphasis on methylmalonic acid as a diagnostic aid. Am. J. Clin. Nutr. **20:** 573.
28. Oski, F. A., R. Myerson, L. A. Barness & W. J. Williams. 1966. A possible relationship between vitamin E and vitamin B_{12}. Am. J. Clin. Nutr. **18:** 307.
29. Pappu, A. S., P. Fatterpaker & S. Sreenivasan. 1978. Possible relationship between vitamin E and B_{12} in the disturbance in methylmalonate metabolism in vitamin E deficiency. Biochem. J. **172:** 115.
30. Dinning, J. S. 1962. Nucleic acid metabolism in vitamin E deficiency. Vitam. Horm. N.Y. **20:** 511.
31. Chvapil, M., S. L. Elias, J. M. Ryan & C. F. Zukoski. 1972. Pathophysiology of zinc. Int. Rev. Neurobiol. **1:** 105.
32. Chvapil, M., Y. M. Peng, A. L. Aronsan & C. Zukoski. 1974. Effect of zinc on lipid peroxidations and metal content in some tissues of rats. J. Nutr. **104:** 434.
33. Bettger, W. S., T. J. Fish & B. L. O'Dell. 1978. Effects of copper and zinc status on erythrocyte stability and superoxide dismutase activity. Proc. Soc. Exp. Biol. Med. **158:** 279.
34. Molenaar, I., C. E. Hulstaert & M. J. Hardonk. 1980. Role in function and ultrastructure of cellular membranes. *In* Vitamin E. L. J. Machlin, Ed.: 372–389. Marcel Dekker, Inc. New York, N.Y.
35. Lucy, J. A. 1978. *In* Tocopherol, Oxygen, and Biomembranes. D. De Duve & O. Hayashi, Eds.: 109–120. Elsevier/North Holland. Amsterdam and New York.
36. Brewer, G. J., L. F. Brewer & A. S. Prasad. 1977. Suppression of irreversibly sickled erythrocytes by zinc therapy in sickle cell anemia. J. Lab. Clin. Med. **90:** 549.

37. MACHLIN, L. J., C. NATTA & M. BRIN. 1979. Vitamin E and sickle cell anemia. Fed. Proc. Fed. Am. Soc. Exp. Biol. **38:** 609.
38. BIERI, J. G. & E. L. PRIVAL. 1966. Effect of deficiencies of tocopherol, retinol, and zinc on the lipid composition of rat testes. J. Nutr. **89:** 55.
39. BETTGER, W. J., P. G. REEVES, J. E. SAVAGE & B. L. O'DELL. 1980. Interaction of zinc and vitamin E in the chick. Proc. Soc. Exp. Biol. Med. **163:** 432.
40. CHVAPIL, M., D. MONTGOMERY, J. C. LUDWIG & C. F. ZUKOSKI. 1979. Zinc in erythrocyte ghosts. Proc. Soc. Exp. Biol. Med. **162:** 480.

DISCUSSION

P. MARFEY (*State University of New York, Albany, N.Y.*): In one of your slides, you showed in a cyclic representation the reduction of a vitamin C free radical to vitamin C. The donor of electrons was NADH going to NAD^+. Now what is needed is only a one-electron reduction, but NADH provides two electrons. In other words, it's a hydride ion containing two electrons that is the reducing equivalent in that case. Did you mean to represent, not reduction of the free radical vitamin C to vitamin C, but rather oxidized vitamin C to reduced vitamin C, which would indeed require two electrons rather than one? Or do you imply that there is a free radical produced on NADH?

L. J. MACHLIN: The mechanism isn't known, but the slide was meant to imply that perhaps two ascorbate radicals are reduced by one mole of NADH.

E. BARRETT (*Interesting Medicine, New York, N.Y.*): You mentioned that vitamin C might increase the absorption of selenium or reduce the need for selenium. I think you put it both ways. What kind of doses are you talking about? And does the vitamin C get used up in that process?

L. J. MACHLIN: In answer to the second question, we don't know whether it is used up. These studies were done in the chicken, which is an ascorbic acid–synthesizing animal, so that it is hard to translate values to humans. One hundred parts per million in the diet would probably translate to a fairly robust level in man.

H. SPRINCE (*Veterans Administration Medical Center, Coatesville, Penn.*): I notice that you have not discussed the interaction between vitamin C and vitamin B_{12}. I wonder if you would care to add some comments about that controversy.

L. J. MACHLIN: There were two reports by Dr. Herbert showing increased destruction of vitamin B_{12} in the presence of high levels of vitamin C. Since then, three different laboratories have reported that if one uses cyanide in the extractions, no such losses are present.

My interpretation is that Dr. Herbert's results were largely an artifact of the particular methodology used and that there are no good data to suggest that there is any problem with B_{12} destruction in the presence of high levels of ascorbic acid.

J. G. BIERI. (*National Institutes of Health, Bethesda, Md.*): Dr. Machlin, in your last slide, you showed the relation of hemolysis and zinc content of the red cells. How do these levels relate to the dietary level?

L. J. MACHLIN: The zinc content of the red cells was not given. The diets contained 6, 18, and 500 parts per million of zinc.

INTERACTIONS OF FAT-SOLUBLE VITAMINS IN HYPERVITAMINOSES

Lotte Arnrich and Veronica A. Arthur

Department of Food and Nutrition
Iowa State University
Ames, Iowa 50011

Introduction

Well-recognized states of hypervitaminosis with toxic manifestations are associated with the two fat-soluble vitamins A and D. In most instances, lipid-soluble vitamins E and K have not led to adverse effects when consumed in pharmacological quantities over prolonged periods, although vitamin E may be antagonistic to vitamin K functions.

Lipid solubility and occurrence in nature with lipid systems are common characteristics of these micronutrients. They are unrelated chemically, except that isoprene units are basic to the synthesis of their structure. From a biochemical aspect, a precise function—analogous to the coenzyme function of many B-vitamins—has not been established for the fat-soluble vitamins in the animal organism. An exception is the role of retinol in vision. The lack of understanding of functions at the molecular level has often been the underlying reason for controversy in interpretation of data pertaining to mechanisms involving fat-soluble vitamins.

Through their common physical characteristic of lipid solubility, certain interactions occur between fat-soluble vitamins in lipid-related systems and structures. This paper is limited to a discussion of the interactions between vitamins A and E where at least one of the members occurs in excess, either at the dietary or at the tissue level. Most of the information comes from research with experimental animals in which hypervitaminosis A has been produced with high dosage levels, leading to frank toxicities manifested in mortality, growth depression, and a range of morphological changes.

The following discussion will focus on three major topics:

1. Effects of tocopherol supplementation in hypervitaminosis A;
2. Excess vitamin A and plasma and tissue levels of tocopherol;
3. Excess tocopherol in the metabolism of physiological amounts of retinol or β-carotene.

Experimental approaches cover the range from overall effects in the whole animal to interactions at the cellular and subcellular level and in model systems.

Much of the research on interactions of vitamin E in hypervitaminosis A dates from the 40s and 50s, when work related to the role of tocopherol in vitamin A metabolism was pursued actively. The controversy surrounding the antioxidant function of tocopherol *in vivo* brought renewed interest to the problem in the 60s, especially in the laboratories of Green and associates in England.[1,2] In recent years, work with model systems has focused on the mechanism of tocopherol interactions with excess vitamin A in biomembranes.

0077-8923/80/0355-0109 $01.75/0 © 1980, NYAS

Effects of Tocopherol Supplementation in Hypervitaminosis A

Effect of Tocopherol on Mortality, Growth Rate, and Pathological Manifestations of Hypervitaminosis A

Experimental animals show severe derangements of many systems in hypervitaminosis A. Where tested, tocopherol administration has usually led to full or partial reversal.

For example, chicks fed 1,000 × the required amount of vitamin A had a survival rate of only 25% compared to controls.[3] This manifestation of severe vitamin A toxicity was completely reversed when large amounts of tocopherol, again amounting to 1,000 × the requirement, were added simultaneously to the birds' diet. Parallel to this, growth rate of chicks on excess vitamin A, which had fallen to 40% of that of controls, was almost normalized with tocopherol supplements.

Similar beneficial effects on rate of growth were reported from a study where varying amounts of tocopherol were used in hypervitaminosis A.[4] During an eight-week feeding period, addition of 2.9×10^6 IU vitamin A/kg diet caused a 25% reduction in weight gain. Growth rates were restored to control levels by raising the tocopherol intake 10 or 100 fold over the basal level.

These two studies are examples of an antagonistic interaction between the two vitamins, where toxicity manifested by excess of one was ameliorated by an excess of the other.

Vitamin E may also act synergistically in toxic manifestations of vitamin A. Testicular degenerative changes in rats fed excess vitamin A were actually potentiated with a large excess of vitamin E.[5] With excess vitamin A alone, testicular weight fell from control values, and moderate testicular damage was ascertained on histological examination. Rats fed excess amounts of both vitamins A and E, separated by approximately eight hours, had more severe testicular damage than was found with excess vitamin A alone. Mortality rates also increased in the doubly supplemented group.

Effect of Tocopherol on Body Reserves of Vitamin A

The concept of the sparing effect of vitamin E on body stores of vitamin A has been under discussion since the experiments of Davies and Moore drew attention to this relationship.[6] In discussing this interaction, several points have to be taken into account. In experiments where investigators have looked at hepatic stores of retinol following supplementation of the ration with the two vitamins, it is not possible to differentiate between (a) reactions occurring in the gastrointestinal tract prior to absorption (*in vitro* reactions); (b) metabolic reactions during utilization of vitamin A for growth and maintenance; and (c) reactions involving depletion of hepatic stores of retinol. Furthermore, it is important to differentiate among experimental results based on a correction of a deficiency of vitamin E and those from excess intakes of vitamin E.

In early observations of Davies and Moore, depletion of large initial hepatic vitamin A stores was accelerated in the absence of dietary vitamin E.[6] After 222 days, vitamin E–deficient rats were also vitamin A deficient, while considerable hepatic vitamin A reserves were left in vitamin E sufficiency. These experimental results were confirmed in the late 60s, but only when initial hepatic vitamin A stores were as large as those in the early study.[2]

The underlying mechanisms for the beneficial effect of vitamin E in this relationship are not fully understood. Interpretations of various investigators differ and are difficult to resolve because of the existing uncertainty of an exclusive antioxidative function of tocopherol *in vivo*.[7,8] Peroxidation of unsaturated lipids, presumably unchecked with vitamin E-deficient diets, could be the cause for the accelerated losses of hepatic retinol, possibly through simultaneous oxidative destruction of vitamin A. However, even with the exclusion of dietary fatty acids, the sparing action of tocopherol in small amounts on initially high hepatic retinol reserves was still evident.[9] In the same experiment, substitution of synthetic antioxidants for vitamin E was ineffective.

Other investigators have used large excesses of tocopherol together with massive doses of vitamin A.[4] The data supported the concept of the sparing action of tocopherol, though the approach differed from the previous ones in that both absorption and metabolic utilization may have affected the results. Hepatic deposits from a 2.9×10^6 IU vitamin A/kg diet with adequate tocopherol were only one-third as large as those formed after simultaneous consumption of tocopherol amounting to 10 or 100 × the basic level.

Of some value in the interpretation of the role of excess vitamin E on high intakes of vitamin A are results of a human study.[10] In India, emergency measures to combat severe vitamin A deficiencies in children have led to a program of supplementation with single massive doses of vitamin A at six-month intervals. It was of interest to explore the value of simultaneous supplementation of vitamin A with 500 mg vitamin E. The effectiveness of the procedure was tested by tagging the vitamin A dose with tritium. Vitamin E supplementation increased absorption of the vitamin A dose to 82% from the basal level of 67%. This improvement in absorption was offset, however, by increased urinary losses, so that net retention of vitamin A in the body was not changed significantly by excess vitamin E.

Studies in our laboratory have led to similar conclusions. Young rats were given a single large dose of retinyl acetate by intubation, then fed a vitamin A-free diet with either 1 or 50 mg *dl*-α-tocopheryl acetate daily for 28 days (TABLE 1). Residual retention of hepatic retinol averaged 48 and 41%, respectively, for the two treatments. Differences were not significant, although a trend towards a slightly faster depletion rate with excess tocopherol was apparent over the total period. In this experiment, the gastrointestinal events were excluded.

In general, large retinol stores seem especially vulnerable to degradation in the vitamin E-deficient state, while utilization of moderate hepatic retinol stores is little,

TABLE 1

DEPLETION OF HEPATIC RETINOL STORES IN RATS FED 1 OR 50 mg *dl*-α-TOCOPHERYL ACETATE*

	Hepatic Retinol (μg)		
Days of Depletion	1 mg αT†	50 mg αT	P
0	478 ± 26‡		
14	352 ± 22	277 ± 21	< 0.05
21	305 ± 33	258 ± 23	NS
28	232 ± 26	194 ± 16	NS

* Rats depleted of retinol reserves were intubated with 1,000 μg retinyl acetate. A control group was killed 7 days later to assess maximum hepatic retinol values (day 0). Remaining rats were fed either 1 or 50 mg αT daily. Groups of 10 rats were killed after 14, 23, or 28 days.

† αT = *dl*-α-tocopheryl acetate.

‡ ± standard error of the mean (SEM).

if any, affected by the high vitamin E intakes. That these lead to high tissue levels of tocopherol was shown in our own animal model, where hepatic tocopherol concentrations rose to 10 × the control level with feeding of 50 mg *dl-α*-tocopheryl acetate daily.

Interactions of Vitamins A and E in Biomembranes

A much debated question concerns the interaction of the two vitamins, A and E, *in vivo.* This problem is closely related to that concerning the *in vivo* function of vitamin E, its role as an antioxidant, and an additional structural role leading to membrane stability.[11] Biomembrane instability and disruption occur with excess vitamin A, when circulating retinol exceeds the binding capacity of retinol-binding protein (RBP) and exerts its membrane-lysing effect.[12] Lysing of membranes by excess retinol has been studied in a variety of systems, such as erythrocytes, lysosomes, and cell membranes in general. Isolated erythrocytes and their behavior towards hemolysing agents have been useful models in these studies.[13-15]

In an early study by the British investigators, hemolysis was produced in normal erythrocytes when retinol was added to the incubation medium.[13] The disruption of red cell membranes by retinol was inhibited by the addition of tocopherol or its acetate. Hydroquinone or diphenyl-*p*-phenylenediamine (DPPD) was completely ineffective among the other compounds tested in this system. These results were corroborated with erythrocytes from animals that had been prefed with excess vitamin A.[16] Comparisons were made over 16 weeks with and without dietary vitamin E. By the 10th week, erythrocytes lysed extensively in the presence of hydrogen peroxide after excess vitamin A alone, while hemolysis could be prevented in rats given excess vitamin A with simultaneous feeding of a moderate dose of 2 IU vitamin E daily.

An unresolved question pertaining to membrane interactions of the two vitamins relates to the role of lipid peroxidation as an obligatory reaction to vitamin A–induced hemolysis, and its prevention by tocopherol. Peroxidation was negligible in an *in vitro* system and did not change as hemolysis of erythrocytes increased with increasing amounts of retinol in the medium.[14] Similarly, it was not possible to detect peroxidation of lipids when erythrocytes from rats prefed with excess vitamin A were hemolysed with hydrogen peroxide. Peroxide values were uniformly low with or without supplementation with vitamin E.[15]

From these reports, it appears that the interaction of vitamin E in hypervitaminosis A may be more complex than an antioxidant reaction involving unsaturated lipids of membranes.[5] Aside from acting as antioxidants of unsaturated lipids, tocopherols are also thought to stabilize membranes through other mechanisms. Experiments with model systems involving monolayers of unsaturated phospholipids at air-water interfaces have led to the suggestion that tocopherol may facilitate molecular packing of phospholipids and thus have a structural role in membrane stability.[11,17]

Tissue Levels of Tocopherol in Hypervitaminosis A

The question has been raised whether hypervitaminosis A may lead to vitamin E deficiency or deplete tissue tocopherol levels.[18] Such interaction could be expected if tocopherol were itself degraded in the process of protecting vitamin A from oxidative destruction. The similarity in hemolysis *in vitro* of erythrocytes in vitamin E deficiency and in hypervitaminosis A has stimulated inquiries regarding tocopherol levels in tissues in hypervitaminosis A.[13] For example, plasma tocopherol levels were examined in chicks fed 10^6 IU/kg diet of retinyl palmitate.[19] Plasma tocopherol concentrations were severely depressed to 12–25% of controls on marginal tocopherol intakes. Only when dietary tocopherol was raised to 60 IU/kg did plasma tocopherol concentration normalize in the presence of high intakes of vitamin A. These results corroborate earlier reports that graded amounts of dietary retinyl acetate from 50 to 5,000 mg/kg lowered plasma and hepatic tocopherol concentrations in rats.[18]

Similar conclusions were drawn from an experiment with a different approach, where rats received radioactive tocopherol while consuming a wide range of vitamin A supplements. Recovery of radioactivity in liver was depressed progressively as the intake of vitamin A increased from 500 to 75,000 IU/day.[16] Values of recovery of labeled hepatic tocopherol, as percent of controls, ranged from 63% for the lowest dose to 17% for the highest intake of vitamin A.

The examples cited so far do not allow for differentiation between *in vitro* interactions in the gastrointestinal tract and any reaction in metabolism between the two vitamins. To exclude reactions occurring in the intestinal phase, vitamin E-depleted chicks were given a single intravenous injection of ^{14}C-*d*-α-tocopherol, followed by feeding of a ration with 0.25% vitamin A acetate for 11 days. Carcass analysis failed to give any evidence of destruction of tocopherol by excess vitamin A. These conclusions were supported with data from a rat experiment where rats received a single oral dose of ^{14}C-labeled tocopherol 48 hours prior to treatment with excess vitamin A.[1]

Recent reports regarding the stability of α-tocopherol during the production of thiobarbituric acid-reactive materials *in vivo* may explain the failure of Green and associates to demonstrate a decrease in tissue tocopherol in hypervitaminosis A.[1] Nakamura and Hishinuma recovered 3–6% of the labeled dose in liver homogenates even in vitamin E deficiency; of this, 90% was undegraded α-tocopherol.[20]

Effect of Excess Tocopherol on Utilization of Physiological Levels of Vitamin A and Its Precursor

In the studies cited so far, vitamin A was in excess either in the diet or at tissue levels. In most instances where large amounts of tocopherol were involved, the interaction was to the benefit of the organism, especially in hypervitaminosis A. In instances where excess tocopherol has been combined with physiological doses of vitamin A, not all the results have been beneficial.

In attempts to find the proper balance between the two vitamins, it was apparent that utilization of moderate amounts of vitamin A for growth or hepatic storage could be improved with a change of the animal's vitamin E status from deficient to adequate.[21,22] The effective dose for tocopherol was between 0.5 and 2.0 mg/day for the rat. With preformed vitamin A, additional supplementation with tocopherol was of no value but also had no adverse effects. β-Carotene as the source of vitamin A was, however, especially sensitive to vitamin E. Following improvement of β-carotene utilization with additions of tocopherol of from 0 to 2.0 mg/day, excess supplements of from 5 to 10 mg, corresponding to 5–10 × the requirement for young rats, were antagonistic to physiological amounts of β-carotene. However, reports to the contrary can also be found.[23]

Based on the present practice of certain individuals to consume tocopherol far in excess of dietary recommendations, we extended studies reported in the 40s and 50s by feeding rats as much as 50 mg *dl*-α-tocopheryl acetate (αT) daily, or roughly 50 × the optimum of 1 mg.

TABLE 2

HEPATIC RETINOL DEPOSITION FROM β-CAROTENE OR RETINYL ACETATE WITH VARYING INTAKES OF *dl-α*-TOCOPHERYL ACETATE*

Experiment	Vitamin A Source	Vitamin A μg RE‡/day	αT† (mg/day)	Total Hepatic Retinol (μg)
1	β-carotene	32	1	130 ± 14§
1	β-carotene	32	10	84 ± 8
1	β-carotene	32	50	11 ± 2
2	β-carotene	39	1	227 ± 22
2	β-carotene	39	50	16 ± 6
2	retinyl acetate	34	1	206 ± 14
2	retinyl acetate	34	50	220 ± 16

* Young vitamin A–depleted rats were fed β-carotene or retinyl acetate for 28 days.
† αT = *dl-α*-tocopheryl acetate.
‡ RE = retinol equivalents.
§ ± SEM.

Similar to previous findings,[21,22] we saw a significant reduction in hepatic retinol from β-carotene supplementation with 10 mg αT/day in 28-day feeding studies (TABLE 2). When the tocopherol dose was raised to 50 mg/day, hepatic deposition of retinol was almost completely inhibited. At the same time, fecal excretion of unconverted carotene increased with excess dietary tocopherol, though amounts of β-carotene lost relative to controls were too small to account for the large differences seen in hepatic retinol deposits.

By comparison, hepatic stores of retinol following feeding of preformed vitamin A as retinyl acetate were not affected by large supplements of tocopherol (TABLE 2). These results suggested that the inhibitory effect of excess tocopherol on β-carotene utilization was likely to occur at the intestinal site of β-carotene conversion to retinol, based on the assumption that β-carotene, once converted to retinol, was metabolized by mechanisms similar to those involved in utilization of dietary retinol.

The question to be asked was whether a high tissue level of tocopherol, resulting from prolonged feeding of 50 mg αT/day, would interfere with the enzymatic con-

TABLE 3

In Vivo INTESTINAL CONVERSION OF ^{14}C-β-CAROTENE TO RETINOL METABOLITES FOLLOWING PREFEEDING WITH *dl-α*-TOCOPHERYL ACETATE*

Fraction	Percent Radioactivity Recovered: 1 mg αT† (N = 9)	Percent Radioactivity Recovered: 50 mg αT (N = 7)	P
β-carotene	73 ± 3.5‡	75 ± 0.6	NS
retinyl ester	10 ± 0.7	17 ± 1.1	<0.001
retinol	10 ± 1.9	6 ± 0.9	NS
retinol + retinyl ester	20 ± 1.9	23 ± 0.7	NS
polar fraction	7 ± 1.6	2 ± 0.9	< 0.05

* Vitamin A–depleted rats were prefed with 50 μg β-carotene and 1 or 50 mg αT daily for 28 days. Rats were injected intraduodenally with 10 μg ^{14}C-β-carotene and killed 1 hour later.
† αT = *dl-α*-tocopheryl acetate.
‡ ± SEM.

TABLE 4

In Vitro CONVERSION OF ^{14}C-β-CAROTENE TO RETINOL METABOLITES BY MUCOSAL HOMOGENATES FOLLOWING PREFEEDING WITH 1 OR 50 mg *dl*-α-TOCOPHERYL ACETATE*

	Percent Radioactivity Recovered		
Fraction	1 mg αT† (N = 7)	50 mg αT (N = 7)	P
β-carotene	87 ± 1.0‡	85 ± 2.2	NS
retinyl ester	1 ± 0.2	1 ± 0.3	NS
retinal	7 ± 0.9	10 ± 2.0	NS
polar fraction	5 ± 0.2	4 ± 0.3	NS

* Vitamin A-depleted rats were prefed with 1 or 50 mg αT daily for 28 days. Rats were fasted for eight hours and killed. Homogenized intestinal mucosal scrapings were incubated with ^{14}C-β-carotene.
† αT = *dl*-α-tocopheryl acetate.
‡ ± SEM.

version of β-carotene to retinol. The enzyme responsible for β-carotene conversion to retinol (β-carotene 15,15′-dioxygenase) is located in the intestinal mucosal cell.[24] Metabolites recovered at the site of conversion are retinol and especially retinyl esters. Rats prefed with 1 or 50 mg αT daily for 28 days, and with adequate retinol stores, were fasted overnight, then given a small test meal to insure presence of ingesta in the intestinal tract. After 2.5 hours, ^{14}C-β-carotene was injected into the duodenum under light anesthesia. One hour was allowed for metabolism of the dose. The small intestine was removed under anesthesia. Retinol metabolites were isolated from the intestinal homogenate. Data from this experiment showed that the conversion process at the intestinal level was essentially unaffected by high tissue levels of tocopherol (TABLE 3). The conclusion that the conversion process of β-carotene was not depressed is supported by data from a subsequent experiment where mucosal scrapings from rats, prefed with tocopherol as before, were used in an *in vitro* assay for β-carotene 15,15′-dioxygenase. In this assay, retinal—the first oxidation product—is the major metabolite (TABLE 4). Again, relative amounts of retinol

TABLE 5

In Vivo INTESTINAL CONVERSION OF ^{14}C-β-CAROTENE TO RETINOL METABOLITES FOLLOWING INTRADUODENAL INJECTION OF ^{14}C-β-CAROTENE WITH 0.2 OR 10 mg *dl*-α-TOCOPHERYL ACETATE*

	Percent Radioactivity Recovered		
Fraction	0.2 mg αT† (N = 8)	10 mg αT (N = 8)	P
β-carotene	73 ± 3.3‡	86 ± 0.9	< 0.001
retinyl ester	18 ± 3.1	7 ± 0.3	< 0.001
retinol	7 ± 0.3	4 ± 0.3	< 0.001
retinol + retinyl ester	25 ± 3.3	13 ± 0.9	< 0.001
polar fraction	2 ± 0.2	2 ± 0.1	

* Rats were injected intraduodenally with 10 μg ^{14}C-β-carotene and either 0.2 or 10 mg αT. They were killed 1 hour later. The amount of αT corresponded to 1 or 50 mg αT used in feeding experiments.
† αT = *dl*-α-tocopheryl acetate.
‡ ± SEM.

TABLE 6

In Vitro Conversion of ^{14}C-β-CAROTENE TO RETINOL METABOLITES BY MUCOSAL HOMOGENATES IN THE PRESENCE OF EXCESS *dl*-α-TOCOPHERYL ACETATE*

	Percent Radioactivity Recovered		
Fraction	0.02 mg αT† (*N* = 8)	1.00 mg αT (*N* = 9)	P
β-carotene	78 ± 1.6‡	86 ± 0.6	< 0.001
retinyl ester	2 ± 0.3	1 ± 0.1	NS
retinal	15 ± 0.8	11 ± 0.4	< 0.001
polar fraction	3 ± 0.3	2 ± 0.2	< 0.001

* Aliquots of a composite mucosal homogenate from stock rats were incubated with 1 μg ^{14}C-β-carotene and 0.02 or 1.00 mg αT.
† αT = *dl*-α-tocopheryl acetate in incubation mixture.
‡ ± SEM.

metabolites did not differ with tocopherol status, confirming that the enzyme activity was undiminished in rats fed 50 mg αT/day.

In these two experiments, the last dose of tocopherol had been administered 24 hours before injection with radioactive carotene. However, in the feeding studies that led to depressed hepatic retinol stores, the two vitamins, β-carotene and tocopherol, had been given combined in the corn oil carrier. The next experiments were designed to produce conditions where ^{14}C-β-carotene was injected together with adequate or excessive amounts of αT. In the *in vivo* experiment, recovery of retinol metabolites, especially in the retinyl ester fraction, was significantly depressed in the presence of excess tocopherol (TABLE 5). Results of a subsequent *in vitro* test, where tocopherol was combined with ^{14}C-β-carotene in the medium, confirmed that tocopherol in excess depressed β-carotene 15,15′-dioxygenase (TABLE 6).

Conclusions drawn from these studies are that high tissue levels of tocopherol do not interfere with the activity of carotene dioxygenase or other mechanisms involved in the conversion process, but that the presence of large amounts of tocopherol in the ingesta interferes with the accessibility of β-carotene to the enzyme. The nature of this inhibition is not understood at present. It could be a direct antioxidant action involving the oxidative steps in the conversion process. The interaction of β-carotene and tocopherol could also be of a physical nature, based on differences in β-carotene dispersion with different amounts of tocopherol at the site of mucosal uptake of β-carotene. Whatever the mechanism, it appears that β-carotene and tocopherol have to be present simultaneously during the absorption process for interactions leading to suppression of retinol synthesis from β-carotene by excess tocopherol to occur.

REFERENCES

1. GREEN, J., I. R. MUTHY, A. T. DIPLOCK, J. BUNYAN, M. A. CAWTHORNE & E. A. MURRELL. 1967. Vitamin E and stress. 7. The interrelationships between polyunsaturated fatty acid stress, vitamin A and vitamin E in the rat and the chick. Br. J. Nutr. **21:** 845–864.
2. CAWTHORNE, M. A., J. BUNYAN, A. T. DIPLOCK, E. A. MURRELL & J. GREEN. 1968. On the relationship between vitamin A and vitamin E in the rat. Br. J. Nutr. **22:** 133–143.

3. McCuaig, L. W. & I. Motzok. 1970. Excessive dietary vitamin E: its alleviation of hypervitaminosis and lack of toxicity. Poult. Sci. **49:** 1050–1052.
4. Jenkins, M. Y. & G. V. Mitchell. 1975. Influence of excess vitamin E on vitamin A toxicity in rats. J. Nutr. **105:** 1600–1606.
5. Maddock, C. L., J. Cohen & S. B. Wolbach. 1953. Effect of hypervitaminosis A on the testes of the rat. AMA Arch. Pathol. **56:** 333–340.
6. Davies, A. W. & T. Moore. 1941. Interaction of vitamins A and E. Nature **147:** 794–796.
7. Lucy, J. A. 1972. Functional and structural aspects of biological membranes: a suggested structural role for vitamin E in the control of membrane permeability and stability. Ann. N.Y. Acad. Sci. **203:** 4–11.
8. Diplock, A. T. 1978. Biological function of vitamin E and the nature of the interaction of the vitamin with selenium. World Rev. Nutr. Diet. **31:** 178–183.
9. Sondergaard, E. 1972. The influence of vitamin E on the expenditure of vitamin A from liver. Experientia **28:** 773–774.
10. Kusin, J. A., V. Reddy & B. Sivakumar. 1974. Vitamin E supplements and the absorption of a massive dose of vitamin A. Am. J. Clin. Nutr. **27:** 774–776.
11. Maggio, B., A. T. Diplock & J. A. Lucy. 1977. Interactions of tocopherols and ubiquinones with monolayers of phospholipids. Biochem. J. **161:** 111–121.
12. Mallia, A. K., J. E. Smith & DeW. S. Goodman. 1975. Metabolism of retinol-binding protein and vitamin A during hypervitaminosis A in the rat. J. Lipid Res. **16:** 180–188.
13. Lucy, J. A. & J. T. Dingle. 1964. Fat-soluble vitamins and biological membranes. Nature **204:** 156–160.
14. Krishnamurthy, S. & V. N. R. Kartha. 1973. Vitamin A induced hemolysis and lipid peroxidation. Effect of vitamin E, D and antioxidants. Curr. Sci. **42:** 225–227.
15. Kartha, V. N. R. & S. Krishnamurthy. 1978. Effect of hypervitaminosis A on hemolysis and lipid peroxidation in the rat. J. Lipid Res. **19:** 332–334.
16. Brubacher, V. G., K. Schärer, A. Studer & O. Wiss. 1965. Über die gegenseitige Beeinflussung von Vitamin E, Vitamin A und Carotinoiden. Z. Ernährungswiss. **5:** 190–202.
17. Lucy, J. A. 1978. Structural interactions between vitamin E and polyunsaturated lipids. World Rev. Nutr. Diet. **31:** 184–189.
18. Pudelkiewicz, W. J., L. Webster & L. D. Matterson. 1964. Effects of high levels of dietary vitamin A acetate on tissue tocopherol and some related analytical observations. J. Nutr. **84:** 113–117.
19. Combs, G. F., Jr. & M. L. Scott. 1974. Antioxidant effects on selenium and vitamin E function in the chick. J. Nutr. **104:** 1297–1303.
20. Nakamura, T. & I. Hishinuma. 1978. Protective effect of tocopherol on the formation of TBA-reactive materials in rat liver. *In* Tocopherol, Oxygen, and Biomembranes. C. de Duve & O. Hayaishi, Eds.: 95–108. Elsevier/North Holland Biomedical Press. Amsterdam and New York.
21. Johnson, R. M. & C. A. Baumann. 1948. The effect of alpha-tocopherol on the utilization of carotene by the rat. J. Biol. Chem. **175:** 811–816.
22. High, E. G. 1956. Further antioxidant studies concerned with the metabolism of carotene and vitamin A. Arch. Biochem. Biophys. **60:** 456–462.
23. Guggenheim, K. 1944. The biological value of carotene from various sources and the effect of vitamin E on utilization of carotene and of vitamin A. Biochem. J. **38:** 260–264.
24. Olson, J. A. & O. Hayaishi. 1965. The enzymatic cleavage of β-carotene into vitamin A by soluble enzymes of rat liver and intestine. Proc. Nat. Acad. Sci. **54:** 1364–1370.

Discussion

H. Sprince (*Veterans Administration Medical Center, Coatesville, Penn.*): Have you considered using α-tocopheryl quinone in your system, rather than α-tocopherol, to see if you can accelerate the effect that you have been getting?

L. Arnrich: No, we have not. We have run into vitamin K antagonism with high levels of α-tocopherol and suspect that tissue quinones may be involved. We did not want to complicate the system in that way.

Unidentified Speaker: Have you tried any other antioxidant on the conversion of carotene to vitamin A?

L. Arnrich: We have not. Synthetic antioxidants were tested in the 40s and 50s, when the early experiments were done, with conflicting results. Depending on the method of administration and type of antioxidant used, the results could vary. With a lipid-soluble antioxidant, one might get an effect. If the material is poorly absorbed, investigators may report no effect. It is very difficult to make a distinction between the various reports on this basis.

NUTRITIONAL INTERACTIONS OF VITAMIN B_{12}, FOLIC ACID, AND THYROXINE*

E. L. R. Stokstad, Margaret May-Sheng Chan,
J. E. Watson, and T. Brody

Department of Nutritional Sciences
University of California
Berkeley, California 94720

Introduction

The feeding of thyroid powder has long been known to produce a growth depression that can be partially corrected by feeding of vitamin B_{12}.[1-4] There is also increased excretion of formiminoglutamic acid (FIGlu), which is similar to that occurring in vitamin B_{12} deficiency.[5-7] Evidence of folic acid deficiency has also been observed in thyrotoxicosis in man.[8,9] The experiments presented here were designed to study mechanisms whereby thyrotoxicosis produces a pseudo-vitamin B_{12} deficiency.

Methods

A low-methionine (0.2%) basal diet was used that contained 20% soy assay protein supplemented with 50 μg of vitamin B_{12} and 5 mg of folic acid per kg, together with adequate amounts of the other known vitamins. FIGlu was measured in urine using the enzymatic method of Tabor and Wyngarden.[10] Histidine oxidation was measured by injecting ca. 0.5 μCi [2-^{14}C]-histidine per animal together with 1 μmol of cold histidine per gram body weight and placing the animal in a small respiration chamber. The expired $^{14}CO_2$ was trapped in a 1:2 mixture of ethanolamine and ethyleneglycolmonomethyl ether for two to three hours, and the radioactivity counted using the scintillating fluid described by Jeffay and Alvarez.[11] Hepatic 5,10-methylenetetrahydrofolate reductase activity was measured using the method of Kutzbach and Stokstad;[12] and methionine synthetase was measured by the method of Sauer and Jaenicke.[13] Formiminotransferase was measured by the procedure of Narisawa *et al.*[14] Distribution of folate coenzymes was measured by the intraperitoneal (ip) injection of 25 μCi of purified ^{3}H-pteroylglutamic acid (^{3}H-PteGlu) (0.5 nmol) 24 hours before sacrifice. The livers were homogenized in 5% ascorbate solution (pH 4.2), and polyglutamate forms of folate were hydrolyzed by autolysis at 37 °C for three hours. Distribution of the single-carbon substituent forms of folic acid in the autolyzed liver was carried out using QAE-Sephadex column chromatography by the method of Davidson *et al.*[15]

Results

In the first experiment, the results of which are described in Table 1, the effects of thyroidectomy and hyperthyroidism produced by feeding of thyroid powder were studied. It can be seen that unoperated (intact) animals on this low-methionine diet

* This work was supported in part by U.S. Public Health Service Grant No. AM-08171 from the National Institutes of Health.

0077-8923/80/0355-0119 $01.75/0

TABLE 1

EXPERIMENT I: EFFECTS OF THYROIDECTOMY, THYROID POWDER, T4, AND METHIONINE ON THE METABOLISM OF HISTIDINE AND FOLATE (Three Animals per Group)

		INT*	INT + TP†	$\overline{\text{Th}}$‡	Th + T4§
Group Number		1	2	3	4
Average body weight (g) (27 days)	− Methionine	186	182	77	118
	+ Methionine‖	230	266	87	216
FIGlu excretion¶ (19 days)	− Methionine	321	1,260	2	208
	+ Methionine‖	84	153	2	45
% 2-[^{14}C]-Histidine oxidized to $^{14}CO_2$** (24 days)	− Methionine	6.8	3.8	44.5	9.2
	+ Methionine‖	20.0	10.0	67.3	30.8
% ^{3}H-H_4PteGlu†† (28 days)	− Methionine	37.9	36.8	62.6	33.2
	+ Methionine‖	47.5	44.4	68.2	40.7

*INT stands for intact rats.

† Thyroid powder (TP) supplemented at 3 g/kg diet.

‡ $\overline{\text{Th}}$ indicates surgical thyroidectomy.

§ Thyroxine (T4) replacement administered by ip injection at 5.0 μg L-Na-T4 per rat every other day.

¶ Urinary formiminoglutamic acid (FIGlu) excretion expressed as μmol FIGlu excreted/24 hours/kg body weight of the animal.

‖ *dl*-Methionine supplementation given at 15 g of *dl*-methionine per kg of diet.

** Three-hour respiration period for histidine oxidation.

†† % ^{3}H-H_4PteGlu = [^{3}H-H_4PteGlu/(^{3}H-5-CH_3-H_4PteGlu + ^{3}H-H_4PteGlu)] × 100.

excreted moderate amounts of FIGlu (321 μg per kg body weight per day). This was increased to 1,260 μmol by feeding of thyroid powder and decreased to 2 μmol by thyroidectomy. The addition of 2.5 μg thyroxine (T4) per day (5 μg injected every other day) increased FIGlu excretion to approximately that of the intact control. The addition of methionine to the intact animals on the basal diet decreased FIGlu excretion to 84 μmol and decreased FIGlu excretion in the animals receiving thyroid powder to 153 μmol. Histidine oxidation was affected in the inverse manner to FIGlu excretion. Thyroidectomy increased histidine oxidation from the intact control level of 6.8% up to 44.5%. Thus, thyroidectomy mimics the action of methionine in that it decreases FIGlu excretion and increases histidine oxidation.

Thyroidectomy decreased FIGlu excretion to lower levels than that produced by feeding of methionine. The addition of methionine to thyroidectomized animals further increased histidine oxidation from 44.5% without methionine to 67.3% with methionine. The addition of methionine to the animals receiving thyroid powder increased histidine oxidation from 3.8% to 10.0%. This may be compared with the histidine oxidation rate of 20% on the basal diet (Group 1). Thus, the addition of methionine overcomes part, but not all, of the histidine oxidation–depressing activity of thyroid powder. It should also be noted that histidine oxidation in the thyroidectomized animals receiving 2.5 μg T4 per day did not completely meet the thyroxine requirements of the thyroidectomized animal.

The proportion of methyltetrahydrofolate to other folate forms in the liver was studied because methyltetrahydrofolate is inactive in those folate-dependent reactions involved in the degradation of FIGlu. The chromatographic separation curves for four different treatments are shown in FIGURE 1, and the percent tetrahydrofolate of total

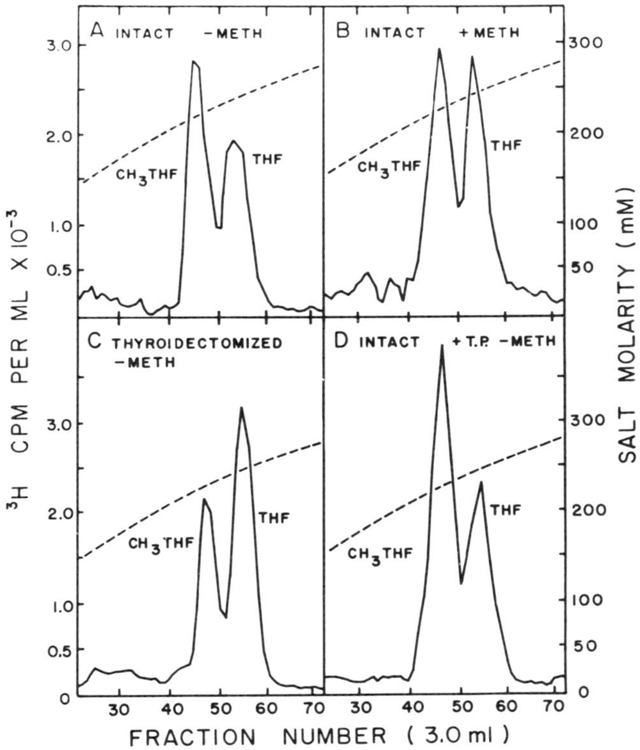

FIGURE 1. QAE-Sephadex column chromatography of autolyzed liver. 2.5 ml of autolysate equivalent to 1 g of liver tissue was chromatographed on a 0.9 × 20-cm column. Elution was effected with an exponential salt gradient using 200 ml 50 mM sodium acetate buffer, pH 5.0, plus 50 mM NaCl in the mixing chamber and 50 mM sodium acetate buffer, pH 5.0, plus 400 mM NaCl. 2% mercaptoethanol was added to both buffers. Animals were sacrificed at 27 days. **(A)** Distribution pattern in intact rat with no methionine; **(B)** Intact rat with methionine; **(C)** Thyroidectomized rat with no methionine; **(D)** Intact rat fed 3 g thyroid powder per kg diet and no methionine. (From Chan and Stokstad.[24] Reproduced by permission of authors and publisher, Elsevier-North Holland Biomedical Press, Amsterdam, The Netherlands.)

folate forms in the liver is also given in TABLE 1. Intact animals on the basal diet contained 37.9% of tetrahydrofolate, which increased to 47.5% on addition of methionine. This is similar to the results previously reported by Noronha and Silverman.[16] The effect of methionine in decreasing the proportion of methyltetrahydrofolate can be accounted for by the effect of *S*-adenosylmethionine (SAM) in inhibiting methylenetetrahydrofolate reductase.[17,18] The inhibition of this enzyme, which forms methyltetrahydrofolate, would be expected to increase the proportion of nonmethyltetrahydrofolates.

Thyroidectomy increased the proportion of tetrahydrofolate to 62.6% (Group 3), which was further increased slightly by addition of dietary methionine to 68.2%. It will be noted that the percentage of tetrahydrofolate parallels the histidine oxida-

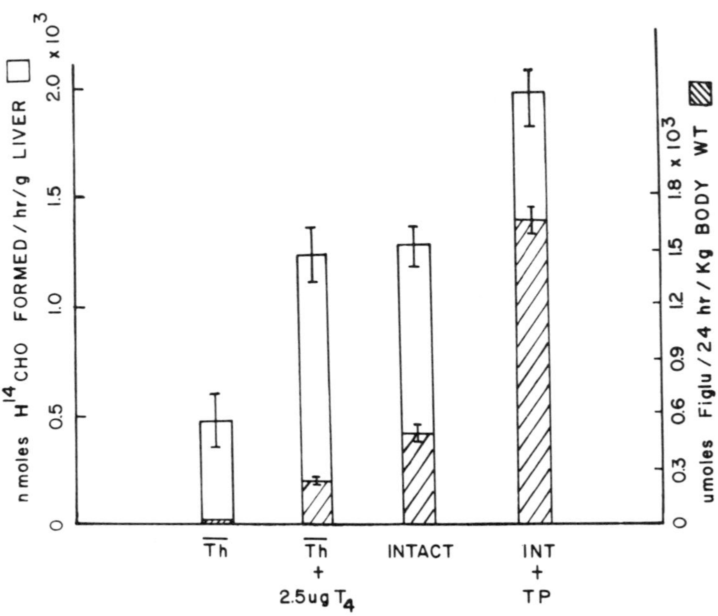

FIGURE 2. Effects of thyroxine (T4) and thyroid powder on formiminoglutamic acid excretion (27 days) and hepatic 5,10-methylenetetrahydrofolic acid reductase levels (33 days). Three animals per group. Bar graphs represent mean ± standard deviation.

tion rate, and those groups that have the highest percentage of tetrahydrofolate also have the highest rate of histidine oxidation.

Since methyltetrahydrofolate is formed from methylenetetrahydrofolate by methylenetetrahydrofolate reductase, it seemed of interest to investigate hepatic levels of this enzyme. The results of this study, presented in FIGURE 2, show that thyroidectomy decreases the level of methylenetetrahydrofolate reductase by 65% and that the feeding of thyroid powder increases this enzyme by ca. 50%. The figure also shows that the levels of methylenetetrahydrofolate reductase in the different groups correspond closely with the level of FIGlu excretion. This decrease in methylenetetrahydrofolate reductase produced by thyroidectomy is consistent with the decreased level of methyltetrahydrofolate found in thyroidectomized animals.

A more extensive study was carried out, in which the effect of thyroxine on three enzymes involved in folate metabolism was examined. Methionine synthetase was studied, since an increase in this enzyme might be expected to increase the level of methionine. Formiminotransferase was measured because this is the first folate-dependent enzyme involved in the degradation of FIGlu. The results, presented in TABLE 2, show that thyroidectomy and thiouracil feeding were equally effective in increasing histidine oxidation to ca. 30% from the intact control level of 4.5%. Feeding of thyroid powder decreased histidine oxidation to 0.6%. Injection of 2.5 μg T4 per day to thyroidectomized animals lowered histidine oxidation to 7.5%, which is a little above the control level. This indicates that this amount was not quite sufficient to normalize histidine oxidation. However, this is in general agreement with previous reports that ca. 2.5 μg T4 per day are required to restore a thyroidectomized rat to the euthyroid state.[19]

TABLE 2

EFFECTS OF HYPER- AND HYPOTHYROID STATES ON HISTIDINE OXIDATION AND HEPATIC LEVELS OF METHYLENE-THF REDUCTASE, METHIONINE SYNTHETASE, AND FORMIMINOTRANSFERASE
(Relative Values Intact Control = 100*)

Type of Rat and Supplement	Number of Survivors	Histidine Oxidation (% in 3 hours)	Methylene-THF Reductase (nmol/hour/g)	Methionine Synthetase (nmol/hour/g)	Formimino-transferase (μmol/hour/g)
Intact Rats (Control)	5	4.5 ± 0.3	100 ± 16 (519)†	100 ± 10 (381)†	100 ± 7 (267)†
TU‡	5	29.4 ± 6.0	73 ± 9	290 ± 31	155 ± 16
TU‡ + 20 mg T4§	5	4.0 ± 1.0	181 ± 18	298 ± 27	109 ± 8
TU‡ + thyroid powder¶	3	1.3 ± 0.2	198 ± 39	149 ± 45	82 ± 8
Thyroid powder¶	4	0.6 ± 0.2	180 ± 36	130 ± 19	91 ± 10
Thyroidectomy	6	29.8 ± 5.0	48 ± 7	170 ± 10	170 ± 12
+ 2.5 μg T4 per day‖	6	7.5 ± 0.5	86 ± 8	161 ± 12	101 ± 8

* Values ± standard error of the mean (SEM).
† Absolute enzyme levels in intact controls. Enzyme activity per g of wet tissue.
‡ 1 g thiouracil per kg diet.
§ 20 mg thyroxine (T4) per kg diet.
¶ 3 g thyroid powder per kg diet.
‖ 5 μg T4 injected every other day.

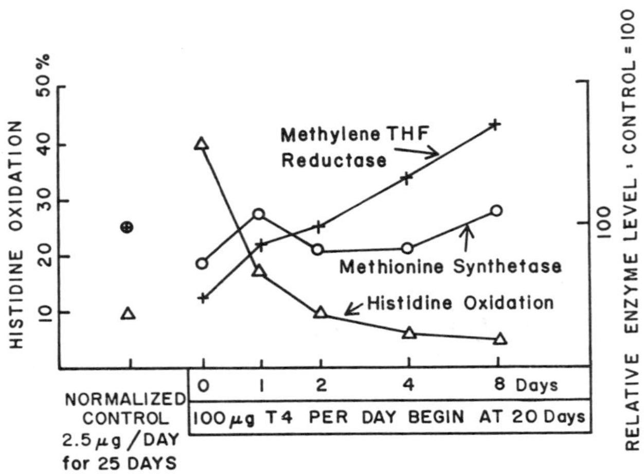

FIGURE 3. Time study of effect of thyroxine injection to thyroidectomized animals on histidine metabolism, methylenetetrahydrofolate reductase, and methionine synthetase. Six animals in each group.

Thyroidectomy reduced methylenetetrahydrofolate reductase to 48% of the control value, while thiouracil decreased it to 73% of the control. In other studies, however, thiouracil produced about the same reduction of this enzyme as did thyroidectomy. Similar increases in reductase activity by administration of thyroxine have been observed by Finkelstein *et al.*[20] The production of a hyperthyroid state either by giving 3 g thyroid powder per kg diet or 20 mg T4 in the diet (equivalent to 200 μg T4 per day) increased methylenetetrahydrofolate reductase to supranormal levels (180–198%). This is consistent with the very low oxidation rate (0.6%) observed with thyroid powder, and with the elevated levels of methyltetrahydrofolate in the liver (FIGURE 1). Both thyroidectomy and thiouracil increased methionine synthetase. However, the feeding of 20 mg of T4 did not lower these to normal levels even though histidine oxidation returned to normal. The feeding of thyroid powder in the

TABLE 3

EFFECT OF METHIMAZOLE ON HISTIDINE OXIDATION AND METHYLENETETRAHYDROFOLATE REDUCTASE IN LIVER*

Group	Treatment† (supplement per kg diet)	Body Weight and Survivors (N) at 22 Days (g)	Histidine Oxidation (%)	Methylene-THF Reductase in Liver (μmol/ hour/g tissue)
1	None	131 (4)	0.8 ± 0.1	711 ± 32
2	0.1 g Methimazole	100 (5)	3.1 ± 0.7	839 ± 62
3	0.3 g Methimazole	96 (5)	6.8 ± 0.4	417 ± 29
4	1.0 g Methimazole	87 (5)	16.6 ± 2.4	168 ± 16
5	Thyroidectomized	74 (3)	20.5 ± 5.7	215 ± 16

* Values = Mean ± SEM.

† Five intact weanling rats were used in Groups 1–4 and four thyroidectomized animals of the same age in Group 5.

presence of thiouracil did decrease methionine synthetase to 149% of control but not quite to the normal level. Although the increase in methionine synthetase occurring in thyroidectomy and with thiouracil is consistent with an increased histidine oxidation, the normalization of histidine oxidation by T4 without reduction of methionine synthetase levels suggests that the change in methionine synthetase is not a dominant factor in influencing histidine oxidation. Also, the failure of thyroid powder to depress methionine synthetase to below normal level shows that changes in this enzyme cannot account for the action of thyroid powder in depressing histidine oxidation below normal. The effects of hypo- and hyperthyroidism on formiminotransferase are consistent with their observed effects on histidine oxidation. Thyroidectomy and thiouracil feeding increased formiminotransferase respectively to 150 and 170% of that for the controls. Thyroid powder depressed formiminotransferase to slightly below normal (82% and 91% of control). It is interesting to note that 20 mg of T4 in the presence of thiouracil normalized formininotransferase, while it did not normalize methionine synthetase.

A time study was made, in which thyroidectomized animals were treated with 100 μg of T4 per day beginning at 20 days after being placed on the experimental diet. A normalized control group consisted of thyroidectomized animals that received 2.5 μg T4 per day for 25 days. Enzyme levels of these euthyroid normalized animals were used as the control (relative value = 100). These results, shown in FIGURE 3, show that histidine oxidation—which was 40% in thyroidectomized animals at 20 days—decreased to the normal level of ca. 10% by the end of the second day of T4 treatment. After 8 days, histidine oxidation had dropped to approximately half the normal level. Methylenetetrahydrofolate reductase levels increased to normal by 2 days, which is the same time at which histidine oxidation became normal. Methionine synthetase, on the other hand, did not change significantly in this experiment and thus bore no consistent relationship to the observed changes in histidine oxidation. This time study further indicates that methylenetetrahydrofolate

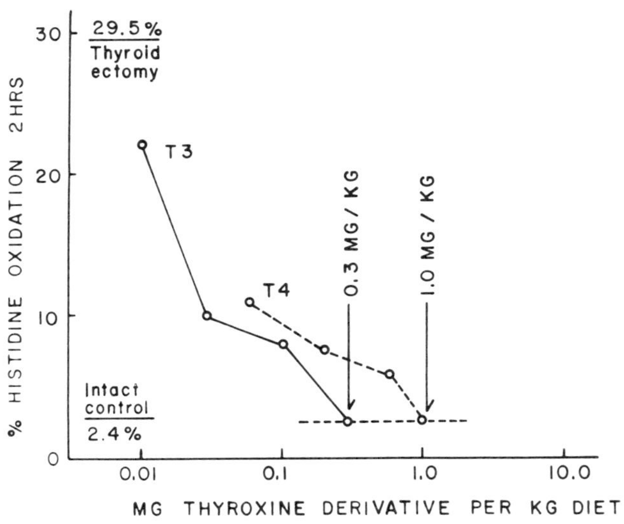

FIGURE 4. Effect of different levels of T3 and T4 in the diet on histidine oxidation in thyroidectomized rats. Time on diet, 23 days; six animals per group.

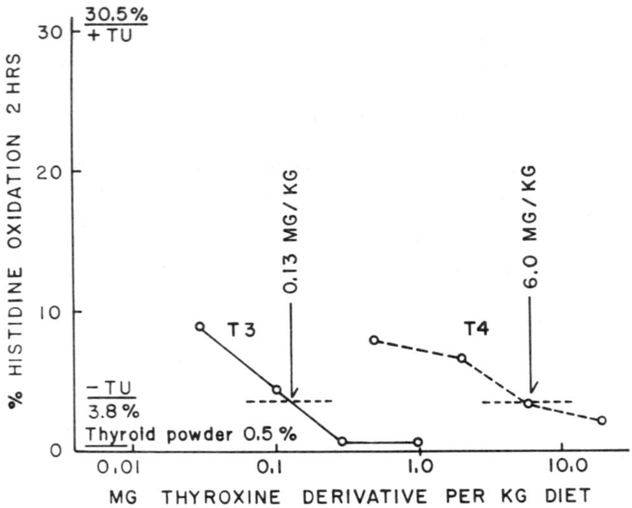

FIGURE 5. Effect of different levels of T3 and T4 in the diet on histidine oxidation in thiouracil-fed (1 g/kg diet) rats. Time on diet, 23 days; six animals per group.

reductase is the primary factor involved in the effect of thyroxine on histidine metabolism.

Methimazole was investigated because this compound inhibits thyroxine production by the thyroid but does not inhibit the extrathyroidal conversion of T4 to T3.[21] It can be seen in TABLE 3 that 1 g of this thyroid inhibitor per kg of diet increased histidine oxidation to approximately the same level (16.6%) as that produced by thyroidectomy (20.5%). Changes in methylenetetrahydrofolate reductase levels in the liver correspond to changes in histidine oxidation. Thus, 1 g of methimazole, which produced the maximum increases in histidine oxidation, also produced the lowest level of methylenetetrahydrofolate reductase. The level of 0.3 g of methimazole, which produced a ca. half-maximum effect on histidine oxidation, also effected ca. 50% of the maximum change in methylenetetrahydrofolate reductase level. This provides further evidence that changes in levels of this enzyme are responsible for the changes in histidine oxidation.

The effects of various levels of T3 and T4 on thyroidectomized animals and thiouracil-fed animals were investigated, since there is evidence that thiouracil inhibits extrathyroidal conversion of T4 to T3.[21,22] The results shown in FIGURE 4 compare the effects of varying levels of T3 and T4 in thyroidectomized rats. The response curves showed that ca. 0.3 mg of T3 and 1.0 mg of T4 (per kg diet) were required to reduce histidine oxidation to the normal level of 2.4%. When the activity of these two forms of thyroxine was compared in a diet containing thiouracil (FIGURE 5), it could be seen that 0.13 mg of T3 and 6 mg of T4 per kg of diet were required for normalization of histidine oxidation. The relative effects of T3 and T4 in these two conditions are summarized in TABLE 4. They are expressed both in the amounts required per mg per kg of diet and approximately as μg consumed per animal per day. This estimate is based on an average feed consumption of 10 g per 100 g of body weight per day. It can be seen that in thyroidectomized animals, T3 is approximately 3 times as effective as T4, while in the presence of thiouracil, T3 is approximately 50 times as active as T4. This may be compared with the report of Stasili

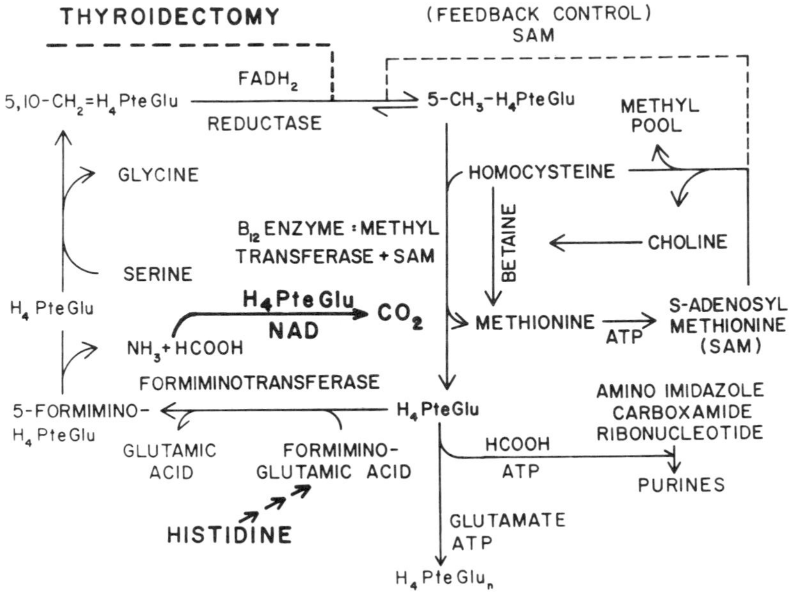

FIGURE 6. Metabolic chart of folate-dependent reactions showing possible sites of thyroxine intervention.

et al., which notes that when T3 and T4 were compared on their calorigenic activity, T3 was 8 times as active as T4, but when compared on a diet containing thiouracil, T3 was 50 times as active as T4.[23]

The ability of 20 mg of T4 in the presence of thiouracil to (a) normalize histidine oxidation, (b) elevate methylenetetrahydrofolate reductase to supranormal levels, but (c) have no effect in reducing methionine synthetase suggests that T4 (without prior conversion to T3) may be active in regulating the reductase but inactive in regulating methionine synthetase.

The main folate-dependent reactions involved in the regulation of forms of folate coenzymes and the metabolism of histidine are shown in FIGURE 6. This shows how the level of methyltetrahydrofolate may be reduced either by inhibition of methylenetetrahydrofolate reductase by SAM (derived from methionine) or by reduction in the level of enzyme by thyroidectomy. While increases in formiminotransferase produced by thyroidectomy might be expected to facilitate FIGlu

TABLE 4

AMOUNTS OF T3 AND T4 REQUIRED TO ACHIEVE EUTHYROID STATE AS MEASURED BY NORMALIZATION OF HISTIDINE OXIDATION

Type of Hypothyroidism	mg/kg diet		μg/day*	
	T3	T4	T3	T4
Thyroidectomized	0.3	1.0	3	10
Thiouracil-fed	0.13	6.0	1.3	60

* Estimated on basis of 10 g food intake per day for 100-g rat.

degradation, there is little evidence to indicate the significance of this factor compared to the effects produced by changes in methylenetetrahydrofolate reductase. The effects of hyperthyroidism in producing supranormal levels of this enzyme, which would increase hepatic levels of methyltetrahydrofolate, can account at least in part for the symptoms of pseudo-B_{12} deficiency that appear in thyrotoxicosis.

References

1. Erschoff, B. H. 1949. Proc. Soc. Exp. Biol. Med. **71:** 209–211.
2. Betheil, J. J. & H. A. Lardy. 1949. J Nutr. **37:** 495–509.
3. Register, U. D., W. R. Ruegamer & C. A. Elvehjem. 1949. J. Biol. Chem. **177:** 129–134.
4. Lewis, U. J., D. U. Tappan, U. D. Register & C. A. Elvehjem. 1950. Proc. Soc. Exp. Biol. Med. **74:** 568–571.
5. Stokstad, E. L. R., R. S. Webb & E. Shah. 1966. Proc. Soc. Exp. Biol. Med. **123:** 752–754.
6. O'Dell, A. & E. L. R. Stokstad. 1967. J. Nutr. **92:** 127–132.
7. Batra, K. K., K. U. Buehring & E. L. R. Stokstad. 1974. Proc. Soc. Exp. Biol. Med. **147:** 72–79.
8. Lindenbaum, J. & F. A. Klipstein. 1964. J. Clin. Pathol. **17:** 666–670.
9. Mohamed, S. D. & M. Roberts. 1965. Lancet **2:** 933–935.
10. Tabor, H. & L. Wyngarden. 1958. J. Clin. Invest. **37:** 824–828.
11. Jeffay, H. & J. Alvarez. 1961. Anal. Chem. **33:** 612–615.
12. Kutzbach, C. & E. L. R. Stokstad. 1967. Biochim. Biophys. Acta **139:** 217–220.
13. Sauer, H. J. & L. Jaenicke. 1972. Klin. Wochenschr. **50:** 986–990.
14. Narisawa, K., T. Tamura, K. Tanno, K. Ohara & T. Arakawa. 1968. Tohoku J. Exp. Med. **94:** 417–430.
15. Davidson, G. E., D. G. Weir & J. M. Scott. 1975. Biochim. Biophys. Acta **392:** 207–215.
16. Noronha, J. M. & M. Silverman. 1962. J. Biol. Chem. **237:** 3299–3302.
17. Kutzbach, C. & E. L. R. Stokstad. 1967. Biochim. Biophys. Acta **139:** 217–220.
18. Kutzbach, C. & E. L. R. Stokstad. 1971. Biochim. Biophys. Acta **250:** 459–477.
19. Reineke, E. P., J. P. Mixner & C. W. Turner. 1945. Endocrinology **36:** 64–67.
20. Finkelstein, J. D., J. J. Martin, W. E. Kyle & J. B. Harris. 1978. Arch. Biochem. Biophys. **191:** 153–160.
21. Laurberg, P. & J. Weeke. 1978. Acta Endocrinol. Copenhagen **87:** 88–94.
22. Escobar del Rey, F. & G. Morreale de Escobar. 1961. Endocrinology **69:** 456–465.
23. Stasili, N. R., R. P. Kroc & R. Edlin. 1960. Endocrinology **66:** 872–885.
24. Chan, M. M.-S. & E. L. R. Stokstad. 1980. Biochim. Biophys. Acta **632:** 244–253.

Discussion

A. B. Eisenstein (*Veterans Administration Medical Center, Brooklyn, N.Y.*): There are several types of anemia that are found in clinical cases of hyperthyroidism. One of them is pernicious anemia. Is that explained by the mechanisms you described?

E. L. R. Stokstad: My understanding is no, because pernicious anemia may be produced by an autoimmune disease that also causes hyperthyroidism. The anemia here would be mainly the result of the vitamin B_{12} deficiency in pernicious anemia rather than of the hyperthyroidism. The anemia I was referring to is that case where there was hyperthyroidism but no evidence of B_{12} deficiency.

C. G. King (*Kennett Square, Penn.*): How are we getting on in the practical accomplishments of keeping the American population supplied with sufficient iodine?

We've had little trouble along the seacoast. We've had very severe trouble through the northern part of our population. Thyroid was a common epidemic, and we brought in iodized salt. Some people think that is dangerous, very few people do. But some people don't take iodized salt because they don't know enough to do it. What is the state of our population now? Are we in good balance?

E. L. R. STOKSTAD: I heard recently that there is a problem with too much iodine being consumed in the diet. This was not due to iodization of salt but rather due to the use of periodates in food formulation, such as in baking. When one adds up all the sources of iodine exclusive of iodized salt, there are cases where there is evidence of an excess iodine intake. Now I don't know how serious the problem is, but apparently there are some individuals who do have a higher intake of iodine than the RDA [recommended dietary allowance] would call for.

C. G. KING: Is there any physician in the audience that would like to comment on that?

UNIDENTIFIED SPEAKER: The evidence is substantial that the average daily intake of iodide and iodine in the U.S. population is several times the RDA at the present time. The American Medical Association Council of Foods and Nutrition sponsored a meeting several months ago examining the question of iodine levels in the U.S. population, and a forthcoming statement will represent a consensus opinion of this group.

I might mention that the greatest single source of iodine intake at the present time is dairy products, which probably arises from the supplementation of feed to dairy cows.

It's somewhat ironic that in the 1920s, we were very concerned about inadequate iodide intake in the U.S. population. As you correctly observed, salt was iodized with a great benefit to the population, especially in those areas where food did not naturally contain iodine, such as our so-called goiter belt and parts of Switzerland. But there is some concern among thyroid specialists that the balance might now be starting to tip the other way.

MICROELEMENT INTERACTIONS OF ZINC, COPPER, AND IRON IN MAMMALIAN SPECIES

George K. Davis

Nutrition Laboratory
University of Florida
Gainesville, Florida 32611

Basic evidence for the routes by which copper and iron, or copper and zinc, or zinc, copper, and iron interact biochemically in mammalian species, including humans, has been slow in accumulating.

From a practical standpoint, it was recognized that anemia developed in animals maintained on an exclusively milk diet; and Hart and coworkers demonstrated that copper additions to the diet prevented the anemia or enabled the animals to synthesize hemoglobin by utilizing the iron that was added to the diet.[1]

The copper toxicity that developed in pigs on high copper levels—given to increase growth performance—was shown by Suttle and Mills to be in part due to an increased requirement for zinc and iron.[2,3]

This apparent interaction of these micronutrients has led to a consideration of the ways in which the interaction may occur biochemically in the living animal. Obviously, the first location in which interaction can occur is the food. The food compounds that are consumed, which have been formed naturally or during processing, may influence the relative availability of the elements. This type of interaction may continue within the lumen of the gastrointestinal tract.

A second location of interaction may be during the process of absorption with competition for binding sites on transport compounds or with action that limits the absorptive capacity of the intestinal mucosal cells.

A third possibility may be that the elements interact either synergistically or antagonistically within the cells of the various organs of the body by promoting or inhibiting reactions that involve the different elements. Since the trace elements appear to exert their metabolic function as part of larger molecules and commonly as part of enzyme systems, the interaction of the elements may be complementary as a result of coordination of cell functions or adverse as a result of interference or substitution in the enzyme structure with resulting altered function.

The transport systems of the body provide additional locations for the elements to interact. Transport mechanisms for one element may involve compounds of another element, or there may be competition for the binding sites by the different elements. Since most metabolic functions are sequential or cyclic, interaction of the elements may be present at various points in the cycle.

Interaction may occur at the site of the target organs or cells at which compounds of the elements exert necessary metabolic functions.

Finally, the interactions may occur during the catabolic phases of metabolism, leading to excretion of the elements with resulting stimulation and acceleration of excretion or, conversely, to suppression of excretion with abnormal storage of the elements.

To add to the complexity of the problem of trace element interaction, Dr. Frieden has suggested that in studies of the interactions of the elements copper, zinc, and iron, many factors may influence the observations that result from the experiments.[4]

0077-8923/80/0355-0130 $01.75/0

1. There are species differences in response.
2. There are individual differences that are genetic.
3. Various compounds of the elements function differently.
4. There are interactions with organic compounds and with other elements.
5. Environmental conditions can affect response.
6. Stage of maturity of the animal can have an effect.
7. Sex differences are often important.
8. The presence of subclinical disease must be considered as a possible factor.
9. The route of exposure to the elements can influence response.
10. Recycling of the elements can influence apparent reaction of the animal to external sources.

These complex interrelationships have made it understandably difficult to establish, with confidence, the interactions that occur among the three elements, zinc, copper, and iron, which are all known to be essential for normal nutrition and metabolism and which have all been identified as having been involved in specific biochemical reactions.

There is no question but that the interaction of iron and copper in hematopoiesis is an obvious one. However, although the pioneering observations were made about 50 years ago and have been confirmed many times since, knowledge concerning the mechanism of the iron-copper interaction still remains to be completely explained.

Gastrointestinal Interactions of Copper, Zinc, and Iron

In normal situations, the requirement for the three metal ions is such that interaction or interference within the gastrointestinal tract reflects the fact that normally the transport mechanism(s) is not completely saturated and that, therefore, adequate binding sites are available for all of the required copper, iron, and zinc.

The early observation that copper was required for normal iron metabolism—and the observation that with a copper deficiency, iron accumulated in the mucosal cells of the intestine as well as in the liver—did not show clearly that iron and copper use a common transport mechanism in the absorption from the gastrointestinal tract.

El-Shobaki and Rummel have noted that copper is preferentially bound to transferrin in the mucosa when compared with iron, so that when iron and copper are administered in excess, iron absorption is inhibited because of the affinity of copper for transferrin.[5] On the other hand, they report that copper is preferentially tied to metallothionein as compared with transferrin. This suggests, of course, that in iron deficiency, copper is taken up in greater proportion by the duodenal mocosa but that transfer to the body tissues is inhibited with the much lower proportion being transferred. These authors also report that copper in excess, approximately 10 times the requirement, inhibits iron absorption because of the affinity of copper to transferrin and that this may be partly responsible for the inhibitory effect of copper on iron absorption.

While copper is necessary for the normal utilization of iron by mammalian species, increasing copper in the diet to toxic or potentially toxic levels has been used as a technique to demonstrate the interaction between copper and zinc and iron. When Suttle and Mills fed to pigs rations containing from 0 to 750 parts per million (ppm) of copper, the higher level resulted in the development of signs of toxicity with jaundice.[2] However, with the addition of 500 ppm of zinc or 750 ppm of iron to the diets containing 750 ppm of copper, the jaundice was eliminated and serum copper and aspartate transaminase values returned to levels similar to those of the control animals. The iron was necessary for the protection against anemia.

Later experiments demonstrated that addition of 150 ppm of zinc and 150 ppm of iron to diets containing 250 ppm or more of copper eliminated all signs of the copper toxicosis that developed when the zinc and iron supplements were not added. This suggested that the signs of copper toxicity that developed in pigs given 250 ppm of copper as a growth stimulant were actually due to the interference of copper with zinc and iron utilization.[3]

Other studies have confirmed these findings and demonstrated that the addition of zinc and iron counteracts the effect of high copper levels in the diet apparently through reduction of absorption, since accumulation in the liver is sharply reduced when zinc and iron are added with the copper to the diet.[6]

There have been many studies in which various levels of iron, copper, and zinc have been administered to different species; they indicate that either very high or very low levels of any of these elements have an influence on the metabolism and utilization of the other two.

Thus, when excessive oral iron was administered to sheep, i.e., levels of 350, 1,000, or 1,750 mg/kg dry concentrate, the iron in the spleen, liver, kidney, and ribs was greatly increased, with most increase evident in the liver and spleen. The copper and zinc were reduced, especially copper in the liver and zinc in the kidneys.[7]

Zinc has been noted to reduce copper absorption in dairy calves, in sheep, in Japanese quail, and in horses, but there does seem to be considerable species, and perhaps even individual, variation.[8-11]

Zinc added at 100 ppm to a diet for horses caused a significant decrease in copper retention, while zinc retention was significantly increased.[11]

While there is some evidence that zinc interferes with absorption and metabolism because of a competition for binding sites on transferrin, the effect of zinc on copper in a competition for binding sites, particularly with metallothionein, would seem to be a more usual site of competition. High levels of zinc—by depressing copper or by causing a functional copper deficiency—would result in poor utilization of iron, with resulting anemia.

As early as 1958, Grant-Frost and Underwood reported that zinc toxicity anemia apparently was due to a creation of a copper deficiency.[12] They noted that the addition of zinc to an otherwise adequate diet for rats markedly reduced the growth, food consumption, hemoglobin levels, copper retention, and body fat content of rats; they had added 0.5% zinc as the oxide. This confirmed earlier work by Van Reen, who had noted that the addition of 0.5 to 0.7% zinc as the carbonate to a diet containing 8 ppm of copper reduced the growth, food consumption, and hemoglobin levels in young rats and produced a marked reduction in liver catalase and cytochrome oxidase activities.[13] Feeding of additional copper at the rate of 0.2 or 0.4 mg daily as the sulfate maintained the liver catalase and cytochrome oxidase activity of the zinc-fed rats at normal levels, but had no effect on the reduced growth of the animals caused by the excess zinc.

Grant-Frost and Underwood concluded that the depressing effect of zinc on growth was due largely, if not entirely, to the reduced food consumption that they believed was due to unpalatability of the diet.[12] They proposed that the anemia caused by zinc was due to an induced copper deficiency that resulted in reduced copper and copper concentrations in the blood and tissues. Probably the high zinc not only reduced copper absorption but also had an antagonistic effect upon absorbed copper, further intensifying the copper deficiency.

It has been suggested that high levels of zinc affect iron metabolism in two ways:

(1) zinc may affect ferritin such that the incorporation of iron into or release from ferritin is impaired; (2) zinc may impair iron absorption and limit the storage of iron as ferritin. High levels of zinc also cause a shortened life span of the red blood cells, resulting in a faster turnover of iron.[14]

Workers at Pennsylvania State University have investigated the effect of levels of zinc in the maternal diet on the zinc, iron, and copper content of the postnatal rat when high levels of the elements were fed during gestation and lactation.[15] Diets containing 0.2%, 0.5%, and 9 ppm of zinc were fed to adult female rats beginning at age 0 of the fetus and continuing through the 14th day of lactation. Total zinc and zinc concentrations were elevated in the newborn and 14-day-old young by both high zinc diets. The mothers given high zinc diets had young with significantly less total body iron and concentration of iron but with livers containing significantly more iron. Copper and copper concentration levels in the whole animal body were not altered due to the high zinc levels. The copper in liver was significantly lower only in the newborn from mothers fed the 0.5% zinc levels in the diet. When animals were analyzed after 14 days of lactation, total copper and concentrations of copper were significantly lower in the whole animal body and in the liver of the young from mothers fed either high level of zinc in the diet as compared with those from mothers on the basal diet. This suggested that the young were receiving both a low copper intake and a high level of zinc from the dams' milk.

Grant-Frost and Underwood noted that the effect of zinc is to increase the excretion of absorbed copper, but they also noted that the timing and the form of copper supplementation may be of considerable significance.[12] The copper that they added entered the alimentary tract at a time when the tract was relatively free of zinc, and the copper could have been absorbed before any effect of zinc on copper availability at the absorption site occurred. They suggest that besides reducing copper absorption, there is an indication—from the low blood and tissue copper concentrations and amounts—that zinc also had an effect on copper at the cellular level. The zinc toxic animal was unlikely to utilize its copper reserves because of an antagonistic effect of the zinc absorbed from the diet.

Support for the observation that nursing young are influenced by the zinc and copper content of the diet of the dam because of the influence upon the trace element content of the milk comes from Kirchgessner and associates, who, working with dairy cows, observed that the copper, iron, and zinc contents of milk and serum were interrelated.[16] A deficiency of zinc at 6 mg/kg of dry feed, which was later supplemented by providing an extra allowance of zinc, demonstrated that there was a close connection between zinc and copper in the milk. With a deficiency, zinc level of milk was decreased and copper was increased. However, when zinc was added as a supplement, zinc in the milk increased and copper decreased. The negative correlation was apparent more in the milk than in the serum, where the level of serum zinc reflected the level of dietary zinc but the copper levels were not changed. Under the conditions of these experiments, the iron in serum and milk showed no correlation to the zinc supply.

The relationship between zinc and iron was recognized early by workers at North Carolina State University, where they examined the effect of excess zinc on the induction of rat liver ferritin synthesis *in vivo*.[17] Coleman and Matrone presented evidence that in high zinc-fed rats, the amount of ferritin was about one-third that found in rats fed a normal zinc diet. The excess dietary zinc resulted in the formation of an "iron poor ferritin."[17] Zinc toxicity did not appear to interfere with the incorporation of amino acids into the ferritin. There was some suggestion that the turnover rate of ferritin iron and ferritin protein in the zinc-fed rats may have been faster than in rats fed the control diet.

The interest in transport mechanisms as a factor in zinc and copper interrelations and their interrelation with iron has resulted in a very considerable examination of the formation of metallothionein.

There is evidence that copper stimulates the synthesis of the metallothioneins that bind copper and zinc and that when zinc is deficient in the diet, there is an increased ratio of copper to zinc in the thioneins of the liver.[18]

Evans and Johnson suggest that it is the metallothioneins that regulate the passage of copper through the intestinal cells.[19] They noted that in the mucosa, cytosol copper is bound to the metallothionein and that therefore the metallothionein would appear to have a function similar to that for zinc transfer.

There are many factors that may influence the interaction of copper, zinc, and iron in the intestine—including the presence of organic molecules; other elements, such as calcium, that influence the pH; compounds of the elements themselves that are presented for absorption from the intestine; and the sequential or concurrent offering of the trace elements. These three elements, which have vital functions that are both independent and interrelated, interact in the intestine primarily insofar as they have common binding sites on transport compounds. Consequently, the interaction at this level of metabolism is demonstrated when one or more of the elements is present in the diet at excessive or deficient levels.

There is some indication that copper and iron compete for binding sites on transferrin, with copper being preferentially bound. On the other hand, it would appear that copper stimulates the formation of thionein(s) and that copper is preferentially bound to metallothionein rather than to transferrin.

Zinc also would appear to be bound to transferrin and, with excess zinc in the diet, may compete with iron and depress iron absorption or, more exactly, iron transfer from the mucosal cells. Zinc also appears to be tied to metallothionein and to compete with copper for binding sites on the protein(s), interfering with copper absorption.

It is interesting that if the ratios of copper, iron, and zinc are maintained at approximately the ratios of the requirement levels for normal nutrition, then the absolute amounts of the elements in the diet can vary over rather wide ranges. Absolute amounts absorbed may vary, but the ratios of the elements absorbed will not be significantly different from that observed with requirement levels.[2,9,13,19]

Postabsorption Metabolism

It must be obvious that in the absorption of copper, zinc, and iron, there appear to be several mechanisms for the absorption of these elements, and the interaction or antagonism probably occurs in specific pathways rather than in all pathways. One of the ways in which zinc affects iron metabolism is the action of zinc on the incorporation of iron into or its release from ferritin. In addition, high levels of zinc seem to shorten the life span of red blood cells, resulting in a faster turnover of iron.[14]

Although there are many hundreds of papers reporting the analysis of various tissues for copper, zinc, and iron, information on the interrelationship of these elements after absorption from the gastrointestinal tract is quite limited in terms of biochemical pathways in which the interactions may occur.

Lower values of copper are found in the liver and other tissues when high levels of zinc are made available in the diet, and it may be suggested that this is a result of the interference with copper. Reduced zinc levels found in various tissues may be a function of the effect of copper on zinc absorption and transfer from the intestinal mucosa. In the case of iron, the relationship between copper and iron, early noted as related to hematopoiesis, has been more thoroughly explored; and the role of ceruloplasmin, as a copper protein functioning as a ferroxidase, has been extensively explored. Although there appears to be some competition between zinc and copper for metallothionein, intravenous injection of copper will result in a copper-induced metallothionein that will also bind zinc. An interaction also occurs in the enzyme superoxide dismutase, which contains both copper and zinc. There is the suggestion that high levels of copper in the diet may be reflected by high levels of copper in the liver, with consequent suppression of the zinc levels. Conversely, high levels of zinc in the diet may result in high levels of zinc in the liver, with depression of copper and therefore a depressed synthesis of ceruloplasmin.

However, the published research clearly demonstrating the interaction between zinc and copper postabsorption is very limited.

The evidence for a function of ceruloplasmin in converting ferrous iron to ferric iron and in the release of the iron so that it may be incorporated into the hemoglobin molecule appears to be reasonably well established, although observations with Wilson's disease suggest that this should not exclude the possibility of an alternate pathway in iron metabolism.[20] Hsieh and Frieden have convincingly advanced evidence for the role of ceruloplasmin in the release of iron from ferritin and conversion to transferrin, with the subsequent movement of ferrous iron to heme and the formation of hemoglobin.[21] It is certain that ceruloplasmin plays an important role in the transfer of iron from the reticuloendothelial cells to plasma. It is probable that the same or a similar mechanism may be the mechanism whereby iron is released from the duodenal mucosal cells and from hepatic parenchymal cells. This would account for the defective iron absorption in copper deficiency. Reduced levels of ceruloplasmin accompanying the copper deficiency would also account for the buildup of iron in the mucosa and in the hepatic cells of the copper-deficient animal.

Although it seems clear that ceruloplasmin is required and does function with respect to the release and incorporation of iron from and into cells and various compounds, the actual way in which it accomplishes this still is uncertain. This pathway has been presented in detail by Frieden and Osaki and the group at Florida State University.[22]

Summary

Practical nutrition and experimental investigations have demonstrated that diets that are either deficient in or contain excessive levels of zinc, iron, or copper will cause changes in the absorption of the other elements from the gastrointestinal tract and that as a result, the tissues of the mammalian species under observation will show distortion of the normal zinc-iron or copper composition and consequent aberrations of the metabolism of the animal.

The great bulk of the published literature has demonstrated that a high level of zinc will cause a depression of iron and copper, especially when the intakes of the copper and iron are marginal or below normal requirements. A high level of copper will cause a depression of zinc, but a high level of iron in the diet will have a much less marked effect on zinc and copper. A deficiency of copper will result in an increased concentration of iron in the mucosal cells and in the liver, with a decrease in hematopoiesis that now appears to be the result of lowered ceruloplasmin resulting from unavailability of sufficient copper for incorporation into this ferroxidase.

There is abundant evidence from published analyses of animals and tissues that the content of zinc, iron, and copper can be greatly altered by many different factors, ranging from the composition of the diet and the compounds of the elements in the diet to environmental changes, including the influence of clinical or subclinical disease.

Good evidence has been presented that the interaction of zinc, copper, and iron in absorption from the gastrointestinal tract is primarily a competition for binding sites on transferrin and the metallothioneins.

The evidence for postabsorption interactions is strong in that the copper protein ceruloplasmin is essential for the release of iron from ferritin, for iron incorporation into transferrin, and for the subsequent release to the heme molecule in the formation of hemoglobin.

It is well known that zinc and copper function together as part of the enzyme superoxide dismutase and that the activity of this enzyme is dependent on the presence of four atoms of the metals per molecule of enzyme.[23,24]

In an attempt to explain the apparent interaction of the trace elements, workers at North Carolina State University examined the chemical parameters of many of the trace elements and pointed out the similarities that enabled the elements to compete for common metabolic sites.[25] Excessive levels of any single element can have the effect of preventing the other elements from obtaining those sites, with resulting distortion of metabolism. The common observation that this distortion can be ameliorated if the other elements are increased in the diet emphasizes that the adverse interaction, which has been reported numerous times, is most conveniently demonstrated when one or another of the elements is present in the diet in deficient or excessive quantities.

The experience of investigators is that if the quantities of the trace elements zinc, copper, and iron are increased in proportion to their normal requirements, the adverse interactions are much less apparent, if they occur at all.

It has been demonstrated numerous times that under normal dietary conditions, the binding sites for transport of the trace elements are far from completely saturated, so that the direct competition for these sites is not a significant factor in the interaction of the elements.

However, it must be evident that since these elements all have vital functions, distortions of the levels of any one of them will result in adverse changes in the others. The biochemical changes that occur, either complementary or adverse, are still poorly understood and offer a fertile field for investigation.

References

1. Hart, E. B., H. Steenbock, J. Waddell & C. A. Elvehjem. 1928. Iron in nutrition. VII. Copper as a supplement to iron for hemoglobin building in the rat. J. Biol. Chem. **77:** 797–812.
2. Suttle, N. F. & C. F. Mills. 1966. Studies of the toxicity of copper to pigs. 1. Effects of oral zinc and iron salts on the development of copper toxicosis. Br. J. Nutr. **20:** 135–148.
3. Suttle, N. F. & C. F. Mills. 1966. Studies of the toxicity of copper to pigs. 2. Effects of protein source and other dietary components on the response to high and moderate intakes of copper. Br. J. Nutr. **20:** 149–161.
4. Frieden, E. 1978. Modes of metal metabolism in mammals. *In* Trace Element Metabolism in Man and Animals. M. Kirchgessner, Ed. **3:** 8–14. Arbeitskreis fur Tierernahrungsforschung. Weihenstephan, Federal Republic of Germany.
5. El-Shobaki, F. L. & W. Rummel. 1979. Binding of copper to mucosal transferrin and inhibition of intestinal iron absorption in rats. Res. Exp. Med. **174:** 187–195.
6. DeGoey, L. W., R. C. Walstrom & R. J. Emerick. 1971. Studies of high level copper supplementation to rations for growing swine. J. Anim. Sci. **33:** 52–57.

7. GRUEN, M., M. ANKE, A. HENNIG, W. SEFFNER, M. PARLSSCHEFELD, G. FALCHOWSKY & B. GROPPEL. 1978. Excessive oral iron applications to sheep. 2. Effect of iron, copper, zinc and manganese contents in different organs. Arch. Tierernaehr. **28:** 341–347.
8. IVAN, M. & C. M. GRIEVE. 1976. Effects of zinc, copper and manganese supplementation of high concentrate rations on gastrointestinal absorption of copper and manganese in Holstein calves. J. Dairy Sci. **59:** 1764–1768.
9. BREMNER, I., B. W. YOUNG & C. F. MILLS. 1976. Protective effect of zinc supplementation against copper toxicosis in sheep. Br. J. Nutr. **36:** 551–561.
10. HAMILTON, R. P., M. R. S. FOX, B. E. FRY, JR., A. O. L. JONES & R. M. JACOBS. 1979. Zinc interference with copper, iron and manganese in the young Japanese quail. J. Food Sci. **44:** 738–741.
11. SPAIS, A. G., A. PAPASTERIADIS, N. ROUBIES, A. AGAINNIDES, N. YANTIS & S. ARGYROUDIS. 1978. Studies on iron, manganese, zinc, copper and selenium retention and interaction in horses. *In* Trace Element Metabolism in Man and Animals. M. Kirchgessner, Ed. **3:** 501–505. Arbeitskreis fur Tierernahrung. Weihenstephen, Federal Republic of Germany.
12. GRANT-FROST, D. R. & E. J. UNDERWOOD. 1958. Zinc toxicity in the rat and its interrelation with copper. Aust. J. Exp. Biol. Med. Sci. **36:** 339–346.
13. VAN REEN, R. 1953. Effects of excessive zinc in the rat and the interrelationship with copper. Arch. Biochem. Biophys. **46:** 337–344.
14. SETTLEMIRE, C. T. & G. MATRONE. 1967. *In vivo* effect of zinc on iron turnover in rats and life span of the erythrocyte. J. Nutr. **92:** 159–164.
15. KETCHESON, M. R., G. P. BARRON & D. H. COX. 1969. Relationship of maternal dietary zinc during gestation and lactation to development and zinc, iron and copper content of the post-natal rat. J. Nutr. **98:** 303–311.
16. KIRCHGESSNER, M., F. J. SCHWARZ, H. P. ROTH & W. A. SCHWARZ. 1978. Interactions between the trace elements zinc, copper and iron after zinc depletion in dairy cows. Arch. Tierernaehr. **28:** 723–733.
17. COLEMAN, C. B & G. MATRONE. 1969. *In vivo* effect of zinc on iron induced ferritin synthesis in rat liver. Biochim. Biophys. Acta **177:** 106–112.
18. HOEKSTRA, W. G., I. BREMNER & N. T. DAVIES. 1978. Effect of zinc status of rats on the synthesis and degradation of copper induced thioneins. *In* Trace Element Metabolism in Man and Animals. M. Kirchgessner, Ed. **3:** 52–56. Arbeitskreis fur Tierernahrsforschung. Weihenstephan, Federal Republic of Germany.
19. EVANS, G. W. & P. E. JOHNSON. 1978. Copper and zinc binding ligands in the intestinal mucosa. *In* Trace Element Metabolism in Man and Animals. M. Kirchgessner, Ed. **3:** 98–105. Arbeitskreis fur Tierernahrsungsforschung. Weihenstephan, Federal Republic of Germany.
20. LEE, G. R., D. M. WILLIAMS & G. E. CARTWRIGHT. 1976. Role of copper in iron metabolism and heme biosynthesis. *In* Trace Elements in Human Health and Disease. Zinc and Copper. A. S. Prasad, Ed. **1:** 373–390. Academic Press, Inc. New York, N.Y.
21. HSIEH, H. S. & E. FRIEDEN. 1975. Evidence for ceruloplasmin as a copper transport protein. Biochem. Biophys. Res. Commun. **67:** 1326–1331.
22. FRIEDEN, E. & S. OSAKI. 1973. Ferroxidases and ferrireductases: their role in iron metabolism. *In* Protein Metal Interactions. Advances in Experimental Medicine and Biology. M. Friedman, Ed. **48:** 235–265. Plenum Press. New York, N.Y.
23. FEE, J. A. & R. G. BRIGGS. 1975. Studies on the reconstitution of bovine erythrocyte superoxide dismutase. V. Preparation and properties of derivatives in which both zinc and copper sites contain copper. Biochim. Biophys. Acta **400:** 430–450.
24. RIGO, A., P. VIGLINO, M. BONORI, D. COCCO, L. CALABRESE & G. ROTILIO. 1978. The binding of copper ions to copper-free bovine superoxide dismutase. Kinetic aspects. Biochem. J. **169:** 277–280.
25. HILL, C. H., G. MATRONE, W. L. PAYNE & C. W. BARBER. 1963. *In vivo* interactions of cadmium with copper, zinc and iron. J. Nutr. **80:** 227–235.

DISCUSSION

E. L. R. STOKSTAD (*University of California, Berkeley, Calif.*): In the late 1950s, some people were adding 200 parts per million of copper sulfate to rations of swine to make them grow faster, based upon an idea similar to an antibiotic growth effect. Could this have been due to the fact that the copper was antagonizing zinc toxicity?

G. K. DAVIS: Dr. Stokstad, I think not, because I doubt very much that there were levels of zinc in the diet at that time that might have been considered an excess—more likely they were deficient. Certainly it was a big help to the swine industry when Dr. Suttle and Dr. Mills were able to show that if you added zinc and iron to the diet, you were able to have those high levels and still have the growth-promoting effect.

There is still a big debate in this country about the value of high copper diets because you don't always get that growth response. But I think it is more likely that that high level of copper has an effect on microorganisms and perhaps gets rid of the roundworms and a few other parasites.

I. BREMNER (*Rowett Research Institute, Bucksburn, Aberdeen, United Kingdom*): I got the impression you were suggesting that the decrease in copper absorption that you get in zinc-treated animals results from displacement of copper from metallothionein. I would suggest that this is the wrong explanation. The work that we have done shows that increasing the dietary zinc intake increases the amount of metallothionein present in the mucosa. We know that copper has a much higher binding affinity than zinc does for the protein, so that what we get is an increase in the amount of copper metallothionein in mucosa, and we have reason to suspect that this forms a type of mucosal block for copper absorption. The fact is that zinc, in essence, increases the amount of copper metallothionein, and it sticks there and isn't available for onward passage into the blood. I think this is the opposite of what you were suggesting.

G. K. DAVIS: Dr. Hoekstra, on his sabbatical in Rowett, demonstrated that when he injected some copper, he got a big increase in metallothionein as well. So that apparently both of these elements have the effect of increasing metallothionein, but it certainly is true that copper is not absorbed when you increase the zinc. Now, whether it is because of the competition for metallothionein or whether there is still a further biochemical transport mechanism that interferes, I'm interested in your comment.

I. BREMNER: I think we must be careful when we speak about induction of metallothionein synthesis by copper. What Bill Hoekstra did with Arden shows quite clearly that copper will induce synthesis in the liver and in the kidneys. No one has ever shown to my satisfaction that you get induction of metallothionein synthesis by copper in the mucosa. We have fed rats diets containing large amounts of copper, Bill has injected rats with copper, and in neither of these cases did we detect a significant increase in the amount of metallothionein in the gut.

G. K. DAVIS: Well, thank you.

J. M. NAVIA (*University of Alabama, Birmingham, Ala.*): I have a little comment with regard to interactions and a plea for the use of appropriate experimental design.

I think that interactions are a reality and that we have to detect them in the experiments we do. In the past, many times, we have done one-way designs and comparisons with two groups and things of this sort. But there are statistical procedures whereby you can do factorial designs and incomplete designs. And there are many different approaches whereby, once you recognize those different factors, you might use experiments where you might detect the main effect and the interactions of many of these factors. We can bring a lot of light once we identify those factors, if we use appropriate experimental designs in our research so that we can actually define and identify, and hopefully later on explain, those interactions.

G. K. DAVIS: I couldn't agree with you more.

E. L. R. STOKSTAD: I just wanted to mention another interaction of copper as a drug.

When I was at Lederle, we had a very good drug, but it was hemolytic. Using a crude diet, we got a normal hemoglobin. Using a purified diet, we got anemia with this drug, so I said that there is an unknown factor in the crude diet that will protect against anemia. We forgot to add copper to our purified diet, and the hemolytic drug simply increased the copper requirement to the point where we had a deficiency. I was wondering if you had ever seen any other cases where a hemolytic agent would increase the requirement for either iron or copper or other minerals involved in red cell formation.

G. K. DAVIS: Somewhat parallel to that, Dr. Stokstad, we have noted that there are frequently present in diets what we've called chelating agents, which have tied up copper to the point where it is no longer available, and this is particularly true of young, growing grass. We have noted that, often, the grass juices that we have expressed were so tightly combined with the copper that the animals fed the expressed juices were not able to, shall I say, hydrolyze the compound(s) and therefore absorb the copper. We actually created a copper deficiency by giving what appeared to be fresh, nutritious grass. This effect disappeared when the grass was mature. I think that the people at the Rowett Institute have also demonstrated that the cured forage does not have this property whereas the fresh forage does.

L. HOWARD (*Albany Medical College, Albany, N.Y.*): It is not clear to me at this point how much of the copper-iron interaction is mediated through ceruloplasmin. I wanted to ask you whether we know what happens to iron absorption and iron transport and iron incorporation in people who have Wilson's disease and have very low ceruloplasmin.

G. K. DAVIS: I think I mentioned that this is the exception to this little story about ceruloplasmin, and I have mentioned in my manuscript that there seems to be no question that this is not the whole story. There must be other mechanisms that are not as efficient as is ceruloplasmin because we know that in Wilson's disease, you do have a problem with copper accumulation.

L. HOWARD: What happens to iron absorption?

G. K. DAVIS: Well, it is absorbed, it is utilized; but we say with Dr. Frieden and Oski and others that this is not the whole story because obviously in Wilson's disease, you must have another mechanism.

INTERACTIONS OF COPPER AND ZINC IN CARDIOVASCULAR DISEASE

Leslie M. Klevay

Human Nutrition Laboratory
U.S. Department of Agriculture
Science and Education Administration
Grand Forks, North Dakota 58202

There are many examples in nutrition of the requirement for a nutrient being partially dependent on the amount of another nutrient in the diet. Amino acid imbalances provided my introduction to this topic.[1] Macronutrients, such as fat or carbohydrate, affect the requirements for vitamins; vitamins affect the requirements for other vitamins; vitamins affect the requirements for minerals; minerals affect the requirements for other minerals and for protein. These alterations of the requirement of a nutrient that are caused by another nutrient are called interactions.

Information on an interaction between copper and zinc has accumulated since Smith and Larson discovered that anemia in rats produced by 0.7% zinc in the diet could be alleviated by feeding of 0.2 mg copper per day.[2] High dietary zinc can increase copper requirements and lessen copper toxicity; high dietary copper can increase zinc requirements and lessen zinc toxicity.[3] Frieden has outlined 10 steps in metal metabolism in mammals, beginning with dietary availability and ending with excretion.[4] It has been suggested that interactions could occur at any of these steps.[5] Davis has discussed some of these.[6] It is not surprising that elements adjacent in the periodic table should interact (for additional sources, see Reference 7). Perhaps nutritional interactions affect human health.

Ischemic (coronary) heart disease is the leading cause of death in the United States and in much of the industrialized world. Often the terms ischemic heart disease and coronary heart disease are used interchangeably. This disease causes about 35% of deaths in the United States, about twice as many as are caused by malignant neoplasms, or cancer. About 10% of the people in the United States between the ages of 45 and 79 have definite or suspected ischemic heart disease. In 1967 the direct cost of treatment of arteriosclerotic heart disease in the United States was about 2 billion dollars, with indirect costs of about 13 billion dollars (for additional sources, see References 8–10). Surely the cost is now greater.

Risk of this disease is not randomly distributed throughout the population; risk increases with age, and men are more susceptible than are women. Hypercholesterolemia, glucose intolerance, hypertension, electrocardiographic abnormalities, and the smoking of cigarettes are so strongly associated with risk of ischemic heart disease that they are called risk factors.[11] Many other associations with risk of ischemic heart disease have been made; because these associations are weaker than the five listed, or because the associations have not been widely accepted as true, these other associations have not been called risk factors.

Experiments with animals plus epidemiologic observations, iatrogenic maneuvers, and experiments of nature are the basis of the zinc/copper hypothesis about the etiology of ischemic heart disease.[5,8–10,12] This hypothesis states that "a metabolic imbalance in regard to zinc and copper is a major factor" in the etiology of ischemic heart disease. This imbalance, either a "relative or absolute deficiency of copper characterized by a high ratio of zinc to copper," results in hypercholesterolemia, myocardial and arterial damage, and increased mortality.

0077-8923/80/0355-0140 $01.75/0

The zinc/copper hypothesis initially was based on the production of hypercholesterolemia in rats by an increase in the ratio of zinc to copper ingested.[12] A relationship was developed between the observations on rats and certain epidemiologic characteristics of people.[12] Then a wide variety of apparently dissimilar characteristics of individuals and populations were shown to be related to the experiment with rats;[5,8,9] similar data on mice and swine also were found.

Among the phenomena associated with a high ratio of zinc to copper and either high risk of mortality or hypercholesterolemia are diets high in fat or sucrose, pregnancy, nephrotic syndrome, chronic hemodialysis, hypertension, and the low amounts of copper found in the presumably normal areas of infarcted hearts. Associated with a low ratio of zinc to copper and either low risk of mortality or hypocholesterolemia are diets high in fiber, hepatic cirrhosis, infectious hepatitis, strenuous exercise, and the availability of hard water.[5,8-10,12]

Because ischemic heart disease is usually associated with atherosclerotic coronary arteries, because lipids are found in atherosclerotic plaques, and because the concentration of cholesterol in blood plasma is predictive of risk of ischemic heart disease, many people view ischemic heart disease as a problem of lipid metabolism. Whatever it is that initiates the atherosclerotic process—and many agents have been proposed—the process begins early in life, perhaps in infancy or *in utero*.[13-17] The process progresses relentlessly; most deaths from ischemic heart disease occur between ages 35 and 64.[13] Abnormalities of connective tissue and uric acid metabolism, thrombosis, etc., precede the abnormalities of the electrocardiogram and the arterial occlusion that often cause death. Recently I have turned my attention to nonlipid abnormalities of ischemic heart disease, as I believe that a hypothesis that attempts to explain the etiology of ischemic heart disease also must address these other aspects of the disease. Data germane to both this hypothesis and this conference can be divided into three categories.

Zinc Effects

Hypocholesterolemia has been produced in pigs, rats, and women and men by zinc deficiency.[18-21] In rats, zinc deficiency results in increased excretion of bile acids.[22] A linear decline in plasma cholesterol was found in two men during a period of zinc deprivation.[21] The basal respiratory quotient of the men decreased from about 1 to about 0.8 even though the carbohydrate intake was substantial.[21]

Interactive Effects

The definition of nutrient interactions in the first paragraph (above) is quite strict. However, nonnutritive materials present in food or that come in contact with foods can alter requirements or dietary availability. In addition, there are statistical associations between analytical characteristics of foods, risk of mortality, environmental characteristics, etc., which can be treated together in this section.

There is a positive correlation ($r = 0.354$, $P < 0.02$) between the ratio of zinc to copper of milk available in 47 cities of the U.S. and the mortality due to coronary heart disease in the cities.[14] Only ethanol and the ratio of zinc to copper of milk have been associated with the risk of death due to heart disease in an epidemiologic study in the continental United States.

There is a positive association ($\chi^2 = 13.5$, $P < 0.001$) between the amount of fat in and the ratio of zinc to copper of 71 foods.[23] Thus, if one decreases the amount of fat in a diet, on the average, the ratio of zinc to copper will decrease too.

The zinc/copper hypothesis initially was based on experiments with rats in which hypercholesterolemia was produced by an increase in the ratio of zinc to copper ingested.[12] Mice with meat anemia, a disease caused by a high dietary ratio of zinc to copper, are hypercholesterolemic.[24]

In adolescent girls, an increase in daily dietary zinc from 11 to 15 mg by the consumption of lemonade containing zinc sulfate produced an increased fecal loss of copper.[25] This effect is more subtle than the hypocupremia produced with larger doses of oral zinc in a patient with sickle-cell anemia.[26]

Phytic acid (*myo*-inositol hexaphosphate) is a naturally occurring chelating agent found in plants. Sodium phytate fed to rats produced hypocholesterolemia and a decrease in the ratio of zinc to copper in hair.[27] Perhaps phytates contribute to the decreased mortality from ischemic heart disease that is associated with habitual consumption of fibrous diets described by Trowell.[28] (For additional sources, see References 27 and 29.)

Ascorbic acid impairs the absorption of copper from the intestinal tract of several species.[30] Ascorbic acid fed to rats produced hypercholesterolemia.[31] Depending on how one compares the effective dose for rats (150 mg/kg of diet) with amounts of ascorbic acid ingested by people, the effective dose for a 70-kg man would be about 82 to 630 mg/day greater than that in the normal diet. These are amounts well in the range of doses taken by people in search of respiratory benefit. Hypercholesterolemia in rats due to ascorbic acid is consonant with the effect on cholesterolemia of a depletion-repletion experiment in men.[32]

The relationship between hard water or high dietary calcium and low risk due to ischemic heart disease, and the several experiments in which increased ingestion of calcium produced decreased cholesterol in serum of men and women, have been reviewed.[33] The mechanism by which these phenomena are related may have been clarified by Romasz *et al.*, who fed rats a wide range of dietary calcium.[34] As dietary calcium increased, the concentration of cholesterol in serum decreased and the concentrations of copper and zinc in liver increased and decreased, respectively. In adult rats, there is an inverse correlation between plasma cholesterol and copper in liver microsomes.[35] Copper in liver may influence the metabolism of cholesterol.

Elkins mentioned the "well known" reaction between copper from foods and the tin-plated surface of cans under acidic conditions to explain the apparent removal of 50% of the copper from canned peaches during 18 months of storage.[36] He attributed the 23% decline of copper in canned beans during 12 months of storage to an interchange of minerals in the beans with those in the blanching water and canning brine. If they apply to other canned foods (apparently enameled cans do not undergo the "well known" reaction), these data complement the apparent decline in copper in fresh foods between 1942 and 1966.[37] This latter period is almost contemporaneous with a 44% increase in the death rate due to arteriosclerotic heart disease (1949–1967), and a period (1940–1965) in which there was no change in availability of fat per capita (for sources, see Reference 37).

The hypercholesterolemia caused by the feeding of L-histidine, first described by Waisman *et al.* (see Reference 38) can be nearly abolished by adding extra copper to the histidine-supplemented diet.[39] The result of this experiment, which shows that the hypercholesterolemia of histidine feeding is due to an alteration of copper metabolism, is not surprising on consideration of the tenacity with which histidine binds copper.[8,12] It may explain the hypercholesterolemia of normal human pregnancy and of the rare, human, inborn error of histidinemia.[8,12] It may extend the zinc/copper phenomenon to two more species: rabbits and rhesus monkeys.

Copper Effects

There are many similarities between people with atherosclerosis and ischemic heart disease and animals deficient in copper. Some characteristics common to both are shown in TABLE 1.

Hypercholesterolemia and Hyperlipoproteinemia

In the initial experiment on which the zinc/copper hypothesis is based, it was noted that although high ratios of zinc to copper produced hypercholesterolemia, the onset of hypercholesterolemia could be delayed by higher absolute amounts of dietary copper when the ratio of zinc to copper was held constant.[12] As the mechanisms by which a high ratio of zinc to copper and copper deficiency produce hypercholesterolemia are likely to be similar, it is advantageous to make dietary copper as low as possible. Experiments can be shortened from 6–21 weeks to 5–6 weeks.[12,40,41] Other experiments have shown hypercholesterolemia in copper deficiency.[40–45] In some of these experiments, part of the effect may be attributable to the relatively large amounts of zinc in the diet.[43,44]

Copper deficiency produces an increase in the incorporation of radioactivity given as mevalonate into plasma cholesterol.[41] The increased biliary excretion of bile acids and cholesterol was insufficient to prevent hypercholesterolemia.[41] Liver cholesterol is not increased;[41,44] sometimes it is decreased.[43,44] Copper deficiency produces an increase in cholesterol in the major classes of lipoproteins;[45] high density lipoprotein cholesterol decreases as a percent of total cholesterol. Thus, the excess cholesterol of copper deficiency is found mainly in plasma.

Hess *et al.* studied the effects of an oral contraceptive agent on young women consuming a formula diet low in zinc, copper, and iron but adequate in other nutrients.[20] During a 35-day period, serum cholesterol declined in both the group

TABLE 1

SOME CHARACTERISTICS OF PEOPLE WITH ISCHEMIC HEART DISEASE AND OF ANIMALS DEFICIENT IN COPPER

Ischemic Heart Disease	Animals Deficient in Copper
1. hypercholesterolemia*	1. hypercholesterolemia
a. increased LDL/HDL†	a. decreased % HDL
2. arterial damage	2. arterial damage
3. myocardial damage	3. myocardial damage
a. fibrosis	a. fibrosis
b. rupture	b. rupture
c. hypertrophy	c. hypertrophy
d. decreased myocardial copper	d. decreased myocardial copper
4. sudden death	4. sudden death
5. abnormal electrocardiograms*	5. abnormal electrocardiograms
a. ST abnormalities	a. ST abnormalities
b. bundle branch block	b. bundle branch block
6. hyperuricemia	6. hyperuricemia
7. abnormal blood clotting	7. blood hypercoaguable

* Risk factor.

† Low density (LD) and high density (HD) lipoproteins (L).

taking the agent and the control group. Hess *et al.* attributed the declines to zinc deficiency.[20] Perhaps the lesser decline in the group taking the agent was due to a decrease in liver copper due to estrogen and relative deficiency of copper in that organ.[46] In copper-deficient rats, cholesterol in plasma correlated negatively with liver copper.[40] In a similar experiment with a wider range of copper intakes, plasma cholesterol correlated negatively with copper in liver microsomes.[35]

Arterial Damage

Atherosclerotic arteries of humans have degenerated elastic tissue and damage of the internal elastic lamina, intramural hemorrhage, fibrous tissue proliferation, necrosis, and an increase in mucopolysaccharides.[13] All of these lesions have been produced in animals by copper deficiency.[40,47,48] To my knowledge, no atherosclerotic plaque identical to that found in people has been produced in animals by copper deficiency.

Myocardial Damage

Hearts of people who die of ischemic heart disease are hypertrophied and fibrotic; they contain increased collagen and have focal hemorrhages. Associated with infarction are edema, neutrophilic infiltration, and loss of cellular outline; the hearts often rupture.[13] All of these pathological changes are found in animals deficient in copper.[40,47,49-53]

Ruptured hearts with hemopericardium and hemothorax have been produced by copper deficiency.[40,47,50] About 24% of those people who die of acute myocardial infarction die of myocardial rupture; 7% of those dying of coronary heart disease have ventricular aneurysm.[54]

Hearts of people who died of myocardial infarction are low in copper.[55-57] Uninfarcted myocardium from infarction victims was compared with myocardial samples from accident victims and others who died of causes unrelated to ischemic heart disease.

Sudden Death

People with ischemic heart disease often die suddenly; 30 to 80% die within 1 hour of the onset of symptoms.[58] It is assumed that abnormal cardiac electrophysiology contributes to these deaths. Cattle and rats deficient in copper die suddenly.[49,53,40,59] Copper deficiency decreased the median longevity of rats by 73%.[59]

Abnormal Electrocardiograms

Insull listed the finding of tall R waves and ST depression or T wave inversion as being associated with left ventricular hypertrophy and increased risk of coronary heart disease.[11] Goldstein noted that ST segment depression, bundle branch block, and persistent Q waves were predictors of sudden death.[58]

The electrocardiographic abnormalities produced in rats by copper deficiency are quite similar to those predictive of risk in people.[59] Tall R waves, ST depression, bundle branch block, and Q waves are shown in FIGURE 1. Some normal electrocardiograms of rats are shown for comparison.

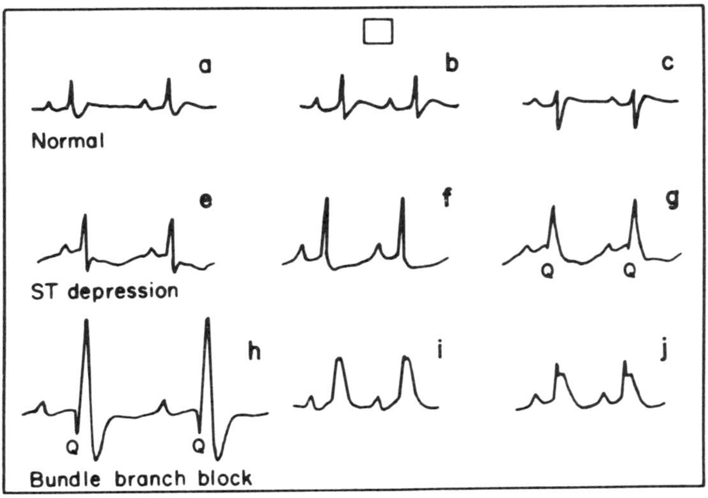

FIGURE 1. □ 50 msecond by 7.1 mV. Normal electrocardiograms on rats supplemented with copper, **a–c**. Abnormal electrocardiograms on rats deficient in copper: ST depression, **e–g**; bundle branch block, **h–j**. Data are from Reference 59.

Hyperuricemia

In the Framingham population, risk of coronary (ischemic) heart disease was related to serum uric acid; men with gout had double the normal risk.[60] Kannel stated that the reason for the apparent association of hyperuricemia with atherogenic traits has yet to be established.[60] Newland has traced the association of uric acid and heart disease and has hypothesized that uric acid may be involved in the pathogenesis of coronary heart disease by promoting thrombosis through the stabilization of platelet aggregates and contributing to the development of hypertension.[61] The hypothesis of Newland and the zinc/copper hypothesis are placed in harmony by the production of hyperuricemia in rats by copper deficiency.[62]

Thrombosis

The thrombotic process is important in atherogenesis.[63] About 14% of those who die of acute myocardial infarction die of thromboembolism.[54] The incorporation and organization of mural thrombi are significant factors in the evolution of atherosclerotic plaques.[64,65] The blood of copper-deficient rats is hypercoaguable; the coagulation time of copper-deficient rats was about 55% of that of supplemented rats.[66]

Dietary Copper

The implication of copper metabolism in ischemic heart disease may seem incongruous, as nutrition textbooks generally state that daily diets contain 2–5 mg of copper. These statements are based on limited data, decades old.[9] The daily amount of dietary copper required to compensate for urinary and fecal losses of adults is 2 mg according to the Food and Nutrition Board of the National Academy of Sciences of the United States.[67] An expert committee of the World Health Organization expressed the requirement as a function of body weight and arrived at 2.1 mg for the average man.[68] Our estimate of the requirement of men, 1.55 mg, includes compensation for surface loss of copper.[69]

Actually, diets in the United States and other industrialized parts of the world may frequently contain less copper than the daily adult requirement of 2 mg.[25,70-83] Amounts of copper exceeding the requirement seem to be unusual.[84-86] The geometric mean (0.82 mg) for daily intake of copper for 20 diets plus one standard deviation equals 1.67 mg;[77] 84% of U.S. diets probably contain less than this amount. This estimate is slightly higher than that of Holden *et al.,* who found that 81% of their subjects consumed less than 1.33 mg of copper per day.[76] Milne *et al.* found that 75% of the intakes of their subjects were less than 2 mg of copper per day.[79] The requirements of infants are not as well defined; however, they seem to be relatively greater.[67,68] Thus, exposure to the atherogenic diet may begin very early in life.[13-17]

Conclusions

The zinc/copper hypothesis on the etiology of ischemic heart disease initially was based on the hypercholesterolemia of rats due to the ingestion of a high ratio of zinc to copper. Later many associations were made between the metabolism of copper and zinc and epidemiology and human cholesterol metabolism in a wide variety of physiological states. Now the hypothesis can be broadened because copper deficiency in several species has produced anatomical, chemical, and physiological abnormalities similar to those found in ischemic heart disease.

For example, animals deficient in copper and people with ischemic heart disease are likely to die suddenly, to be hypercholesterolemic and hyperuricemic, to have arteries with abnormal connective tissue, and to have fibrotic, hypertrophied hearts low in copper with abnormal electrocardiograms. Hypercholesterolemia and abnormal electrocardiograms are two of five risk factors predictive in people. In the continental United States, only ethanol and the ratio of zinc to copper of milk have been associated with risk of death due to coronary (ischemic) heart disease. I conclude that the hypothesis relating absolute or relative deficiency of copper to the etiology of ischemic heart disease is consonant with more facets of the disease than is any other hypothesis.

References

1. Harper, A. E. 1958. Balance and imbalance of amino acids. Ann. N.Y. Acad. Sci. **69:** 1025–1041.
2. Smith, S. E. & E. J. Larson. 1946. Zinc toxicity in rats. J. Biol. Chem. **163:** 29–38.
3. Underwood, E. J. 1977. Trace Elements in Human and Animal Nutrition. 4th edit.: 61, 226, 231. Academic Press, Inc. New York, N.Y.
4. Frieden, E. 1978. Modes of metal metabolism in mammals. *In* Trace Element Metabolism in Man and Animals. M. Kirchgessner, Ed. **3:** 8–14. Institut fur Ernahrungsphysiologie, Technische Universitat Munchen. Freising-Weihenstephan. Federal Republic of Germany.
5. Klevay, L. M. Ischemic heart disease: updating the zinc/copper hypothesis. Proceedings

of the American College of Nutrition Meeting, Minneapolis, Minn., June, 1978. (In press.)
6. DAVIS, G. K. 1980. Microelement interactions of zinc, copper, and iron in mammalian species. Ann. N.Y. Acad. Sci. (This volume.)
7. NIELSEN, F. H., C. D. HUNT & E. O. UTHUS. 1980. Interactions between essential trace and ultratrace elements. Ann. N.Y. Acad. Sci. (This volume.)
8. KLEVAY, L. M. 1975. Coronary heart disease: the zinc/copper hypothesis. Am. J. Clin. Nutr. **28:** 764–774.
9. KLEVAY, L. M. 1977. The role of copper and zinc in cholesterol metabolism. *In* Advances in Nutritional Research. H. H. Draper, Ed. **1:** 227–252. Plenum Publishing Corporation. New York, N.Y.
10. KLEVAY, L. M. 1977. Elements of ischemic heart disease. Perspect. Biol. Med. **20:** 186–192.
11. INSULL, W., JR. 1973. Coronary Risk Handbook: 3. American Heart Association. New York, N.Y.
12. KLEVAY, L. M. 1973. Hypercholesterolemia in rats produced by an increase in the ratio of zinc to copper ingested. Am. J. Clin. Nutr. **26:** 1060–1068.
13. SCOTTI, T. M. 1977. Heart. *In* Pathology. W. A. D. Anderson & J. M. Kissane, Eds.: 737–855. C. V. Mosby Co. St. Louis, Mo.
14. KLEVAY, L. M. 1974. The ratio of zinc to copper in milk and mortality due to coronary heart disease: an association. *In* Trace Substances in Environmental Health. D. D. Hemphill, Ed. **8:** 9–14. University of Missouri Press. Columbia, Mo.
15. OSBORN, G. R. 1968. Stages in development of coronary disease observed from 1500 young subjects. Relationship of hypotension and infant feeding to aetiology. *In* Le Rôle de la Paroi Artérielle dans l'Athérogénèse. M. J. Lenègre, L. Seebat & J. Renais, Eds.: 93–139. Centre National de la Recherche Scientifique. Paris, France.
16. KLEVAY, L. M. & K. G. D. ALLEN. 1977. Vitamin B_6, copper, and atherosclerosis. Lancet **1:** 1209.
17. LEVINE, C. I. & J. C. MURRAY. 1977. The aetiological role of maternal vitamin-B_6 deficiency in the development of atherosclerosis. Lancet **1:** 628–630.
18. BURCH, R. E., R. V. WILLIAMS, H. K. J. HAHN, M. M. JETTON & J. F. SULLIVAN. 1975. Serum and tissue enzyme activity and trace-element content in response to zinc deficiency in the pig. Clin. Chem. N.Y. **21:** 568–577.
19. PATEL, P. B., R. A. CHUNG & J. Y. LU. 1975. Effect of zinc deficiency on serum and liver cholesterol in the female rat. Nutr. Rep. Int. **12:** 205–210.
20. HESS, F. M., J. C. KING & S. MARGEN. 1977. Effect of low zinc intake and oral contraceptive agents on nitrogen utilization and clinical findings in young women. J. Nutr. **107:** 2219–2227.
21. SANDSTEAD, H., L. KLEVAY, J. MAHALKO, L. INMAN, W. BOLONCHUK, H. LUKASKI, G. LYKKEN, T. KRAMER, L. JOHNSON, D. MILNE & J. WALLWORK. Marginal Zn nutriture: effects on lipid metabolism and plasma zinc. Am. J. Clin. Nutr. (In press.)
22. TOPPING, D. L., R. J. ILLMAN, I. E. DREOSTI, R. P. TRIMBLE & I. R. RECORD. 1978. Effects of zinc deficiency on bile acid secretion in the rat. Nutr. Rep. Int. **18:** 631–637.
23. KLEVAY, L. M. 1974. An association between the amount of fat and the ratio of zinc to copper in 71 foods: inferences about the epidemiology of coronary heart disease. Nutr. Rep. Int. **9:** 393–399.
24. JACOB, R. A., L. G. BAESLER, L. M. KLEVAY, D. E. LEE & P. L. WHERRY. 1977. Hypercholesterolemia in mice with meat anemia. Nutr. Rep. Int. **16:** 73–79.
25. GREGER, J. L., S. C. ZAIKIS, R. P. ABERNATHY, O. A. BENNETT & J. HUFFMAN. 1978. Zinc, nitrogen, copper, iron and manganese balance in adolescent females fed two levels of zinc. J. Nutr. **108:** 1449–1456.
26. PRASAD, A. S., G. J. BREWER, E. B. SCHOOMAKER & P. RABBANI. 1978. Hypocupremia induced by zinc therapy in adults. J. Am. Med. Assoc. **240:** 2166–2168.
27. KLEVAY, L. M. 1977. Hypocholesterolemia due to sodium phytate. Nutr. Rep. Int. **15:** 587–595.
28. TROWELL, H. 1975. Ischaemic heart disease, atheroma and fibrinolysis. *In* Refined Carbohydrate Foods and Disease. D. P. Burkitt & H. C. Trowell, Eds.: 195–226. Academic Press. London, England.
29. KLEVAY, L. M. 1976. Ischemic heart disease: the fiber hypothesis. *In* Proceedings of the

Miles Symposium '76 on "Dietary Fibre": 33–39. Nutrition Society of Canada. Halifax, Nova Scotia, Canada.
30. Evans, G. W. 1973. Copper homeostasis in the mammalian system. Physiol. Rev. **53:** 535–570.
31. Klevay, L. M. 1976. Hypercholesterolemia due to ascorbic acid. Proc. Soc. Exp. Biol. Med. **151:** 579–582.
32. Hodges, R. E., J. Hood, J. E. Canham, H. E. Sauberlich & E. M. Baker. 1971. Clinical manifestations of ascorbic acid deficiency in man. Am. J. Clin. Nutr. **24:** 432–443.
33. Klevay, L. M. The influence of copper and zinc on the occurrence of ischemic heart disease. J. Environ. Pathol. Toxicol. (In press.)
34. Romasz, R. S., E. A. Lemmo & J. L. Evans. 1977. Diet calcium, sex and age influences on tissue mineralization and cholesterol in rats. *In* Trace Substances in Environmental Health. D. D. Hemphill, Ed. **11:** 289–296. University of Missouri Press. Columbia, Mo.
35. Jacob, R. A., L. M. Klevay & G. M. Logan, Jr. 1978. Hair as a biopsy material. V. Hair metal as an index of hepatic metal in rats: copper and zinc. Am. J. Clin. Nutr. **31:** 477–480.
36. Elkins, E. R. 1979. Nutrient content of raw and canned green beans, peaches and sweet potatoes. Food Technol. **33:** 66–70.
37. Klevay, L. M. & J. Forbush. 1976. Copper metabolism and the epidemiology of coronary heart disease. Nutr. Rep. Int. **14:** 221–228.
38. Geison, R. L. & H. A. Waisman. 1970. Plasma and tissue cholesterol and lipid levels in rabbits on L-histidine-supplemented diets. Proc. Soc. Exp. Biol. Med. **133:** 234–237.
39. Harvey, P. W., H. A. Hunsaker & K. G. D. Allen. 1980. Histidine induced cholesterolemia due to copper changes. Fed. Proc. Fed. Am. Soc. Exp. Biol. **39:** 786.
40. Allen, K. G. D. & L. M. Klevay. 1978. Cholesterolemia and cardiovascular abnormalities in rats caused by copper deficiency. Atherosclerosis **29:** 81–93.
41. Allen, K. G. D. & L. M. Klevay. 1978. Copper deficiency and cholesterol metabolism in the rat. Atherosclerosis **31:** 259–271.
42. Allen, K. G. D. & L. M. Klevay. 1978. Cholesterol metabolism in copper deficient rats. Life Sci. **22:** 1691–1697.
43. Lei, K. Y. 1977. Cholesterol metabolism in copper-deficient rats. Nutr. Rep. Int. **15:** 597–605.
44. Lei, K. Y. 1978. Oxidation, excretion, and tissue distribution of [26-^{14}C] cholesterol in copper-deficient rats. J. Nutr. **108:** 232–237.
45. Allen, K. G. D. & L. M. Klevay. 1978. Influence of dietary copper deficiency on cholesterol content of rat plasma lipoproteins. (abst.). Clin. Res. **26:** 695A.
46. Evans, G. W., N. F. Cornatzer & W. E. Cornatzer. 1970. Mechanism for hormone-induced alterations in serum ceruloplasmin. Am. J. Physiol. **218:** 613–615.
47. Shields, G. S., W. F. Coulson, D. A. Kimball, W. H. Carnes, G. E. Cartwright & M. M. Wintrobe. 1962. Studies on copper metabolism. XXXII. Cardiovascular lesions in copper-deficient swine. Am. J. Pathol. **41:** 603–621.
48. Linker, A., W. F. Coulson & W. H. Carnes. 1964. Cardiovascular studies on copper-deficient swine. VI. The mucopolysaccharide composition of aorta and cartilage. J. Biol. Chem. **239:** 1690–1693.
49. Bennetts, H. W., R. Harley & S. T. Evans. 1942. Studies on copper deficiency of cattle: the fatal termination ("Falling Disease"). Aust. Vet. J. **18:** 50–63.
50. Kelly, W. A., J. W. Kesterson & W. W. Carlton. 1974. Myocardial lesions in the offspring of female rats fed a copper deficient diet. Exp. Mol. Pathol. **20:** 40–56.
51. Leigh, L. C. 1975. Changes in the ultrastructure of cardiac muscle in steers deprived of copper. Res. Vet. Sci. **18:** 282–287.
52. Gubler, C. J., G. E. Cartwright & M. M. Wintrobe. 1957. Studies on copper metabolism. XX. Enzyme activities and iron metabolism in copper and iron deficiencies. J. Biol. Chem. **224:** 533–546.
53. Davis, G. K. 1976. Copper and cardiac integrity. *In* The Biomedical Role of Trace Elements in Aging. H. M. Hsu, R. L. Davis & R. W. Neithamer, Eds.: 81–90. Eckerd College Gerontology Center. St. Petersburg, Fla.
54. Spiekerman, R. E., J. T. Brandenburg, R. W. P. Achor & J. E. Edwards. 1962. The spectrum of coronary heart disease in a community of 30,000. Circulation **25:** 57–65.

55. WESTER, P. O. 1965. Trace elements in human myocardial infarction determined by neutron activation analysis. Acta Med. Scand. **178:** 765–788.
56. ANDERSON, T. W., L. C. NERI, G. B. SCHREIBER, F. D. F. TALBOT & A. ZDROJEWSKI. 1975. Ischemic heart disease, water hardness and myocardial magnesium. Can. Med. Assoc. J. **113:** 199–203.
57. CHIPPERFIELD, B. & J. R. CHIPPERFIELD. 1978. Differences in metal content of the heart muscle in death from ischemic heart disease. Am. Heart J. **95:** 732–737.
58. GOLDSTEIN, S. 1974. Sudden Death and Coronary Heart Disease: 24–32. Futura Publishing Company, Inc. Mt. Kisco, N.Y.
59. KLEVAY, L. M. & K. E. VIESTENZ. 1979. Abnormal electrocardiograms in rats deficient in copper. Am. J. Clin. Nutr. **32:** 932.
60. KANNEL, W. B. 1976. Some lessons in cardiovascular epidemiology from Framingham. Am. J. Cardiol. **37:** 269–282.
61. NEWLAND, H. 1975. Hyperuricemia in coronary, cerebral and peripheral arterial disease: an explanation. Medical Hypotheses **1:** 152–155.
62. KLEVAY, L. M. 1980. Hyperuricemia in rats due to copper deficiency. Fed. Proc. Fed. Am. Soc. Exp. Biol. **39:** 429.
63. CHANDLER, A. B., K. EURENIUS, G. C. MCMILLAN, C. B. NELSON, C. J. SCHWARTZ & S. WESSLER. 1978. The thrombotic process in atherogenesis. Adv. Exp. Med. Biol. **104:** 3–546.
64. SCHWARTZ, C. J., A. B. CHANDLER, R. G. GERRITY & H. K. NAITO. 1978. Clinical and pathological aspects of arterial thrombosis and thromboembolism. Adv. Exp. Med. Biol. **104:** 111–126.
65. MUSTARD, J. F., M. A. PACKHAM & R. KINLOUGH-RATHBONE. 1978. Platelets, thrombosis and atherosclerosis. Adv. Exp. Med. Biol. **104:** 127–144.
66. LAU, B. W. C., T. R. KRAMER & L. M. KLEVAY. 1980. Increased coagulability of blood in copper deficient rats. Fed. Proc. Fed. Am. Soc. Exp. Biol. **39:** 429.
67. Food and Nutrition Board. 1974. Recommended Dietary Allowances. 8th edit.: 95–96. National Research Council, National Academy of Sciences. Washington, D.C.
68. DARBY, W. J., L. FRIBERG, C. F. MILLS, J. PARIZEK, V. RAMALINGASWAMI, H. A. RONAGHY, H. H. SANDSTEAD, E. J. UNDERWOOD, N. M. RAO, R. PAR, J. M. BENGOA, E. M. DEMAEYER & W. MERTZ. 1973. Trace Elements in Human Nutrition. Technical Report Series No. 532: 15–19. World Health Organization. Geneva, Switzerland.
69. KLEVAY, L. M., S. J. RECK, R. A. JACOB, G. M. LOGAN, JR., J. M. MUNOZ & H. H. SANDSTEAD. 1980. The human requirement for copper. I. Healthy men fed conventional, American diets. Am. J. Clin. Nutr. **33:** 45–50.
70. WHITE, H. S. 1969. Inorganic elements in weighed diets of girls and young women. J. Am. Diet. Assoc. **55:** 38–43.
71. GORMICAN, A. 1970. Inorganic elements in foods used in hospital menus. J. Am. Diet. Assoc. **56:** 397–403.
72. PRICE, N. O., G. E. BUNCE & R. W. ENGEL. 1970. Copper, manganese, and zinc balance in preadolescent girls. Am. J. Clin Nutr. **23:** 258–260.
73. KLEVAY, L. M., K. P. VO-KHACTU & R. A. JACOB. 1975. The ratio of zinc to copper of cholesterol-lowering diets. *In* Trace Substances in Environmental Health. D. D. Hemphill, Ed. **9:** 131–138. University of Missouri Press. Columbia, Mo.
74. BROWN, E. D., M. P. HOWARD & J. C. SMITH, JR. 1977. The copper content of regular, vegetarian and renal diets. Fed. Proc. Fed. Am. Soc. Exp. Biol. **36:** 1122.
75. VAN BERGE HENEGOUWEN, G. P., T. N. TANGEDAHL, A. F. HOFMANN, T. C. NORTHFIELD, N. F. LARUSSO & J. T. MCCALL. 1977. Biliary secretion of copper in healthy man. Gastroenterology **72:** 1228–1231.
76. HOLDEN, J. M., W. R. WOLF & W. MERTZ. 1979. Zinc and copper in self-selected diets. J. Am. Diet. Assoc. **75:** 23–28.
77. KLEVAY, L. M., S. J. RECK & D. F. BARCOME. 1979. Evidence of dietary copper and zinc deficiencies. J. Am. Med. Assoc. **241:** 1916–1918.
78. SPENCER, H., C. R. ASMUSSEN, R. B. HOLTZMAN & L. KRAMER. 1979. Metabolic balances of cadmium, copper, manganese, and zinc in man. Am. J. Clin. Nutr. **32:** 1867–1875.
79. MILNE, D. B., D. D. SCHNAKENBERG, H. L. JOHNSON & G. L. KUHL. 1980. Trace mineral intake of enlisted military personnel. J. Am. Diet. Assoc. **76:** 41–45.

80. Koivistoinen, P., A. Ahlström, H. Nissinen, M. Pekkarinen & P. Roine. 1970. Mineral element compositions of Finnish diets. Part 1: Fe, Cu, Mn, Zn, Mg, Na, K, Ca and P. Suom. Kemistil. B **43:** 426–430.
81. Hartley, T. F., J. B. Dawson & A. Hodgkinson. 1974. Simultaneous measurement of Na, K, Ca, Mg, Cu and Zn balances in man. Clin. Chim. Acta **52:** 321–333.
82. Guthrie, B. E. & M. F. Robinson. 1977. Daily intakes of manganese, copper, zinc, and cadmium. Br. J. Nutr. **38:** 55–63.
83. Abdulla, M. & S. Svensson. 1979. Copper. *In* Nutrition and Old Age. B. Borgström, A. Nordén, B. Åkesson, M. Abdulla & M. Jägerstad, Eds.: 172–175. Carl Bloms Boktryckeri AB. Lund, Sweden. [Also published in 1979. Scand. J. Gastroenterol. Suppl. **14**(52).]
84. Schroeder, H. A., A. P. Nason, I. H. Tipton & J. J. Balassa. 1966. Essential trace elements in man: copper. J. Chronic Dis. **19:** 1007–1034.
85. Tipton, I. H. & P. L. Stewart. 1969. Analytical methods for the determination of trace elements—standard man studies. *In* Trace Substances in Environmental Health. D. D. Hemphill, Ed. **3:** 305–330. University of Missouri Press. Columbia, Mo.
86. Walker, M. A. & L. Page. 1977. Nutritive content of college meals. J. Am. Diet. Assoc. **70:** 260–266.

Discussion

Unidentified Speaker: Sulfinpyrazone, known as Anturane®, is a uricosuric agent that has recently been shown to prevent sudden death after myocardial infarction for the first six months. Your remarks about copper and uric acid were interesting. Do you know of any connection with sulfinpyrazone, copper, and uric acid?

L. M. Klevay: No, I don't, except that it inhibits tubular reabsorption of uric acid. I've not studied the effects of various drugs effective in heart disease or in lowering lipids in deficient animals. I think it would be interesting for someone to do that. We're more interested in nutrition than in pharmacology; however, the effect of drugs on people may be influenced by nutritional status.

Unidentified Speaker: About a year or two ago, there was a rash of deaths of women who consumed liquid protein diets. Although the potassium hypothesis was evoked to explain the sudden deaths, it was noted that they also occurred in people who had been supplemented with potassium. Is the copper in such diets very low?

L. M. Klevay: Yes, they are notably deficient in copper. As I pointed out in a letter to the *New England Journal of Medicine* [1979. **300:** 48, 328], the maximum copper intake would be less than one-tenth of the adult requirement, if liquid protein were to be a sole source of copper.

N. F. Suttle (*Moredun Research Institute, Edinburgh, Scotland*): In the experimentally copper-depleted animal, you find a low serum copper, a low liver copper, a low copper concentration in heart, and a low level of superoxide dismutase in heart muscle. Do you find any of these changes in ischemic heart disease?

L. M. Klevay: Three studies—in Sweden, Canada, and England—have shown that copper is low in the uninfarcted portion of infarcted hearts. In some cases, other minerals were changed, but the consistent finding seems to be low copper. In rats so deficient in copper that some had ruptured hearts, we have found plasma copper to be 4 to 5% of normal. I do not believe that plasma copper within the normal range is proof that nutritional status is satisfactory. I think analogy with potassium and magnesium is appropriate. Recently we found that men being depleted of zinc had normal or increased plasma zinc.

N. F. Suttle: What is the extent of the reduction in heart copper?

L. M. Klevay: The results for the three studies quoted in the manuscript ranged from 13 to 29% lower than normal.

Unidentified Speaker: A number of people are taking zinc to reduce pain for arthritic conditions, pain for back, etc. Do these people run extra risk of a heart condition?

L. M. Klevay: I don't know. Greger has shown that adolescent girls given lemonade that increased their zinc intake from 11 to 15 mg lost extra copper in feces.

C. H. Hill (*North Carolina State University, Raleigh, N.C.*): In copper deficiency, the elastin in the aorta has specific abnormalities in that the isodesmosines are lower and the lysine is higher. Are these changes also found in ischemic heart disease?

L. M. Klevay: There are changes in the anatomy of elastic tissue in ischemic heart disease. I don't know whether the chemical changes you mention have been found.

M. D. Schneider (*University of Tennessee, Knoxville, Tenn.*): What happens to the collagen and elastin in aortas of copper-deficient animals?

L. M. Klevay: Arterial elastin is disrupted and decreased, probably because of impaired activity of lysyl oxidase, an enzyme containing copper. Collagen is increased.

M. D. Schneider: That brings us around to another question. Are platelets and prostaglandins involved?

L. M. Klevay: Copper metabolism has been implicated in prostaglandin synthesis. This is not surprising, considering the chemistry of prostaglandins.

H. G. Petering (*University of Cincinnati Medical Center, Cincinnati, Ohio*): In answer to Dr. Suttle's question, in cooperation with Dr. Klaus Stemmer, we have been able to produce myocardial damage in animals on diets low in copper with very little, if any, change in myocardial copper.

Dr. Klevay, I wonder whether we shouldn't modify the zinc/copper hypothesis and talk about copper deficiency. We think zinc is only modifying the copper, and there are many other ligands in the environment, or heavy metals that can do the same thing. I think we can unify the hypothesis by focusing it more on copper than on the zinc to copper ratio.

L. M. Klevay: I agree that copper is probably important in the control of cholesterol metabolism. For example, we've found that in adult rats, the concentration of cholesterol in plasma had a negative correlation with copper in liver microsomes. However, if one eliminates the consideration of zinc, one can't explain the hypocholesterolemia found in rats, swine, women, and men deficient in zinc. Dr. George Davis mentioned that we don't know how these things work intracellularly. Consequently, I'm reluctant to discard the ratio concept.

Unidentified Speaker: If the persons or animals were copper sufficient, would the zinc/copper ratio still hold?

L. M. Klevay: One of the difficulties of studying ratios is that the possibilities are infinite. Unfortunately, we do not know how much copper is required by either rats or people. The phenomenon we're discussing exists with rat diets containing as high as 2 μg copper per gram of diet. I haven't seen data at higher amounts. The amounts of copper and zinc used in our experiments are similar to those found in dried human diets.

INTERACTIONS BETWEEN ESSENTIAL TRACE AND ULTRATRACE ELEMENTS

Forrest H. Nielsen

Human Nutrition Laboratory
U.S. Department of Agriculture
Science and Education Administration
Grand Forks, North Dakota 58202

Curtiss D. Hunt* and Eric O. Uthus†

University of North Dakota
Grand Forks, North Dakota 58202

INTRODUCTION

Since 1970, a number of reports have suggested that several elements present in minute quantities in animal tissues are essential nutrients. These trace elements include arsenic, nickel, and vanadium. Highly sophisticated methods were required to produce deficiencies of those trace elements in animals. This suggests that arsenic, nickel, and vanadium nutrition would not be of practical significance because spontaneous deficiency states would be unlikely in man or animals. However, situations other than a simple deficiency might make these elements of nutritional significance. For example, the interaction of these ultratrace elements (dietary requirement, 50 ng/g or less) with other essential trace elements might adversely affect an organism. Because some recent findings support that possibility, interactions between nickel and iron, nickel and copper, arsenic and zinc, and vanadium and chromium are described.

NICKEL-IRON INTERACTION

The first indication that nickel and iron may interact was reported by Lederer and Lourau in 1948.[1] They suggested that nickel was indispensable for hematopoiesis because nickel apparently activated an enzyme that was needed for hematopoiesis. In 1972, Lange found that the intraperitoneal (ip) injection of nickel accelerated and intensified erythropoiesis in rabbits with induced hemolytic anemia.[2] Shortly thereafter, it was found that nickel toxicity in rats depressed packed cell volume and hemoglobin and elevated the iron level in plasma, serum, red blood cells, heart, liver, testes, spleen, kidney, and all major cellular fractions of the liver and kidney.[3,4] Schnegg and Kirchgessner reported that the signs of nickel deficiency—depressed hematocrits, hemoglobin, and erythrocyte counts—in rats could be reduced in severity by increasing dietary iron from 50 μg/g to 100 μg/g.[5-8] Apparently, nickel deficiency impaired iron absorption but had little influence on iron's metabolic efficiency.[6] Schnegg and Kirchgessner also found that nickel deprivation in rats depressed the iron content in liver, spleen, and kidney.[7,8] On the other hand, Spears *et al.* reported that nickel deprivation increased the iron concentration in liver, spleen,

* Department of Anatomy.
† Department of Biochemistry.

0077–8923/80/0355–0152 $01.75/0 © 1980, NYAS

and lung of sheep.[9] Recently we found that the iron status of the rat has a major influence on the extent and severity of the signs of nickel deprivation.[10] Severe iron deficiency was more detrimental to nickel-supplemented than to nickel-deficient rats, as growth was more severely depressed and perinatal mortality was higher in nickel-supplemented rats. However, when the diet contained marginally deficient or adequate levels of iron, nickel-deprived rats did not perform as well as nickel-supplemented controls. Also, the number and severity of the signs of nickel deprivation, especially in F_2 generation rats, increased when dietary iron was supplied at 45 μg/g as ferric sulfate instead of at 30 μg/g as ferric chloride.

We confirmed the interaction between nickel and iron in factorially arranged experiments. Nickel and/or iron nutriture affects growth; hematocrit; hemoglobin level; plasma concentration of alkaline phosphatase, total lipids, phospholipids, and cholesterol; and liver contents of total lipids, phospholipids, cholesterol, copper, iron, nickel, manganese, and zinc.[3-11] Thus, we examined those parameters to ascertain the nickel-iron interaction.

In three fully crossed, two-factor, completely randomized experiments, female weanling rats were fed a diet supplemented with iron at levels of 0, 25, 50, and 100 μg/g and nickel at levels of 0, 5, and 50 μg/g.[12] In experiment 3, an additional level of iron—12.5 μg/g—was used. In experiments 1 and 3, iron was supplemented as $Fe_2(SO_4)_3 \cdot nH_2O$; in experiment 2, as a mixture of 40% $FeSO_4 \cdot nH_2O$ and 60% $Fe_2(SO_4)_3 \cdot nH_2O$.

After 9–10 weeks, when dietary iron was supplemented as ferric sulfate only, the interaction between iron and nickel affected hematocrit, hemoglobin, plasma alkaline phosphatase activity, plasma phospholipid level, liver weight/body weight ratio, liver lipid extract yellow pigment, and liver copper concentration.[12] However, when dietary iron was supplemented as a ferric and ferrous sulfate mixture, nickel and iron did not interact to affect any parameter examined.

The hemoglobin data are shown in TABLE 1. In experiments 1 and 3, when the dietary ferric sulfate level was low, hemoglobin levels were lower in nickel-deprived than in nickel-supplemented rats. When iron/g of diet was 25 μg in experiments 1 and 3, nickel-deprived rats had average hemoglobins of 10.09 and 6.19 g/100 ml respectively; whereas those fed a nickel supplement of 5 or 50 μg/g had hemoglobins of 11.77 and 12.09, and 8.31 and 8.92 g/100 ml respectively. Dietary nickel apparently had no effect on hemoglobin when the diet contained 100 μg of iron/g. The data for hemoglobin gave no evidence of an interaction between nickel and iron when dietary iron was supplied as ferric and ferrous sulfate.

When the interaction between nickel and iron affected other parameters, it generally did so in a manner similar to that found with hemoglobin.[12] That is, signs of nickel deprivation were more severe when dietary iron, as ferric sulfate, was low; or the signs of moderate iron deficiency were more severe when dietary nickel was deficient. Thus, the findings suggest a synergistic relationship between nickel and iron when dietary iron is supplied as ferric sulfate only.

The apparent dependence of the nickel-iron interaction upon the presence of only the relatively insoluble ferric sulfate suggests that nickel has a role in the absorption of the ferric ion but not in that of the ferrous ion. In other words, nickel apparently converts the unavailable ferric ion into a form that can be absorbed. Perhaps nickel enhances the complexation of the ferric ion to a lipophilic molecule. Some evidence shows that both active and passive transport mechanisms play a role in iron absorption.[13] Active transport to the serosal surface is relatively specific for the divalent cation, which indicates that the ferric ion is absorbed by passive transport.[14] Passive transport is diffusion controlled and only permits the transit of lipophilic molecules. Possibly nickel acts in an enzymatic reaction that forms the

TABLE 1

EFFECTS IN RATS OF NICKEL, IRON, AND THEIR INTERACTION ON HEMOGLOBIN LEVELS

Treatment* (μg/g)		Hemoglobin Level (g/100 ml)		
Ni	Fe	Experiment 1	Experiment 2	Experiment 3
0	0	2.65	3.73	2.55
0	12.5	—	—	4.90
0	25	10.09	13.27	6.19
0	50	12.65	13.42	10.85
0	100	13.05	13.23	11.61
5	0	3.03	4.08	3.36
5	12.5	—	—	5.81
5	25	11.77	13.15	8.31
5	50	12.98	13.26	10.92
5	100	13.07	13.13	11.41
50	0	3.88	4.46	2.95
50	12.5	—	—	5.01
50	25	12.09	13.01	8.92
50	50	12.62	13.29	11.13
50	100	12.80	13.26	11.65
		Analysis of Variance—P Values		
Nickel effect		0.003	0.003	0.0002
Iron effect		0.0001	0.0001	0.0001
Nickel × iron		0.0001	NS	0.0002
Error mean square (df)		0.31 (7)	0.16 (58)	0.56 (75)

* Amounts of Ni (nickel chloride) and Fe (ferric sulfate in experiment 1 and 3; mixture of 40% ferrous sulfate and 60% ferric sulfate in experiment 2) supplemented to diet.

lipophilic iron transport molecule or makes more of a transport ligand available for the ferric ion. For example, nickel may inhibit the catabolism of a transport molecule by combining with it or with an enzyme involved in its breakdown. On the other hand, nickel may be essential for the enzymatic formation or the structural integrity of a molecule involved in ferric ion transport.

The hypothesis that nickel functions in the passive diffusion of the ferric ion is supported by the data for hemoglobin. Dowdle *et al.* suggested that the active transport mechanism for iron becomes important if passive diffusion is restricted.[15] Thus, at the lower levels of iron supplementation, when iron was supplied as a ferric-ferrous mixture, some ferrous ions were available for active transport and nickel deprivation did not affect hemoglobin levels. On the other hand, when ferric iron only was fed, the active transport mechanism could not operate and, in nickel deprivation, the passive diffusion of lipophilic ferric complexes was inhibited. As a result, significant differences occurred between nickel-deprived and nickel-supplemented rats at low levels of iron supplementation.

NICKEL-COPPER INTERACTION

Cuprous and cupric ions have a preferred coordination number of four and form tetrahedral and square coplanar complexes, respectively. Nickel can possess inner orbital bonding, in which the preferred coordination number is four, and form either tetrahedral or square coplanar complexes. Thus, if nickel is present in biological systems with a coordination number of four, nickel and copper would have similar chemical parameters and a nickel-copper interaction probably would be competitive according to the chemical interaction hypothesis of Hill and Matrone.[16] Reports indicative of a competitive interaction are that of Roslyakov *et al.*, who found that copper prevented blindness caused by excess nickel in sheep, and that of Schroeder *et al.*, who found that dietary nickel supplementation decreased lung and spleen copper.[17,18] Spears *et al.* reported that supplementing nickel to rats alleviated copper deficiency signs of growth retardation and depressed hematocrit and hemoglobin.[19] Spears *et al.* speculated that nickel substituted for copper at certain biological sites, thus preferentially sparing copper for some vital functions. This speculation was supported by the finding that nickel tended to decrease the copper content in some tissues of copper-deficient rats.[19]

Some findings indicate that nickel and copper also interact noncompetitively. In rats, nickel toxicity elevated the copper level in serum, liver, kidney, and spleen;[4] whereas nickel deprivation depressed the copper level in liver, spleen, and kidney of rats and in liver in sheep.[7-9]

As with the nickel-iron studies, we decided to confirm the interaction between nickel and copper by using factorially arranged experiments. Because iron nutriture apparently affects the response of rats to nickel deprivation, three fully crossed factors—variable levels of copper, iron, and nickel—were used in the experiments. In addition to determining the parameters determined in the nickel-iron interaction studies, we also determined heart, liver, kidney, and spleen weight and plasma ceruloplasmin. In experiment 1, female weanling rats were fed a diet (containing about 10 ng of nickel, 0.44 μg of copper, and 2.3 μg of iron/g) supplemented with copper at levels of 0, 0.5, and 5 μg/g; nickel, 0, 5, and 50 μg/g; and iron, 15 and 45 μg/g.[12] The iron supplement was a mixture of 40% ferrous sulfate and 60% ferric sulfate. In experiment 2, the diet was supplemented with copper at levels of 0, 0.5, and 12 μg/g; nickel, 0, 1, and 10 μg/g; and iron, 25 and 100 μg/g. The iron supplement was ferric sulfate only. The rats were killed after 11 weeks in experiment 1 and after 9 weeks in experiment 2.

In experiment 1, when dietary iron was supplemented as the ferric and ferrous sulfate mixture, the interaction between copper and nickel affected the ratios of liver wt/body wt, spleen wt/body wt, kidney wt/body wt, and heart wt/body wt; hematocrit and hemoglobin; plasma alkaline phosphatase activity, cholesterol, phospholipids, and lipids; and liver contents of iron, manganese, and nickel. In experiment 2, when dietary iron was supplemented as ferric sulfate only, nickel and copper did not interact to affect any parameter examined.

The hemoglobin data are shown in TABLE 2. In experiment 1, when the ferric-ferrous sulfate mixture was fed, the anemia was less severe in the copper- and nickel-deficient rats than in copper-deficient rats given supplemental nickel. In experiment 2, when ferric sulfate only was fed, dietary nickel apparently did not affect the anemia caused by copper deficiency.

The data for heart wt/body wt ratio in TABLE 3 show that nickel deprivation alleviated the enlarged heart in severe copper deficiency when dietary iron was supplied as the ferric and ferrous sulfate mixture. In experiment 2, when ferric sulfate only was fed, dietary nickel apparently did not affect the enlarged heart caused by copper deficiency.

When the interaction between nickel and copper affected other parameters, it did so in a manner generally similar to that found with hemoglobin and heart wt/body wt ratio. That is, signs of copper deficiency were more severe when nickel was supplemented to the diet. Thus, the findings suggest an antagonistic relationship between nickel and copper when dietary iron is supplied in a relatively available form

TABLE 2

EFFECT IN RATS OF COPPER, IRON, NICKEL, AND THEIR INTERACTIONS ON HEMOGLOBIN LEVELS

Experiment 1				Experiment 2			
Treatment* (μg/g)			Hemoglobin Level	Treatment* (μg/g)			Hemoglobin Level
Fe	Cu	Ni	(g/100 ml)	Fe	Cu	Ni	(g/100 ml)
15	0	0	9.31	25	0	0	3.87
15	0	5	7.13	25	0	1	4.61
15	0	50	7.22	25	0	10	3.85
15	0.5	0	11.74	25	0.5	0	7.17
15	0.5	5	11.37	25	0.5	1	7.60
15	0.5	50	11.84	25	0.5	10	8.49
15	5	0	12.01	25	12	0	7.61
15	5	5	12.08	25	12	1	8.55
15	5	50	12.19	25	12	10	9.05
45	0	0	10.12	100	0	0	10.03
45	0	5	10.51	100	0	1	11.31
45	0	50	9.22	100	0	10	10.65
45	0.5	0	11.90	100	0.5	0	11.74
45	0.5	5	12.14	100	0.5	1	12.40
45	0.5	50	12.01	100	0.5	10	12.25
45	5	0	12.11	100	12	0	12.57
45	5	5	12.50	100	12	1	12.70
45	5	50	12.50	100	12	10	12.21

Analysis of Variance—P Values	Experiment 1	Experiment 2
Copper effect	0.0001	0.0001
Iron effect	0.0001	0.0001
Nickel effect	0.0001	0.005
Cu × Fe	NS	NS
Cu × Ni	0.006	NS
Fe × Ni	0.005	NS
Cu × Fe × Ni	NS	NS
Error mean square (df)	0.55 (87)	0.81 (87)

* Amounts of iron (mixture of 40% ferrous sulfate and 60% ferric sulfate in experiment 1; ferric sulfate in experiment 2), Cu (copper sulfate), and Ni (nickel chloride) supplemented to diet.

(ferric and ferrous sulfate mixture). We found that dietary nickel or a nickel-copper interaction did not affect the copper content of the liver, the only tissue tested, of copper-deficient rats. This indicates that the interaction between nickel and copper does not occur mainly at the absorption level but occurs at various metabolic sites.

We are not certain whether the interaction between copper and nickel depends upon the availability of dietary iron or upon the severity of iron deficiency. The data in TABLES 2 and 3 show that the effect of increasing dietary nickel on hemoglobin and heart wt/body wt ratio in copper-deficient rats was similar when the diet contained 45 μg of iron/g as a ferric and ferrous sulfate mixture or 100 μg of iron/g as ferric sulfate only. It was at the low levels of iron supplementation that differences appeared. In rats with severe iron deficiency anemia (25 μg of iron/g of diet as ferric sulfate only), copper deficiency signs were not affected by nickel. On the other hand, in moderate iron deficiency (15 μg of iron/g of diet as a ferric and ferrous sulfate mixture), nickel supplementation exacerbated copper deficiency. Further studies with levels of a ferric and ferrous sulfate mixture that cause severe iron deficiency or

TABLE 3

EFFECT IN RATS OF COPPER, IRON, NICKEL, AND THEIR INTERACTIONS ON HEART WEIGHT/BODY WEIGHT RATIO

Experiment 1				Experiment 2			
Treatment* (μg/g)			Heart Wt/ Body Wt	Treatment* (μg/g)			Heart Wt/ Body Wt
Fe	Cu	Ni	Ratio × 100	Fe	Cu	Ni	Ratio × 100
15	0	0	0.499	25	0	0	0.699
15	0	5	0.636	25	0	1	0.627
15	0	50	0.913	25	0	10	0.714
15	0.5	0	0.373	25	0.5	0	0.404
15	0.5	5	0.378	25	0.5	1	0.400
15	0.5	50	0.362	25	0.5	10	0.402
15	5	0	0.330	25	12	0	0.382
15	5	5	0.331	25	12	1	0.363
15	5	50	0.343	25	12	10	0.355
45	0	0	0.497	100	0	0	0.513
45	0	5	0.530	100	0	1	0.486
45	0	50	0.596	100	0	10	0.571
45	0.5	0	0.363	100	0.5	0	0.348
45	0.5	5	0.366	100	0.5	1	0.370
45	0.5	50	0.358	100	0.5	10	0.372
45	5	0	0.324	100	12	0	0.348
45	5	5	0.334	100	12	1	0.359
45	5	50	0.325	100	12	10	0.349

Analysis of Variance—P Values

	Experiment 1	Experiment 2
Copper effect	0.0001	0.0001
Iron effect	0.02	0.0001
Nickel effect	0.01	NS
Cu × Fe	0.04	0.0005
Cu × Ni	0.002	NS
Fe × Ni	NS	NS
Cu × Fe × Ni	NS	NS
Error mean square (df)	0.012 (70)	0.004 (88)

* Amounts of iron (mixture of 40% ferrous sulfate and 60% ferric sulfate in experiment 1; ferric sulfate in experiment 2), Cu (copper sulfate), and Ni (nickel chloride) supplemented to diet.

with levels of ferric sulfate only that cause moderate iron deficiency are needed to clarify the question.

An interesting sidelight in these experiments was the finding that interactions between copper and iron were highly significant only in experiment 2. However, as for the nickel-copper interactions, we do not know whether this was due to the form of the iron supplement or to the degree of iron deficiency when low levels of iron were fed.

ARSENIC-ZINC INTERACTION

We found that arginine supplementation made signs of arsenic deprivation in chicks appear earlier and more severe.[20] One of these signs was an elevation in the zinc content of liver. Arginine supplementation also made some zinc-deprivation signs in chicks more severe.[21] This suggested to us that there may be an interrelationship between arsenic and zinc.

Day-old cockerels were fed the diet shown in TABLE 4 (containing about 5 ng of arsenic and 7 μg zinc/g) supplemented with two levels of arsenic and zinc. The supplements were arsenic as $Na_2HAsO_4 \cdot 7H_2O$, 0 and 2 μg/g; zinc as $Zn(C_2H_3O_2)_2 \cdot 2H_2O$, 5 (zinc deficient) and 40 μg/g.

After 32 days, an interaction between arsenic and zinc affected growth, leg development, liver wt/body wt ratio, hematocrit, and plasma alkaline phosphatase (TABLE 5). Spleen wt, gonad wt, shank skin dermatitis, and feathering were not affected by an interaction between arsenic and zinc.

When dietary zinc was 40 μg/g, the arsenic-deprived chicks exhibited leg abnormalities that differed from those of the zinc-deficient chicks. Although the legs were twisted and appeared weak, they were not extremely short and thick with swollen hocks. The arsenic-supplemented chicks fed 40 μg of zinc/g of diet did not exhibit any obvious leg abnormalities. Dietary arsenic apparently had little effect on the leg abnormalities of zinc-deficient chicks.

The effect of dietary arsenic on growth and hematocrits was dependent upon the zinc status of the chick (TABLE 5). When dietary zinc was 40 μg/g, the arsenic-deprived chicks exhibited depressed growth and elevated hematocrits. During zinc

TABLE 4

COMPOSITION OF BASAL CHICK DIET FOR ARSENIC-ZINC INTERACTION STUDIES*

Ingredient	g/kg Diet
Casein, high protein	160.00
Ground corn, acid washed†	673.70
Corn oil	75.00
Fat-soluble vitamins†	0.11
Vitamin mix‡	4.89
Choline chloride	1.30
Arginine	4.00
Glycine	5.00
Methionine	0.50
Cholecalciferol mix§	0.50
Mineral mix¶	25.00
KH_2PO_4	25.00
$CaCO_3$	25.00
	1000.00

* Diet analyzed about 5 ng of arsenic and 7 μg zinc/g on an air-dried basis.

† See Nielsen *et al.* for acid washing procedure and fat-soluble vitamins.[29]

‡ The vitamin mix supplied (in mg/kg diet): retinyl acetate (500,000 IU/g), 8; retinyl palmitate (250,000 IU/g), 16; thiamin·HCl, 16; pyridoxine·HCl, 12; niacin, 60; calcium pantothenate, 20; vitamin B_{12} (0.1% triturate with mannitol), 20; folic acid, 2; biotin, 1; riboflavin, 16; menaquinone, 1; and glucose, 4,740.

§ The cholecalciferol mix contained (in g): cholecalciferol (40,000,000 IU/g), 0.0005; and glucose, 10. Mix contained 2000 IU cholecalciferol/g.

¶ The mineral mix supplied (in g/kg diet): NaCl, 3.75; $Mg(C_2H_3O_2)_2 \cdot 4H_2O$, 4.35; Mn $(C_2H_3O_2)_2 \cdot 4H_2O$, 0.225; iron sponge dissolved in HCl, 0.038; $CuSO_4 \cdot 5H_2O$, 0.06; KI, 0.0004; Na_2SeO_3, 0.0003; $(NH_4)_6Mo_7O_{24} \cdot 4H_2O$, 0.004; Cr $(C_2H_3O_2)_3 \cdot H_2O$, 0.002; NH_4VO_3, 0.0002; acid-washed ground corn, 16.5701.

deficiency, however, growth was more markedly depressed and hematocrits more markedly elevated in the arsenic-supplemented than in the arsenic-deficient chicks.

In contrast to effects on growth and hematocrits, effects of dietary zinc on liver wt/body wt ratio and plasma alkaline phosphatase activity apparently depended upon the arsenic status of the chick (TABLE 5). Zinc deficiency did not affect the liver wt/body wt ratio of arsenic-supplemented chicks. When the chicks were arsenic deprived, zinc deficiency elevated the liver wt/body wt ratio. Plasma alkaline phosphatase activity was elevated in zinc-deficient chicks that were fed supplemental arsenic. On the other hand, zinc-deficiency slightly depressed plasma alkaline phosphatase activity in arsenic-deprived chicks.

The findings indicate that the interaction between arsenic and zinc is noncompetitive. This would be expected because they exist in biological systems in dissimilar form—arsenic as an anion, zinc as a cation. The findings seem to indicate that arsenic is necessary for the efficient utilization or metabolism of zinc. Many of the signs of arsenic deprivation are similar to signs of zinc deprivation—depressed growth, leg abnormalities, and elevated hematocrits and plasma alkaline phosphatase activity.[11] These signs were found even though the diet supposedly contained an adequate amount of zinc (40 μg/g). On the other hand, arsenic deprivation appeared to alleviate some zinc-deprivation signs but exacerbate others. Perhaps arsenic enhanced the utilization of zinc at some metabolic sites, thus removing zinc from others. This could explain the divergent effects of arsenic deprivation on zinc-deprivation signs. Obviously, more studies are needed to determine how and at which metabolic sites the interaction between arsenic and zinc occurs.

VANADIUM-CHROMIUM INTERACTION

Based on the physicochemical properties of their ions, vanadium and chromium should antagonistically interact in biological systems.[16] In the anions of both elements, the oxygen atoms are attached to the central atom in an sp^3 arrangement and thus form a tetrahedral structure. In both anions, the 4s and 4p orbitals are used.

TABLE 5

EFFECTS ON CHICKS OF ARSENIC, ZINC, AND THEIR INTERACTION

Treatment* As (μg/g)	Treatment* Zn (μg/g)	Body Weight† (g)	Liver Wt/ Body Wt Ratio × 100	Hematocrit (%)	Plasma Alkaline Phosphatase Activity (units)‡
0	5	783	2.39	31.3	1.381
0	40	904	2.03	30.9	1.632
2	5	746	2.08	32.0	2.012
2	40	979	2.07	29.8	1.464
		Analysis of Variance—P Values			
Arsenic effect		NS	0.01	NS	NS
Zinc effect		0.0001	0.0006	0.01	NS
As × Zn		0.06	0.002	0.05	0.003
Error mean square (df)		19821 (84)	0.06 (83)	4.9 (84)	0.368 (84)

* Amounts of arsenic (sodium arsenate) and zinc (zinc acetate) supplemented to diet.

† Weight of chicks at age four weeks.

‡ Units were μmoles *p*-nitrophenyl phosphate split/minute/ml of plasma.

TABLE 6

EFFECTS ON CHICKS OF VANADIUM, CHROMIUM, AND THEIR INTERACTION

Treatment* V (μg/g)	Treatment* Cr (μg/g)	Body Weight† (g)	Hematocrit (%)	Plasma Cholesterol (mg/100 ml)	V Content, Calcified Cartilage‡ (ng/g)
0	0	1066	30.3	124	ND§
0	500	1044	30.4	120	69
5	0	1070	31.3	118	110
5	500	235	24.7	178	713
		Analysis of Variance—P Values			
Vanadium effect		0.0001	0.0001	0.0001	0.0001
Chromium effect		0.0001	0.0001	0.0001	0.0001
Vanadium × chromium		0.0001	0.0001	0.0001	0.0003

* Amounts of V (ammonium metavanadate) and Cr (chromium acetate) supplemented to diet.

† Weight of chicks at age four weeks.

‡ From proximal tibiae.

§ Not detected.

Wright reported findings supporting the concept that chromium and vanadium competitively interact.[22] He found that chromium was effective in overcoming growth depression and mortality associated with feeding 20 μg of vanadate/g of diet. In other studies, chromium partially overcame the uncoupling of oxidative phosphorylation caused by vanadate *in vivo* and *in vitro*.[22]

The studies of Wright encouraged us to test the possibility that high dietary chromium would enhance the signs of vanadium deprivation in chicks. Thus, in a fully crossed, two-factor experiment, day-old cockerels were fed a diet (containing 8 ng of vanadium and 1 μg of chromium/g) supplemented with vanadium at levels of 0 and 5 μg/g as NH_4VO_3 and chromium at levels of 0 and 500 μg/g as $Cr(C_2H_3O_2)_3 \cdot H_2O$. After 32 days, those chicks fed 500 μg of chromium and 5 μg of vanadium/g of diet exhibited depressed growth and hematocrits and elevated plasma cholesterol, kidney (Na,K) ATPase, liver wt/body wt ratio, gall bladder size, and vanadium content in some tissues. Examples of the data are given in TABLE 6. The proximal tibiae morphology was also drastically altered in the chicks supplemented with vanadium plus chromium. The growth plate was abnormally thick, and the zone of calcified cartilage abnormally thin. Metaphyseal bone was nonexistent. Transmission electron microscopic examinations revealed a disorganized growth plate and the presence of an abnormal electron-dense matrix component around the chondrocytes in the proliferative zone. Five μg of vanadium/g of diet without chromium supplementation had no obvious effect on chicks.

The addition of 500 μg of chromium/g of diet apparently made 5 μg of vanadium/g of diet toxic to chicks. Many of the abnormalities exhibited in those chicks were similar to the signs of vanadium toxicity. These include depressed growth and hematocrits, enlarged livers, distended gall bladders, and elevated plasma cholesterol.[24-28]

An attempt to repeat the previous findings was unsuccessful. Chromium supplementation of the vanadium-supplemented chicks gave similar findings, but the apparent vanadium toxicity signs were very mild. Thus, we became concerned about the possibility that the supplementation with vanadium plus chromium destroyed some labile dietary ingredient. A vitamin analysis of the diet that gave the severe abnormalities described indicated that some of the vitamins—including niacin, thiamine, and riboflavin—were destroyed, perhaps by the vanadium and chromium supplementation. Whether destruction of the vitamins accounted for the abnormalities was unclear. Thus, further studies are needed to ascertain whether high dietary chromium makes relatively small amounts of dietary vanadium toxic for chicks. Until then, any discussion of the interaction between vanadium and chromium in biological systems seems inappropriate.

Summary

Fully crossed, factorially arranged experiments showed that, under defined conditions, interactions occur between nickel and iron, nickel and copper, arsenic and zinc, and possibly vanadium and chromium. Nickel and iron interacted when dietary iron was supplemented as ferric sulfate only. Signs of nickel deprivation were more severe when dietary iron was low; or the signs of moderate iron deficiency were more severe when dietary nickel was deficient. When iron was supplemented to the diet as a 60% ferric–40% ferrous sulfate mixture, nickel and iron apparently did not interact. The findings suggested a synergistic relationship between nickel and iron when dietary iron was in a relatively unavailable form. An antagonistic interaction between nickel and copper was found when dietary iron was supplemented as a 60% ferric–40% ferrous sulfate mixture. Signs of copper deficiency were more severe in nickel-supplemented than in nickel-deprived rats. When the rats were made severely iron deficient by feeding of low levels of ferric sulfate only, no apparent interaction between nickel and copper was found. The interaction between arsenic and zinc apparently was noncompetitive. When dietary zinc was 40 μg/g, arsenic-deprived chicks exhibited depressed growth and elevated hematocrits. In zinc deficiency, growth was more markedly depressed and hematocrits more markedly elevated in arsenic-supplemented than in arsenic-deficient chicks. Arsenic might be necessary for the efficient utilization or metabolism of zinc. Findings indicating an interaction between vanadium and chromium were tentative. In one experiment, the addition of 500 μg of chromium/g of diet apparently made 5 μg of vanadium/g of diet toxic for chicks. Thus, the interactions between essential trace and ultratrace elements might be of nutritional significance.

References

1. Lederer, E. & M. Lourau. 1948. Action antagoniste de certains cations divalents sur un enzyme secrété par la muqueuse gastrique et jouant un rôle dans l'hématopoiese. Biochim. Biophys. Acta **2:** 278–285.
2. Lange, E. R. 1972. Effect of nickel on hemopoiesis in rabbits and fish. Uch. Zap. Latv. Gos. Univ. **176:** 63–79. (In Russian.)
3. Whanger, P. D. 1973. Effects of dietary nickel on enzyme activities and mineral contents in rats. Toxicol. Appl. Pharmacol. **25:** 323–331.
4. Schnegg, A. & M. Kirchgessner. 1976. Zur toxizität von alimentär verabreichtem Nickel. Landwirtsch. Forsch. **29:** 177–185.
5. Schnegg, A. & M. Kirschgessner. 1975. Veränderungen des Hämoglobingehaltes, der Erythrozytenzahl und des Hämatokrits bei Nickelmangel. Nutr. Metab. **19:** 268–278.
6. Schnegg, A. & M. Kirchgessner. 1976. Zur Absorption und Verfügbarkeit von Eisen bei Nickel-Mangel. Int. Z. Vitam. Ernährungsforsch. **46:** 96–99.

7. Schnegg, A. & M. Kirchgessner. 1976. Zur Inter Aktion von Nickel mit Eisen, Kupfer und Zink. Arch. Tierernähr. **26:** 543–549.
8. Schnegg, A. & M. Kirchgessner. 1978. Ni deficiency and its effects on metabolism. *In* Trace Element Metabolism in Man and Animals. M. Kirchgessner, Ed. **3:** 236–243. University of Munchen. Freising-Weihanstephan, Federal Republic of Germany.
9. Spears, J. W., E. E. Hatfield & G. C. Fahey, Jr. 1978. Nickel depletion in the growing ovine. Nutr. Rep. Int. **18:** 621–629.
10. Nielsen, F. H., T. J. Zimmerman, M. E. Collings & D. R. Myron. 1979. Nickel deprivation in rats: nickel-iron interactions. J. Nutr. **109:** 1623–1632.
11. Underwood, E. J. 1977. Trace Elements in Human and Animal Nutrition. 4th edit. Academic Press, Inc. New York, N.Y.
12. Nielsen, F. H., T. R. Shuler, T. J. Zimmerman, M. E. Collings & E. O. Uthus. 1979. Interaction between nickel and iron in the rat. Biol. Trace Element Res. **1:** 325–335.
13. May, P. M., D. R. Williams & P. W. Linder. 1978. Biological significance of low molecular weight iron (III) complexes. *In* Metal Ions in Biological Systems. Iron in Model and Natural Compounds. H. Sigel, Ed. **7:** 29–76. Marcel Dekker, Inc. New York, N.Y.
14. Manis, J. G. & D. Schachter. 1962. Active transport of iron by intestine: features of the two-step mechanism. Am. J. Physiol. **203:** 73–80.
15. Dowdle, E. B., D. Schachter & H. Schenker. 1960. Active transport of Fe^{59} by everted segments of rat duodenum. Am. J. Physiol. **198:** 609–613.
16. Hill, C. H. & G. Matrone. 1970. Chemical parameters in the study of in vivo and in vitro interactions of transition elements. Fed. Proc. Fed. Am. Soc. Exp. Biol. **29:** 1474–1481.
17. Roslyakov, A. K., M. A. Baiturin & Z. U. Izbasarov. 1972. Prevention of nickel blindness of sheep in the Abtyubinsk region. Tr. Alma-At. Zoovet. Inst. (24): 142–144. (In Russian.)
18. Schroeder, H. A., M. Mitchener & A. P. Nason. 1974. Life-term effects of nickel in rats: survival, tumors, interactions with trace elements and tissue levels. J. Nutr. **104:** 239–243.
19. Spears, J. W., E. E. Hatfield & R. M. Forbes. 1977. Nickel-copper interrelationship in the rat. Proc. Soc. Exp. Biol. Med. **156:** 140–143.
20. Nielsen, F. H. & T. R. Shuler. 1978. Arsenic deprivation studies in chicks. (abst.). Fed. Proc. Fed. Am. Soc. Exp. Biol. **37:** 893.
21. Coleman, B. W., E. M. Reimann, R. H. Grummer, M. L. Sunde & W. G. Hoekstra. 1971. Antagonistic effect of arginine on zinc metabolism in chicks. J. Nutr. **101:** 1695–1702.
22. Wright, W. R. 1968. Metabolic interrelationship between vanadium and chromium. Ph.D. Thesis. North Carolina State University. Raleigh, N.C.
23. Hunt, C. D. 1979. The effect of dietary vanadium on ^{48}V metabolism and proximal tibial growth plate morphology in the chick. Ph.D. Thesis. University of North Dakota. Grand Forks, N. Dak.
24. Proescher, F., H. A. Seil & A. W. Stillians. 1917. A contribution to the action of vanadium with particular reference to syphillis. Amer. J. Syph. **1:** 347–405.
25. Berg, L. R. 1963. Evidence of vanadium toxicity resulting from the use of certain commercial phosphorus supplements in chick rations. Poult. Sci. **42:** 766–769.
26. Hathcock, J., C. H. Hill & G. Matrone. 1964. Vanadium toxicity and distribution in chicks and rats. J. Nutr. **82:** 106–110.
27. Hafez, Y. S. M. & F. H. Kratzer. 1976. The effect of diet on the toxicity of vanadium. Poult. Sci. **55:** 918–922.
28. Chakbraborty, D., A. Bhattacharyya, K. Majumdar & G. C. Chatterjee. 1977. Effects of chronic vanadium pentoxide administration on L-ascorbic acid metabolism in rats: influence of L-ascorbic acid supplementation. Int. J. Vitam. Nutr. Res. **47:** 81–87.
29. Nielsen, F. H., D. R. Myron, S. H. Givand, T. J. Zimmerman & D. A. Ollerich. 1975. Nickel deficiency in rats. J. Nutr. **105:** 1620–1630.

Discussion

W. R. Holub (*Life Systems, Inc., Melville, N.Y.*): You seem to be the right person to ask a philosophic question, or a three-part philosophic question, since you are venturing beyond permutations of two.

First, on the basis of your experience, would you conjecture about the possibility that probably all elements in the periodic table are, at least in one degree or another, essential and also that probably all interact with each other directly or indirectly. Also, probably all vitamins interact with each other directly or indirectly. If such interactions are occurring, should not we reevaluate single element or single vitamin intervention because such intervention may be upsetting the stack of cards?

F. H. Nielsen: There is no doubt that single element or single vitamin intervention must be closely evaluated. Single nutrient intervention may have an adverse effect on health through a detrimental interaction with another nutrient or nutrients. I suspect there are many interactions occurring between elements and vitamins, about which very little is known. There is an urgent need for more knowledge about the extent and type of interactions occurring between nutrients.

I do not believe that every element on the periodic table will be found essential. Also, I am not as enthusiastic as Dr. Klaus Schwarz was about the possibility of the existence of a large number of undiscovered essential trace elements. Actually, I think more evidence is needed to establish the essentiality of some trace elements that have been accepted as essential by some people, such as vanadium and tin.

J. C. Smith, Jr. (*Beltsville Human Nutrition Research Center, U.S. Department of Agriculture, Beltsville, Md.*): Dr. Nielsen, I wonder if you would elaborate briefly on the interaction between arsenic and zinc. You suggested that arsenic may be making zinc utilization or absorption more efficient?

F. H. Nielsen: That is correct. Perhaps arsenic is necessary for some enzyme or metabolic process that affects the metabolism of zinc.

J. C. Smith, Jr.: Have you thought about the possibility that you are feeding enough arsenic to affect the microflora of the gut and thus affect zinc metabolism?

F. H. Nielsen: I doubt that the microflora of the gut were affected by the arsenic supplemented to the diet. The arsenic supplement was sodium arsenate. Pentavalent arsenic is relatively innocuous at the level used in our experimental diets, 2 μg/g. Many foods contain a much larger level of pentavalent arsenic. For example, some seafoods, such as shrimp, can contain 10 to 12 μg of arsenic/g.

J. C. Smith, Jr.: I am suggesting that perhaps some microflora that normally inhibit zinc absorption were eliminated by the arsenic supplementation. There is more efficient utilization of zinc in germfree animals. Also, I recall that it was suggested that arsenic supplementation elevated growth in swine by acting as an antimicrobial agent.

F. H. Nielsen: Nonetheless, I do not believe arsenic was exerting its action in my studies by altering gut microflora. This belief is supported by the fact that arsenic supplementation exacerbated some signs of zinc deficiency. If arsenic were just changing gut microflora and thus improving absorption of zinc, arsenic supplementation should have alleviated most all signs of zinc deficiency.

C. H. Hill (*North Carolina State University, Raleigh, N.C.*): I have two comments. First, you may be interested in knowing that we have found that the growth depression caused by nickel toxicity can be alleviated by adding zinc to the diet. The other comment is that I was relieved you could not duplicate your finding that high levels of dietary chromium induce an apparent vanadium toxicity in chicks fed 5 μg of vanadium/g of diet. I am relieved because that finding wrecked a beautiful hypothesis, and because we could not repeat your finding.

F. H. Nielsen: I feel fortunate that I was able to state first that perhaps the adverse effects found in the original vanadium-chromium experiment were not due to just a vanadium-chromium interaction.

J. M. Navia (*University of Alabama, Birmingham, Ala.*): I'd like to make a comment and a suggestion in regard to your very fine experimental designs. I compliment you on your approach to identifying different interactions. My comment is in regard to the ability to reproduce various experiments in different laboratories. I noticed your experimental diets contained corn and skim milk. Recently, much progress has been made in developing adequate purified diets. I believe that if we resorted to a purified diet that could be reproduced in different laboratories, some problems in reproducing experiments between laboratories would be eliminated. I wonder whether the use of purified diets would be appropriate. Also, did you use distilled, deionized, or tap water in your studies?

F. H. Nielsen: Because of time limitations, I could not describe in detail the experimental methods and materials used in my studies. The water used in our latest experiments was purified in two steps. The first step was passing the water through a reverse osmosis system. Then the water was further deionized by passing it through activated carbon and ion exchange columns. The resistivity of the final water was approximately 18 megohm-cm.

The use of purified diets is not always possible. For example, the conventional method of using purified ingredients apparently is not the best method for obtaining nickel-deficient diets. Some purified ingredients, especially minerals, are too contaminated with nickel. Thus, a preferable method is to use a diet made mainly of natural feedstuffs that are low in nickel and contain most vitamins and minerals in amounts such that no major addition of chemicals is necessary.

In our studies, all feedstuffs used were analyzed for the trace element under study. When a certain lot of an ingredient, such as skim milk or ground corn, was found to contain a suitable low level of contamination, most or all of that lot was purchased. Thus, when experiments were duplicated, the animals in the second experiment usually were fed a diet made of ingredients used in the first experiment. To further assure that there was a low level of trace-element contamination in the diet, one major ingredient, ground corn, was acid washed. We have published the procedure for acid washing ground corn. Also, some of my recent publications described the sources of the ingredients used in my experimental diets.

H. G. Petering (*University of Cincinnati Medical Center, Cincinnati, Ohio*): Did you say that the interaction between zinc and arsenic was dependent upon the arginine level in the diet?

F. H. Nielsen: No. We decided to ascertain whether zinc interacts with arsenic because both zinc and arsenic deficiencies in chicks apparently are exacerbated by excess dietary arginine. This finding suggested to us that both zinc and arsenic may affect the same metabolic pathway. In the arsenic-zinc interaction studies, the diet contained 1.2% arginine. This level of arginine was not particularly high because the chick requirement for arginine is about 1% of the diet.

H. G. Petering: Do you have any problem in removing nickel contamination from the iron supplements?

F. H. Nielsen: We could not obtain iron salts commercially in a suitable noncontaminated form. Thus, we made the iron salts in our laboratory. The starting materials were specially purified iron sponge and mineral acids.

MAGNESIUM, CALCIUM, AND PARATHYROID HORMONE INTERACTIONS

Maurice E. Shils

Memorial Sloan-Kettering Cancer Center
and
Cornell University Medical College
New York, New York 10021

INTRODUCTION

The first published observations concerning magnesium (Mg) deficiency in man were those of Hirschfelder; in a relatively small number of hypomagnesemic patients with renal insufficiency or hypoparathyroidism, he noted twitching and convulsions, some of which improved with magnesium.[1] Flink and his associates advanced knowledge of human Mg depletion with their studies in patients with acute alcoholism superimposed on chronic alcoholism and in others who had been maintained on prolonged intravenous fluids without Mg.[2] Flink *et al.* described personality changes, tremors, athetoid movements, and convulsions and made certain observations relative to Mg and potassium levels. Nevertheless, the symptomatology and biochemical abnormalities ascribable to deficiency of Mg were not adequately defined and were a matter of some disagreement despite various individual case reports. This lack of clarity was attributable to two major facts: firstly, despite various attempts, experimental *symptomatic* human deficiency had not been induced; and secondly, the accounts of symptomatic depletion in patients always occurred in the setting of predisposing diseases and clinical situations that were usually complex (TABLE 1). In such circumstances, associated complex and uncontrollable variables—such as multiple dietary inadequacies, metabolic abnormalities, manifestations of basic disease, severe infection, and treatments given in close proximity to the Mg supplementation—made it difficult and potentially misleading to ascribe certain clinical manifestations specifically to Mg deficiency. Furthermore, at that time, the clinical literature was in disagreement concerning the relation of Mg deficiency to serum calcium (Ca) levels and to the occurrence of latent or overt tetany—defined here as a positive Trousseau sign or spontaneous carpopedal spasm. Some investigators expressed the opinion that tetany was not a manifestation of Mg deficiency, per se, and that a coexisting hypocalcemia was not related to the Mg depletion. Others suggested that there was a relationship, since hypomagnesemia, hypocalcemia, and neurological symptoms improved in relation to Mg therapy but not to Ca. Still another type of clinical picture was reported in which hyperirritability, tetany, and other neuromuscular abnormalities occurred in the setting of hypomagnesemia but where the serum Ca was normal; this syndrome was claimed to respond to Mg but not to Ca salts.

EXPERIMENTAL OBSERVATIONS

Experimental Symptomatic Magnesium Deficiency in Man

In an attempt to develop a better understanding of the role of this ion, an effort was made to induce Mg depletion by dietary means in adult human volunteers with

0077-8923/80/0355-0165 $01.75/0

TABLE 1

CLINICAL CONDITIONS ASSOCIATED WITH MAGNESIUM DEFICIENCY

1. Severe malabsorption of various etiologies
2. Chronic alcoholism with malnutrition
3. Prolonged infusion of Mg-free solutions
4. Renal tubular disorders secondary to disease or drugs
5. Endocrine disorders (especially of parathyroid)
6. Genetic defect in absorption
7. Uncommon miscellaneous causes

normal absorption and renal function who were under close clinical supervision. In this study, individuals were maintained on a highly purified, tube-fed diet supplemented with Mg during a control period. The basal diet supplied 800 mg of Ca per day throughout the study and adequate amounts of vitamin D. Observations were made during the control period, in the depletion period when Mg was omitted from the diet, and during the subsequent repletion period. All subjects became markedly hypomagnesemic. Six of the seven subjects became significantly hypocalcemic. The serum phosphorus was normal or slightly low in most of the patients, but it was elevated in one of the patients; following repletion, three of the patients had a marked fall in phosphorus. Despite the adequacy of intake of Ca and vitamin D, all of the patients who became symptomatic had developed hypocalcemia. The time to obvious neurological changes varied greatly, signs appearing in anywhere from 25 to 110 days. These signs included positive Chvostek and Trousseau signs, tremor, and muscle fibrillations and spasticity.

The following observations made in this study are pertinent to this paper:

1. Serum Ca decreased when serum Mg declined to moderately low levels.
2. There was an association in time between the low serum Ca and Mg in the onset of neurological signs.

TABLE 2

THE INFLUENCE OF EXPERIMENTAL Mg DEPLETION ON SERUM Ca LEVELS IN VARIOUS SPECIES—LITERATURE REFERENCES

	Ca Level Compared to Controls		
Species	Increased	Normal	Decreased
Rat	*†	*†	51‡†
Mouse		9	8
Guinea Pig		52	7
Chick			16, 17
Dog		53, 55, 56, 57	6, 10, 18, 19, 43, 54
Pig			58
Sheep			59, 60
Cow		61	62, 63, 64, 65, 66
Monkey			6, 10, 20
Man		67	3

* Numerous references.
† See text.
‡ Reference number.

3. Administration of Ca intravenously raised the serum Ca only as long as the infusion lasted; cessation of the infusion was followed by a prompt fall in serum Ca and a prompt return of neurological signs.

4. Although serum Mg increased rapidly with the administration of Mg, there was a lag period of two or more days before there was a significant rise in the serum calcium.

5. Most of the clinical signs cleared or improved before the serum Ca reached normal levels.

6. The balance studies performed during the deficiency experiment indicated that the patients were absorbing Ca quite well and that they were in positive Ca balance.

7. Urinary Ca fell to very low levels. The infusion of Ca intravenously did not result in a significant increase in the excretion of Ca.

It was concluded that Mg was somehow essential for the mobilization of Ca from bone, but the exact mechanism was not apparent from these studies. These experimental observations have been increasingly confirmed in patients with symptomatic Mg deficiency of various etiologies.

Observations in Other Species

The rat had been the species given major attention in earlier studies of Mg deficiency. As increasing numbers of observations have been made with other species, it has become apparent that the rat is not a representative species with respect to serum Ca alterations. The rat is not even typical of other rodents either in this respect or in certain aspects of symptomatology.

TABLE 2 summarizes changes noted in the level of serum Ca in experimentally induced Mg deficiency in various species, including rodents, chicks, ruminants, dogs, pigs, primates, and man. I have reviewed the literature over a 14-year period and found reports from 14 different laboratories (many having more than one published paper on the subject) reporting on serum Ca levels in the Mg-depleted rat. Five laboratories noted either no change or variable changes as compared to control values in the deficient animals and 8 observed consistent hypercalcemia; only 1 reported hypocalcemia. Comments on this isolated report of hypocalcemia have been made elsewhere, where it was suggested that the calcium change was secondary to renal dysfunction.[4]

When the dietary level of Ca is severely restricted, the Mg-deficient rat develops hypocalcemia.[5,6] The reports on changes in serum Ca in the deficient guinea pig and mouse are contradictory. The development of hypocalcemia in the guinea pig as noted by Morris and O'Dell is complicated by the development of a decrease in creatinine clearance.[7] Alcock and Shils found that deficient male Swiss mice became hypocalcemic rapidly.[8] Goldman *et al.,* using females of the same strain, reported normal Ca levels;[9] in this study, the dietary Ca level was high (1.2%), whereas the diet of Alcock and Shils provided 0.14%. The latter diet resulted in normocalcemia or hypercalcemia in the deficient rat, so that a true species difference unrelated to diet is apparent. The data obtained in the dog are also conflicting, but the more recent studies seem to agree that hypocalcemia develops consistently, especially if the animals are not old. Experimental deficiencies in the chick, pig, sheep, calf, and monkey resulted in hypocalcemia in almost all studies. When the identical diet was fed to rats, mice, dogs, monkeys, and man, only the rat failed to develop hypocalcemia.[10] When hypocalcemia developed in the monkey, successive increases in dietary Ca did not prevent or overcome the hypocalcemia of Mg deficiency, whereas a single intramuscular injection of Mg (17 mEq) caused a marked rise in plasma Ca that persisted for one week or more (FIGURE 1).

Interrelationships among Magnesium, Calcium, Parathyroid Hormone, and Bone Metabolism

Although Mg-deficient rats often develop the biochemical changes indicative of hyperparathyroidism (hypercalcemia, hypophosphatemia, hypocalciuria, and hyperphosphaturia) and although parathyroidectomy eliminated the relative hypercalcemia in this species,[11-14] other species develop changes suggestive of a relative hypoparathyroid state. These observations have led to efforts to clarify these interrelations.

Effect of Parathyroid Extract In Vitro

Raisz and Niemann found that when parathyroid extract (PTE) was added to fetal rat bones *in vitro,* less Ca was released from the bone when the medium was low in Mg than when the Mg was normal.[15] When PTE was added *in vitro* to nonfetal bone derived from both magnesium-deficient and normal rats, it did not result in as

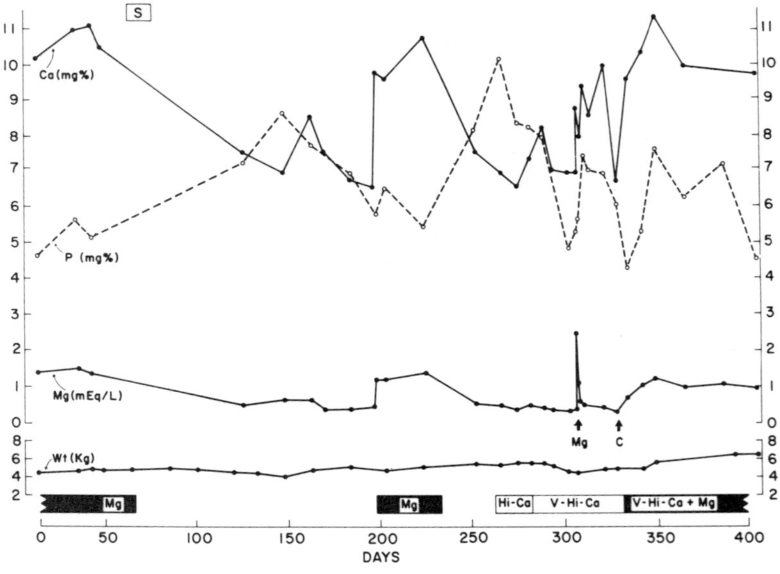

FIGURE 1. Failure of increased calcium intake to overcome hypocalcemia in a magnesium-deficient monkey. Two periods of magnesium depletion are indicated; each was associated with development of hypomagnesemia, hypocalcemia, and behavioral changes. During the first depletion period, the calcium content of the diet was 140 mg %; this was then increased to 235 mg % (Hi-Ca diet) and then increased again to 542 mg % (very Hi-Ca diet). Despite the increased calcium intake, hypocalcemia was present with the magnesium deficiency. On day 308, when the animal was having spasticity and tremor, 17 mEq magnesium were injected intramuscularly, with a transient response of magnesium and calcium. Twenty-two days later, there was a convulsion. Magnesium was reinstituted, with a sustained rise in plasma magnesium and calcium and disappearance of symptoms.

large a release of Ca, phosphate, and hydroxyproline from bone derived from deficient animals as it did from control bone.[13] These studies suggest that Mg deficiency induces a degree of refractoriness of bone to the action of parathyroid hormone (PTH). These observations with rat tissues create an apparent contradiction, since serum Ca tends to be elevated in the deficient rat; they suggest that other factors operate in the intact animal.

Effect of Parathyroid Extract In Vivo

The effectiveness of PTE in raising the level of serum Ca has been compared in control and Mg-deficient rats and other species. Intact, parathyroidectomized, or thyroparathyroidectomized animals have been utilized. TABLE 3 compares the responses of deficient animals to Mg-fed controls. Experimental conditions differed

TABLE 3

RESPONSE OF SERUM Ca TO PARATHYROID EXTRACT (PTE) INJECTION IN Mg-DEFICIENT ANIMALS AS COMPARED TO Mg-FED CONTROLS

	Surgical Status*		
Species	Intact	PTX	T-PTX
Rat	S (11)†	S (14)	R (13)‡
Dose (units & period)	200 at 0, 12, & 24 hr (ip)	150/kg (ip)	50 (ip)
Test at (hr)	6	3	2 & 6
	S (50)		
Dose (units & period)	50/100 g BW × 1 (sc)		
Test at (hr)	5		
Chick	R (16)		
Dose (units & period)	15/100 g BW × 1 (iv)		
Test at (hr)	¼–1½		
	R (17)		
Dose (units & period)	50, 100, or 200 × 1 (sc)		
Test at (hr)	4		
Dog	PR (19)§		S (18)
Dose (units & period)	2/kg × 8 hr (iv)		various¶; also 0.3/hr × 40 (iv)
Test at (hr)	8		‖
	S (18)		
Dose (units & period)	various¶		
Test at (hr)	‖		
Monkey	S (20)		
Dose (units & period)	2 or 4/kg/hr × 24 hr (iv) 15/kg BID × 2 days		
Test at (hr)	4, 7, and 24		

* Abbreviations: **PTX** = parathyroidectomized; **T-PTX** = thyroparathyroidectomized; **S** = similar response to PTE between Mg-deficient and control animals; **PR** = Mg-deficient animals partially refractory to PTE; **R** = Mg-deficient animals refractory to PTE; **ip** = intraperitoneal; **sc** = subcutaneous; **iv** = intravenous; **BW** = body weight; **BID** = twice a day.

† Reference numbers are given in parenthesis.

‡ Significant, but small, rise in Ca in controls.

§ Dogs acted as own controls.

¶ PTE given continuously iv with stepwise graduations every 48 hours to attain level of normocalcemia.

‖ Ca levels determined at 12, 24, 41, and 48 hours at each dose.

from one study to another in the amount and rate of PTE administration and time of blood collection for Ca determination. Very unphysiologic doses of PTE were given in some instances.

Three of four studies with rats revealed no inhibitory effect of Mg deficiency in the response; the exception is of interest in that there was only a slight, but significant, increase in controls.[13] In the study of Hahn *et al.*, serum Ca also rose in deficient rats with dibutyryl cyclic adenosine 3′,5′-monophosphate (cyclic AMP) in deficient as well as control rats.[14] Mg-deficient chicks proved resistant to PTE in the two reported studies. This responsiveness to PTE following Mg administration was then investigated. In one study, Mg was injected in an amount sufficient to raise the serum Mg level to normal in one hour, at which time the PTE at 30 u/100 g body weight was injected; there was no response in the newly treated chicks.[16] In the other study, following three days of Mg depletion, the birds were again responsive to PTE.[17]

Two studies have been reported on dogs. In the experiments of Suh *et al.* using dogs of various ages, no significant difference was noted in the amount of PTE required to attain normal serum Ca levels between deficient and control intact animals when the PTE was infused stepwise until the normal plasma Ca level was reached.[18] Comparison of the response to PTE of magnesium-deficient thyroparathyroidectomized and intact dogs revealed no difference; this experiment indicates that excess calcitonin secretion was not a factor in the hypocalcemia occurring in the intact deficient dogs. The authors concluded that hypocalcemia in Mg-deficient dogs is not due to resistance of end organ (bone) to the Ca-mobilizing action of PTE, but rather, it is a result of defective synthesis or diminished secretion of PTH.

Levi *et al.,* using adult female mongrel dogs, obtained somewhat different results.[19] Their animals acted as their own controls in the course of control, depletion, and repletion periods. Significant hypocalcemia developed with the depletion, and PTE produced an increase of serum Ca. However, the magnitude of the increments in serum Ca with PTE was greater during the control and repletion periods than during the depletion period. Reduced calcemic response was shown during the infusion when the serum Mg reached 1.0 mg % or less, and there was no significant correlation between the calcemic response to PTE when serum Mg was reduced further. Immunoreactive parathyroid hormone (iPTH) was present in normal amounts in the two animals studied and remained stable during Mg depletion despite the hypocalcemia. These authors concluded that there was both an impaired responsiveness to PTH and a reduced secretion of the hormone consequent to the hypocalcemia developing during Mg deficiency.

Rhesus monkeys gave calcemic responses to PTE when depleted of Mg similar in amount to those observed when Mg was given.[20] In experiments using the stumptailed monkey, I have also noted an excellent response to PTE in hypocalcemic Mg-deficient monkeys.[6]

Thus, with exception of the chick, other laboratory species tested—including the rat, dog, and monkey—appear to be capable of responding to PTE with respect to elevation of serum Ca levels during Mg deficiency. The responsiveness of the latter three species suggests that abnormality occurring in these Mg-deficient mammals would appear to reside primarily in the inability of the parathyroid gland to secrete an amount of hormone appropriate to the serum Ca level. Direct evidence in laboratory animals for this belief has been obtained only in the study of Levi *et al.,* where the immuno-cross-reactivity between canine and bovine PTH was utilized to detect circulating PTH in canine serum.[19] However, this same study also indicated a relative refractoriness of bone. Data obtained from Mg-depleted human subjects suggest the occurrence of both events.

TABLE 4 summarizes serum Ca responses to PTE given to Mg-deficient adult pa-

TABLE 4

EFFECT OF PARATHYROID EXTRACT (PTE) INJECTION ON SERUM CALCIUM IN ADULT MAN: COMPARISON OF RESPONSES BEFORE AND AFTER MAGNESIUM REPLETION

	Pre-Mg			Post-Mg			
Patients*	PTE (units)	Δ Ca† (mg %)	Hour	PTE (units)	Δ Ca† (mg %)	Hour	Reference
10A	200 q6h × 2d‡	1	48	200 q6h × 2d	3§	48	21
1M	200 q6h × 2d	0.3	48	200 q6h × 2d	3.1	48	21
1M	1/kg/hr × 10 hr iv	0§	12 & 24	1/kg/hr × 10 hr iv	0§	24	22
1M	1/kg/hr × 10 hr iv	> 0.5§	12 & 24	1/kg/hr × 10 hr iv	0§	12	22
					0.5	24	
1M	300 q6h × 3d	0.3	24	300 q6h × 1d	3.3	24	23
		2.9	72				
1M	200 q6h × 3d	2.0	72	—	—	—	27
1M	200 q6h × 3d	1.4	72	—	—	—	27
1M	300 iv in ¼ hr then 200 q6h × 8 im¶	2	48	—	—	—	25

* A = alcoholic; M = malabsorber.
† Increase in serum Ca above baseline values at the hour indicated following initial injection of PTE.
‡ q6h × 2d means every 6 hours for 2 days.
§ Changes estimated from graph in original publication.
¶ im means intramuscular.

tients. Since Estep *et al.* first reported that Mg-deficient individuals (primarily alcoholics who were hypocalcemic) were refractory to PTE until they have been given Mg,[21] data have been published on additional adult patients, all of whom had malabsorption of some type. In three of these studies, Ca rose slowly or inappropriately in response to PTE in the presence of hypomagnesemia.

Note should be taken of certain methodologic problems associated with most of these studies. The amount of PTE given by Muldowney *et al.* appears to have been inadequate to give positive responses in their two subjects in the repleted state;[22] therefore, the absence of response in the depleted state has no significance. Estep *et al.* and Connor *et al.* retested the effect of PTE relatively early in the repletion period, i.e., at a time when serum Ca should have been starting to rise in response to Mg alone;[21,23] hence, it is not possible to delineate the relative contributions of PTE and of Mg during this critical period. Others did not retest their subjects following Mg administration. Hypoparathyroid patients given PTE have a rise in serum Ca that is marked in the first 24 hours.[24] The deficient patient of Anast *et al.* responded with an increase of Ca that was two-thirds that of a patient with idiopathic hypoparathyroidism.[25] These data provide some basis for concluding that Mg depletion in adults results in varying degrees of resistance of bone to the effects of PTE.

Data have been reviewed on the responses to PTE of five children—four of whom were young infants—with hypomagnesemia resulting from an isolated defect in intestinal Mg absorption.[4] Each was treated differently, and there were differing stages of deficiency, thus making comparison hazardous. With the exception of one patient, there was a response to PTE during the deficiency period, although perhaps with a prolonged lag period in two patients. Only two patients were retested after Mg repletion; both responded to PTE with a more rapid rise and higher Ca levels. Unlike those in the adult repletion studies, these two subjects had achieved normal serum Ca levels prior to retesting.

The Mg-deficient patients of Estep *et al.*, Muldowney *et al.*, Connor *et al.*, and Rude *et al.* were refractory in their renal responses (urinary phosphate, and/or hydroxyproline and/or cyclic AMP excretion) to PTE.[21-23,26] Two adult patients, an 8-year-old patient, and a 24-year-old patient (the latter two with primary hypomagnesemia) had good renal responses to PTE.[27,28,25] The reason for these contradictory results is unclear but may relate to differences in degree of Mg depletion.

Roles of Calcium and Magnesium in Synthesis and Secretion of Parathyroid Hormone

In Vitro *Studies*

Considerable advances have been made recently in the understanding of the sequence of events leading to the secretion of PTH; these have been summarized recently.[29] Pre-proparathyroid hormone is very rapidly converted into proparathyroid hormone by cleavage of amino acids, and this form in turn loses its NH_2 terminal hexapeptide to form PTH, which is presumably stored in secretory granules; this process is estimated to take somewhat less than one hour. PTH is secreted in response to a fall in blood concentration of Ca. Secretion appears to be dependent on cyclic AMP production, which in turn requires Mg. If the serum Ca is elevated, secretion is stopped and stored PTH is partially degraded and its biosynthesis suppressed.

Studies in perfused parathyroid glands *in vivo* and with organ culture, viable tissue slices, or isolated parathyroid cells give clear evidence that the concentrations of Mg ions and Ca ions affect PTH secretion in the same direction.[30]

In studying the formation of PTH in cultured explants of normal bovine parathyroid glands, Targovnik *et al.* found that over 18 hours, Ca and Mg were equivalent in decreasing the release of the hormone; as one was decreased and the other increased so that the total divalent ion concentration remained constant, PTH secretion remained unchanged.[31] However, when Mg concentration was very low, the hormone was diminished regardless of the total cation concentration. The data of Oldham *et al.*, using bovine parathyroid gland slices *in vitro,* suggest that Mg is at least as potent as Ca in blocking PTH release.[32] However, more recent observations indicate that Mg is appreciably less effective on a molar basis than is Ca in suppressing PTH release.[33-35] In bovine tissue slice preparations, Mg was approximately 40% as potent as Ca.[33] In *in vivo* studies in calves where PTH was measured in parathyroid vein blood, variations in plasma Mg concentration had approximately one-third to one-half the effect of similar changes in plasma Ca (FIGURE 2).[35]

The relative effectiveness of Ca and Mg appears different with respect to their influences on PTH synthesis. Hamilton and colleagues found increased incorporation of amino acids in PTH isolated from the tissue or from the medium when the concentration of Ca was lowered in the medium, but Mg was without effect on biosynthesis.[36] While DNA synthesis in rat parathyroid glands in organ culture was

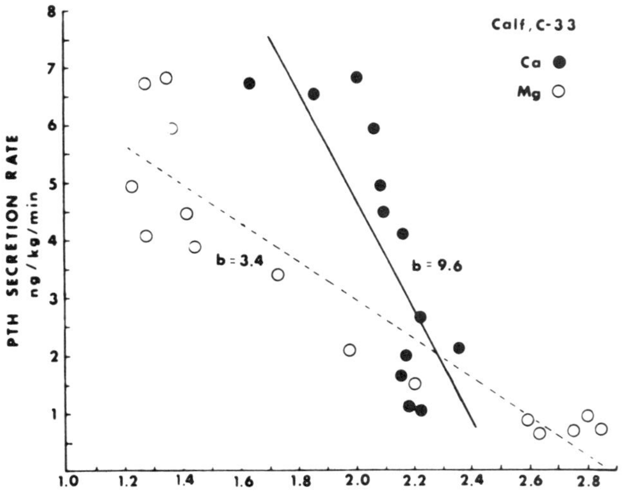

FIGURE 2. Relative effects of calcium and magnesium on iPTH secretion rate. Alterations in plasma calcium concentration in the calf were induced by a constant infusion of either calcium chloride or Na_2EDTA into the jugular vein or by infusion of various solutions of $MgCl_2$ into a contralateral jugular vein. iPTH was measured in venous blood draining the superior parathyroid gland. The concentration of magnesium or calcium in the plasma was varied during periods in which the other was kept constant. The iPTH secretion rate is related to the concentration of each ion during the period in which the concentration of the ion was varied. Note that variations in plasma magnesium concentration had less effect on the iPTH secretion rate than that observed with changes in plasma calcium concentration. In this particular calf, magnesium had approximately one-third the effect of calcium; in other studies, the effect was approximately one-half. (From Mayer and Hurst, Reference 35. Reprinted with permission of the Endocrine Society.)

affected by the Ca concentration of the medium, Mg was without effect.[37] In tissue slices, Mg had no effect on hormone biosynthesis and Ca altered synthesis by only approximately 15%; neither cation affected conversion of proPTH to PTH.[32]

In perfusion studies of goat or sheep parathyroid glands *in vivo,* there was a marked increase in PTH when the perfusion fluid had a low Mg content and the Ca level remained constant.[30] This result suggests to this author that the Ca level per se was not at a level to maximally suppress PTH secretion; when the Mg concentration fell, stimulation of secretion occurred.

Immunoreactive Parathyroid Hormone Levels in Magnesium Deficiency

A resolution to the problem of the etiology of the variations in serum Ca with Mg deficiency appeared to be at hand with the advent of immunoassays for PTH, and in fact, considerable insight has been gained by such determinations. At the same time, it has become apparent that the assay procedures are more complex than originally postulated because of the nature of the antigens—usually bovine and porcine extracts of PTH—and the metabolism of PTH. Berson and Yallow had discovered that circulating PTH existed in more than one form, and other studies have provided further evidence on this point.[37,38] In addition to the intact PTH, lower weight hormonal fragments are present from both the carboxyterminal and aminoterminal portions of the PTH molecule, with the carboxyterminal fragments being present in larger amounts.

Fragments in peripheral blood appear to be derived from those secreted and those formed by metabolism of the intact hormone by specific organs after secretion. The relative amounts contributed by these two processes are affected by such factors as Ca level and clearance rates. Circulating intact hormone is only 5% to perhaps 25% of the total plasma iPTH. The predominant circulating forms are fragments, consisting of approximately two-thirds of the intact sequence, that contain the middle and carboxyterminal portions of the molecule; these fragments have no known biologic activity. Assays have been developed for both terminal fragments, and these have been employed clinically in different laboratories, with discordant results obtained when the same samples are analyzed by the various methods. Because of

TABLE 5

SUMMARY OF iPTH LEVELS IN Mg-DEFICIENT SUBJECTS

Patient	Etiology*	iPTH in Relation to Normal	Method	Reference
1 F	M	elevated	?	23
1 F	1°	undetectable	intact & COOH terminal	42
1 M	1°	undetectable	?	28
3 M&F	M; A	normal	?	27
12 M&F	M	low or normal, 7; elevated, 5	primarily NH_2 terminal	4
1 F	1°	low normal	intact & COOH terminal	25
1 F	M	normal	?	68
16	A(6); M(5) iv Rx(5)	undetectable, 7; normal, 3; elevated, 6	primarily NH_2 terminal	41

* A = alcoholic; M = malabsorber; 1° = primary hypomagnesemia; iv Rx = on Mg-free iv fluids; (*x*) = number of patients.

methodologic problems existing at present, most assays may provide only a semiquantitative index of the biologically active hormone. Nevertheless, in comparing the iPTH in identical samples by four commercially available radioimmunoassays, patients with hyperparathyroidism, for example, as a group have significantly higher mean values for iPTH than do those with hypercalcemia associated with malignancy.[40] While recognizing that there are methodological problems with the assay, nevertheless, interesting and instructive data have been accumulating on iPTH levels in Mg-deficient dogs and human subjects. TABLE 5 summarizes data on iPTH levels in serum of 32 different Mg-deficient patients. Considerable variation occurred in these studies. Two individuals with primary hypomagnesemia had either undetectable or low normal levels. Various adults with deficiency related to alcoholism, intestinal malabsorption, or infusion of Mg-low parenteral solutions had low, normal, or elevated levels.

Serial determinations of iPTH have been made following intravenous administration of Mg to deficient patients. The results of various investigators are consistent on the following points:

1. Serum Mg rises rapidly with a single quick injection of Mg.
2. Serum iPTH also rises rapidly; by the end of one minute after Mg, the level is manyfold that of the baseline value;[25,26,41] the peak levels may be achieved in approximately 5 to 10 minutes and then decline (FIGURE 3).[25,41]

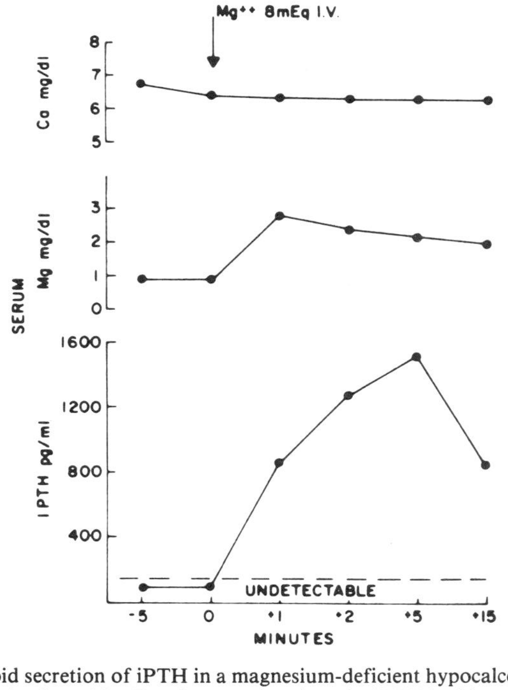

FIGURE 3. Rapid secretion of iPTH in a magnesium-deficient hypocalcemic patient. Prior to the intravenous injection of 8 mEq of magnesium ion, the iPTH had been undetectable, and it rose rapidly to very high levels within one minute. (From Rude *et al.*, Reference 41. Reprinted with permission of the Endocrine Society.)

3. With continued Mg injections, iPTH levels remain high and decline after serum Ca begins to rise.[3,26,42]

4. Serum Ca stays constant or may even fall transiently following initiation of Mg repletion and does not rise significantly toward normal until a lapse of two or more days.[3,25,26]

The effect of Mg depletion on the responsiveness of bone to PTH has been studied directly in the isolated perfused tibia of control dogs and those with chronic moderate Mg depletion.[43] The markedly decreased uptake of infused synthetic bovine PTH-34 by the bone in deficient dogs together with a much lower cyclic AMP production as compared to controls indicates skeletal resistance to PTH.

Vitamin D

Lack of a calcemic response to vitamin D during Mg deficiency has been reported in rats.[44] Pharmacologic doses of this vitamin have resulted in contradictory reports with either little or no calcemic effect or a good response in Mg-deficient hypocalcemic patients with malabsorption or alcoholism.[45,46] Earlier reports indicate that small amounts of vitamin D enhance Mg absorption in various experimental animals (cf., Reference 47), and large doses had a similar effect in a few subjects. More recent data indicate that moderate doses of vitamin D_2 given to patients with various disorders of Ca metabolism or bone disease had only a small positive effect on net Mg absorption despite the large increase in Ca absorption.[47] Others were unable to find any significant correlation between Mg or phosphate absorption and plasma 1,25-$(OH)_2$ cholecalciferol concentrations, although net intestinal Ca absorption was positively correlated.[48] Significant amounts of Mg and phosphate were absorbed in the absence of detectable plasma 1,25-$(OH)_2$-D concentrations.

It is known that PTH plays a role in experimental animals in the conversion of 25-OH-D_3 to 1,25-$(OH)_2$-D_3 by virtue of the stimulation of the hydroxylase in the kidney and that PTH is required for 1,25-$(OH)_2D_3$ to exert its function on bone.[49] Similarly, the presence of some form of vitamin D is necessary for PTH to exert its effect on mobilization of Ca from bone. To this author's knowledge, there are no published data on the levels of 1,25-$(OH)_2$-D in Mg deficiency when serum iPTH levels are low. If formation of this vitamin D metabolite is impaired when iPTH levels are low, it may explain some of the discordant results of the effects of vitamin D administration in Mg deficiency.

Summary

Sequence of Effects of Magnesium Deficiency on Calcium and Parathyroid Hormone and Response to Magnesium Repletion

Sequence I: The Initiation of Hypocalcemia

When there is an adequate intake of Ca, negative Ca balance does not occur with Mg deficiency. Consequently, Ca depletion can be ruled out as a cause of the hypocalcemia of Mg deficiency. There must develop, as a primary factor, a failure of Ca to leave the metabolically labile bone mineral. This defect is accompanied by a deposition in bone mineral and/or in soft tissues of absorbed dietary Ca, with a resultant progressive fall in serum Ca. In the deficient rat and in older animals of certain species fed relatively large amounts of Ca who do not become hypocalcemic, the failure to mobilize Ca from bone may be counterbalanced by increased absorption of

Ca from the intestine with a resultant maintenance of serum Ca. There are at least two major mechanisms responsible for the failure of Ca release from bone as Mg deficiency progresses: (1) the decreased heteroionic exchange of Mg for Ca at the bone surface and (2) impairment of the normal metabolic activity of osteocytes in maintaining mineral homeostasis by active bone resorption; this cellular change may be related in whole or in part to the development of resistance to PTH (which may operate through impaired cyclic AMP generation) and possibly to alterations in 1,25-$(OH)_2$ cholecalciferol formation and function.

Sequence II: The Perpetuation of Hypocalcemia

With the development of hypocalcemia, one would expect PTH production and secretion to increase. At this stage of Mg depletion, some individuals do have elevated levels of the hormone; nevertheless, their serum Ca levels remain depressed, indicating a resistance to the hormone. Other subjects have low levels of hormone or "normal" levels that are inappropriate to the circulating calcium level; this situation indicates an inadequacy of PTH secretion that might possibly be associated with more rapid degradation of the hormone after secretion. Thus, there is a failure at two levels in the PTH mechanism designed to maintain Ca homeostasis. It is tempting to speculate that these two stages are related to the degree of Mg deficiency, with bone resistance occurring first, followed by failure of PTH secretion as the deficiency becomes more severe. Excessive calcitonin does not appear to be to be involved in the hypocalcemia. At present, there is no evidence for or against involvement of a failure of formation or function of the metabolically active form(s) of vitamin D, although resistance to vitamin D has been reported to occur in Mg deficiency.

Sequence III: The Regression of Hypocalcemia

Following administration of Mg, an increase in PTH occurs; the rapidity of its rise depends upon the rate and amount of Mg given. Presumably, in the early interval after repletion starts, Mg ions are entering the hydration shell of bone, permitting a heteroionic Ca exchange to begin; this early exchange may explain the rapid improvement that occurs in some of the neuromuscular and other symptoms with little or no detectable change in circulating Ca levels. The end-organ insensitivity to PTH recedes as Mg concentration increases at sites on the osteocytes, inducing increased responsiveness to PTH with resultant bone resorption. This may be a relatively slow process and may account for the lag period of several days between the time of initiating Mg repletion and an appreciable rise in serum Ca. With or without end-organ resistance, an elevated PTH level occurs and remains high until serum Ca has achieved a normal range, at which time the hormone level declines.

References

1. Hirschfelder, A. D. 1934. J. Am. Med. Assoc. **102:** 1138.
2. Fink, E. B., F. L. Stutzman, A. R. Anderson *et al.* 1954. J. Lab. Clin. Med. **43:** 169–183.
3. Shils, M. E. 1964. Am. J. Clin. Nutr. **15:** 133–143; 1969. Medicine **48:** 61–85.
4. Shils, M. E. 1976. *In* Trace Elements in Human Health and Disease. A. S. Prasad, Ed. **2:** 23–46. Academic Press, Inc. New York, N.Y.
5. Macmanus, J. & F. W. Heaton. 1969. Clin. Sci. **36:** 297–306.
6. Shils, M. E. Unpublished data.
7. Morris, E. R. & B. I. O'Dell. 1969. Proc. Soc. Exp. Biol. Med. **132:** 105–110.

8. Alcock, N. W. & M. E. Shils. 1974. Proc. Soc. Exp. Biol. Med. **146:** 137–141.
9. Goldman, R. H., R. E. Kleiger, E. Schweizer & D. C. Harrison. 1971. Proc. Soc. Exp. Biol. Med. **136:** 747–749.
10. Shils, M. E. 1966. Fed. Proc. Fed. Am. Soc. Exp. Biol. **25:** 609.
11. Heaton, F. W. 1965. Clin. Sci. **28:** 543–553.
12. Gitelman, H. J., S. Kukolj & L. G. Welt. 1969. J. Clin. Invest. **47:** 118–126.
13. MacManus, J., F. W. Heaton & P. W. Lucas. 1971. Endocrinology **49:** 253–258.
14. Hahn, T. J., L. R. Chase & L. V. Avioli. 1972. J. Clin. Invest. **51:** 886–891.
15. Raisz, L. G. & I. Niemann. 1969. Endocrinology **85:** 446–452.
16. Breitenbach, R. P., W. A. Gonnerman, W. L. Erfling & C. S. Anast. 1973. Am. J. Physiol. **225:** 12–17.
17. Reddy, C. R., J. W. Coburn, D. L. Hartenbower *et al.* 1973. J. Clin. Invest. **52:** 3000–3010.
18. Suh, S. M., A. Csima & D. Fraser. 1971. J. Clin. Invest. **50:** 2668–2678.
19. Levi, J., S. G. Massry, J. W. Coburn *et al.* 1974. Metabolism **23:** 323–335.
20. Dunn, M. J. 1971. Clin. Sci. **41:** 333–344.
21. Estep, H., W. A. Shaw, C. Watlington *et al.* 1969. J. Clin. Endocrinol. Metab. **29:** 842–848.
22. Muldowney, F. P., J. T. McKenna, L. H. Kyle *et al.* 1970. J. Med. **28:** 61–68.
23. Connor, T. B., P. Toskes, J. Mahaffey *et al.* 1972. Johns Hopkins Med. J. **131:** 100–117.
24. Bethune, J. E., R. A. Turpin & H. Inove. 1968. J. Clin. Endocrinol. **28:** 673–678.
25. Anast, C. S., J. L. Winnacher, L. R. Forte & T. W. Burns. 1976. J. Clin. Endocrinol. Metab. **42:** 707–717.
26. Rude, R. K., S. B. Oldham & F. R. Singer. 1976. Clin. Endocrinol. **5:** 209–224.
27. Chase, L. R. & E. Slatapolsky. 1974. J. Clin. Endocrinol. Metab. **38:** 363–371.
28. Suh, S. M., A. H. Tashjian, Jr., N. Matsuo *et al.* 1973. J. Clin. Invest. **52:** 153–160.
29. Habener, J. & J. T. Potts. 1978. New Engl. J. Med. **299:** 580–585.
30. Buckle, R. M., A. D. Care, C. W. Cooper & H. J. Gitelman. 1968. J. Endocrinol. **42:** 529–534.
31. Targovnik, J. H., J. S. Rodman & L. M. Sherwood. 1971. Endocrinology **88:** 1477–1482.
32. Oldham, S. B., J. A. Fischer, C. C. Capen *et al.* 1971. Am. J. Med. **50:** 650–657.
33. Habener, J. F. & J. T. Potts, Jr. 1976. Endocrinology **98:** 197–202.
34. Brown, E. M., S. Hurwitz & G. D. Aurbach. 1976. Endocrinology **99:** 1582–1588.
35. Mayer, G. P. & J. G. Hurst. 1978. Endocrinology **102:** 1803–1807.
36. Hamilton, J. W., F. W. Spierto, R. R. MacGregor & D. V. Cohn. 1971. J. Biol. Chem. **246:** 3224–3233.
37. Lee, M. J. & S. I. Roth. 1975. Lab. Invest. **33:** 72–79.
38. Martin, K. J., K. A. Hruska, J. J. Freitag *et al.* 1979. New Engl. J. Med. **301:** 1092–1098.
39. Habener, J. F. & G. V. Segre. 1979. Ann. Intern. Med. **91:** 782–785.
40. Raisz, L. G., C. H. Yajnik, R. S. Bockman & B. B. Bower. 1970. Ann. Intern. Med. **91:** 739–740.
41. Rude, R. K., S. B. Oldham, C. F. Sharp, Jr. & F. R. Singer. 1978. J. Clin. Endocrinol. Metab. **47:** 800–806.
42. Anast, C. S., J. M. Hohs, L. S. Kaplan & T. W. Burns. 1972. Science **177:** 606–608.
43. Freitag, J. J., K. J. Martin, M. B. Conrades *et al.* 1979. J. Clin. Invest. **64:** 1238–1244.
44. Lifshitz, F., H. C. Harrison & H. E. Harrison. 1967. Endocrinology **81:** 849–853.
45. Medalle, R., C. Waterhouse & T. J. Hahn. 1976. Am. J. Clin. Nutr. **29:** 854–858.
46. Petersen, V. P. 1963. Acta Med. Scand. **173:** 285.
47. Hodgkinson, A., D. H. Marshall & B. E. C. Nordin. 1979. Clin. Sci. **57:** 121–123.
48. Wilz, D. R., R. W. Gray, J. G. Dominquez & J. Leman, Jr. 1979. Am. J. Clin. Nutr. **32:** 2052–2060.
49. DeLuca, H. F. 1979. Nutr. Rev. **37:** 161–193.
50. Rayssiguier, Y. & P. Larvor. 1974. Horm. Metab. Res. **6:** 91.
51. Carillo, B. J., W. G. Pond, L. Krook *et al.* 1961. Proc. Soc. Exp. Biol. Med. **107:** 793–796.

52. MORRIS, E. R. & B. L. O'DELL. 1963. J. Nutr. **81:** 175.
53. HOOBLER, S. W., H. D. KRUSE & E. V. MC COLLUM. 1937. Am. J. Hyg. **25:** 86–106.
54. BUNCE, G. E., K. J. JENKINS & P. H. PHILLIPS. 1962. J. Nutr. **76:** 17–22.
55. BUNCE, G. E., Y. CHIEMCHAISRI & P. H. PHILLIPS. 1962. J. Nutr. **76:** 23–29.
56. WENER, J., K. PINTAR, M. A. SIMON *et al.* 1964. Am. Heart J. **67:** 221–231.
57. SETA, K., R. KLEIGER, E. E. HELLERSTEIN *et al.* 1966. Am. J. Cardiol. **17:** 516–519.
58. MILLER, E. R., D. E. ULBREY, C. L. ZUTANT *et al.* 1965. J. Nutr. **85:** 13–20.
59. MCALEESE, D. M. & R. M. FORBES. 1959. Nature **184:** 2025–2026.
60. L'ESTRANGE, J. L. & R. F. E. AXFORD. 1964. J. Agric. Sci. **62:** 353–368.
61. BLAXTER, K. L., B. COWLISHAW & J. A. F. ROOK. 1960. Anim. Prod. **2:** 1–15.
62. PARR, W. H. 1957. Vet. Rec. **69:** 71–76.
63. SMITH, R. H. 1958. Biochem. J. **70:** 201–205.
64. SMITH, R. H. 1961. Nature **191:** 181–182.
65. LARVOR, P., A. GIRARD, M. BROCHHART *et al.* 1964. Ann. Biol. Anim. Biochem. Biophys. **4:** 345–369.
66. RAYSSIGUIER, Y., J. M. GAREL, M. J. DAVICCO & J. P. BARLET. 1977. Horm. Metab. Res. **9:** 438–439.
67. DUNN, M. J. & M. WALSER. 1966. Metabolism **15:** 884–895.
68. WIEGMANN, T. & M. KAYE. 1977. Arch. Intern. Med. **137:** 953–955.

DISCUSSION

W. R. HOLUB (*Life Systems, Inc., Melville, N.Y.*) Do you know if any work has been done on manganese in this interaction, particularly at the lamella layer of bone?

M. E. SHILS: In relation to magnesium deficiency, you mean? No, I'm not aware of any.

L. HOWARD (*Albany Medical College, Albany, N.Y.*): Dr. Shils, is the delayed effect in any part related to the requirement for magnesium in the hydroxylation steps of vitamin D?

M. E. SHILS: Magnesium-deficient animals seem to be resistant to vitamin D given in large amounts. You heard Dr. DeLuca say that for the conversion of 25-OH cholecalciferol to the 1,25-$(OH)_2$ form, one must have parathyroid hormone. It may well be that if one had a severely depleted individual with little or no secretion of parathyroid hormone, then there could be a hindrance in the conversion to the most active metabolic form of vitamin D. But as far as I know, nobody has ever done this experiment.

H. SPENCER (*Veterans Administration Hospital, Hines, Ill.*): I should like to ask you about chronic alcoholics. As you mentioned, they are low in magnesium. We have noted that their serum calcium is low and that serum phosphorus is high. I wonder whether this is due to the fact that PTH secretion is inhibited. Is the PTH [parathyroid hormone] low in magnesium-deficient alcoholics?

M. E. SHILS: If they are sufficiently deficient, they can be at a stage where their PTH is high or low depending on the given individual and the degree of deficiency.

H. SPENCER: This would explain the changes in serum calcium and phosphorus in these patients. I could never explain why their serum phosphorus is about 5–5½ for some time and the serum calcium would be about 8½–9, serum magnesium low.

M. E. SHILS: The first study showing unresponsiveness to parathyroid extract was done mostly in alcoholics who were hypomagnesemic and hypocalcemic.

UNIDENTIFIED SPEAKER: Have any *in vitro* experiments been done with parathyroid gland, incubating it with various concentrations of calcium and magnesium? What happens when the magnesium goes low?

M. E. SHILS: There have been a number of studies. One of the first studies was done with explants of bovine parathyroid glands in organ culture by Targovnik and associates. When the magnesium concentration was very low, parathyroid hormone did not appear in normal amounts in the fluid. They thought that the synthesis of parathyroid hormone was suppressed, but more recent data suggest that production is not suppressed in this situation. They were very probably dealing with depressed secretion as the result of the very low magnesium. At somewhat higher levels of magnesium, you reach the certain level (still low) such that varying the calcium and magnesium independently causes an identical response as long as the total divalent concentration is the same. Whether it is low calcium and high magnesium or low magnesium and high calcium, the secretion of the hormone is the same.

Since that experiment, there have been more sophisticated studies with isolated cells of pig or cow parathyroid glands and also studies *in vivo* in cattle in which serum calcium had been depressed by a chelating agent. These later studies indicate that magnesium has about one-third the effect of equivalent amounts of calcium in depressing parathyroid hormone secretion. They both can affect secretion, but calcium is the more potent.

M. D. SCHNEIDER (*University of Tennessee, Knoxville, Tenn.*): At the time that you observed the symptoms in the magnesium deficiency, did you observe also a fall in magnesium in red cells?; and furthermore, did you look at the cerebrospinal fluid magnesium?

M. E. SHILS: We did do red cell magnesium measurements frequently. They fell more slowly and to a lesser degree than did serum or plasma magnesium. We did spinal fluid on one patient. Spinal fluid in normal man tends to be higher in magnesium than is blood even though there is much less protein present. Spinal fluid magnesium also decreased, but not a great deal. But we only did one individual.

EFFECT OF CALCIUM, PHOSPHORUS, MAGNESIUM, AND ALUMINUM ON FLUORIDE METABOLISM IN MAN*

Herta Spencer, Lois Kramer, Dace Osis,
Emilie Wiatrowski, Clemontain Norris, and Menahem Lender

Metabolic Section
Veterans Administration Hospital
Hines, Illinois 60141

Introduction

Small amounts of fluoride in water have been shown to be beneficial in preventing dental caries.[1,2] Fluoride may also be important for the maintenance of the integrity of the skeletal structure, as the incidence of osteoporosis has been reported to be lower in naturally high fluoride areas than in areas where the fluoride content of the water is low.[3] Fluoride that has entered the body is primarily excreted via the kidney. This pathway of fluoride excretion in man was described many years ago and has been recently confirmed in strictly controlled studies.[4,5]

The availability of fluoride for absorption may depend on the presence of certain minerals in the intestine. Studies in animals have shown that calcium, phosphorus, magnesium, and aluminum reduce the intestinal absorption of fluoride. A high calcium intake decreased the absorption of fluoride in dogs and in rats.[4,6,7] The concurrent use of both calcium and phosphorus reduced the skeletal uptake of fluoride in rats more than did a high calcium intake alone.[8] With regard to the effect of calcium and phosphorus on fluoride metabolism in man, the absorption of fluoride from bone meal, cryolite, or calcium fluoride was considerably lower than from sodium fluoride.[9,10] Fish protein concentrate, which contains relatively large amounts of calcium and phosphorus, decreased the absorption of fluoride in weanling rats, but this could not be confirmed in man.[11,12] Regarding the effect of magnesium, this mineral decreased the intestinal absorption of fluoride in rats, and the combined use of magnesium and calcium reduced the deposition of fluoride in bone.[13]Aluminum decreased the absorption of fluoride in cattle and ameliorated the severity of fluorosis.[14,15] As the human diet contains a variety of minerals that may interfere with the intestinal absorption of fluoride, the effect of some of these were investigated in man in this research unit.

Materials and Methods

Metabolic balance studies of fluoride were carried out in adult males under constant and strictly controlled dietary conditions in the Metabolic Research Ward in control studies and during the addition of various minerals. Metabolic balances of calcium, phosphorus, and magnesium were also carried out. The constant, analyzed diet contained an average 1.5 mg fluoride, 230 mg calcium, 800 mg phosphorus, 250 mg magnesium, and 2 mg aluminum per day. Due to the intake of certain amounts of fluoridated water, containing 1 part per million (ppm) fluoride, the total daily fluoride intake was greater than that contained in the diet and averaged 4.2 mg per

* Supported by U.S. Public Health Service Grant No. DE-02486.

0077-8923/80/0355-0181 $01.75/0

TABLE 1

EFFECT OF CALCIUM AND PHOSPHORUS ON FLUORIDE METABOLISM IN MAN

Number of Studies	Study Condition	Study Days	Fluoride (mg/day) Intake	Urine	Stool	Balance
	Effect of Calcium, Low Phosphorus Intake					
7	Low Ca	26	4.0	2.9	0.13	+0.9
4	High Ca*	30	3.9	2.9	0.20	+0.7
	Effect of Phosphorus, Low Calcium Intake					
7	Low P	26	4.0	2.9	0.13	+0.9
7	High P†	25	4.1	3.2	0.13	+0.7
	Effect of Phosphorus, High Calcium Intake					
4	Low P	32	3.9	2.9	0.20	+0.7
4	High P†	32	4.4	2.9	0.31	+1.2

* High calcium intake = 2,000 mg/day due to addition of calcium gluconate tablets to the constant low calcium diet containing 220 mg/day.

† High phosphorus intake = 2,000 mg/day due to the addition of sodium glycerophosphate to the low calcium diet containing 800 mg phosphorus.

day. The daily fluid intake was kept constant. The diet and the excretions in urine and stool were analyzed for fluoride, calcium, phosphorus, and magnesium in each six-day metabolic study period.

In studies of the effect of calcium, the intake was increased from 200 mg to 2,000 mg per day by adding calcium as the gluconate to the constant diet. In studies of the effect of phosphorus, the intake was increased from 800 mg to 2,000 mg per day by adding sodium glycerophosphate. In studies of the effect of magnesium, the intake was increased from 250 to 850 mg per day by adding magnesium as the oxide. In studies of the effect of aluminum on fluoride metabolism, relatively small doses of the antacid aluminum hydroxide, i.e., 30 ml three times daily, were used.

Some of the studies of the effects of the various minerals were also carried out during a high fluoride intake that was due to the addition of sodium fluoride, which increased the total fluoride intake from about 4 mg to 14 and 50 mg per day. These fluoride supplements were given to patients with osteoporosis. Complete collections of urine and stool were obtained for several weeks in all studies.

Total fluoride in the diet, the drinking water, the excretions, and the sodium fluoride tablets was analyzed by an adaptation of the method of Singer and Armstrong.[16-18] Recoveries of fluoride added to the diet ranged from 90% to 100%; to stool, from 91% to 96%; and to urine, from 93% to 99%. Recoveries of standards averaged 99%. Calcium and magnesium were determined by atomic absorption spectroscopy, and phosphorus by a modification of the method of Fiske and SubbaRow.[19,20] The preparation of the diet, urine, and stool aliquots for fluoride analysis and for calcium, phosphorus, and magnesium analyses has been previously described from this laboratory.[16,21]

RESULTS

Effect of Calcium on Fluoride Metabolism in Man

TABLE 1 shows data of fluoride balances determined in the same subjects during a low calcium intake of 200 mg/day and during a high calcium intake of 2,000 mg/

TABLE 2

EFFECT OF FLUORIDE ON THE CALCIUM AND PHOSPHORUS BALANCE

Number of Studies	Fluoride Intake (mg/day)	Study Days	Calcium (mg/day)				^{47}Ca Absorption (% Dose)‡	Phosphorus (mg/day)			
			Intake	Urine	Stool	Balance		Intake	Urine	Stool	Balance
3	3.2*	24	2009	196	1685	+128	22	825	416	314	+95
3	44.2†	86	2005	159	1753	+ 93	22	791	390	338	+63

* Fluoride intake was due to the fluoride content of the diet and drinking water.
† High fluoride intake was due to the addition of sodium fluoride.
‡ A tracer dose of $^{47}CaCl_2$ was given orally in each study.

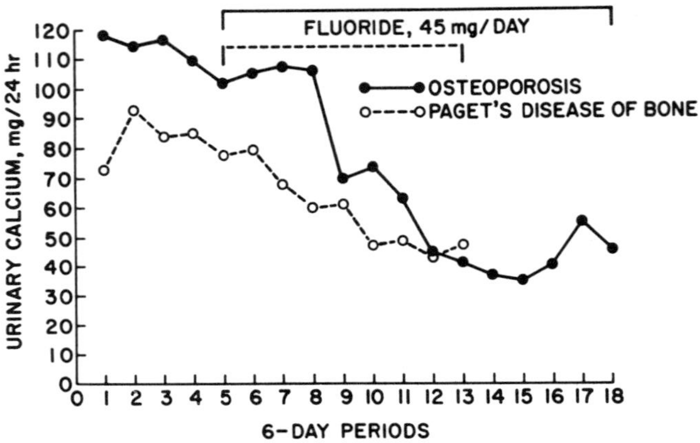

FIGURE 1. Effect of fluoride on urinary calcium in osteoporosis and Paget's disease of bone. Each point depicting the urinary calcium excretion in the control and high fluoride studies is an average of the calcium excretion in a six-day study period.

day. The fluoride balance data show that the main pathway of fluoride excretion is via the kidney, approximately 70% of the fluoride intake, while the fecal fluoride is very low, corresponding to 3–7% of the intake. Increasing the calcium intake 10-fold had no effect on the urinary fluoride excretion, increased the fecal fluoride only slightly and not significantly, and did not change the fluoride balance.

Effect of Fluoride on Calcium Metabolism in Man

TABLE 2 shows the effect of increasing the fluoride intake on the calcium and phosphorus balance. These studies were carried out during a high calcium intake of 2,000 mg/day in patients with osteoporosis. Increasing the fluoride intake 14-fold resulted in a decrease of the urinary calcium, while the stool calcium remained approximately the same and the calcium balance became slightly less positive. These results indicate that a high fluoride intake does not increase the intestinal absorption of calcium. This was confirmed in ^{47}Ca studies, which showed that the intestinal absorption of ^{47}Ca was the same during the low and high fluoride intakes.

FIGURE 1 shows the effect of fluoride on the urinary calcium in a patient with osteoporosis and in a patient with Paget's disease of bone. In both cases, the urinary calcium decreased moderately but distinctly with time. The urinary calcium excretion of the patient with osteoporosis started to decrease after four six-day periods of fluoride administration, while the urinary calcium of the patient with Paget's disease of bone started to decrease within the first six days of fluoride administration, and this decrease continued with time thereafter.

With the exception of the effect of fluoride in decreasing the urinary calcium, fluoride had no effect on any other parameter of the metabolism of calcium, such as the intestinal absorption of calcium or the endogenous fecal calcium excretion.

Effect of Phosphorus on Fluoride Metabolism

TABLE 1 shows that increasing the phosphorus intake by a factor of 2.5—from 800 to 2,000 mg/day—had no effect on either the urinary or fecal fluoride excretions or on the fluoride balance when fluoride was given during a low calcium intake of 220 mg/day. During a high calcium intake of 2,000 mg/day, the increase in phosphorus intake did not affect the urinary fluoride, while the fecal fluoride increased, i.e., from 0.20 mg to 0.31 mg/day. However, the fluoride balance did not become more negative during the high phosphorus intake. The slight increase in fecal fluoride in this study was most likely the result of the slight increase of the fluoride intake during the high phosphorus intake.

Effect of Fluoride on the Phosphorus Balance

TABLE 2 shows that increasing the fluoride intake from an average of 3.2 mg to 44.2 mg/day did not affect the urinary or fecal phosphorus excretion or the phosphorus balance.

Effect of Magnesium on the Fluoride Balance

TABLE 3 shows fluoride balance data obtained during a relatively low dietary magnesium intake, averaging 282 mg/day, and during the addition of 538 mg magnesium as the oxide to the constant intake. Increasing the magnesium intake to 820 mg/day from an average of 282 mg, during a low calcium intake of 220 mg/day, did not result in a change of the urinary fluoride, while the fecal fluoride barely increased and the fluoride balance became slightly less positive. During a high calcium intake of 2,000 mg/day, the high magnesium intake again had no effect on the urinary fluoride, while the fecal fluoride approximately doubled; however, these excretions were very low, and therefore, the fluoride balance remained unchanged.

Effect of Fluoride on the Magnesium Balance

Two levels of added fluoride were used in this study, so that the total fluoride intake was raised to approximately 13 mg and 45 mg/day, respectively, compared to an intake ranging from 3.1 to 4.1 mg/day, respectively, in the control study. The ef-

TABLE 3

EFFECT OF MAGNESIUM ON THE FLUORIDE BALANCE

Number of Studies	Magnesium Intake (mg/day)	Study Days	Fluoride (mg/day) Intake	Urine	Stool	Balance
				Low Calcium Intake*		
5	282	32	4.7	3.6	0.2	+0.9
	820†	28	4.8	4.0	0.3	+0.5
				High Calcium Intake‡		
1	287	16	3.9	2.3	0.2	+1.4
	903†	42	4.1	2.3	0.5	+1.3

* Low calcium intake = 220 mg/day.

† High magnesium intake was due to the addition of magnesium oxide to the constant diet containing approximately 250 mg magnesium.

‡ High calcium intake = 2,000 mg/day.

fect of the 13-mg fluoride intake was studied during three calcium intake levels of 200, 1,400, and 2,000 mg/day (TABLE 4). The magnesium balance data in the control studies show that neither of these calcium intakes had any effect on the urinary magnesium excretions. The fecal magnesium excretions also changed very little, except for the slight increase in the group that received a calcium intake of 2,000 mg/day. Increasing the fluoride intake by approximately 9 mg/day to a total of 13 mg/day during the different calcium intakes vs. 4 mg/day did not appreciably change the magnesium balances. Increasing the fluoride intake further—about 15-fold, to 45 mg/day—also did not affect the urinary or fecal magnesium excretions or the magnesium balance.

Effect of Aluminum on the Fluoride Balance

TABLE 5 shows data on the effect of aluminum given as the antacid aluminum hydroxide on the fluoride metabolism of two groups of patients, namely, patients with normal renal function and patients with chronic renal failure.

Patients with Normal Renal Function

In the control studies, the fluoride balances were similar to those of the control studies carried out during a low calcium and low phosphorus intake shown in TABLES 1 and 3. Adding a relatively small amount of aluminum hydroxide, i.e., 30 ml three times daily, which contained a total of 1.8 g aluminum and approximately 1 mg fluoride, resulted in a significant increase of the fecal fluoride excretion that far exceeded the fluoride content of the aluminum hydroxide. The urinary fluoride decreased significantly and the fluoride balance became less positive during the intake of aluminum hydroxide.

TABLE 4

EFFECT OF FLUORIDE ON THE MAGNESIUM BALANCE

Number of Studies	Calcium Intake* (mg/day)	Fluoride Intake† (mg/day)	Study Days	Magnesium (mg/day)			
				Intake	Urine	Stool	Balance
5	200	4.1	28	263	111	133	+19
	200	13.2	20	239	110	130	− 1
3	1,400	4.1	18	259	108	135	+16
	1,400	13.5	22	259	116	154	−11
3	2,000	3.6	26	260	108	160	− 8
	2,000	13.9	26	278	104	181	− 7
3	2,000	3.1	30	242	88	144	+10
	2,000	45.9	90	221	94	127	0

* The low calcium intake of 200 mg was that contained in the constant metabolic diet. All higher calcium intakes were due to the addition of calcium gluconate tablets to the constant low calcium diet.

† The low fluoride intake was due to the fluoride content of the diet and drinking water. The higher fluoride intakes were due to the addition of sodium fluoride.

Patients with Chronic Renal Failure

The fluoride balance of these patients differs significantly from those of patients with normal renal function, primarily because of the significantly lower urinary fluoride excretion (TABLE 5). Although the fecal fluoride excretion was slightly, but significantly, greater than the excretion of patients with normal renal function, this increase was very small and the fluoride balance was markedly positive, +2.3 mg/day compared to +1.4 mg/day for patients with normal renal function. The intake of the relatively small dose of aluminum hydroxide (30 ml three times daily) had a similar effect as in patients with normal renal function, i.e., the fecal fluoride increased significantly, the urinary fluoride decreased, and the fluoride balance of the patients with chronic renal failure became considerably less positive than in the control study. This decrease of the fluoride balance, induced by the intake of aluminum hydroxide, resulted in a fluoride balance that was the same as the fluoride balance of patients with normal renal function in the control study (TABLE 5).

FIGURE 2 shows the marked decrease in the intestinal absorption of fluoride of patients with normal renal function and of patients with chronic renal failure during the intake of aluminum hydroxide. The absorption of fluoride in the control study was high, exceeding more than 90% of the intake, and was similar in both groups of patients. During the use of relatively small doses of the antacid aluminum hydroxide, the intestinal absorption of fluoride of the patients with normal renal function and of the patients with chronic renal failure decreased markedly.

DISCUSSION

The present studies have shown that the added amounts of calcium and phosphorus had only a limited effect on the intestinal absorption of fluoride in man. Increasing the intake 10-fold, from about 200 mg to 2,000 mg calcium per day, during a low fluoride intake resulted only in a very slight increase in fecal fluoride excretion (TABLE 1); there was no change in urinary fluoride, and the fluoride balance was not affected. Similar results have been previously reported by this group.[22] The results obtained in man contrast with those obtained in animal studies, which have

TABLE 5

EFFECT OF ALUMINUM AS THE HYDROXIDE ON FLUORIDE METABOLISM IN MAN

Number of Studies	Study Condition	Study Days	Fluoride (mg/day) Intake	Urine	Stool	Balance
				Normal Renal Function		
5	Control	26	4.4	2.8	0.2	+1.4
	Aluminum Hydroxide*	22	5.4	2.2	3.2	0
				Chronic Renal Failure		
7	Control	32	3.8	1.2	0.3	+2.3
	Aluminum Hydroxide*	26	4.6	0.9	2.3	+1.4

* 90 ml aluminum hydroxide per day containing 1.8 g aluminum. Aluminum content of the diet in the control study is approximately 2 mg.

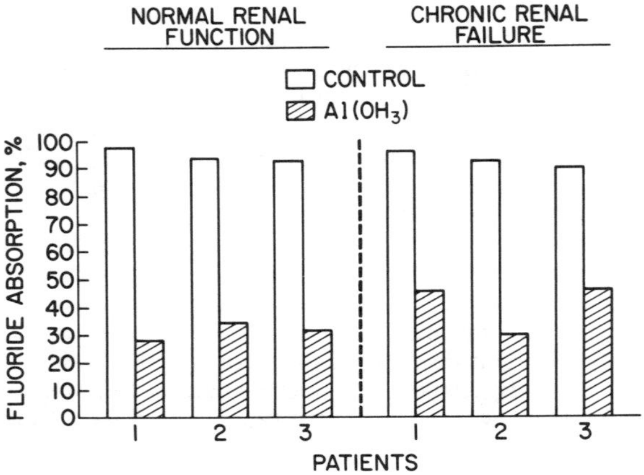

FIGURE 2. Effect of aluminum hydroxide on the intestinal absorption of fluoride in man. The intestinal absorption of fluoride in the control and aluminum hydroxide studies has been determined as the net absorption from fluoride balance data.

shown that a high calcium intake decreases the availability of fluoride for absorption in dogs and rats.[4,6–8]

Increasing the phosphorus intake in man in the present study did not increase the fecal fluoride excretion during a low calcium intake, irrespective of the fluoride intake, and therefore, the absorption of fluoride did not decrease. This is probably due to the fact that calcium-phosphate precipitates did not form in the intestine during a low calcium intake, which would be expected to bind fluoride and thereby increase the fecal fluoride. During the concomitant use of a high calcium and high phosphorus intake, the increase in fecal fluoride may in part be due to this mechanism. However, this increase represented only a very small amount of fluoride in relation to the much higher fluoride intake, and therefore, the fluoride balance did not change. Others have reported that the urinary and fecal fluoride excretions of two subjects were greater when fluoride was ingested with milk, which contains both calcium and phosphate, than of two others who received fluoride in water.[23] This would indicate that the decrease in intestinal absorption of fluoride was due to the presence of calcium and phosphate in milk. However, another study reported that the incidence of dental caries of children decreased when fluoride was given in milk for prolonged periods of time, indicating that fluoride was well absorbed from milk despite its high calcium and phosphorus content.[24]

In contrast to results obtained in man, phosphate inhibited the absorption of fluoride in animals. In rats, both calcium and phosphorus decreased the uptake of fluoride in bone and the combined use of calcium and phosphorus was more effective than was calcium alone.[7,8] Also, when fluoride was given in milk instead of in water, the bone uptake of fluoride in rats decreased, presumably as a result of decreased intestinal absorption of fluoride due to the calcium and phosphorus content of milk.[25] On the other hand, it has been reported that phosphorus promotes the intestinal absorption of fluoride in animals and that the combined use of phosphorus and fluoride was more effective than fluoride alone in preventing osteoporosis induced in rats, presumably due to increased absorption of fluoride.[13,26] With regard to the effect of fluoride on the intestinal absorption of phosphorus, fluoride has been reported to enhance the absorption of phosphate.[27] Phosphorus balances determined in the present study in man did not indicate such an effect (TABLE 2).

Regarding the effect of fluoride on calcium metabolism, a study in rats showed that neither the transport, the absorption, the utilization, nor the deposition of calcium in bone was affected by fluoride.[28] However, studies in man reported that fluoride increased the intestinal absorption of calcium and improved the calcium balance in patients with osteoporosis.[29] Other studies, including our own, could not confirm this observation.[30-32] A decrease of the urinary calcium, as shown in FIGURE 1, has been observed in several studies.[29-32] This decrease may reflect inhibition of bone resorption induced by fluoride, and this effect may be the basis of the beneficial effect of fluoride therapy in patients with osteoporosis, in whom the rate of bone resorption is increased. It is of interest that the decrease in urinary calcium was observed to coincide with the onset of clinical improvement of patients with osteoporosis receiving fluoride therapy.[32] Improvement of the crystal structure of bone by fluoride has been demonstrated by x-ray diffraction;[33] and many *in vitro* studies have shown that fluoride decreases the solubility of bone. Increased bone formation during fluoride therapy has also been reported.[34-37] In our studies of patients with osteoporosis and in studies by others, the high fluoride intake was given during a high calcium intake.[32,37] The combined use of both a high calcium and a high fluoride intake is indicated, as fluoride given during a low calcium intake tends to enhance the development of fluorosis. Therefore, a problem appears to arise as to whether calcium interferes with the intestinal absorption of fluoride in man, since animal studies have shown that calcium inhibits the absorption of fluoride.[6,7] Extensive fluoride balance studies carried out in man in this research unit showed that increasing the calcium intake 10-fold, from 200 mg to 2,000 mg/day, given as calcium gluconate in divided doses, did not decrease the intestinal absorption of fluoride.[22] This aspect of the administration of calcium is pointed out because a study by others reported that the plasma levels of fluoride were lower when sodium fluoride was given together with calcium carbonate than during the intake of fluoride alone, indicating inhibition of fluoride absorption by calcium carbonate.[38] The difference in results obtained in the latter study and in our study may be due to the concurrent use of both fluoride and calcium carbonate versus the use of divided doses of calcium throughout the day. Also, it is not certain whether the form of calcium used plays a role.

The lack of change of the fluoride balance during the high magnesium intake in man is the result of the small increase of the fecal fluoride in relation to the much higher fluoride intake. This result again contrasts with results obtained with magnesium in animals.[39] In the rat, magnesium decreased the availability of fluoride for absorption.[13,40] Also, fluoride has been reported to be less toxic in the presence of magnesium in the guinea pig;[41] and these authors have suggested that a high magnesium intake may be beneficial in areas where fluorosis is endemic. The incidence of fluorosis has indeed been reported to be lower in areas in India where the drinking water contained relatively large amounts of both magnesium and calcium, possibly a result of decreased availability of fluoride for absorption under these conditions.[42]

The lack of effect of calcium, phosphorus, and magnesium on the intestinal absorption of fluoride in man, which contrasts with the effect of these minerals in animals, may be explained by the difference in the amounts of these minerals used in animals and in man in relation to body weight. Inordinately greater amounts of these inorganic elements were used in animals than in man.

Aluminum has been reported to interfere with the intestinal absorption of fluoride in animals. The severity of fluorosis in rats was reduced by aluminum;[43] the intestinal absorption of fluoride in sheep and cattle was reduced, and the fluoride content of bone was lower than in control animals.[14,15] The possibility that aluminum may also decrease the intestinal absorption of fluoride in man has been suggested, but no data were reported.[44] In one study in man, the urinary fluoride excretion was lower when both fluoride and Al-ethylenediaminetetraacetic acid (Al-EDTA) were given together than following the use of a single dose of sodium fluoride alone.[45] This decrease in urinary fluoride was interpreted to be due to a decrease of the intestinal absorption of fluoride induced by aluminum, but the fecal fluoride excretion was not determined.

The present studies have shown that the antacid aluminum hydroxide, which is widely used in clinical medicine, increased significantly the fecal fluoride excretion and thereby markedly inhibited the intestinal fluoride absorption, similar to previous observations made in this laboratory.[46] The aluminum-induced inhibition of fluoride absorption may cause changes of the bone structure, as the lack of fluoride may contribute to the development of skeletal demineralization as indicated by a survey on osteoporosis.[3] In addition to the complexing action of aluminum for fluoride, aluminum combines with phosphate in the intestine and induces phosphorus depletion, which is associated with increased bone resorption.[47,46,48] These two factors may have a synergistic, adverse effect on bone and may contribute to the development of skeletal demineralization. It should also be considered that this dual effect of aluminum may counteract the beneficial therapeutic effect of fluoride for osteoporosis if aluminum-containing antacids are used in order to alleviate gastric irritation caused by the use of large amounts of sodium fluoride.[29-32,37]

Little is known about fluoride metabolism of patients with chronic renal failure, in whom the function of the main pathway of fluoride excretion, the kidney, is impaired. Most communications report on increased levels of fluoride in plasma and bone of dialyzed patients.[49] Bone pain and skeletal fractures of patients undergoing dialysis have been ascribed to prolonged exposure to high fluoride levels in the dialysate.[50] The present study of patients with chronic renal failure, who did not undergo dialysis, shows that urinary fluoride of patients with chronic renal failure is significantly lower than that of patients with normal renal function. The small increase in fecal fluoride did not compensate for the decrease in urinary fluoride, and the fluoride retention—determined in fluoride balance studies—was therefore greater than that of patients with normal renal function. Aluminum hydroxide, which is commonly used therapeutically for patients with chronic renal failure, markedly increased the fecal fluoride excretion, resulting in a significant decrease of the fluoride retention of these patients. Whether this decrease is desirable or not is not known, as fluoride therapy has been shown to be beneficial for osteoporosis, and patients with chronic renal failure—especially those undergoing hemodialysis—tend to develop osteoporosis in addition to bone changes of renal osteodystrophy.[29-32,37,51] The increased fluoride retention in chronic renal failure may possibly protect against the development and/or progression of osteoporosis in these patients.

Summary

The studies of the interaction of fluoride with minerals in man have shown that:

1. in contrast to observations made in animals, the high intake of calcium, phosphorus, and magnesium in amounts that can be used in humans did not inhibit the intestinal absorption of fluoride in man;

2. the lack of effect of added calcium, given in divided doses, on the intestinal absorption of fluoride has relevance for the use of a high calcium intake during fluoride therapy for osteoporosis;

3. aluminum as the hydroxide, commonly used as an antacid in clinical medicine, significantly decreases the intestinal absorption of fluoride. This in-

hibitory effect, in conjunction with the known effects of aluminum-containing antacids in causing calcium loss as a consequence of phosphorus depletion, may contribute to the development of skeletal demineralization.

References

1. McClure, F. J. & R. C. Likins. 1951. Fluorine in human teeth studied in relation to fluorine in the drinking water. J. Dent. Res. **30:** 172–176.
2. Hayes, R. L., N. W. Littleton & C. W. White. 1957. Posteruptive effects of fluoridation in first permanent molars of children in Grand Rapids, Michigan. Am. J. Public Health **217:** 192–199.
3. Bernstein, D., N. Sadowsky, D. M. Hegsted, C. Guri & F. Stare. 1966. Prevalence of osteoporosis in high- and low-fluoride areas in North Dakota. J. Am. Med. Assoc. **193:** 499–504.
4. Largent, E. J. 1954. Metabolism of inorganic fluorides. *In* Fluoridation as a Public Health Measure. J. H. Shaw, Ed.: 49–78. American Association for the Advancement of Science. Washington, D.C.
5. Spencer, H., I. Lewin, E. Wiatrowski & J. Samachson. 1970. Fluoride metabolism in man. Am. J. Med. **49:** 807–813.
6. Greenwood, D. A., J. R. Blaney, O. K. Skinsnes & P. C. Hodges. 1946. Comparative studies of the feeding of fluorides as they occur in purified bone meal powder, defluorinated phosphate and sodium fluoride in dogs. J. Dent. Res. **25:** 311–326. (As quoted by Largent, E. J. 1961. Fluorosis: The Health Aspects of Fluoride Compounds: 74–89. Ohio State University Press. Columbus, Ohio.)
7. Wagner, M. J. & J. C. Muhler. 1960. The effect of calcium and phosphorus on fluoride absorption. J. Dent. Res. **39:** 49–52.
8. McClure, F. J. & H. H. Mitchell. 1931. The effect of fluorine on the calcium metabolism of albino rats and the composition of bones. J. Biol. Chem. **90:** 297–320.
9. Machle, W. & E. J. Largent. 1943. The absorption and excretion of fluoride. II. The metabolism at high levels of intake. J. Ind. Hyg. Toxicol. **25:** 112–123.
10. McClure, F. J., H. H. Mitchell, T. S. Hamilton & C. A. Kinser. 1945. Balances of fluoride ingested from various sources in food and water by five young men. J. Ind. Hyg. Toxicol. **27:** 159–170.
11. Zipkin, I., S. M. Zucas & B. R. Stillings. 1970. Biological availability of the fluoride of fish protein concentrate in the rat. J. Nutr. **100:** 293–299.
12. Spencer, H., D. Osis, E. Wiatrowski & J. Samachson. 1970. Availability of fluoride from fish protein concentrate and from sodium fluoride in man. J. Nutr. **100:** 1415–1424.
13. Stookey, G. K., D. B. Crane & J. C. Muhler. 1964. Further studies on fluoride absorption. Proc. Soc. Exp. Biol. Med. **115:** 295–298.
14. Greenwood, D. A., J. L. Shupe, G. E. Stoddard, L. E. Harris, H. M. Nielsen & L. E. Olson. 1964. Fluorosis in cattle. Special Report No. 17: 31. Utah State Agricultural Experiment Station. Logan, Utah.
15. Hobbs, C. S., R. P. Moorman, Jr., J. M. Griffith, J. L. West, G. M. Merriman, S. L. Hansard, C. C. Chamberlain, W. H. MacIntire, L. J. Hardin & L. S. Jones, Eds. 1954. Bulletin No. 235: 87–101, 119–143, 144–152. The University of Tennessee Agricultural Experiment Station. Knoxville, Tenn.
16. Osis, D., E. Wiatrowski, J. Samachson & H. Spencer. 1974. Fluoride analysis of the human diet and of biological samples. Clin. Chim. Acta **51:** 211–216.
17. Osis, D., L. Kramer, E. Wiatrowski & H. Spencer. 1974. Dietary fluoride intake in man. J. Nutr. **104:** 1313–1318.
18. Singer, L. & W. D. Armstrong. 1965. Determination of fluoride. Anal. Biochem. **10:** 495–500.
19. Willis, J. B. 1961. Determination of calcium and magnesium in urine by atomic absorption spectroscopy. Anal. Chem. **33:** 556–559.
20. Fiske, C. H. & Y. T. SubbaRow. 1925. The colorimetric determination of phosphorus. J. Biol. Chem. **66:** 375–400.

21. Osis, D., K. Royston, J. Samachson & H. Spencer. 1969. Atomic-absorption spectrophotometry in mineral and trace-element studies in man. Dev. Appl. Spectrosc. **7A:** 227–235.
22. Spencer, H., D. Osis, L. Kramer, E. Wiatrowski & C. Norris. 1975. Effect of calcium and phosphorus on fluoride metabolism in man. J. Nutr. **105:** 733–740.
23. Muhler, J. C., G. K. Stookey, L. B. Spear & D. Bixler. 1966. Blood and urinary fluoride studies following the ingestion of single dosages of fluoride. J. Oral Ther. Pharmacol. **2:** 241–260.
24. Rusoff, L. L., B. S. Konikoff, J. B. Frye, Jr., J. E. Johnston & W. W. Frye. 1962. Fluoride addition to milk and its effect on dental caries in school children. Am. J. Clin. Nutr. **11:** 94–101.
25. Ericsson, Y. 1958. The state of fluorine in milk and its absorption and retention when administered in milk. Investigations with radioactive fluoride. Acta Odontol. Scand. **16:** 51–77.
26. Shambaugh, G. E., Jr. & A. Petrovic. 1968. Effects of sodium fluoride on bone. J. Am. Med. Assoc. **204:** 969–973.
27. Alcock, N. W. 1965. The relation of fluoride to other inorganic substances in vivo. Proc. Soc. Exp. Biol. Med. **120:** 150–154.
28. Singer, L., M. D. Dale & W. D. Armstrong. 1965. Effects of high fluoride intake on utilization of dietary calcium and on solubility of calcified tissues. J. Dent. Res. **44:** 582–586.
29. Rich, C., J. Ensinck & P. Ivanovich. 1964. The effects of sodium fluoride on calcium metabolism of subjects with metabolic bone diseases. J. Clin. Invest. **43:** 545–556.
30. Rose, G. A. 1965. A study of the treatment of osteoporosis with fluoride therapy. Proc. R. Soc. Med. **58:** 436–440.
31. Spencer, H., I. Lewin, J. Fowler & J. Samachson. 1969. Effect of sodium fluoride on calcium absorption and balances in man. Am. J. Clin. Nutr. **22:** 381–390.
32. Spencer, H., I. Lewin, D. Osis & J. Samachson. 1970. Studies of fluoride and calcium metabolism in patients with osteoporosis. Am. J. Med. **49:** 814–822.
33. Zipkin, I., A. S. Posner & E. D. Eanes. 1962. The effect of fluoride on the X-ray diffraction pattern of the apatite of human bone. Biochim. Biophys. Acta **59:** 255–258.
34. Cass, R. M., J. D. Croft, P. Perkins, W. Nye, C. Waterhouse & R. Terry. 1966. New bone formation in osteoporosis following treatment with sodium fluoride. Arch. Intern. Med. **118:** 111–116.
35. Manzke, E., R. Rawley, G. Vose, M. Roginsky, J. I. Rader & D. J. Baylink. 1977. Effect of fluoride therapy on nondialyzable urinary hydroxyproline, serum alkaline phosphatase, parathyroid hormone, and 25-hydroxyvitamin D. Metabolism **26:** 1005–1010.
36. Reutter, F. W. & A. J. Olah. 1970. Bone biopsy findings and clinical observations in longterm treatment of osteoporosis with sodium fluoride and vitamin D_3. *In* Fluoride in Medicine. T. L. Vischer, Ed.: 249–255. Hans Huber Publishers. Bern, Switzerland.
37. Jowsey, J., B. L. Riggs, P. J. Kelly & D. L. Hoffman. 1972. Effect of combined therapy with sodium fluoride, vitamin D and calcium in osteoporosis. Am. J. Med. **53:** 43–49.
38. Jowsey, J. & B. L. Riggs. 1978. Effect of concurrent calcium ingestion on intestinal absorption of fluoride. Metabolism **27:** 971–974.
39. Spencer, H., L. Kramer, E. Wiatrowski & D. Osis. 1978. Magnesium-fluoride interrelationships in man. II. Effect of magnesium on fluoride metabolism. Am. J. Physiol. **234**(4): E343–E347.
40. Weddle, D. A. & J. C. Muhler. 1954. The effects of inorganic salts on fluorine storage in the rat. J. Nutr. **54:** 437–444.
41. O'Dell, B. L., R. I. Moroni & W. O. Regan. 1973. Interaction of dietary fluoride and magnesium in guinea pigs. J. Nutr. **103:** 841–850.
42. Jolly, S. S., B. M. Singh, O. C. Mathur & K. C. Malhotra. 1968. Epidemiological, clinical and biochemical study of endemic dental and skeletal fluorosis in Punjab. Br. Med. J. **16:** 427–429.
43. Becker, D. E., J. M. Griffith, C. S. Hobbs & W. H. MacIntire. 1950. The alleviation of fluorine toxicosis by means of certain aluminum compounds. J. Anim. Sci. **9:** 647.

44. HODGE, H. C. 1961. Metabolism of fluorides. J. Am. Med. Assoc. **177:** 313–316.
45. MELLBERG, J. R. 1965. Stabilization of fluoride solutions in glass containers by aluminum. J. Pharm. Sci. **54:** 615–616.
46. SPENCER, H. & M. LENDER. 1979. Adverse effects of aluminum-containing antacids on mineral metabolism. Gastroenterology **76:** 603–606.
47. BRUDEVOLD, F., E. MORENO & Y. BAKHOS. 1972. Fluoride complexes in drinking water. Arch. Oral Biol. **17:** 1155–1163.
48. LOTZ, M., E. ZISMAN & F. C. BARTTER. 1968. Evidence for a phosphorus-depletion syndrome in man. N. Engl. J. Med. **278:** 409–415.
49. TAVES, D. R., R. TERRY, F. A. SMITH & D. E. GARDNER. 1965. Use of fluoridated water in long-term hemodialysis. Arch. Intern. Med. **115:** 167–172.
50. POSEN, G. A., D. R. TAVES, J. R. MARIER *et al.* 1968. Renal osteodystrophy in long-term hemodialysis with fluoridated water. Abstr. Am. Soc. Nephrol.: 51.
51. JOWSEY, J. & P. J. KELLY. 1968. Effect of fluoride treatment in a patient with osteoporosis. Mayo Clin. Proc. **43:** 435–443.

DISCUSSION

H. H. SANDSTEAD (*Human Nutrition Center, U.S. Department of Agriculture, Grand Forks, N. Dak.*): I realize that you have used older patients. Since fluoride incorporation into bone is dependent on the age of bone and also on whether these patients have been consuming fluoridated water, I would like you to comment on the possibility that if you had younger human subjects, you might observe some changes. In the case of the rat, these animals are weanling animals and are rapidly growing, and perhaps that might be a factor. We have done the studies on aluminum, and we get the same interference with absorption and utilization of fluoride.

H. SPENCER: The average age of our patients in the fluoride balance studies is about 45 years. We had the occasion to study one or two patients who were younger, 37–38 years old, and we found no difference in their pattern of fluoride metabolism. The intestinal absorption of fluoride is very high. The main problem in terms of fluoride metabolism is whether the function of the kidney is normal or abnormal.

H. H. SANDSTEAD: Have you done any studies with aluminum cookware? A lot of people use aluminum cookware. What is the significance of that or of fluoride enrichment in the water supply on long-term effects of the population? Do you have any thoughts on that?

H. SPENCER: I cannot answer this question because I don't know how much of the aluminum comes off the cookware. One would have to assume that boiling water or food in an aluminum pan would release aluminum, but it is not known how much aluminum would become available. We analyzed quite a number of diets and found that they contain 2 to 2½ mg of aluminum, but I don't know the effect of cooking food in aluminumware.

H. BHAGAVAN (*Hoffmann-La Roche, Inc., Nutley, N.J.*): Do you have any information on how much aluminum is absorbed from aluminum hydroxide?

H. SPENCER: We recently published a paper on aluminum metabolism in man, and the absorption of aluminum is rather low. However, when you give aluminum-containing antacids, the aluminum balance becomes positive; and we have calculated that over 10 weeks of intake of aluminum-containing antacids, the aluminum retention can be as high as a total of 200 to 300 mg. It is known that aluminum is deposited in brain and bone and in other tissues, including the lungs.

E. L. R. STOKSTAD (*University of California, Berkeley, Calif.*): I was interested in your comment about the effects of calcium on fluoride balance. Those who are opposed to the fluoridation of water will say that fluoride added to soft water is absorbed much more than fluoride that occurs naturally in water, which is usually associated with calcium in water. Now, your data suggest that there is no effect, but specifically, did you have any data?

H. SPENCER: No, I have no data on the difference in fluoride absorption from these different sources of fluoride. The calcium content of the water in Chicago is high, 36 mg calcium per liter. However, we have done studies using demineralized water, which has a low calcium content of 1 mg or less, as well as with tap water, which contains 36 mg calcium per liter. Our patients drink a large amount of fluid, maybe two or three liters of water per day. We did not find any difference in percent fluoride absorption when using the two types of water.

W. MERTZ (*Beltsville Human Nutrition Research Center, U.S. Department of Agriculture, Beltsville, Md.*): We know that the iodide ion is not very different from the fluoride ion. Have you ever seen or suspected an effect of the antacids on iodine absorption?

H. SPENCER: No, we have not studied this aspect. This is a very interesting point.

THE ROLE OF THIOMOLYBDATES IN THE NUTRITIONAL INTERACTIONS OF COPPER, MOLYBDENUM, AND SULFUR: FACT OR FANTASY?

N. F. Suttle

Moredun Research Institute
Edinburgh EH17 7JH, Scotland

Introduction

It is rare for an interaction between nutrients to attract more attention than do the nutrients themselves, but this could be said of the interaction between Cu, Mo, and S, at least insofar as ruminant nutrition is concerned. Interest was aroused by the fact that the interaction in ruminants differs radically from that in rats. In ruminants, the antagonism of Cu metabolism by Mo (as MoO_4^{2-}) is potentiated by dietary S, occurs at low Mo concentrations [< 10 parts per million (ppm)], and results in tissue Cu depletion, whereas in rats, it is alleviated by S, occurs at high concentrations (> 100 ppm Mo), and results in tissue Cu accretion (for recent reviews, see Suttle, Pitt, and Mason).[1-3] Interest in the ruminant interactions is sustained by the fact that they occur under grazing conditions in many countries and are responsible for losses of production through the induction of Cu deficiency.[4]

During the last decade, the seemingly irreconcilable differences between species in their responses to Mo have been rationalized into a single hypothesis that proposes that the Cu antagonism is effected through a product—thiomolybdate (TM)— of an interaction between S and MoO_4^{2-} and that species differences arise because the principal site of TM formation may be located in the gut in ruminants and systemically in rats. The "TM hypothesis" is given experimental support through observations that when rats are given Mo as TM, the antagonism takes on what were hitherto regarded as specifically ruminant characteristics.[5] The hypothesis provides a useful model for integrating the profuse experimental data on the interaction, although it will undoubtedly be refined in the course of time. The objects of this review are therefore to trace the origins of the TM hypothesis and to evaluate the largely indirect evidence that takes it from the realms of fantasy towards those of fact.

Origins of the Thiomolybdate Hypothesis

The mechanism of the Cu × Mo × S interaction was conceived initially as a phenomenon of membrane transport by Dick, who proposed that in ruminants, the transport of MoO_4^{2-} across membranes was blocked by SO_4^{2-} and that Cu transport was impaired during this process.[6]

Following up the chance observation that an insolurble Cu:Mo complex was formed when Cu^{2+} and MoO_4^{2-} were mixed *in vitro,* Dowdy and Matrone suggested that similar complexes might also form in the gut, i.e., that the interaction was a chemical one rather than a physiological one.[7,8] The preformed complex—2 $CuMoO_4$, $Cu(OH)_2$—was shown to contain Cu of low biological availability; though absorbable, it was poorly utilized for ceruloplasmin synthesis by piglets. Their initial hypothesis had an obvious drawback in that it made no allowance for the effects of SO_4^{2-} on the course of the antagonism. Subsequently, the protective effect of S

0077-8923/80/0355-0195 $01.75/0 © 1980, NYAS

against the Cu × Mo antagonism in nonruminants was explained by an SO_4^{2-} × MoO_4^{2-} interaction of the type observed by Dick that enhanced urinary MoO_4^{2-} excretion;[6] this would reduce the opportunity for systemic formation of unavailable Cu:Mo complexes, although there was no experimental evidence that such complexes could be formed in the tissues.[9] The exacerbative effect of S in ruminants was explained in terms of a separate interaction between Cu and S^{2-} in the rumen, leading to the formation of insoluble CuS;[9] but this made no allowance for the fact that the effects of S and Mo together were far greater than were their independent effects on Cu metabolism.

Matrone eventually produced a hypothesis that was consistent with the characteristics of the interaction in ruminants.[10] It involved a further interaction between the Cu:Mo complex and an unspecified degradation product (*X*) of S in the rumen, which yielded a triple unabsorbable complex of Cu, Mo, and S. This idea was elaborated by Suttle, who suggested that *X* was in fact S^{2-} and that another chemical reaction known to occur *in vitro*, whereby S^{2-} and MoO_4^{2-} combined to form MoS_4^{2-}, also occurred in the rumen, yielding unabsorbable $CuMoS_4$.[1] Furthermore, the presence of Cu- and Mo-containing proteins in the plasma of ewes given MoO_4^{2-} + SO_4^{2-} was interpreted as possible evidence that Cu:Mo complexes form systemically. Dick and his associates in the meantime had been studying the biological properties of TM given to sheep and rats, and they duly published a brief summary of results indicating that TM formed in MoO_4^{2-}-rich cultures of rumen microorganisms.[11] When given orally, TM mimicked the effects of MoO_4^{2-} + SO_4^{2-} on plasma Cu distribution in sheep and induced Cu deficiency in the rat.

The TM hypothesis thus evolved into a concept similar to that proposed originally by Dick and one consistent with the characteristics of the Cu × Mo × S interaction in ruminants.[6] It would, however, be an inappropriate model for species, such as the rat, with limited capacity for S^{2-} production in the gut. It remained for Mason to propose that TM might be formed in the tissues of nonruminants as a consequence of the inhibition of sulfite oxidation by MoO_4^{2-}, thus giving a similar basic mechanism for the interaction in nonruminants.[3] If TM were generated systemically, the path would be clear for SO_4^{2-} to alleviate the Cu × Mo antagonism by reducing MoO_4^{2-} absorption and retention as earlier hypotheses had suggested.

EVIDENCE FOR THIOMOLYBDATE FORMATION *In Vivo*

An important step in validation of the TM hypothesis would be confirmation of TM formation *in vivo* at Mo concentrations known to be antagonistic to Cu. The only approach so far made to this problem has involved identification of the characteristic spectral absorption of the MoS_4^{2-} ion (TM_4) in supernatants of *in vitro* rumen cultures.[12,5,11] The presence of the related MoO_2S_2 (TM_2) and MoO_1S_3 (TM_3) ions has been similarly detected.[11] However, Mills *et al.* estimated that spectral techniques would only detect TM_4 *in vivo* at dietary Mo concentrations above 100 mg/kg dry matter (DM), i.e., at levels characteristic of the nonruminant rather than the ruminant interaction.[5] In nonruminants, proof is one step further away in that the accumulation of endogenous S^{2-} has not been found in rats showing Mo-induced inhibition of sulfite oxidase activity.[13] Validation of the TM hypothesis therefore rests largely on indirect evidence that ruminants respond to preformed TM in much the same way as they do to dietary MoO_4^{2-} + SO_4^{2-}.

THE VALIDITY AND SIGNIFICANCE OF INDIRECT EVIDENCE OF TM FORMATION

Much of the indirect evidence supporting the TM hypothesis concerns alterations in the plasma distribution of Cu and Mo. Since some of the separative techniques used in obtaining this evidence identify physicochemical, rather than physiological, compartments in the plasma Cu, it is important to discuss them in some detail before using data in evidence. Work at our laboratory showed that the addition of MoO_4^{2-} + SO_4^{2-} to the diet of ewes markedly increased the fraction of the plasma Cu that was extractable with sodium diethyldithiocarbamate [direct reacting (DR) Cu] and led to the appearance of a nonextractable fraction other than ceruloplasmin.[14] This "residual" Cu, unlike ceruloplasmin Cu, was not released by treatment with trichloracetic acid (TCA).[15] Subsequently, it was found that the TCA-insoluble and DR Cu compartments partly overlapped, that the former consisted of proteins that concomitantly and firmly bound Cu and Mo, and that TCA-insoluble Mo was also induced.[16,17] The credentials of TCA-insoluble Cu as a measure of plasma Cu distribution *in vivo* were called into question by other workers, who noted that when TM_4 was given intravenously to sheep, it caused ceruloplasmin Cu to precipitate quantitatively as TCA-insoluble Cu.[18] The artifact may, however, be confined to situations in which relatively large amounts of preformed TM are mixed directly with plasma. TCA-insoluble Cu must reflect an *in vivo* interaction because it cannot be induced by MoO_4^{2-} *in vitro* and its formation *in vivo* is enhanced by adding SO_4^{2-} as well as MoO_4^{2-} to the diet.[19] TCA-insoluble Cu therefore reflects a systemic consequence of the $MoO_4^{2-} \times SO_4^{2-}$ interaction.

INDIRECT EVIDENCE FOR THE TM HYPOTHESIS IN RUMINANTS

Systemic Effects of TM and Molybdate

If the systemic effects of dietary Mo are attributable to TM formation in the rumen, TM must be absorbable and administration of preformed TM prior to the sites of absorption should induce changes in plasma Cu and Mo distribution similar to those induced by dietary MoO_4^{2-}. The administration of TM_4 to sheep via the duodenum leads to the appearance in the plasma of TCA-insoluble Cu and low molecular weight proteins, possibly modified albumin, containing Cu and Mo;[5,11] these anomalies are similar to those produced by the addition of MoO_4^{2-} to the diet.[16,19] Bremner and Young found that cytosol preparations of kidney cortex from sheep given dietary MoO_4^{2-} + SO_4^{2-} also contained TCA-insoluble Cu and that Cu and Mo accumulated in the same protein fraction.[19] When TM is added to the diet of lambs, the response is similar to that obtained with MoO_4^{2-} + SO_4^{2-} in that there is generalized tissue Cu depletion, the exception being the kidney, in which both Cu and Mo accumulate (TABLE 1).[40] It would appear that TM and MoO_4^{2-} can both induce protein complexes in the plasma, which accumulate in the kidney in an unsuccessful excretory process.

Proof that the systemic effects of dietary MoO_4^{2-} have their origins in the gut was found in an unexpected way. Grace and Suttle found that when $^{99}MoO_4^{2-}$ was infused continuously into the blood of ewes on diets supplemented with MoO_4^{2-} + SO_4^{2-}, it did not exchange freely with the Mo being absorbed from the gut.[30] The protein-bound Mo pool in plasma retained a particularly low specific activity (SA),

TABLE 1

TISSUE CU AND MO CONCENTRATIONS IN LAMBS GIVEN AMMONIUM TETRATHIOMOLYBDATE (ATM_4)* OR NO SUPPLEMENT IN A CEREAL-BASED DIET FOR 14 WEEKS†

	Tissue Cu (mg/kg DM)		Tissue Mo (mg/kg DM)	
Tissue	No Supplement	ATM_4	No Supplement	ATM_4
Liver	60.2	8.3	3.4	9.7
Fleece	3.8	1.3	0.4	3.7
Cecal Mucosa	5.1	2.8	1.5	6.5
Muscle	2.7	1.6	0.6	1.6
Kidney	16.7	29.2	2.8	27.3

* 20 mg Mo/kg DM.
† The diet contained 3.5 mg Cu and 1.7 g S/kg DM.[42]

suggesting that it had been supplied with Mo—already in a complexed, poorly exchangeable form—from the low SA milieu of the gut. The fact that the low SA complexes did not readily cross the glomerular membrane underlines how close Dick was in his initial hypothesis for the Cu × Mo × S interaction in ruminants.[6]

There is no evidence that Cu is absorbed in a complexed form with Mo. The fact that Cu given intravenously or subcutaneously accumulates as DR Cu in sheep given dietary Mo indeed suggests that anomalies in plasma Cu distribution are purely systemic in origin.[31,32]

Although the above conclusions are based on data for three different physicochemical Cu compartments, they probably reflect a common biochemical anomaly in the binding of Cu to plasma proteins. It would follow that changes in TCA-insoluble Cu reflect an interaction between MoO_4^{2-} and SO_4^{2-} that originates in the gut and that they can therefore be used as semiquantitive criteria of the effects of MoO_4^{2-} and TM on Cu absorption.

Effect of TM and Molybdate on Cu and Mo Absorption

The interactions between Cu, Mo, and S that are located in the gut influence Cu and Mo absorption, but their effects must be inferred largely from data on hepatic Cu retention and plasma Cu or Mo distribution. In a continuation of an experiment in which TM_4 (2.7 or 5.4 Mo/kg DM) was added to the diet of lambs, the rate of depletion of hepatic Cu was not affected when the diet was low in Cu, but when Cu was added, the hepatic accumulation of Cu was decreased by about 30% (FIGURE 1).[20] This suggests that TM_4 reduced the absorption but had little effect on the endogenous loss of Cu. Previous experiments with ewes had shown that MoO_4^{2-} + SO_4^{2-} markedly reduced Cu absorption at similar Mo concentrations.[21]

TCA-insoluble Cu accumulated in the plasma during the depletion phase of the above experiment (FIGURE 1) but disappeared during the repletion phase, suggesting that the addition of Cu limited the absorption of TM and hence its ability to exert a systemic effect on Cu metabolism. Mason *et al.* found that dietary Cu supplementation reduced TCA-insoluble Mo concentrations in plasma and reduced the absorption of Mo^{99} in sheep on an MoO_4^{2-} + SO_4^{2-}-supplemented diet.[22] Together, these results confirm the similarity of responses to TM_4 and to MoO_4^{2-} + SO_4^{2-} in sheep and the likelihood that Cu and Mo can be bound together in an unabsorbable form in the gut during both treatments.

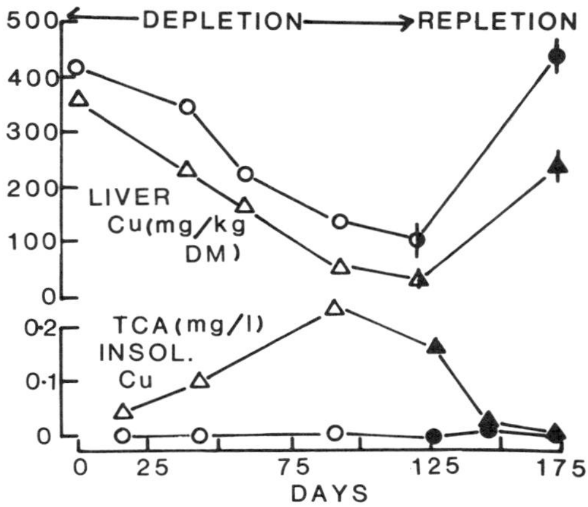

FIGURE 1. Changes in liver copper and plasma TCA-insoluble Cu concentrations in lambs given ammonium tetrathiomolybdate (△, ▲ providing 5.4 mg Mo/kg DM) or no supplement (○, ●) in their cereal-based diet during initial periods of Cu depletion (open symbol) and final periods of Cu repletion (closed symbol). The diets contained 3.5 and 15.5 mg Cu/kg DM respectively and 1.7 g S/kg DM.[20,41]

Sites of Interaction Affecting Absorption

Evidence on the site of the Cu × Mo × S interaction in ruminants has been obtained by administering Mo by different routes into the alimentary tract. Mason *et al.* showed that if Mo^{99} was given via the duodenum, its absorption was no longer impaired by dietary S.[22] It had previously been shown that the absorption of Cu and Mo from an S-rich diet was enhanced by giving Mo via the abomasum instead of in the diet.[21] It would thus appear that Mo must pass through the rumen in order to interact with S and impair both its own absorption and that of Cu. This localization of the initial interaction is consistent with the TM hypothesis, which assumes that MoO_4^{2-} is converted to TM in the S^{2-}-rich environment of the rumen.

The involvement of Cu in the gut interaction, however, occurs at sites beyond the rumen. This inference is drawn from an experiment in which initially hypocupremic ewes on diets high or low in MoO_4^{2-} + SO_4^{2-} were given Cu orally as $CuSO_4$ or CuO needles; the latter lodge in the abomasum and there slowly release absorbable Cu.[23] The supplement reduced by about 65% the period of protection from hypocupremia afforded by each Cu source. Although the two Cu sources gave contrasting patterns of fecal Cu excretion (FIGURE 2), with both, there was a clear correlation between fecal Cu and Mo excretion. It would therefore appear that, even when Cu was released postrumenally, MoO_4^{2-} + SO_4^{2-} simultaneously lowered the absorption of Cu and Mo by inducing the formation of unabsorbable Cu:Mo complexes.

INDIRECT EVIDENCE FOR THE TM HYPOTHESIS IN NONRUMINANTS

Systemic Effects of TM and MoO_4 in Rats

The evidence so far provides a strong case that TM formation plays an important part in both the gut and systemic interactions between Cu and Mo in ruminants,

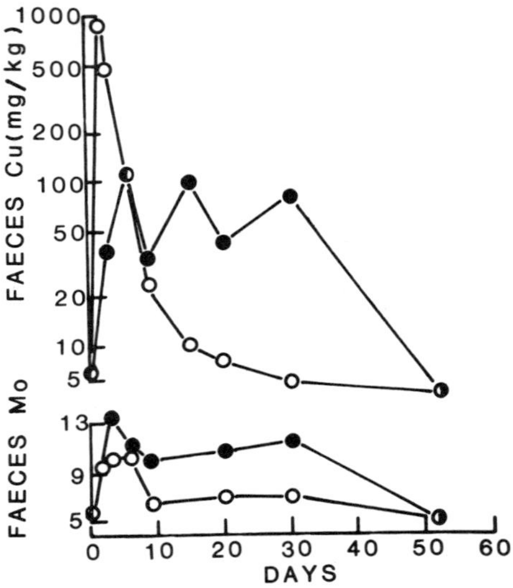

FIGURE 2. Changes in the fecal concentrations (mg/kg DM) of Cu and Mo in ewes following the administration of single oral doses of 0.5 g Cu as $CuSO_4$ (○) or cupric oxide needles (●). The basal diet contained 1.2 mg Cu, 3.5 mg Mo, and 3 g S/kg DM.[43]

and it is based on both the qualitative and quantitative similarities in the responses to TM_4 and MoO_4^{2-}. In moving to the rat, most of the qualitative and quantitative similarities are lost. The addition of as little as 1 mg Mo as TM/kg diet can induce anomalies in plasma Cu distribution, whereas > 50 mg Mo/kg as MoO_4^{2-} are required.[5,24] The anomaly induced by MoO_4^{2-} does, however, resemble that induced by TM_4 insofar as it consists of Cu and Mo firmly bound to protein, probably via SH groups.[24]

The effects of small supplements of TM_4 on liver Cu concentrations in rats resemble those in lambs, i.e., there is depletion of reserves.[5] The early onset of severe pathological changes in the gut and skeleton, however, precludes the investigation of larger supplements, which, when given as MoO_4^{2-}, cause liver Cu accretion.[25,26]

The quantitative differences in systemic responses to TM_4 and to MoO_4^{2-} suggest that if substances resembling TM_4 are part of the Cu × Mo × S interaction, they require a much higher threshold of dietary Mo concentration for their formation in rats than in ruminants.

Effects of TM and MoO_4 on Cu and Mo Absorption in Rats

The comparisons again are remarkable for their contrasts rather than for their similarities. While small supplements of TM_4 markedly reduce Cu absorption, there are no reports of impaired Cu absorption in MoO_4^{2-}-supplemented rats.[5] There are, therefore, no grounds for suggesting that formation of TM in the gut plays a part in the Cu × Mo antagonism in this species.

Reservations about the TM Hypothesis

In Ruminants

Experiments using preformed TM_4 are open to a number of objections. Studies using *in vitro* buffer solutions to simulate the rumen environment have shown that when K_2MoS_4 is added, hydrolysis occurs, giving an equilibrium mixture of 0.67 TM_4:0.26 TM_3:0.06 TM_2, together with the formation of HS^- and H_2S.[27] It was therefore suggested that the effects of TM_4 *in vivo* might be attributable to any one of these five species. It is, however, inconceivable that the release of micronutrient amounts of HS^- and H_2S will have a significant effect on interactions occurring in the rumen. The affinity of TM_4 for binding groups on protein will, however, mean that TM_4 formed *de novo* or added to the diet is likely to enter a variety of complexes with organic as well as inorganic species. Furthermore, such factors as S^{2-} concentrations in the rumen may determine the equilibrium ratios of TM_4:TM_3:TM_2. It would, therefore, be unrealistic to propose that the addition of TM_4 simulates completely the interaction of $MoO_4^{2-} \times SO_4^{2-}$ *in vivo* or that the gut and systemic effects of TM given as TM_4 are solely attributable to that ion.

The isolation of the active constituent of a suspected nutrient or active product of a nutrient interaction is usually confirmed by the enhanced biological activity of that constituent or product, compared with the unprocessed nutrient or mixture of nutrients. In the case of TM_4 in ruminants, it is not so. The changes in Cu absorption implied by the results for hepatic Cu retention indicated by Figure 1 are less than those anticipated from the addition of a corresponding amount of MoO_4^{2-} to a high S diet, and the effects on TCA-insoluble Cu are unremarkable relative to those produced by MoO_4^{2-}.[28,16] Such results could only be explained in terms of a quantitative conversion of MoO_4^{2-} to TM_4. The alternative—that TM_4 is degraded to MoO_4^{2-}—is unlikely, since MoO_4^{2-} would not be expected to impair Cu metabolism under the dietary conditions at which TM_4 was effective (Figure 1).[20] Two factors may favor the quantitative transformation of MoO_4^{2-} to TM_4 in ruminants: first, the levels of S^{2-} in the rumen are those of a macronutrient, and this would drive the reaction towards completion; and second, MoO_4^{2-} that escapes conversion during its first passage through the rumen may be recycled via the saliva, thus increasing the potential for TM formation.[29]

If there is quantitative conversion of MoO_4^{2-} to TM and the latter forms insoluble complexes with cations, such as Cu, the consequences in terms of Mo depletion might be as physiologically important as those for Cu depletion. Furthermore, MoS_4^{2-} may substitute for MoO_4^{2-} at systemic sites and inhibit Mo-dependent enzymes, such as xanthine oxidase. Acceptance of the TM hypothesis therefore carries with it acceptance of the possibility that some of the clinical and pathological abnormalities previously considered to be attributes of induced Cu deficiency may in fact be those of an induced Mo deficiency. Responses to Cu supplementation could still arise through the formation of unabsorbable complexes, which would limit the extent of systemic TM effects.

In Nonruminants

Since there is no evidence that TM_4 is formed in significant amounts in the rat gut, the responses of rats to dietary TM_4 are unlikely to simulate the physiological responses of this species to MoO_4^{2-}. They may serve as a model for those reactions in ruminants that occur postrumenally, provided that there are no dietary or species differences. Unfortunately, the limited data available suggest that such differences exist. In rats given TM_4 (4–6 mg Mo/kg DM) in a semipurified diet for 5 weeks, all the plasma Cu was TCA-insoluble and ceruloplasmin levels fell to zero when the diet contained 3 mg Cu/kg DM.[5] With lambs given diets of similar Cu and TM concentrations (FIGURE 1), only 20% of the plasma Cu was TCA-insoluble after 18 weeks. In similar experiments with rats, gross pathological abnormalities developed in the gut and in the skeleton within 7–14 days;[25,26] whereas in lambs, hypertrophy of the cecal mucosa was the only pathological abnormality found.[42] The effects of TM_4 in weanling rats given a semisynthetic diet are thus more extreme than those in the preruminant and ruminant lamb and are likely to exaggerate the systemic responses of sheep to TM formed in the gut. One contributory factor to these differences may be that on the highly digestible rat diet, TM_4 attains higher concentrations in the gut and forms less unabsorbable complexes with organic constituents of the diet.

The Relative Importance of Gut and Systemic Effects

The responses of sheep to MoO_4^{2-} clearly reflect interactions located at gut and systemic sites. Assuming that TM formation is involved, the relative importance of systemic effects will increase as the production of TM increases, provided that the process of insoluble complex formation in the gut is saturated. The factors determining the quantity of TM that is available for absorption seem unbelievably complex and interwoven. Mo, for example, is important in determining the amount of S^{2-} as well as MoO_4^{2-} available for TM formation. Mo inhibits the production of S^{2-} from sulfate by rumen cultures at relatively low concentrations *in vitro* (0.33 μM,) but the effect diminishes logarithmically up to 1.33 μM.[33] The effect at high dietary Mo concentrations (50 mg/kg DM) is dependent on the dietary S source, however, with Mo enhancing S^{2-} production from methionine and inhibiting its production from SO_4^{2-}.[34] At those high dietary levels, an additional effect is introduced *in vivo,* that of inhibition of S^{2-} absorption across the rumen wall.[35] Cu, too, may have a twofold effect, countering the Mo inhibition of S^{2-} production from sulfide and forming unabsorbable complexes with TM.

It follows that the appearance of systemic effects of TM is likely to bear a complex relationship with dietary Cu, Mo, and S concentrations, and this is seen in the three experiments with sheep in which effects of several increments in Mo on plasma Cu distribution were studied. The concentrations of dietary Mo (mg/kg DM) required to increase plasma DR Cu were < 8.5 with adequate dietary S and limited Cu in the diet, between 8 and 16 with inadequate dietary S, and > 16 with excess dietary Cu.[36,16,37]

If the changes in plasma Cu distribution are seen as "the visible part of the iceberg" of the Cu $\times$ Mo $\times$ S interaction, then the "invisible part"—the changes in Cu and Mo absorption—is likely to show quantitative relationships with dietary Cu, Mo, and S concentration that are equally complex. Within a restricted range of dietary Cu and Mo concentrations, it has proved possible to predict the absorbability of Cu with some precision on a single type of diet (semipurified).[38] It would, however, be unwise to use such relationships to predict the effects of high Mo concentrations ($>$ 8 mg/kg DM). Furthermore, current studies indicate that Cu absorbability in other types of diet, such as fresh and conserved forages, may be determined by distinctly different relationships.[39]

All the experimental observations on ruminants that have been quoted so far in this review have referred exclusively to sheep. Limited studies with calves have indicated that for a given dietary Mo and S concentration, Cu is absorbed with an efficiency that is approximately 1% unit lower than that of the sheep.[38] It is possible that the quantitative relationships between Cu, Mo, and S will differ between cattle and sheep, but it seems unlikely that differences in the site of interaction will be found.

Guinea pigs respond to MoO_4^{2-} in ways that are closer to those of the sheep than to those of the rat. Hepatic Cu accumulation is decreased by Mo concentrations as low as 4 mg/kg DM, and changes in plasma DR Cu appear with as little as 26 mg Mo/kg DM.[36] The guinea pig presumably has a greater capacity to generate S^{2-} in its cecum than does the rat, and the differences between species in their susceptibility to the Cu × Mo antagonism may be related to their ability to produce S^{2-}, and therefore TM, in the gut. It would appear that the guinea pig provides a more appropriate model for studying the Cu × Mo interaction in ruminants than does the rat because the gut effect predominates.

Conclusions

The similarities in the physiological effects of TM_4 and MoO_4^{2-} + SO_4^{2-} in ruminants suggest strongly that TM is formed at an early stage of the MoO_4^{2-} × SO_4^{2-} interaction in the S^{2-}-rich environment of the rumen. The subsequent absorption and metabolism of TM and its effects on Cu and Mo metabolism are, however, likely to involve species more complex than the MoS_4^{2-} ion. Qualitative similarities in the anomalies in plasma Cu distribution caused by high MoO_4^{2-} levels in the rat and TM in ruminants suggest that TM-like species may also be formed at systemic sites in nonruminants. The contrasting features of the Cu × Mo antagonism in ruminants and rats, notably the effects of S and the changes in tissue Cu status, may be explained in terms of the relative importance of gut and systemic sites of TM formation in the two classes of animal. When the gut site predominates (as in ruminants), Cu and Mo absorptions are concurrently impaired, causing tissue depletion that dietary S aggravates by increasing TM formation. When the systemic site predominates (as in the rat), Cu and Mo excretion is impaired, causing tissue accretion that dietary S ameliorates by lowering the absorption of Mo and decreasing TM formation.

References

1. Suttle, N. F. 1974. Proc. Nutr. Soc. **33:** 299–305.
2. Pitt, M. A. 1976. *In* Agents and Actions **6/6:** 758–769. Birkauser Verlag. Basel, Switzerland.
3. Mason, J. 1978. Vet. Sci. Commun. **2:** 85–94.
4. Underwood, E. J. 1977. *In* Trace Elements in Human and Animal Nutrition. 4th edit.: 123–127. Academic Press, Inc. New York, N.Y.
5. Mills, C. F., I. Bremner, T. T. El-Gallad, A. C. Dalgarno & B. W. Young. 1978. *In* Proceedings, Third International Symposium on Trace Element Metabolism in Man and Animals. M. Kirchgessner, Ed.: 150–158. Arbeitskreis Tierernahrung. Weihenstephan, Federal Republic of Germany.
6. Dick, A. T. 1956. *In* Inorganic Nitrogen Metabolism. W. D. McElroy & B. Glass, Eds: 445–473. Johns Hopkins Press. Baltimore, Md.
7. Dowdy, R. P. & G. Matrone. 1968. J. Nutr. **95:** 191–196.
8. Dowdy, R. P. & G. Matrone. 1968. J. Nutr. **95:** 197–201.
9. Huisingh, J., G. G. Gomez & G. Matrone. 1973. Fed. Proc. Fed. Am. Soc. Exp. Biol. **32:** 1921–1925.
10. Matrone, G. 1973. *In* Proceedings, First International Symposium on Trace Element

Metabolism in Animals. C. F. Mills, Ed.: 354–362. E & S Livingstone. Edinburgh, Scotland.
11. Dick, A. T., D. W. Dewey & J. M. Gawthorne. 1975. J. Agric. Sci. Cambridge **85:** 567–568.
12. Tridot, G. & J. C. Bernard. 1962. Acta Chim. Acad. Sci. Hung. **34:** 178–191.
13. Cardin, C. J., A. Dennehy, J. Mason & C. Roberts. 1976. Biochem. Soc. Trans. **4:** 873–877.
14. Suttle, N. F. & A. C. Field. 1968. J. Comp. Pathol. **78:** 351–362.
15. Smith, B. S. W. & H. Wright. 1973. (abst.). Proc. Nutr. Soc. **32:** 25.
16. Smith, B. S. W. & H. Wright. 1975. J. Comp. Pathol. **85:** 299–305.
17. Smith, B. S. W. & H. Wright. 1975. Clin. Chim. Acta **62:** 55–63.
18. El-Gallad, T. T., I. Bremner & C. F. Mills. 1977. (abst.). Proc. Nutr. Soc. **36:** 104.
19. Bremner, I. & B. W. Young. 1978. Br. J. Nutr. **39:** 325–336.
20. Suttle, N. F. 1979. (abst.). Proc. Nutr. Soc. **38:** 58.
21. Suttle, N. F. 1975. *In* Trace Elements in Soil-Plant-Animal Systems. D. J. D. Nicholas & A. R. Egan, Eds.: 271–289. Academic Press, Inc. New York, N.Y.
22. Mason, J. M., M. Lamand, J. C. Tressol & C. Lab. 1978. Ann. Rech. Vet. **9:** 577–586.
23. Dewey, D. W. 1977. Search **8:** 326–327.
24. Nederbragt, H. 1977. *In* Copper-molybdenum interaction in the rat. Ph.D. Thesis. University of Utrecht. Utrecht, The Netherlands.
25. Fell, B. F., D. Dinsdale & T. T. El-Gallad. 1979. J. Comp. Pathol. **89:** 495–514.
26. Spence, J. A., N. F. Suttle, G. Wenham, T. T. El-Gallad & I. Bremner. 1980. J. Comp. Pathol. **90:** 139–153.
27. Weber, K. M., D. D. Leaver & A. G. Wedd. 1979. Br. J. Nutr. **41:** 403–405.
28. Suttle, N. F. & M. McLauchlan. 1976. (abst.). Proc. Nutr. Soc. **35:** 22.
29. Suttle, N. F. & N. D. Grace. 1978. (abst.). Proc. Nutr. Soc. **37:** 68.
30. Grace, N. D. & N. F. Suttle. 1978. Br. J. Nutr. **41:** 125–136.
31. Smith, B. S. W., A. C. Field & N. F. Suttle. 1968. J. Comp. Pathol. **78:** 449–461.
32. Suttle, N. F. & A. C. Field. 1974. Vet. Rec. **95:** 166–169.
33. Huisingh, J. & G. Matrone. 1972. Proc. Soc. Exp. Biol. Med. Sci. **139:** 518–521.
34. Huisingh, J., D. C. Milholland & G. Matrone. 1975. J. Nutr. **105:** 1199–1205.
35. Gawthorne, J. M. & D. J. Nader. 1976. Br. J. Nutr. **35:** 11–23.
36. Suttle, N. F. 1973. *In* Proceedings, Seventh Annual Conference on Trace Substances in Environmental Health, Columbia, Missouri. D. D. Hemphill, Ed.: 245–249. University of Missouri. Columbia, Mo.
37. Suttle, N. F. 1977. Anim. Feed Sci. Technol **2:** 235–246.
38. Suttle, N. F. 1978. *In* Proceedings, Symposium on Sulphur in Forages, Wexford, Ireland. J. C. Brogan, Ed.: 197–211. An Foras Tabuntais. Dublin, Ireland.
39. Suttle, N. F. 1980. Proc. Nutr. Soc. (In press.)
40. Suttle, N. F. & A. C. Field. 1969. J. Comp. Pathol. **79:** 453–464.
41. Suttle, N. F. 1980. (Unpublished results.)
42. Suttle, N. F., K. W. Angus & J. A. Spence. 1980. (Unpublished data.)
43. Suttle, N. F. 1980. (Unpublished data.)

Discussion

H. Spencer (*Veterans Administration Hospital, Hines, Ill.*): Could the bone changes that you have shown be an effect of thiomolybdate causing copper deficiency because of the decrease in copper absorption? Osteoporosis does occur in copper-deficient animals.

N. F. Suttle: Yes, our first inclination was to think that this was a straightforward effect of a particularly severe copper deficiency and that it involved a defect in the maturation of collagen, which became incompletely mineralized.

H. SPENCER: Do you have a control study on low copper alone?, and do you see the same bone changes?

N. F. SUTTLE: We've done various studies with simple copper deficiency and also with molybdenum and sulfate supplements and have found a matrix osteoporosis in lambs but nothing as severe as that which we induce with thiomolybdate in rats. It appears that thiomolybdate has exaggerated systemic effects in the rat, and we are not quite sure why this is. It could be that on the semipurified rat diet, much more thiomolybdate is getting absorbed than from the ruminant diet. Another possibility is that rats, with their much higher relative rate of bone development, are more susceptible to the skeletal effects of thiomolybdate.

W. MERTZ (*Beltsville Human Nutrition Research Center, U.S. Department of Agriculture, Beltsville, Md.*): Do you see exostoses in regular copper deficiency? You saw them with your thiomolybdate.

N. F. SUTTLE: In cattle, there is a widening of the epiphysis at the hock joint as the cartilage overgrows and spills over, but nothing like the proliferation, or the exostoses, at many sites that we found in the thiomolybdate-treated rat.

W. MERTZ: The reason why I'm asking is that there is a syndrome called genu valgum in people living in some areas in India. It is a very serious disease that incapacitates people, that is endemic in certain areas, and that occurs only when four factors coincide, namely, low calcium intake (usually less than 200 mg per day), high fluoride intake (drinking water with 3 to 4 mg fluoride per liter or more and high water intakes that translate into 10–12 mg of fluoride per day just from water), high molybdenum intake, and low copper intake. This disease, which is different from the classical picture of fluorosis, occurred only after the building of a big water reservoir, which apparently raised the molybdenum levels in the food and drinking water that were consumed. Exostoses are part of this syndrome, and I wonder whether one could look at animal models to study this picture more clearly.

N. F. SUTTLE: The Rowett group has looked at an experimental rat model along these lines. They used thiomolybdate as a copper antagonist in the presence of relatively low levels of fluoride and found antagonistic effects in the form of a decrease in bone strength and deleterious effects on other bone parameters. If Ian Bremner is here, he might be able to say whether they have an explanation for those effects.

I. BREMNER (*Rowett Research Institute, Bucksburn, Aberdeen, United Kingdom*): I'm afraid the short answer is no. This work is being done by John Quarterman, and experiments are still in progress to try and identify exactly what is happening.

Can I be devil's advocate for a moment and ask why, in experiments where you have shown that dietary molybdenum levels as low as 2 ppm in the ruminant produce a copper deficiency state, you never find any signs of your anomalous copper fractions, yet in all experiments done with rats given low levels of thiomolybdate, you always get an increase in plasma copper concentration and you always find TCA-insoluble copper?

N. F. SUTTLE: What we have in ruminants is a mixture of gut and systemic effects. As you increase the amount of thiomolybdate that's formed, you will eventually saturate the process of insoluble complex formation in the rumen and at sites farther down the tract. Once thiomolybdate formation has exceeded that threshold, you will start to get systemic effects. In most of our earlier work with relatively low levels of molybdenum and sulfate, we were dealing with predominantly gut effects, whereas in the rat for some reason or other, this threshold is rapidly passed and systemic effects predominate.

L. M. KLEVAY (*Human Nutrition Laboratory, U.S. Department of Agriculture, Grand Forks, N. Dak.*): I've not been able to find any estimates of molybdenum in human diets. Do you have any ideas on that? Dr. Mertz's is the first mention of it that I've noticed.

N. F. SUTTLE: In 1973, at the seventh Trace Substances in Environmental Health conference at Columbia, Missouri, I did—as a ruminant nutritionist—dare to suggest that there might be implications for the copper:molybdenum antagonism in nonruminants and in man. There are some figures in my paper for molybdenum in different foodstuffs [see Reference 36].

W. MERTZ: There are figures on molybdenum in foods from the USA, namely, from the Colorado group, and there are quite extensive figures from India. The people at the Nutrition Institute in India are very much concerned with molybdenum intake. And there are some quite extensive figures from Russia, where they also have described a syndrome in humans, endemic in high-molybdenum provinces, that resembles gout in some ways and apparently is caused by an imbalance between molybdenum and copper intake. However, in order to get that syndrome, they have to have molybdenum intakes of 5 and 10 mg per day, which is much more than we have.

H. H. SANDSTEAD (*Human Nutrition Center, U.S. Department of Agriculture, Grand Forks, N. Dak.*): As I understand it, the water supply in Denver is very high in molybdenum because there is a large molybdenum mine not too far from there and a lot of the water that is used in Denver comes from the same area. Has anything abnormal been reported in Denver?

W. MERTZ: To the best of my knowledge, no health effects have been found; but that leaves us still with the two reports of health effects at higher intakes than we find in this country—one from India and one from Russia.

M. S. SEELIG (*New York University Medical Center, New York, N.Y.*): Some years ago I looked into the question of copper and molybdenum in terms of possible molybdenum deficiencies in American and other diets. One of the things that came out was that deficiencies seemed possible during pregnancy and during infancy, especially in infants who did not get milk. Molybdenum is present in the milk factor, which was discovered by DeRenzo. The response to iron was much improved when they gave milk or, strangely enough, when it was given as molybdenized iron. That was an accidental observation, and we wondered whether the activation of xanthine oxidase might have played a role here, both in absorption of iron and in the utilization of tissue iron.

I've been treating patients with D-penicillamine to pull out copper, and a common response has been a profound increase in hemoglobin. I wondered whether we might have been breaking up the copper molybdenum biocomplex and conceivably could have made molybdenum available to activate xanthine oxidase.

N. F. SUTTLE: If we're dealing with copper:molybdenum relationships at the low molybdenum concentrations in most human diets, thiomolybdate formation is an unlikely mechanism for the interaction. Although I concentrated on thiomolybdates for obvious reasons, we cannot yet rule out the possibility that straightforward copper:molybdenum complexes of the type described by Dowdy and Matrone [1968] might be formed, and there are some data for rats that suggest that this is so. Whichever theory we are looking at, the implications for molybdenum are the same as those for copper: both are rendered unabsorbable, and the consequences of an induced molybdenum deficiency can become important.

G. K. DAVIS (*University of Florida, Gainesville, Fla.*): You've been working primarily with ovine species. In our cattle, we found the bone changes that you saw in rats, and additionally fractures, but it always was accompanied by a rather low phosphorus intake, and I suspect that the relationship in bone may be related to a phosphorus metabolism problem rather than to a strictly copper:molybdenum relationship. We always have to consider that when we alter one variable, we are probably altering several and that this interferes with our interpretation.

INTERACTIONS OF ESSENTIAL MINERALS: GENERAL DISCUSSION

Moderator: W. Mertz

Beltsville Human Nutrition Research Center
U.S. Department of Agriculture
Science and Education Administration
Beltsville, Maryland 20705

M. S. Belsky (*New York University School of Medicine, New York, N.Y.*): I would like to ask Dr. Klevay some questions. What is the role that he sees for magnesium in ischemic heart disease? Many people have postulated that magnesium may be important since it also has been found to be low in heart disease patients. Also, Fleck has demonstrated that following heart attacks, magnesium is lowered and then subsequently rises. Are these consistent with the hard water–soft water hypothesis?

The next question is about a letter to the editor of the *American Journal of Clinical Nutrition* on the use of copper in some patients who had arrhythmias. The final question is, Have you found copper to affect HDL/LDL [high density lipoproteins/low density lipoproteins] in man as it does in rats?

L. M. Klevay (*Human Nutrition Laboratory, U.S. Department of Agriculture, Grand Forks, N. Dak.*): I think magnesium is important; however, I don't know how it works. Perhaps it has an effect similar to calcium. If one varies the calcium intake of rats, as calcium intake increases, cholesterol in plasma falls. Along with this fall, liver zinc decreases and liver copper increases. People fed extra calcium have a fall in cholesterol.

The arrhythmia letter to the *American Journal of Clinical Nutrition* is fascinating. Three people—including one with a lifelong history of ventricular premature beats and one who had had several premature beats per minute for several years—were cured of their premature beats by 4 mg of copper (as gluconate) per day. One of them had noted an increase in premature beats when he had increased his zinc intake before taking copper.

L. J. Machlin (*Hoffmann-La Roche, Inc., Nutley, N.J.*): I'd like to ask Dr. Spencer if she could tell us about the possible hazards of aluminum in regard to Alzheimer's disease and senile dementia.

H. Spencer (*Veterans Administration Hospital, Hines, Ill.*): I can only state that an association has been reported between a high aluminum content in brain and Alzheimer's disease. I don't believe there is information available on the extent of aluminum exposure that causes increased deposition of aluminum in brain in this disease.

M. S. Seelig (*New York University Medical Center, New York, N.Y.*): Dr. Belsky raised the question about magnesium, an area in which I am most interested. I think that there is a great deal of evidence for the correlation of marginal deficiencies of magnesium with the high incidence of sudden death from ischemic heart disease, which is believed to be electrical in nature. How this interrelates with the copper, I really don't know. Dr. Klevay and I have been studying some of the patients that I mentioned in regard to the D-penicillamine. Very preliminary results show that people who have had their copper depleted and who were supplemented with zinc for taste loss developed hyperlipidemia. One developed multiple xan-

0077-8923/80/0355-0208 $01.75/0 © 1980, NYAS

thomata. Dr. Klevay has very kindly done the hair analyses. Two of the patients had a drop in pre–beta lipoprotein and a change from type IV to normal after copper was repleted and zinc withheld. The man who had the multiple xanthomata had these disappear.

W. G. HOEKSTRA (*University of Wisconsin, Madison, Wis.*): I have a question and comment concerning the general area of cardiovascular disease and nutritional insult.

I gather that one can induce atherosclerotic lesions by a variety of methods of injuring or damaging arteries. One wonders if one might create transient damage from nutritional deficiency that can be perpetuated despite correction of the deficiency. For example, in magnesium deficiency, where calcification of major blood vessels occurs, the lesions are very difficult to reverse.

My question is, What do we know about reversibility of the aortic damage from copper deficiency? Could you comment on the problems one might run into in surveying cardiovascular patients near the end of their lives if the deficiency may have occurred much earlier.

W. MERTZ: Thank you. I think Dr. Klevay would answer that from the clinical point of view, and perhaps we could ask Dr. Davis and Dr. Suttle to answer this from another viewpoint.

L. M. KLEVAY: Ischemic heart disease generally kills people over age 40. The initial lesion, which must exist a priori but which has not been defined, may begin *in utero,* in infancy, or in childhood. Certainly atherosclerosis is present by the third decade. Generally, people consider a heart attack to be the result of a lengthy, inexorable process that probably results from continual insult. The early insult that you suggest or a similar, intermittent insult seems quite reasonable. However, these insults probably would complicate measurements made near death.

I don't know about the reversibility of arterial damage due to copper deficiency. However, some of the abnormal electrocardiograms that we have produced are reversible.

W. MERTZ: Okay, thank you Dr. Klevay. Dr. Davis?

G. K. DAVIS (*University of Florida, Gainesville, Fla.*): The answer really is in two parts. First, the lesions that have occurred with functional copper deficiency include calcification of the large vessels. In our experiments, at least, we have carried animals as long as two years on adequate diets trying to reverse the lesions, without any signs of reversal. On the other hand, the Hawaiian workers reported that they did get reversal. Now there has been work reported from California and elsewhere in humans where they thought that they were getting reversal. We have not been able to see it. Second, with respect to the copper deficiency, there is a replacement of the elastic fibers with a lipid type of deposit. We can see no repair in terms of increasing the elastic fibers. This has been with smaller animals and with cattle, so I can't say that this is true in all species, but at least it is the case in those we've examined.

One of the things that first came out in our studies was an apparent change in the bone and what appeared to be a degeneration of the cartilaginous tissue in the joints. Our animals began to assume abnormal gaits, as we called it, apparently due to pain. This suggested a relationship to arthritis, whereupon I began to get all kinds of letters, even people offering themselves as guinea pigs so that we would study aspects of arthritis. Of course, we were not able to do this in our work.

More recent work reported from Australia suggests that the copper bracelet that people have used so often and that we have deprecated as worthless may be giving relief from arthritis. The suggestion was made that the normal acid reaction of the skin on these bracelets may result in some copper absorption. This is probably very uncertain. I'm sure other people are going to look at this, and we would like to have definite data. It is very interesting that we've gone such a complete circle.

N. F. SUTTLE (*Moredun Research Institute, Edinburgh, Scotland*): I would like to make a comment about the development of cardiovascular lesions during experimental copper deficiency and to point out the enormous effects that there are both of species and of age on the development of these lesions. If we take a species, such as the chick, with a rapid rate of elastin formation and we look at it just after hatching, the effect is spectacular. If we look at the rat, then things are a little bit more difficult. If we go to the ruminant, then our studies of copper deficiency have yet to produce any cardiovascular lesions even though they've produced many other signs of abnormality.

Now we are also finding that as the animal matures, its copper requirement diminishes, and it's going to be far more difficult to induce cardiovascular lesions in an adult than in a rapidly growing animal. I think we should bear these species and age effects in mind before we extrapolate too much from our experimental depletion situations to the state of adult man.

L. M. KLEVAY: Most of our experiments have been done with growing animals. We have preliminary results on rats made deficient in copper as adults. Some of these rats, after about a year of deprivation, got abnormal electrocardiograms without becoming anemic or hypercholesterolemic.

J. C. SMITH, JR. (*Beltsville Human Nutrition Research Center, U.S. Department of Agriculture, Beltsville, Md.*): I wonder if someone would elaborate upon magnesium in regard to sudden infant death.

M. S. SEELIG: I was happy that Dr. Suttle raised the question about age differences. We find that marked arterial lesions occur predominantly in animals that are purely magnesium deficient and not loaded in calcium as most rats are. Most rats are given a lot of calcium and a lot of vitamin D in their normal diets, and when they are given magnesium-deficient diets, it markedly intensifies the problem. But in many species of animals—such as rats, cats, dogs, monkeys, and cattle—the major changes are intimal, with intimal proliferation and intimal medial thickening, if the animals are on a diet that is not imbalanced and that is magnesium depleted with the other elements normal. But the very first change is elastin degeneration, with lipid droplets appearing along the course of the degenerated and reduplicated elastin. You usually get microfocal lesions in the myocardium in this instance, because the very small intramyocardial arteries are affected first. With the high dose of calcium and vitamin D, there tends to be a more generalized arteriosclerosis.

As regards sudden infant death, certainly Joan Caddell has considered this a good deal from the standpoint of respiratory disorders. I think that it is quite possible that the electrical sudden death may be at least partially due to magnesium deficiency of the infant. This is particularly true in infants of women who have had multiple pregnancies and who are young and therefore have not met their own magnesium requirements.

Finally, I would like to refer to an old piece of work by Burch and Lazzarra, who showed that the Mg-28 exchange is most rapid in the septum. It would be exceedingly interesting to see whether magnesium-deficient infants have lost more magnesium from the septum and whether there might be a conduction abnormality as a result. This requires investigation.

W. MERTZ: I would like to ask one question, a brief one, since it follows Dr. Klevay's presentation and Dr. Seelig's. Does either one of your hypotheses have room for other factors? In other words, does the copper hypothesis have room for things like magnesium and vice versa?

L. M. KLEVAY: One of my approaches to the problem of atherosclerosis and heart disease is to find out if some of the many observations are not mutually exclusive. In other words, there's a tendency among students of heart disease to fragment the field—some people study lipids, some people study hard water, some people study fiber, some people study clotting, some people study exercise, etc. Referring to my slide on pellagra, many of those observations still have a grain of truth. Some had common attributes. Repeatedly in my papers I used my phrase "apparently dissimilar" observations; they may not be dissimilar at all. Perhaps in addition to the mechanisms for magnesium action reviewed by Dr. Seelig, magnesium has an effect on copper and zinc metabolism similar to that of calcium.

W. MERTZ: That's a good statement. Dr. Davis?

G. K. DAVIS: The question was raised about the changes that may occur in the heart. When we saw our first cases of what we called quick death, or falling disease as it was called in Australia, our first reaction was, How do we produce this so that we are on hand when it happens? Frankly, heart failure doesn't occur when you say it is going to occur at 8 o'clock in the morning, and consequently, I started a group of experiments in which I attempted to produce this at will. I was able to do so when I supplemented very small amounts of copper and the animal started to respond very rapidly and then I withdrew it. In other words, I just gave it to them for about 30 days and then, on the 31st day, completely eliminated the copper from their diet. Within a period of about three weeks, I had the animals dropped, and of course we went through their hearts with a fine-tooth comb and found essentially what Mildred Seelig is reporting. That is, very numerous particular ecchymosis type of hemorrhages within the myocardium, and that was about all we could find.

But you must also have a minimal amount of phosphorus in the diet at the same time. So here we are saying, Alright it's copper, but it is influencing other parameters of metabolism that may be as important as the copper itself.

W. MERTZ: Thank you Dr. Davis. Are there additional comments?

M. S. SEELIG: I would just like to say that I was very studiously supplementing the patients I mentioned earlier wth magnesium, despite which they developed their changes in the lipid distribution and also developed myocardial infarctions. These findings are very disconcerting.

W. MERTZ: I think it's important to realize, as we have today, that the interactions among essential trace elements are very numerous; the unidirectional approach many of us follow is all right for increasing our knowledge, but it's probably very dangerous to apply this knowledge without great restraints until we know a good deal about interactions. This has come out many times today.

I would just like to mention that the Committee on Recommended Dietary Allowances, in the latest edition, has recognized this danger of interactions by oversupplementation with one element. It has stated in its table the estimated ranges of safe and adequate intakes for six of the new trace elements: copper, manganese, molybdenum, selenium, chromium, and fluoride. These ranges are given with a warning that when these ranges are exceeded by self-supplementation, the risk of creating imbalance is increased. We can be very glad that this idea of interactions has been recognized in the recommended allowances. I just wanted to bring out again this word of caution.

INTERACTIONS OF VITAMIN E AND SELENIUM WITH MERCURY AND SILVER

Howard E. Ganther

Department of Nutritional Sciences
University of Wisconsin
Madison, Wisconsin 53706

Introduction

The theme of this conference is fully reflected in the subject of this paper, which discusses some well-established interactions between a vitamin, an essential trace element, and two hazardous metals. With metals, interactions are the rule rather than the exception, and since selenium is a close relative of sulfur, interactions of selenium with metals are also to be expected. It is more difficult to see how a fat-soluble substance like vitamin E can interact with metals, from the purely chemical standpoint. Perhaps the most puzzling aspect to be explained is how rather modest levels of selenium, and vitamin E, can be so effective in modifying the toxicity produced by substantially larger amounts of silver or mercury in a target tissue. A nutritional approach can be taken. To undertake such an approach to these micronutrient:metal interactions, we would like to know (1) what the micronutrients do, i.e., their biological functions; (2) what the micronutrients do to the metals; and (3) what the metals do to the micronutrients. Exploration of these questions may in turn lead to a better understanding of how the toxic metals actually exert their toxic effects.

The functions of vitamin E and selenium in the control of peroxidative damage have been generally accepted. Vitamin E can give up a hydrogen atom to a free radical and thereby inhibit propagation of radical chain reactions.[1] Vitamin E may also play a role in membrane structure beyond that of an antioxidant.[2] The discovery by Rotruck and Hoekstra that glutathione peroxidase was a selenoprotein, catalyzing hydroperoxide decomposition (Equation 1), greatly clarified the biochemical

$$\mathrm{ROOH + 2\,GSH \rightarrow ROH + HOH + GSSG} \qquad (1)$$

basis for the nutritional interactions of vitamin E, selenium, and sulfur amino acids.[3] This topic was reviewed by Hoekstra and is discussed elsewhere at this conference by Tappel.[4]*

There may well be other functions in animals for selenium and for vitamin E, but for the present, we may ask whether the interactions of silver and mercury with these micronutrients can be explained in terms of radical-induced peroxidative damage. It is known that metals that undergo univalent redox reactions can initiate peroxidative destruction. Historically, it was the idea that silver could have a prooxidant effect that led to the work by Shaver and Mason 30 years ago that first demonstrated the strong protective effect exerted by vitamin E against silver toxicity.

Vitamin E and Silver

In 1951, Shaver and Mason reported in an abstract that weanling rats fed a

* See page 18 for Tappel's paper.

0077-8923/80/0355-0212 $01.75/0

vitamin E–deficient diet and given 0.15% (1,500 parts per million) $AgNO_3$ in the drinking water showed signs of toxicity and muscular dystrophy and died within 18–40 days, whereas animals given the same diet plus vitamin E survived.[5] In 1958, Dam *et al.* found that 20 ppm of Ag as $AgNO_3$ promoted exudative diathesis in vitamin E–deficient chicks.[6] By this time it was known that liver necrosis in rats and exudative diathesis in chicks were caused by a combined deficiency of vitamin E and selenium. A decade later, Diplock and coworkers demonstrated the ability of silver to induce liver necrosis in rats and exudative diathesis in chicks fed diets low in vitamin E, protein, and presumably Se.[7-8] Vitamin E, Se, sulfur amino acids, and antioxidants were able to prevent these deficiency signs to varying degrees. The effects of Ag were observed even in fat-free diets, leading Diplock *et al.* to conclude that lipid peroxidation was not the basis for the stress induced by Ag.[7] Other workers have demonstrated the induction of lesions of vitamin E or selenium deficiency in turkey poults, chicks, ducklings, and pigs by silver added to the diet or drinking water.[9-13] If high enough levels of Ag are used, such signs can be induced even in practical-type diets adequate in vitamin E and Se.[10,11,13]

Silver seems to be especially effective at inducing vitamin E–selenium deficiency. Bunyan *et al.* found that gold, copper, or arsenic did not duplicate the effects of silver.[8] Whanger and Weswig found that of 19 elements tested, silver, zinc, and vanadium promoted liver necrosis in rats at the levels tested, and silver was by far the most effective.[14] High levels of zinc and copper induced deficiency signs in chicks.[15] Arsenic, cadmium, and tellurium had no effect in increasing Se–vitamin E deficiency in pigs;[12] but tellurium was found to induce deficiency signs in ducklings.[11] Silver is not exclusively an antagonist of vitamin E and Se, since signs of copper deficiency have also been observed in chicks given silver.[16]

On a weight basis, selenium is more effective than is vitamin E in overcoming the effects of silver, as would be expected considering that the nutritional requirement for selenium is below 1 ppm. However, it appears that in the reduction of Ag-induced mortality, vitamin E at 100 or 200 IU/kg of diet may be more effective than 1 ppm of Se in experiments with chicks, pigs, and ducklings.[10,13,11] The diets used in these experiments, however, were commercial rations or were formulated from crude feedstuffs and therefore were adequate in selenium, not deficient. The effect of vitamin E against silver may be greater when selenium is present.

Selenium and Heavy Metals

Selenium, like sulfur, has a high affinity for heavy metals.[17] There is now considerable evidence for biological interactions between various heavy metals and selenium. With few exceptions, the interactions lead to decreased biological activity of both the metals and the selenium. Dietary levels of selenium of the same order of magnitude as the nutritional requirement for this essential trace element are highly effective in reducing the toxicity of methylmercury, a toxicant accumulated in fish; thus, the interactions are of practical importance.[18] Metals may also be useful probes for investigating biological functions of selenium. One underlying basis for such interaction is probably found in the chemical nature of the elements. Interesting scientific or technological applications of the mercury:selenium interaction have appeared from time to time.[19,20]

A biological interaction of mercury with selenium metabolism in animals was noted almost 40 years ago.[21] The first toxicological interactions to be recognized involved acute toxicity effects of the injected metal, which could be prevented by injecting approximately equimolar amounts of a selenium salt, such as sodium selenite.

$$H_2SeO_3 \xrightarrow{GSH} GSSeSG \xrightarrow[\text{glutathione reductase}]{NADPH} GSSeH \xrightarrow[\text{glutathione reductase}]{NADPH} H_2Se$$

FIGURE 1. Glutathione:glutathione reductase pathway for reduction of selenium. GSSeSG = selenotrisulfide derivative of glutathione; GSSeH = glutathione selenopersulfide. (See Reference 53.)

Cadmium-induced testicular necrosis was the first lesion shown to be prevented by selenium.[22,23] Later, Parizek and collaborators demonstrated that sodium selenite and other selenium compounds were highly effective in preventing lethality of mercuric chloride or cadmium chloride.[24,25]

When approximately equimolar doses of selenium and heavy metals are employed, the interaction probably involves the formation of complexes that reduce the availability of the components. The interacting components may be simply the metal and the selenium, or ternary complexes involving proteins may also be involved when selenium is built into a protein. Inorganic salts of selenium are rapidly reduced in tissues of animals to selenotrisulfides (-S—Se—S-), selenopersulfides (-S—SeH), hydrogen selenide, di- and trimethyl selenide, and probably other low-molecular-weight metabolites and protein derivatives (FIGURE 1). Such complexing generally results in increased retention of the metal and the selenium in the animal and decreased elimination via excretory pathways, milk, or offspring.[26-29] The distribution of the metal and selenium between tissues and within the components of tissues can also be altered dramatically. In the case of Cd-induced testicular necrosis, selenium increases testicular uptake to some extent but greatly decreases the uptake in the soluble fraction; within the soluble fraction, however, selenium caused a large decrease in the amount of Cd bound in a 30,000-molecular-weight peak and a corresponding increase in Cd binding to larger proteins.[30]

SILVER, SELENIUM AND GLUTATHIONE PEROXIDASE

From the work of Diplock and others, it appeared that silver might induce a conditioned deficiency of selenium by interfering with the conversion of selenium to the biologically active form, effectively increasing the dietary requirement. Following the discovery that glutathione peroxidase contained selenium, it was possible to investigate the effect of silver on the level of this biologically active form of selenium in tissues of animals given 0.5 ppm of Se in the diet.[31] This amount of Se normally would be more than adequate for development of maximum enzyme activity. These experiments were conducted by Ms. Patricia Wagner in collaboration with Dr. Hoekstra. Weanling rats were fed basal diets containing 20% casein so that liver necrosis would not occur in the absence of added vitamin E or selenium. Upon addition of 75 or 750 ppm of Ag as $AgNO_3$ to the drinking water, depressed growth and some mortality were observed in rats given a basal diet (containing 2% cod-liver oil) low in vitamin E and selenium.[32] Selenium (0.5 ppm, as sodium selenite) prevented the growth depression observed with 75 ppm Ag and markedly improved growth and survival of rats given 750 ppm Ag, even though the Ag concentration of liver and kidney was higher.[32] A number of other experiments with 750 ppm Ag showed that either 0.5 ppm of Se or 100 IU/kg of vitamin E largely prevented the growth depression.[32,33] Liver glutathione peroxidase activity in rats given 0.5 ppm Se plus 75 ppm Ag for 52 days was 30% of that for rats given 0.5 Se without Ag, and was practically undetectable when 750 ppm Ag were given.[32] Ag also decreased glutathione (GSH) peroxidase in erythrocytes and kidney.[32]

A time-course study of the levels of GSH peroxidase, Se, and Ag in rats given 750 ppm Ag plus 0.5 ppm Se showed that for liver, there was an initial rise in liver Se concentration during the first week, paralleled by a rise in liver Ag.[33] After that, liver Se and Ag concentrations fell to a minimum at 22 days and rose slowly thereafter. Glutathione peroxidase activity in liver fell progressively throughout the 22-day period and remained at very low levels. This study shows that liver accumulated a biologically inactive form of selenium, possibly complexed to Ag, during the first week. By increasing dietary selenium from 0.5 ppm to 5 ppm, the effect of silver on liver GSH peroxidase was partially overcome.[33] The effect of Ag on liver GSH peroxidase was reversible; in rats receiving 0.5 ppm Se, enzyme activity returned to normal levels within five weeks when Ag administration was discontinued.[33] These results indicate that Ag probably induces a conditioned deficiency of Se and makes selenium unavailable for the synthesis of glutathione peroxidase. The effectiveness of low levels of Se against Ag toxicity is thus explained in terms of overcoming the conditioned deficiency of Se. It is not necessary for Se to decrease tissue levels of Ag, nor is a significant fraction of the total Ag complexed by Se.

Vitamin E was as effective as Se in overcoming the growth depression produced by Ag but did not prevent the depression in glutathione peroxidase.[33] Thus, it appears that the growth depression is not related to the Ag-induced decrease in glutathione peroxidase.

Methylmercury, Selenium, and Vitamin E

One of the most interesting and widely explored interactions is that of mercury and selenium. It is observed in both acute and chronic studies, with either inorganic or methylmercury salts, and with both inorganic and organic forms of selenium.[18,24,29,34–36] Collaborative studies at the University of Wisconsin have demonstrated protection by 0.5 ppm of selenium as sodium selenite against toxic effects of much larger quantities of methylmercury fed to rats, Japanese quail, and cats.[18,37–39] Vitamin E also protects against methylmercury toxicity if large amounts of vitamin E (several hundred ppm in the diet) are given, as first reported by Welsh, and the combination can give rather remarkable prolongation of survival, as shown in an experiment conducted by Dr. Mahmoud El-Begearmi (Table 1).[40,64] Vitamin E does not seem to duplicate the ability of selenium to overcome growth depression in rats given methylmercury, in contrast to the ability of both to overcome growth depression in rats given silver.[17,32]

Table 1

Delay of Methylmercury Toxicity in Rats by Selenium and Vitamin E Added to Crude Diet*

Additions (mg/kg)			Days to First Toxic Signs	Days to 50% Toxic Signs	Days to 50% Mortality
Hg	Se	E			
—	—	—	—	—	—
30	—	—	21	24	44
30	0.5	—	48	56	70
30	—	500	28	56	70
30	0.5	500	98	112	117

* Corn-soy diet. Se content 0.10 mg/kg by fluorometric analysis; vitamin E 15.6 IU/kg by calculation. (From M. M. El-Begearmi, Reference 64, with permission of the author.)

The protective effect of selenium against methylmercury has been confirmed in many laboratories, and mechanisms have been discussed elsewhere.[41,42] It is clear that selenium does not decrease mercury or methylmercury concentrations in tissues.[41,42] Selenium-treated animals may remain unaffected even when they have reached tissue mercury levels otherwise associated with toxic effects. Brain mercury levels above 10 ppm are generally lethal, but Japanese quail survived with total Hg levels averaging 58 ppm in brain after long-term feeding of 15 ppm Hg as methylmercury plus 6 ppm of Se as sodium selenite.[38] Similarly high levels were reported when methylmercury, rather than total mercury, was analyzed in brain of quail.[43] The level of Se in the brain under such conditions is higher than normal but is far below a stoichiometric ratio in relation to the mercury.[38]

The effect of selenium on tissue mercury levels is somewhat dependent on the dose of methylmercury. In rats fed graded levels of methylmercury plus or minus 0.5 ppm Se for 16 weeks, the presence of selenium had no effect on tissue Hg levels at low levels of methylmercury; at higher levels of methylmercury, selenium increased the accumulation of mercury in brain and kidney but not in liver (FIGURES 2–4). It is believed that the presence of selenium may allow a greater transformation of methylmercury to the inorganic form, which is then accumulated in certain organs. In Se-deficient rats, kidney Hg levels reached a maximum at a dose of 5 ppm methylmercury in the diet and did not rise with a further increase in dose, whereas rats given methylmercury plus Se showed a progressive rise in Hg level with dose (FIGURE 3).

The effect of increasing methylmercury dosage on tissue selenium levels is to

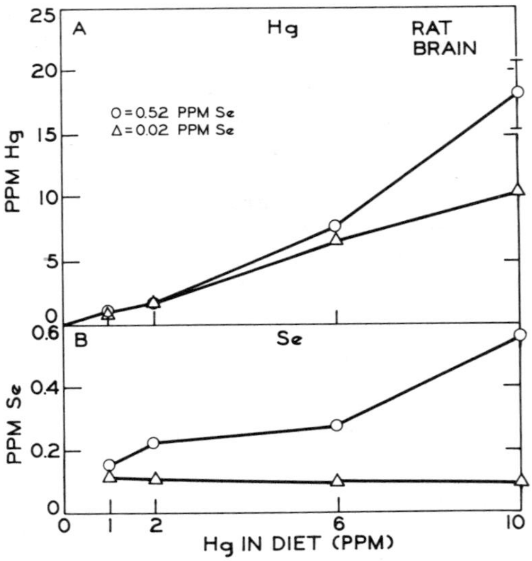

FIGURE 2. Mercury and selenium concentrations in brain of rats after 16 weeks of feeding various levels of methylmercury chloride in a diet containing 20% of casein, supplemented with 100 IU of vitamin E per kg, plus or minus 0.5 ppm of Se added as sodium selenite (experiment performed by Ms. Patricia Wagner). Hg was analyzed by flameless atomic absorption after acid digestion. Se was analyzed by a fluorometric procedure after acid digestion. Each value represents the mean concentration (ppm, fresh basis) for tissues from 8–10 animals analyzed in duplicate by Peggy Kroll.

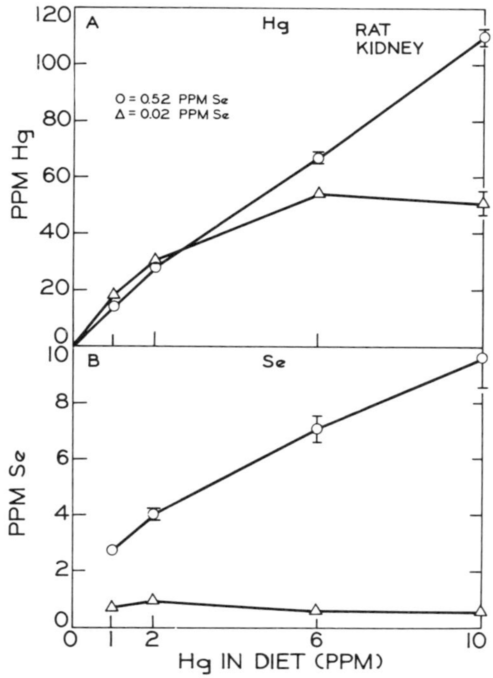

FIGURE 3. Mercury and selenium concentrations in kidney of rats fed graded levels of methylmercury ± 0.5 ppm Se. (See FIGURE 2.)

cause increased accumulation if selenium is available, but if selenium is lacking, there is no accumulation of selenium despite the rise in mercury levels (FIGURES 2–4).

Glutathione peroxidase activity is not affected by methylmercury in the manner observed with silver, especially in liver. In rats, some tissues may show a decline in glutathione peroxidase activity when animals are fed methylmercury for several months (FIGURE 5). It is possible that a decrease in glutathione peroxidase activity caused by methylmercury might be critical in target organs, such as brain, that have rather low levels of glutathione peroxidase. In cats, glutathione peroxidase activity in brain (and muscle) was decreased when methylmercury was fed for long periods, whereas liver was unchanged and kidney tended to be slightly higher.[65] Dr. Wagner has observed that rats fed 40 ppm Hg as methylmercury for 3 weeks or 20 ppm for 15 weeks had increased levels of glutathione peroxidase in liver when assayed using GSH and HOOH (FIGURE 5).[33]

METHYLMERCURY TOXICITY AND PROTECTIVE FACTORS IN FISH

Fish—particularly predators at the end of the food chain—contain elevated levels of methylmercury. Levels in muscle of marine food fish, such as tuna, are usually below 1 ppm;[44] but fish exposed to Hg-polluted inland waters may contain 10 to 20 ppm. Marine fish also contain selenium, averaging 0.4–0.9 ppm in most species.[44] The weight ratio of Hg to Se is less than 1 for tuna;[18,44] however, in fish ex-

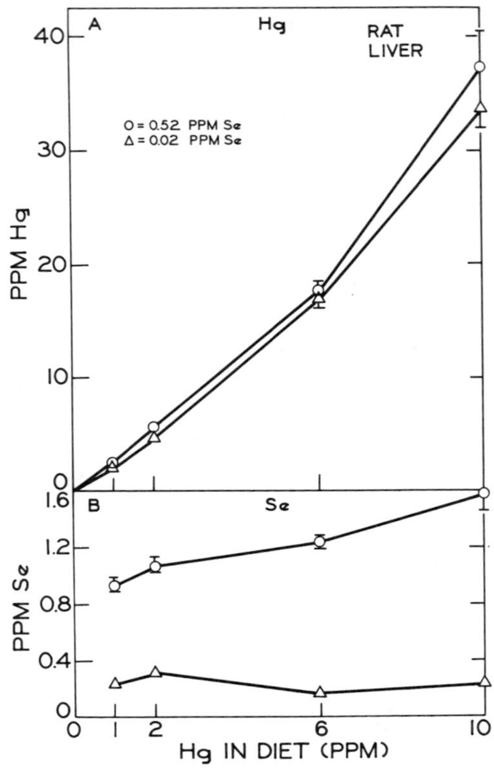

FIGURE 4. Mercury and selenium concentrations in liver of rats fed graded levels of methylmercury ± 0.5 ppm of Se. (See FIGURE 2.)

posed to Hg-polluted waters in Japan and Sweden, the Hg:Se ratio is 10:1 or more, showing that the uptake of Se in such fish does not keep pace with the uptake of Hg.[45,46]

It is important to distinguish the toxicological situation for mercury in marine fish from that for mercury in fish from polluted waters. First, there is the difference in Hg levels. It appears that marine fish have always contained some mercury, because mercury of natural origin has always been present at relatively constant levels in the ocean.[47,48] Fish in waters locally polluted with mercury take up more mercury because more mercury is available. Second, concentrations of Se in the ocean are such that selenium may be taken up by marine fish to a greater extent than by fish in inland waters, particularly for freshwater fish in geographical regions where selenium is relatively deficient. The concentration of selenium in the oceans is about 0.09 ppb, approximately the same as that of Hg.[48,49] It is therefore possible for marine fish, such as tuna, to accumulate both mercury and selenium quite easily, reflecting the availability of the elements in the ocean. In comparing batches of high-mercury tuna to low-mercury tuna, the increase in mercury was matched by an equimolar increase in selenium.[18] More extensive surveys indicate that this is not necessarily true for the general case, however.[44] Studies with rats fed purified diets plus methylmercury and sodium selenite showed that uptake of selenium with mer-

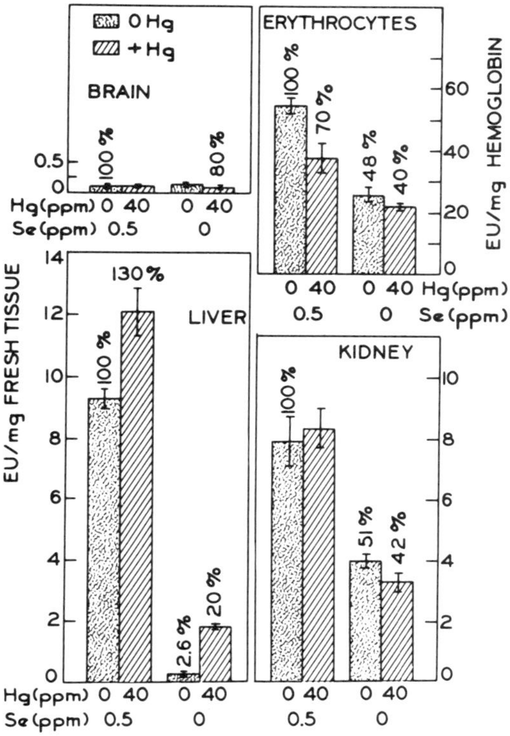

FIGURE 5. Glutathione peroxidase activity of tissues from rats fed 40 ppm of methylmercury chloride for three weeks. (From P. Wagner, Reference 33, p. 126, with permission of the author.) A 20% casein purified basal diet containing 100 IU/kg of vitamin E and 0.017 ppm Se was fed, with or without 0.5 ppm of Se as sodium selenite. Values are means of five rats per group ± standard error, determined with H_2O_2 as substrate. During the third week, three out of five rats fed 40 ppm Hg without supplemental Se showed signs of neurotoxicity.

cury is not an obligatory process (FIGURES 2–4). Mercury was accumulated to high levels even when a selenium-deficient diet was fed, and the uptake of selenium did not match the uptake of mercury even when the diets contained 0.5 ppm of selenium as selenite. In the practical situation, fish from Hg-polluted inland waters probably take up larger amounts of mercury in relation to selenium because there is a greater supply of mercury in relation to selenium compared to marine waters. Thus, the toxicological picture can be different in the two cases because of the modifying effect of selenium, as discussed earlier.

The presence of a factor or factors in marine fish that can decrease methylmercury toxicity is well established.[18,34,37,50] This was first shown with Japanese quail fed diets containing a toxic level of mercury (20 ppm) added as methylmercury hydroxide.[18] Quail fed diets containing 17% of tuna as the protein source survived longer than did quail fed corn-soybean diets. It was shown that the Se content of tuna was high enough (about 3 ppm) that 17% of tuna in the diet furnished 0.5 ppm of Se, and 0.5 ppm Se significantly reduced methylmercury toxicity. Is Se in tuna responsible for its protective effect, or is some other factor involved? We hope to isolate and identify the chemical forms of selenium in tuna to get at this question directly.

Although the circumstantial evidence points to selenium as the main protective factor in tuna, other nutrients in tuna might play some role as well, such as sulfur amino acids or vitamin E.[51,40] Arsenic is also found in tuna, probably in an organic form.[44] Sodium arsenite is known to modify selenium toxicity and metabolism, as reviewed elsewhere, so there is the possibility of an arsenic:selenium interaction.[53] It is interesting that a three-way combination of arsenite, selenite, and sulfur amino acids is more effective against methylmercury toxicity than are these substances fed alone or in two-way combinations.[51,52] Arsenite does not appear to interfere with the protective effect of selenite against methylmercury but instead may enhance it.

The action level for mercury in fish was set at 0.5 ppm by the Food and Drug Administration in 1969 and was raised to 1.0 ppm in 1979, based on more recent evidence relating to the toxic dose of methylmercury in humans and on the intake of methylmercury achieved by eating various amounts of marine fish. However, the presence of selenium or other protective substances in fish was not factored into the current guideline, so there is probably an additional margin of safety.

Mercury and Selenium in Cats Fed Fish

A study was conducted at the University of Wisconsin, in collaboration with Drs. L. Chang, A. Dudley, and M. L. Sunde, to investigate the possible modifying effects of tuna on methylmercury toxicity and metabolism in cats. (A preliminary account of some aspects of this study is published.)[39] Cats were fed fish-based diets for 19 months. Two groups of cats were fed basal diets containing 40% of tuna (canned tuna fish) or frozen pike, supplying about 0.3–0.4 ppm of Hg. The pike were from Lake Winnipeg, into which Hg-contaminated rivers flow. The tuna diet contained about 0.3 ppm more Se than did the pike diet, reflecting the lower content of Se in the freshwater fish. Another group of cats received a commercial fish-flavored cat food having a low level of mercury (below 0.01 ppm). Cats fed the 40% pike or tuna basal diets thrived and grew faster than did the group fed commercial cat food. Levels of Hg in blood and brain of cats fed fish were higher than for those fed commercial cat food but were well below toxic levels. Liver Hg levels (Table 2) were considerably higher for cats fed tuna (22 ppm), as compared to 4 ppm in cats fed pike and 0.6 ppm in control cats. Liver Se levels in cats fed tuna were all higher than 2 ppm, and reached 20 ppm in one cat. A striking correspondence between the level of

Table 2

Mercury and Selenium Accumulation in Liver of Cats Fed Diets Containing Northern Pike or Tuna

Diet*	N	Hg†	Se†	Hg/Se Weight Ratio	Hg/Se Molar Ratio
40% Pike‡	12	4.0 ± 0.53	0.69 ± 0.04	5.8	2.3
40% Tuna§	7	22.3 ± 7.6	5.3 ± 2.1	4.2	1.7
Cat Food¶	7	0.6 ± 0.1	1.2 ± 0.1	0.5	0.2

* Diets fed for 19 months; no Hg or Se was added.
† ppm wet weight; mean ± standard error.
‡ Complete diet contained 0.30 ppm Hg, 0.17 ppm Se.
§ complete diet contained 0.37 ppm Hg, 0.45 ppm Se.
¶ "Fish flavored," contained <0.01 ppm Hg, 0.5 ppm Se.

Hg and Se in liver in individual cats fed tuna or pike was noted, indicating a tendency for both elements to be accumulated in a ratio of between one and two atoms of Hg per atom of Se. No pathological changes could be found in tissues of cats fed tuna or pike for 19 months, in contrast to an earlier report.[54] It appears that Hg and selenium can be accumulated together in a nontoxic, biologically unavailable form, possibly reflecting a direct chemical interaction between mercury and some form of selenium. A similar accumulation of Se and inorganic Hg has been noted in liver of marine mammals.[55] Along the same lines, it is interesting that in men exposed to inorganic Hg in the mines in Yugoslavia, elevated levels of both Hg and Se, in approximately equimolar ratio, were found in brain and other tissues many years after exposure to mercury had ceased.[56]

Possible Role of Free Radicals in Metal Toxicity

It is clear that selenium and vitamin E exert powerful effects in reducing methylmercury and silver toxicity. Levels of selenium normally found in foods (less than 1 ppm) delay the onset of toxic signs caused by much higher levels of the toxic metal. Direct protective effects of both vitamin E and selenium have been observed *in vitro* when methylmercury was added to cultured nervous tissue cells. The only functions established in animals for selenium and vitamin E at micronutrient levels are related to the prevention of oxidative damage in tissues. Can the interactions of silver and methylmercury with these micronutrients be understood in terms of radical-induced peroxidative damage, triggered by the metals and aggravated by their ability to inhibit the various systems defending against peroxidation? This idea has been explored in more detail elsewhere and forms the basis for a new hypothesis regarding the toxicity of methylmercury.[41] Stated in simplest form, the hypothesis is that the neurotoxicity of methylmercury and other alkyl metals may involve free radicals formed by the breakdown of methylmercury and does not result solely from the intact organometallic compound.

The starting point for this hypothesis was the idea that homolytic cleavage of the carbon:metal bond would release an alkyl radical (such as $CH_3\cdot$) and a metal radical (FIGURE 6). There is an abundance of chemical literature documenting the homolytic decomposition of alkyl mercurials and other organometallic compounds.[41]

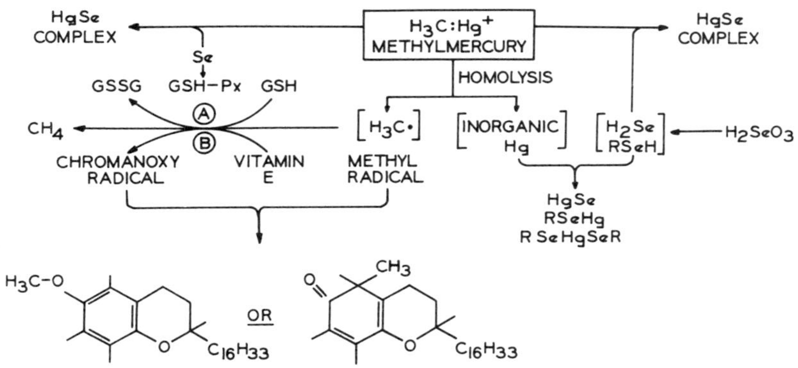

FIGURE 6. Proposed mechanism for biotransformation of methylmercury by a homolytic process, as modified by vitamin E and selenium.

The breakdown of methylmercury can be induced *in vitro* by radicals formed by the Cu-mediated autooxidation of ascorbate.[57] *In vivo,* such a process would probably be initiated by the cytochrome P_{450} system of microsomes. Assuming that the breakdown of methylmercury took place by such a process, the consequences could be either favorable or harmful. If the radicals formed from the alkylmercurial could be converted to less reactive products (methyl radical to methane, for example), rather than reacting with target molecules in cells, such a process could be the first step in detoxification of the alkylmetal. This would have the favorable result of converting the toxicant to less toxic products that could be more readily excreted (methane and Hg^{++}, in the case of methylmercury).

On the other hand, if the radicals reacted with constituents in the tissue, cellular damage would occur, so that homolytic breakdown would be associated with toxic effects, analogous to the activation of a proximate carcinogen to a carcinogen by microsomal drug-metabolizing enzymes.

Methylmercury, owing to its high lipid solubility, would be taken up by membranes in target tissues, such as brain, in close proximity to lipids. Its breakdown would then initiate a chain reaction of peroxidation involving lipids or would result in radical damage to proteins or nucleic acids as well. The onset of neurological changes would be preceded by a lag phase, during which the various systems defending against peroxidation would be overcome. The susceptibility of a tissue to damage would be a function of the methylmercury concentration, the rate at which homolytic breakdown occurred, and the capacity of the tissue to defend against peroxidative damage, as determined by levels of glutathione peroxidase, vitamin E, and other substances.

Vitamin E could modify methylmercury metabolism by acting as a radical scavenger. It might be more efficient than other antioxidants because of its physiochemical properties for interacting with unsaturated fatty acid chains in membranes. Vitamin E could donate a hydrogen atom to the methyl radical, converting it to methane (FIGURE 5), followed by regeneration of vitamin E from the radical. Such mechanisms would involve vitamin E in a catalytic role. The tocopherol radical might also form as a stable adduct with the methyl radical, a mechanism requiring stoichiometric consumption of the tocopherol.[58]

Selenium would be able to aid detoxification in several ways. Its presence in glutathione peroxidase could allow for glutathione-linked reduction of radicals (i.e., conversion of methyl radical to methane, as does vitamin E) or of peroxides. Selenium would have the added capability of complexing tightly with the metallic product of the breakdown. This reaction might help control peroxidation initiated by the metal and could explain the gradual accumulation of mercury and selenium that is often observed in tissues (see above). The function of Se as a catalyst in glutathione peroxidase would be consistent with the fact that selenium is protective against methylmercury toxicity at levels far below the level of methylmercury in the target organ. In addition, especially in chronic toxicity, the presence of vitamin E and selenium might allow for a sustained decomposition of alkylmetals by stabilizing microsomal cytochrome P_{450} systems involved in alkylmetal metabolism. There is some evidence that high doses of methylmercury inhibit the conversion of methylmercury to inorganic mercury.[63] Perhaps this involves damage to the metabolizing system by the products of the breakdown of methylmercury, which vitamin E or glutathione peroxidase would minimize. This would explain why kidney (which serves as a sink for Hg^{++} released from methylmercury)[59] accumulates Hg in a direct ratio to dietary methylmercury up to 10 ppm if 0.5 ppm Se is present in the diet, but not in the case where Se-deficient diets are fed (FIGURE 3).

While this hypothesis is based on the known biological functions of vitamin E and selenium, other mechanisms are not excluded, based on the likelihood that Se has other roles. There is some evidence that dietary selenium has effects in certain phenobarbital-induced transformations that may involve some functional form of Se other than glutathione peroxidase.[60] Phenobarbital increases the rate of ethane and ethylene production from triethyllead and delays its toxic effects.[61,62] Dietary vitamin E and selenium promote increased evolution of ethane following triethyllead injection.[62] These results are consistent with the hypothesis that organometallic compounds in general—and metals, such as silver, that undergo univalent redox reactions—may promote tissue damage through radical-induced mechanisms.

Summary

It is well established that the toxicity of silver and methylmercury is suppressed by the presence of low levels of vitamin E or selenium in the diet, but little is known of the mechanisms involved. Silver induces a conditioned deficiency of selenium in rats, as shown by its effects on tissue levels of selenium and glutathione peroxidase (a selenoprotein), but methylmercury does not. Supplements of selenium do not decrease mercury levels in tissues of animals given methylmercury, and animals given selenium plus methylmercury may accumulate high levels of mercury without signs of toxicity. Although an equimolar accumulation of selenium and mercury in tissues sometimes occurs and could lead to mutual detoxification, such a coaccumulation is not always linked to protection. The only known functions of vitamin E and selenium are related to the prevention of oxidative damage. It is possible that their protective effects against heavy metals may involve such functions, thus accounting for the protection afforded by low levels of the nutrients against high levels of the metal toxicants.

References

1. Tappel, A. L. 1972. Ann. N.Y. Acad. Sci. **203:** 12–28.
2. Lucy, J. A. 1972. Ann. N.Y. Acad. Sci. **203:** 4–11.
3. Rotruck, J. T., A. L. Pope, H. E. Ganther, A. B. Swanson, D. G. Hafeman & W. G. Hoekstra. 1973. Science **179:** 588–590.
4. Hoekstra, W. G. 1975. Fed. Proc. Fed. Am. Soc. Exp. Biol. **34:** 2083–2089.
5. Shaver, S. L. & K. E. Mason. 1951. Anat. Rec. **109:** 382.
6. Dam, H., G. K. Nielsen, I. Prange & E. Sondergaard. 1958. Nature London **182:** 802–803.
7. Diplock, A. T., J. Green, J. Bunyan, D. McHale & I. R. Muthy. 1967. Br. J. Nutr. **21:** 115–125.
8. Bunyan, J., A. T. Diplock, M. A. Cawthorne & J. Green. 1968. Br. J. Nutr. **22:** 165–182.
9. Jensen, L. S., R. P. Peterson & L. Falen. 1974. Poult. Sci. **53:** 57–64.
10. Peterson, R. P. & L. S. Jensen. 1975. Poult. Sci. **54:** 795–798.
11. Van Vleet, J. F. 1977. Am. J. Vet. Res. **38:** 1393–1398.
12. McDowell, L. R., J. A. Froseth & R. C. Piper. 1978. Nutr. Rep. Int. **17:** 19–33.
13. Van Vleet, J. F. 1976. Am. J. Vet. Res. **37:** 1415–1420.
14. Whanger, P. D. & P. H. Weswig. 1978. Nutr. Rep. Int. **18:** 421–428.
15. Jensen, L. S. 1975. Proc. Soc. Exp. Biol. Med. **149:** 113–116.
16. Peterson, R. P. & L. S. Jensen. 1975. Poult. Sci. **54:** 771–775.
17. Ganther, H. E., P. A. Wagner, M. L. Sunde & W. G. Hoekstra. 1973. *In* Trace Substances in Environmental Health. D. D. Hemphill, Ed. **6:** 247–252. University of Missouri. Columbia, Mo.

18. Ganther, H. E., C. Goudie, M. L. Sunde, M. J. Kopecky, P. Wagner, S. H. Oh & W. G. Hoekstra. 1972. Science **175:** 1122–1124.
19. Norlander, B. W. 1927. Ind. Eng. Chem. **19:** 518–521.
20. Teixeira, L. C., K. Kammermeyer & W. W. Johnson. 1970. J. Am. Dent. Assoc. **81:** 1159–1162.
21. Gusberg, S. B., P. Zamechik & J. C. Aub. 1941. J. Pharmacol. Exp. Ther. **71:** 239–245.
22. Kar, A. B. & R. P. Das. 1963. Proc. Nat. Inst. Sci. India Part B **29:** 297.
23. Mason, K. E., J. A. Brown, J. O. Young & R. R. Nesbit. 1964. Anat. Rec. **149:** 135–147.
24. Parizek, J. & L. Ostadalova. 1967. Experentia **23:** 142–143.
25. Parizek, J., I. Benes, I. Ostadalova, A. Babicky, J. Benes & J. Lener. 1969. Physiol. Bohemoslov. **18:** 95–103.
26. Ganther, H. E. & C. A. Baumann. 1962. J. Nutr. **77:** 210–216.
27. Eybl, V., J. Sykora & F. Mertl. 1969. Arch. Toxikol. **25:** 296–305.
28. Moffitt, A. E. & J. J. Clary. 1974. Res. Commun. Chem. Pathol. Pharmacol. **7:** 593–603.
29. Parizek, J., I. Ostadalova, A. Babicky, J. Benes & L. Pavlik. 1974. *In* Trace Element Metabolism in Animals. W. G. Hoekstra, J. W. Suttie, H. E. Ganther & W. Mertz, Eds. **2:** 119–131. University Park Press. Baltimore, Md.
30. Chen, R. W., P. A. Wagner, W. G. Hoekstra & H. E. Ganther. 1974. J. Reprod. Fertil. **38:** 293–306.
31. Oh, S. H., H. E. Ganther & W. G. Hoekstra. 1974. Biochemistry **13:** 1825–1829.
32. Wagner, P. A., W. G. Hoekstra & H. E. Ganther. 1975. Proc. Soc. Exp. Biol. Med. **148:** 1106–1110.
33. Wagner, P. A. 1975. Ph.D. Thesis. University of Wisconsin. Madison, Wis.
34. Stillings, B. R., H. Lagally, P. Bauersfeld & J. Soares. 1974. Toxicol. Appl. Pharmacol. **30:** 243–254.
35. Iwata, H., H. Okamoto & Y. Ohsawa. 1973. Res. Commun. Chem. Pathol. Pharmacol. **5:** 673–680.
36. Potter, S. & G. Matrone. 1974. J. Nutr. **104:** 638–647.
37. Ganther, H. E. & M. L. Sunde. 1974. J. Food Sci. **39:** 1–5.
38. El-Begearmi, M. M., M. L. Sunde & H. E. Ganther. 1977. Poult. Sci. **56:** 313–322.
39. Chang, L. W., A. W. Dudley, Jr., M. A. Dudley, H. E. Ganther & M. L. Sunde. 1977. *In* Neurotoxicology. L. Roizin, H. Shiraki & N. Grcevic, Eds.: 275–282. Raven Press. New York, N.Y.
40. Welsh, S. O. & J. H. Soares, Jr. 1976. Nutr. Rep. Int. **13:** 43–51.
41. Ganther, H. E. 1978. Environ. Health Perspect. **25:** 71–76.
42. Skerfving, S. 1978. Environ. Health Perspect. **25:** 57–65.
43. Stoewsand, G. S., C. A. Bache & D. J. Lisle. 1974. Bull. Environ. Contam. Toxicol. **11:** 152–156.
44. Hall, R. A., E. G. Zook & G. M. Meaburn. 1978. National Marine Fisheries Service Survey of Trace Elements in the Fishery Resource. NOAA Technical Report No. NMFS SSRF-721: 1–6. National Oceanic and Atmospheric Administration. Washington, D.C.
45. Usioka, T. 1960. Kumamoto Igakkai Zasshi **34:** 383–386.
46. Beijer, K. & A. Jernelov. 1978. Environ. Health Perspect. **25:** 43–45.
47. Miller, G. E., P. M. Grant, R. Kishore, F. J. Steinkruger, F. S. Rowland & V. P. Gunn. 1972. Science **175:** 1121–1122.
48. Hammond, A. L. 1971. Science **171:** 788–789.
49. Bowen, H. J. M. 1966. Trace Elements in Biochemistry: 19. Academic Press, Inc. New York, N.Y.
50. Ohi, G., S. Nishigaki, H. Seki, Y. Tamura, T. Maki, H. Konno, S. Ochia, H. Yamada, Y. Shiramura, I. Mizoguchi & H. Yagyu. 1976. Environ. Res. **12:** 49–58.
51. El-Begearmi, M., H. E. Ganther & M. Sunde. 1974. Poult. Sci. **53:** 1921.
52. El-Begearmi, M., H. E. Ganther & M. Sunde. 1975. Poult. Sci. **54:** 1756.
53. Ganther, H. E. 1979. Adv. Nutr. Res. **2:** 107–128.
54. Chang, L. W., S. Yamaguchi & A. W. Dudley, Jr. 1974. Arch. Neuropathol. **28:** 171–176.
55. Koeman, J. H., W. H. M. Peeters & C. H. M. Koudstaal-Hol. 1973. Nature **245:** 385–386.

56. Kosta, L., A. R. Byrne & V. Zelenko. 1975. Nature **254:** 238–239.
57. Gage, J. C. 1975. Toxicol. Appl. Pharmacol. **32:** 225–238.
58. Urano, S. & M. Matsuo. 1976. Lipids **11:** 380–383.
59. Clarkson, T. W. 1972. Ann. Rev. Pharmacol. **12:** 375–406.
60. Correia, M. A. & R. F. Burk. 1976. J. Biol. Chem. **253:** 6203–6210.
61. Ramstoeck, E. R., W. G. Hoekstra & H. E. Ganther. Chem. Biol. Interact. (In press.)
62. Ramstoeck, E. R., W. G. Hoekstra & H. E. Ganther. 1980.Toxicol. Appl. Pharmacol. **54:** 251–257.
63. Ostlund, K. 1969. Acta Pharmacol. Toxicol. Suppl. **27:** 57–62.
64. El-Begearmi, M. M. 1978. Ph.D. Thesis. University of Wisconsin. Madison, Wis.
65. Ganther, H. E., L. W. Chang, A. W. Dudley, Jr. & M. L. Sunde. 1975. (Unpublished data.)

Discussion

A. L. Tappel (*University of California, Davis, Calif.*): Congratulations on the nice work. I have two questions. The first one is about the inhibition of glutathione peroxidase by silver. Now, you measure enzyme activity, so presumably you cannot tell for sure if it is enzyme that is inhibited or if there is a decrease in enzyme concentration?

H. E. Ganther: Perhaps we can answer that in terms of an experiment that we did by mixing liver homogenates from animals given silver and animals that were not given silver. There was no inhibitory effect by the silver-containing homogenate on the activity of the control homogenate. This suggests that there is no direct effect of silver *in vitro.* The decrease in activity probably was caused by decreased synthesis of enzyme *in vivo* caused by interference of silver with selenium metabolism.

W. G. Hoekstra (*University of Wisconsin, Madison, Wis.*): You might add that *in vivo,* the rate of decrease in terms of liver glutathione peroxidase is just what you see if you suddenly initiate the feeding of a selenium-free diet—not an immediate inactivation.

A. L. Tappel: So then the best explanation is the one you gave, namely, that the silver complexes the selenium and effectively removes this from being available for producing glutathione peroxidase.

H. E. Ganther: The time-course data definitely support this explanation.

A. L. Tappel: I have another question. I was impressed by your use of a casein diet. I think you implied, Dr. Ganther, that this diet was very low in selenium and that it could be used for producing a selenium deficiency?

H. E. Ganther: Yes, if you use glutathione peroxidase activity as a measure of deficiency, you will definitely see a deficiency. Selenium in casein is quite low, particularly in that imported from New Zealand and Australia, which is where most of the casein is from. We are using casein that contains 0.1 or 0.2 parts per million Se, so that 20% of casein supplies about 0.02 to 0.04 ppm in the diet. That is below the requirement.

A. L. Tappel: So this would be a much better diet than the usual yeast protein diet.

H. E. Ganther: Except that it does not produce any clinical signs of deficiency, such as liver necrosis.

W. G. Hoekstra: It's a moderate selenium deficiency, and you have to be careful about the reasons for it. You've got to monitor selenium content before you start.

A. L. TAPPEL: Yes, I think that's a very important contribution, thank you.

H. E. GANTHER: I would emphasize that people who use a 20% casein diet without supplementation of selenium are not providing selenium at an adequate level.

UNIDENTIFIED SPEAKER: In your silver experiment, did you look for the interaction between the silver ion and the chloride ion?

H. E. GANTHER: All the animals were given chloride. We did not try variations in dietary chloride levels. So the experiments were done in the presence of chloride, and whatever effect silver has in binding selenium is in competition with the affinity of silver for chloride.

R. HENDERSON (*Olin Corporation, New Haven, Conn.*): In view of the vast differences in toxicity of inorganic salts of mercury, elemental mercury, and methylmercury, have you tried to identify the form of mercury in the brain of quail given increased amounts of selenium? Since you are obviously getting different toxicity, it must be changed from methylmercury as it is deposited in the brain along with selenium.

H. E. GANTHER: We have not done analysis of methylmercury, but a group at Cornell University fed Japanese quail high levels of selenium and high levels of methylmercury (20 ppm Hg). They observed about 38 ppm methylmercury in brain of quail that were kept alive by the administration of large amounts (5 ppm) of selenium [see Reference 43]. So apparently there's more than enough methylmercury in the brain to be toxic under normal conditions, and the presence of selenium somehow prevents the expression of the toxicity.

ERYTHROCYTE DEFORMABILITY AS AFFECTED BY VITAMIN E DEFICIENCY AND LEAD TOXICITY

O. A. Levander, S. O. Welsh, and V. C. Morris

Beltsville Human Nutrition Research Center
U.S. Department of Agriculture
Science and Education Administration
Beltsville, Maryland 20705

Several interactions of lead with various nutrients have now been described.[1,2,3] In some cases, nutritional deficiencies potentiate the toxic effects of lead, whereas in other cases, excess intake of nutrients appears to be of some benefit against lead poisoning.[4]

Our interest in a possible interaction of vitamin E and lead was originally stimulated by the suggestion that vitamin E deficiency might decrease the activity of δ-aminolevulinic acid dehydrase, a key regulatory enzyme in the heme biosynthetic pathway.[5] Since excessive exposure to lead is known to inhibit this enzyme, we reasoned that a long-term deficiency of vitamin E might put rats chronically poisoned with lead in "double jeopardy" by causing a pronounced blockade of heme production, thus leading to a marked anemia.[6]

Increased Anemia in Vitamin E–Deficient Lead-Poisoned Rats

In accord with our working hypothesis, a combination of vitamin E deficiency and lead toxicity caused an anemia more severe than that produced by either insult alone (TABLE 1). However, a pronounced reticulocytosis was observed in our deficient poisoned rats, thereby suggesting that the anemia was hemolytic in nature and due to an increased red cell destruction rather than to an impaired red cell production.[7] Enlargement of the spleen—an observation consistent with the concept of an increased splenic trapping of defective red blood cells—was also seen in the deficient poisoned rats. But the rat may not be a good model for the study of hemolytic congestive hypersplenism, since in this species, the spleen becomes an active center of hematopoiesis in severe anemias and the "filtering" function of the organ may be obscured by the hematopoietic response. Nonetheless, functional defects, such as increased *in vitro* mechanical fragility, were found in the erythrocytes from deficient poisoned rats.[7] This increased mechanical fragility was thought to be the result of a "tanning" of the red cell membrane by lead, thereby making it more "brittle." Additional evidence for a tanning of the red cell membrane was provided by experiments that showed that exposure to lead made erythrocytes from vitamin E–deficient rats "tougher" and more resistant to a combined osmotic and peroxidative stress.[8] If lead indeed reacted with red cell membranes to render them tougher and more brittle, one would expect such erythrocytes to be less deformable. A simple and convenient way to estimate the deformability of erythrocytes is to measure their filterability.

0077-8923/80/0355-0227 $01.75/0 © 1980, NYAS

TABLE 1

EFFECTS OF VITAMIN E DEFICIENCY ON THE TOXIC RESPONSE TO LEAD IN RATS*

Diet	Lead in Water (ppm)	Weight Gain (g)	Spleen Weight (g)	Spleen Weight (% of body wt)	Hematocrit Value (% by volume)	Mechanical Fragility Index
+ Vitamin E	0	195 ± 8^{a}	0.40 ± 0.02^{b}	0.17 ± 0.01^{b}	41.0 ± 0.6^{a}	4.7 ± 0.4^{b}
− Vitamin E	0	177 ± 7^{a}	0.43 ± 0.01^{b}	0.19 ± 0.01^{b}	41.0 ± 0.4^{a}	3.7 ± 0.3^{b}
+ Vitamin E	250	143 ± 7^{b}	0.56 ± 0.04^{b}	0.28 ± 0.01^{b}	36.8 ± 0.7^{b}	3.4 ± 0.3^{b}
− Vitamin E	250	124 ± 4^{c}	1.04 ± 0.14^{a}	0.60 ± 0.07^{a}	33.4 ± 1.0^{c}	16.0 ± 2.7^{a}

* Mean values of four to six animals ± standard error (SE); means in the same column with different superscripts differ significantly at the $P < 0.05$ level (Duncan's multiple range test). For details of methods, see Reference 7. (Reprinted with permission of the American Institute of Nutrition.)

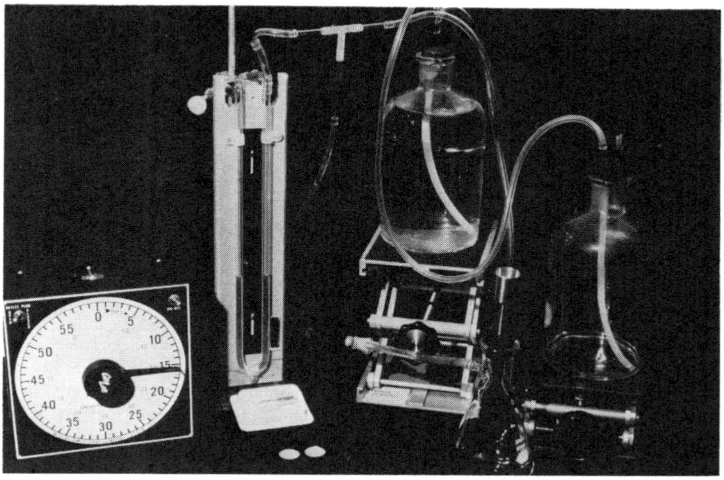

FIGURE 1. Photograph of red blood cell filtration apparatus.

Decreased Filterability of Erythrocytes from Vitamin E-Deficient Lead-Poisoned Rats

The *in vivo* survival of erythrocytes depends upon several factors, including their ability to undergo mechanical deformation in the microcirculation in order to navigate capillaries as narrow as 3 μ in cross section (i.e., less than half the diameter of the typical rat red blood cell).[9] This mechanical deformability can be easily estimated by measuring the ability of rat erythrocytes to pass through polycarbonate membrane filters with 3-μ pores.[10,11] The experimental apparatus that we use to determine erythrocyte filterability is shown in FIGURE 1 and is very similar to that used by others.[10] A schematic drawing of the filtration setup is given in FIGURE 2.

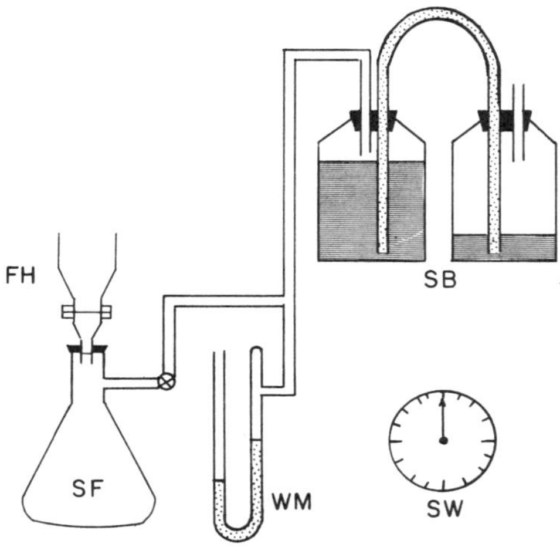

FIGURE 2. Schematic drawing of red blood cell filtration apparatus. **FH** is filter holder; **SF**, suction flask; **WM**, water manometer; **SB**, siphon bottles; and **SW**, stop watch.

TABLE 2

EFFECT OF VITAMIN E DEFICIENCY ON FILTERABILITY OF ERYTHROCYTES FROM LEAD-POISONED AND NONPOISONED RATS*

Diet	Lead in Water (ppm)	Filtration Time after Incubation for 0 Hours (sec)	2 Hours (sec)	4 Hours (sec)	6 Hours (sec)
Basal + vitamin E†	0	12 ± 1[a]	14 ± 0[a]	20 ± 2[a]	40 ± 6[a]
Basal + vitamin E	250	13 ± 1[a]	15 ± 1[a]	20 ± 2[a]	32 ± 10[a]
Basal	0	12 ± 0[a]	15 ± 1[a]	22 ± 1[a]	229 ± 96[b]
Basal	250	17 ± 1[b]	56 ± 11[b]	144 ± 53[b]	453 ± 89[c]

* Mean values of four rats ± SE; means in the same column with different superscript letters differ significantly at the $P < 0.05$ level (Duncan's multiple range test). For details of methods, see Reference 13. (Reprinted with permission of the American Institute of Nutrition.)

† Added at 100 ppm as *dl-α*-tocopheryl acetate.

On the surface, the technique appears quite simple, and in fact, the filtration measurement itself does not even require electricity. However, certain precautions must be taken for the successful application of this method.[12] In particular, the use of filter membranes with low pore density markedly enhances the quality of the data generated. Our experience indicates the desirability of determining under actual laboratory conditions the filtration characteristics of several lots of membranes with low pore density obtained directly from the manufacturer and then purchasing only those lots found to be suitable for hematorheological purposes.

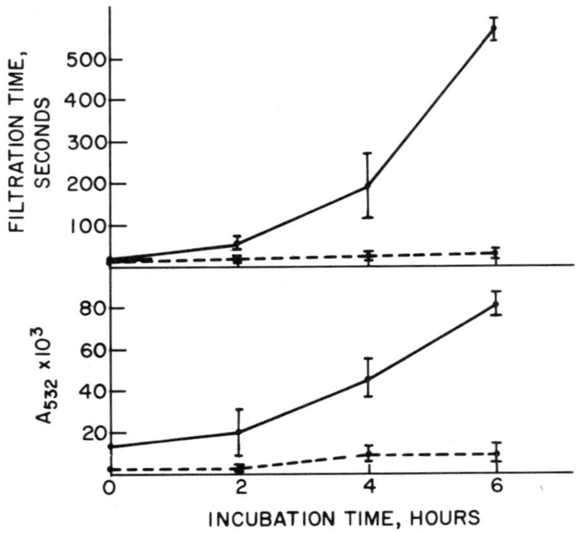

FIGURE 3. Relationship between red blood cell filtration time (upper half) vs. lipoperoxidation as indicated by the thiobarbituric acid reaction (lower half). Solid lines are data from vitamin E-deficient lead-poisoned rats, whereas dashed lines are data from vitamin E-supplemented nonpoisoned rats. (See Reference 13 for details. Reprinted with permission of the American Institute of Nutrition.)

TABLE 3

EFFECT OF CELL AGE ON THE FILTERABILITY OF ERYTHROCYTES FROM VITAMIN E-DEFICIENT RATS POISONED WITH 1,000 ppm LEAD*

Diet	Lead in Water† (ppm)	Red Blood Cell Age	Filtration Time after Incubation for 0 Hours (sec)	3 Hours (sec)	4 Hours (sec)	5 Hours (sec)
Basal + vitamin E‡	0	young	15 ± 1^{a}	21 ± 3^{a}	29 ± 6^{a}	51 ± 6^{a}
		old	16 ± 1^{a}	26 ± 3^{a}	33 ± 5^{a}	54 ± 14^{a}
		unfractionated	16 ± 1^{a}	21 ± 1^{a}	30 ± 2^{a}	45 ± 8^{a}
Basal + vitamin E	1,000	young	17 ± 1^{a}	21 ± 2^{a}	33 ± 8^{a}	50 ± 9^{a}
		old	17 ± 1^{a}	20 ± 1^{a}	34 ± 9^{a}	50 ± 12^{a}
		unfractionated	16 ± 1^{a}	19 ± 1^{a}	22 ± 2^{a}	30 ± 3^{a}
Basal	0	young	15 ± 1^{a}	23 ± 4^{a}	24 ± 2^{a}	34 ± 3^{a}
		old	17 ± 2^{a}	21 ± 2^{a}	91 ± 15^{b}	$>600^{c}$
		unfractionated	17 ± 1^{a}	17 ± 2^{a}	28 ± 5^{a}	369 ± 151^{b}
Basal	1,000	young	16 ± 1^{a}	39 ± 3^{b}	56 ± 10^{ab}	150 ± 24^{a}
		old	29 ± 9^{b}	52 ± 10^{c}	289 ± 50^{d}	$>600^{c}$
		unfractionated	30 ± 6^{b}	43 ± 3^{bc}	145 ± 4^{c}	$>600^{c}$

* Mean values of three pooled blood samples each from two or three rats ± SE; means in the same column not sharing a common superscript letter differ significantly at $P < 0.05$ (Duncan's multiple range test). For details of methods, see Reference 15. (Reprinted with permission of the American Institute of Nutrition.)

† Added as lead acetate.

‡ Added at 100 ppm as *dl*-α-tocopheryl acetate.

We demonstrated that red blood cells from vitamin E–deficient rats lost their filterability after incubation *in vitro* and that this loss was exacerbated by concurrent lead poisoning of the animals (TABLE 2). The decreased filterability of erythrocytes from deficient poisoned rats was correlated with the extent of lipid peroxidation (FIGURE 3) and was prevented by feeding the synthetic organic antioxidant *N, N'*-diphenyl-*p*-phenylenediamine.[13] Incubation with various prooxidants, such as hydrogen peroxide or dialuric acid, markedly decreased the filterability of erythrocytes from vitamin E–deficient rats, and lead poisoning intensified this effect.[14] Fractionation of erythrocytes from deficient rats according to cell age by differential centrifugation revealed that the filterability of incubated old red cells declined much more than that of the young cells, and lead poisoning of the animals exaggerated this age-dependent difference (TABLE 3). It is well documented that as red blood cells age, they gradually lose their normal discocytic shape and become more spherocytic.[16]

Increased Sphericity of Erythrocytes from Vitamin E–Deficient Lead-Poisoned Rats

The deformability, and hence filterability, of red blood cells is determined by three main factors: the viscosity of the cellular contents, the rigidity of the cell membrane, and the shape of the cell itself.[17] The young mature healthy red blood cell is a biconcave disc that has an excess area of membrane surface for the given intracellular volume enclosed. This high surface-to-volume ratio imparts a high degree of mechanical deformability to the cell, thereby allowing it to stretch, bend, and flex as necessary while it courses through the circulatory system. If a red cell loses membrane, it gradually loses its discocytic shape and becomes more spherocytic. In the limiting case, the discocyte loses so much membrane that it becomes a spherocyte. A sphere, of course, is geometrically the most efficient way to enclose a given volume, but in a red cell, this very efficiency renders the spherocyte a hard and rigid body, unable to deform and pass through orifices narrower than its own diameter. Examination of the erythrocytes from our control and deficient poisoned groups by scanning electron microscopy revealed that red cells from both groups exhibited the normal discocytic shape before incubation when both groups were filterable (FIGURE 4). However, after six hours of incubation, the control cells were still highly filterable

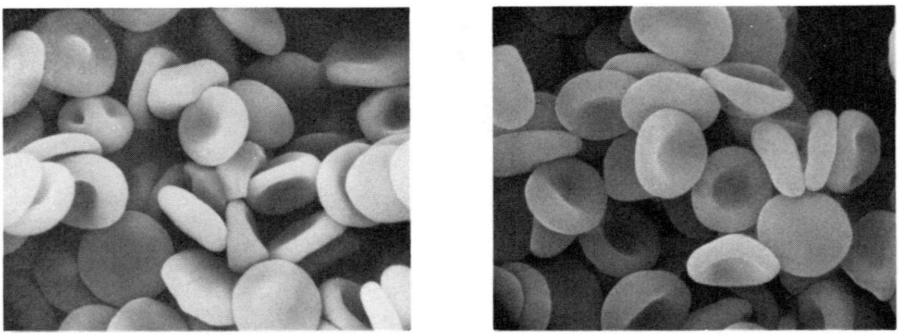

FIGURE 4. Scanning electron micrographs of unincubated red blood cells from vitamin E–supplemented nonpoisoned rats (left) and vitamin E–deficient lead-poisoned rats (right). Cells suspended in tris-buffered saline containing 0.25% bovine serum albumin. (Reprinted from Reference 18, with permission of the American Institute of Nutrition.)

and retained their discocytic morphology, whereas the nonfilterable cells from deficient poisoned rats were undergoing endocytosis, which would ultimately result in spherocytosis (FIGURE 5). We think that this morphological change in the erythrocytes from vitamin E-deficient lead-poisoned rats accounts for their decreased filterability *in vitro*. Presumably, this decreased filterability *in vitro* reflects the decreased survivability of such red cells *in vivo,* which in turn is responsible for the increased hemolytic anemia observed in the deficient poisoned rats.

The Mechanism of the Increased Sphericity of Erythrocytes from Vitamin E-Deficient Lead-Poisoned Rats

Our early experiments showed that lead exposure increased the fragility of erythrocytes from vitamin E-deficient rats when subjected to *in vitro* mechanical trauma but decreased their fragility when subjected to concomitant peroxidative and osmotic stress.[7,8] These seemingly contradictory results were accommodated by the hypothesis that the lead was tanning the red cell membrane, thereby making it brittle but also tougher. Others had shown that various bivalent heavy metal cations could be used to strengthen fragile plasma membranes to aid in their isolation.[19] This concept of membrane tanning, in fact, was the original rationale for investigating erythrocyte filterability, since it was assumed that tanning by lead would result in decreased red cell deformability. However, this original idea had to be abandoned when it was found that lead poisoning per se generally had no effect on the filterability of either unincubated or incubated red cells, whereas vitamin E deficiency alone caused a profound decrease in the filterability of incubated red cells, although lead poisoning always exacerbated this effect. Since vitamin E deficiency itself also caused the spherocytic shape change in the incubated red cells, it became clear that the deficiency was the main factor influencing filterability, with lead poisoning having a secondary, albeit still important, role.[18]

At this point, our working hypothesis was revised to reflect the primary role of lipid peroxidation in determining red cell filterability and shape. Several experimental observations tended to reinforce this shift in thinking. For example, there was a good correlation between the loss of filterability during incubation and the extent of lipid peroxidation;[13] incubation with various prooxidants *in vitro* accelerated the loss of filterability, whereas feeding a synthetic antioxidant protected against it;[14,13] and erythrocytes of old cell age, which were largely responsible for the decreases in

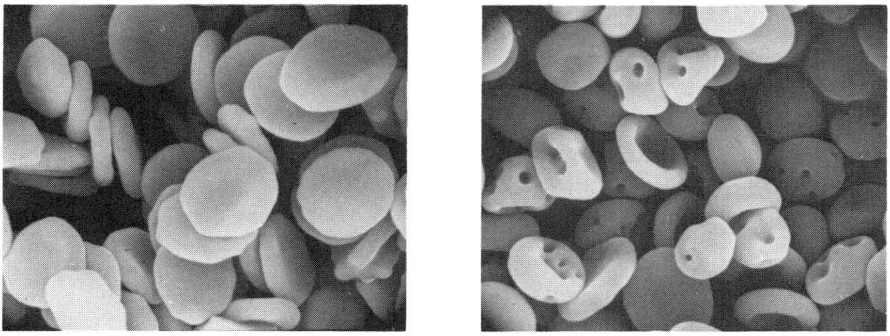

FIGURE 5. Red blood cells as in FIGURE 4 after six hours of incubation. (Reprinted from Reference 18, with permission of the American Institute of Nutrition.)

filterability of mixed red cell populations, also were the most sensitive to the effects of hydrogen peroxide added *in vitro*.[15]

Since the inner half of the lipid bilayer of the erythrocyte membrane contains more polyunsaturated fatty acids than does the outer half, we speculated that more extensive peroxidation occurring in the inner leaflet might expand this half of the bilayer, thereby causing a change to the stomatocytic shape.[18] If this process continued far enough, the end result would be formation of stomatospherocytes or spherocytes. Others had shown that stomatocytes could be produced by selective membrane expansion due to incubation of the red cells with certain cationic drugs that intercalated preferentially in the inner half of the membrane.[20] As an alternate hypothesis for spherocyte formation, we suggested that lipid peroxidation might lead to a generalized membrane loss, possibly as a result of endocytosis and internalization of membrane components.[18]

If increased lipid peroxidation were indeed the explanation for the spherocytosis in red cells from vitamin E-deficient rats, lead poisoning could conceivably stimulate

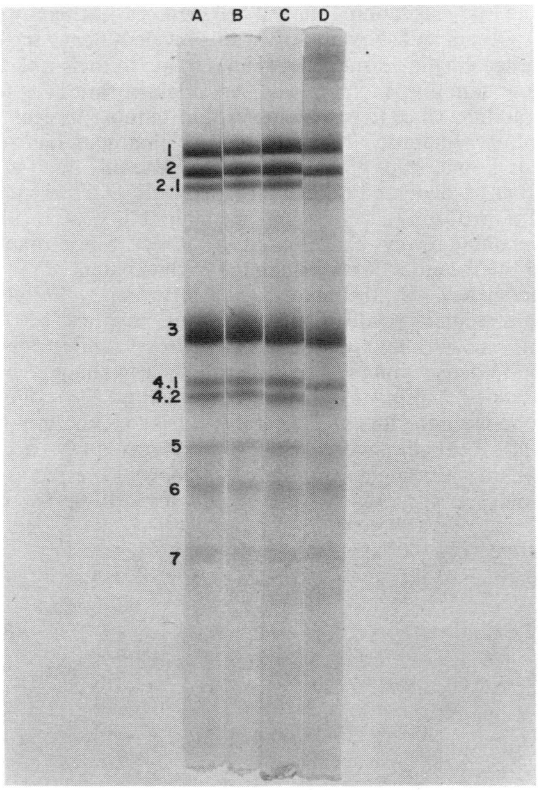

FIGURE 6. Effect of vitamin E deficiency on red blood cell (RBC) membrane proteins separated by SDS electrophoresis. **A**: unincubated RBC from vitamin E-supplemented rats (+E RBC). **B**: same as A but incubated four hours. **C**: unincubated RBC from vitamin E-deficient rats (−E RBC). **D**: same as C but incubated four hours. Only the RBC from sample D were nonfilterable. (For experimental details, see Reference 25).

this process by either of two different mechanisms. First of all, lead could react with certain membrane components, such as the phosphate groups of phospholipids, to disrupt the structure of the lipid bilayer, thereby rendering the polyunsaturated moieties more susceptible to peroxidative attack.[21] On the other hand, lead is known to be a weak, though still effective, catalyst of lipid peroxidation, so its presence in the membrane could promote structural disintegration in that way also.[22]

Although direct peroxidative damage to lipid membrane components still appears to be an attractive explanation for the decreased filterability of red cells from vitamin E-deficient lead-poisoned rats, many researchers working on erythrocyte membrane structure now think that the shape of the red cell probably depends more directly on the state of the membrane proteins, particularly spectrin.[23,24] We found an association between the decreased filterability of incubated red blood cells from vitamin E-deficient rats and an increased cross-linking of erythrocyte membrane proteins as shown by sodium dodecyl sulfate (SDS) electrophoresis, and concurrent lead toxicity exaggerated both of these changes (FIGURES 6 and 7). This appearance

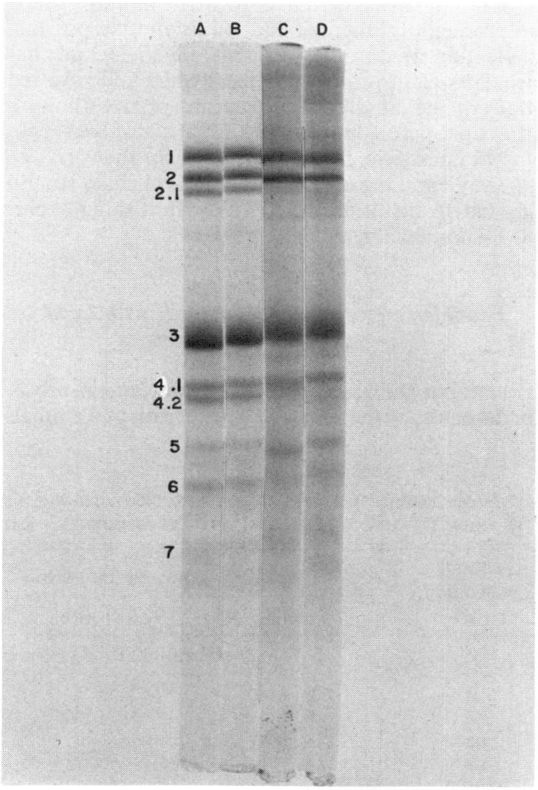

FIGURE 7. Effect of vitamin E deficiency and lead toxicity on RBC membrane proteins separated by SDS electrophoresis. **A**: unincubated +E RBC from lead-poisoned rats. **B**: same as A after four hours incubation. **C**: unincubated −E RBC from lead-poisoned rats. **D**: same as C after four hours incubation. RBC from sample C had impaired filterability, and RBC from sample D were nonfilterable. (For experimental details, see Reference 25.)

of polymerized proteins of molecular weight greater than that of spectrin was accompanied by an increased generalized staining throughout the gel, possibly due to proteolysis, and by a decrease in the staining associated with bands 2.1 and 4.2. The mechanism of this increased aggregation of red cell membrane proteins is not known but apparently does not involve transglutaminase, since neither calcium nor ionophore was present in our incubation medium.[26] Oxidation of protein sulfhydryls to produce disulfide cross-links appears to be a reasonable explanation, since others have shown that sulfhydryl oxidizing agents induced intermolecular disulfide bonds in spectrin and decreased the deformability of human red cells.[27] Red cell deformability was also decreased in patients with glucose-6-phosphate dehydrogenase deficiency and associated chronic hemolytic disease whose cells contained high molecular weight polypeptide aggregates linked by intermolecular disulfide bonds.[28] However, there was a good association between the extent of red cell membrane protein aggregation and the red cell glutathione concentration in these patients, whereas we found no association between glutathione levels and the decreased filterability of red cells from vitamin E–deficient rats treated with *N*-ethylmaleimide (TABLE 4). Formation of Schiff bases by the reaction of protein amino groups with malonyldialdehyde, an end product of lipid peroxidation, is another possible mechanism for the protein polymerization we observe, since malonyldialdehyde has been shown to increase high molecular weight protein polymers when added to red cells *in vitro*.[29] Needless to say, both of the latter two mechanisms of cross-linking are compatible with the concept that lipid peroxidation is the initial causative event of shape change in red cells from vitamin E–deficient rats, which then gives rise to protein polymerization either by "spilling over" of free radical chain reactions into the protein domain (oxidation to disulfide links) or by furnishing a chemically reactive cross-linking agent (malonyldialdehyde).

Possible Interaction of Vitamin E with Lead Intoxication in Humans

Although the research discussed above provides ample proof for the role of vitamin E status in determining the response of experimental animals to lead poison-

TABLE 4

EFFECT OF *N*-ETHYLMALEIMIDE ON FILTERABILITY AND GLUTATHIONE (GSH) LEVELS OF RBC FROM VITAMIN E–DEFICIENT AND -SUPPLEMENTED RATS*

Diet	*N*-Ethylmaleimide (M)	Incubation Period: 0 Hours	3 Hours	5 Hours
		Filtration Time (seconds)		
Control	0	15 ± 1	21 ± 2	22 ± 2
Deficient	0	16 ± 1	68 ± 32	>600
Control	10^{-4}	13 ± 2	16 ± 1	—
Deficient	10^{-4}	14 ± 1	>600	—
		GSH (mg/100 ml RBC)		
Control	0	109 ± 3	—	104 ± 5
Deficient	0	100 ± 2	—	94 ± 4
Control	10^{-4}	14 ± 3	12 ± 5	—
Deficient	10^{-4}	13 ± 3	16 ± 1	—

* Mean values of three rats ± SE; for details of methods, see Reference 25.

ing, there is not much evidence to suggest a similar relationship between vitamin E intake and human lead intoxication. However, an elevated incidence of Heinz bodies, indicative of oxidative stress, was reported in children living near a lead smelter.[30] Patients with sickle-cell anemia have depressed plasma and red blood cell vitamin E levels, and yet children with this disease have elevated levels of lead in their hair.[31-33] Moreover, sickle-cell children appear to be more susceptible to lead-induced neuropathy than are normal children.[34] Vitamin E has been shown to protect rats against the neurotoxicity caused by methylmercury;[35] and it would seem appropriate to investigate its possible value against lead-induced encephalopathy. Persons lacking glucose-6-phosphate dehydrogenase are clearly at risk with regard to oxidative stress, and although there are contradictory reports, administration of vitamin E is thought to have some beneficial effect against the anemia that afflicts certain individuals with this condition.[36,37] Also, black school children deficient in this enzyme have higher blood lead levels than do children not deficient in the enzyme.[38] These reports taken individually provide only weak support for the hypothesis that vitamin E may play a role in human lead poisoning, but taken in combination, they provide a suitable rationale for evaluating vitamin E status in individuals exposed to lead.

REFERENCES

1. LEVANDER, O. A. 1979. Lead toxicity and nutritional deficiencies. Environ. Health Perspect. **29:** 115–125.
2. MOORE, M. R. 1979. Diet and lead toxicity. Proc. Nutr. Soc. **38:** 243–250.
3. MAHAFFEY, K. R. 1974. Nutritional factors and susceptibility to lead toxicity. Environ. Health Perspect. **7:** 107–112.
4. LEVANDER, O. A. 1977. Nutritional factors in relation to heavy metal toxicants. Fed. Proc. Fed. Am. Soc. Exp. Biol. **36:** 1683–1687.
5. CASSI, P. I., J. W. HAUSWIRTH & P. P. NAIR. 1972. Biosynthesis of heme in vitamin E deficiency. Ann. N.Y. Acad. Sci. **203:** 93–102.
6. GRIGGS, R. C. 1964. Lead poisoning: hematologic aspects. Prog. Hematol. **4:** 117–137.
7. LEVANDER, O. A., V. C. MORRIS, D. J. HIGGS & R. J. FERRETTI. 1975. Lead poisoning in vitamin E-deficient rats. J. Nutr. **105:** 1481–1485.
8. LEVANDER, O. A., R. J. FERRETTI & V. C. MORRIS. 1977. Osmotic and peroxidative fragilities of erythrocytes from vitamin E-deficient lead-poisoned rats. J. Nutr. **107:** 373–377.
9. WEED, R. I. 1975. Hereditary spherocytosis—a review. Arch. Intern. Med. **135:** 1316–1323.
10. GREGERSEN, M. I., C. A. BRYANT, W. E. HAMMERLE, S. USAMI & S. CHIEN. 1967. Flow characteristics of human erythrocytes through polycarbonate sieves. Science **157:** 825–827.
11. CHIEN, S. 1977. Principles and techniques for assessing erythrocyte deformability. Blood Cells **3:** 71–99.
12. MORRIS, V. C. 1979. Factors influencing filterability measurements of red blood cells (RBC) from vitamin E-deficient rats. Fed. Proc. Fed. Am. Soc. Exp. Biol. **38:** 875.
13. LEVANDER, O. A., V. C. MORRIS & R. J. FERRETTI. 1977. Filterability of erythrocytes from vitamin E-deficient lead-poisoned rats. J. Nutr. **107:** 363–372.
14. LEVANDER, O. A., V. C. MORRIS & R. J. FERRETTI. 1977. Effect of oxidants, hydrazines, and aminoquinolines on the filterability of erythrocytes from vitamin E-deficient lead-poisoned rats. J. Nutr. **107:** 2135–2143.
15. LEVANDER, O. A., V. C. MORRIS & R. J. FERRETTI. 1978. Effect of cell age on the filterability of erythrocytes from vitamin E-deficient lead-poisoned rats. J. Nutr. **108:** 145–151.
16. LESSIN, L. S., P. P. KLUG & W. N. JENSEN. 1976. Clinical implications of red cell shape. Adv. Intern. Med. **21:** 451–500.

17. LACELLE, P. L. 1970. Alteration of membrane deformability in hemolytic anemias. Semin. Hematol. **7:** 355–371.
18. LEVANDER, O. A., M. FISHER, V. C. MORRIS & R. J. FERRETTI. 1977. Morphology of erythrocytes from vitamin E-deficient lead-poisoned rats. J. Nutr. **107:** 1828–1836.
19. WARREN, L. 1974. Isolation of plasma membranes from tissue culture-L cells. *In* Methods in Enzymology. Biomembranes. S. Fleischer & L. Packer, Eds. **31**(Part A): 156–162. Academic Press, Inc. New York, N.Y.
20. DEUTICKE, B. 1968. Transformation and restoration of biconcave shape of human erythrocytes induced by amphiphilic agents and changes of ionic environment. Biochim. Biophys. Acta **163:** 494–500.
21. PASSOW, H. 1971. The red blood cell: penetration, distribution and toxic actions of heavy metals. *In* Effects of Metals on Cells, Subcellular Elements, and Macromolecules. J. Maniloff, J. R. Coleman & M. W. Miller, Eds.: 291–340. Charles C. Thomas. Springfield, Ill.
22. POKORNY, J., H. ZWAIN & G. JANICEK. 1964. Influence of traces of metals on the activity of phenolic antioxidants. Fette Seifen Anstrichm. **66:** 1059–1062.
23. RALSTON, G. B. 1978. The structure of spectrin and the shape of the red blood cell. Trends Biochem. Sci. **3:** 195–198.
24. PALEK, J., P. A. LIU & S. C. LIU. 1978. Polymerisation of red cell membrane protein contributes to spheroechinocyte shape irreversibility. Nature **274:** 505–507.
25. LEVANDER, O. A. & S. O. WELSH. Cross linking of membrane proteins in red blood cells from vitamin E-deficient lead-poisoned rats. Life Sci. (In press.)
26. LORAND, L., L. B. WEISSMANN, D. L. EPEL & J. BRUNER-LORAND. 1976. Role of the intrinsic transglutaminase in the Ca^{2+}-mediated crosslinking of erythrocyte proteins. Proc. Nat. Acad. Sci. **73:** 4479–4481.
27. FISCHER, T. M., C. W. M. HAEST, M. STOHR, D. KAMP & B. DEUTICKE. 1978. Selective alteration of erythrocyte deformability by SH-reagents. Evidence for an involvement of spectrin in membrane shear elasticity. Biochim. Biophys. Acta **510:** 270–282.
28. JOHNSON, G. J., D. W. ALLEN, S. CADMAN, V. F. FAIRBANKS, J. G. WHITE, B. C. LAMPKIN & M. E. KAPLAN. 1979. Red cell membrane polypeptide aggregates in glucose-6-phosphate dehydrogenase mutants with chronic hemolytic disease—a clue to the mechanism of hemolysis. New Engl. J. Med. **301:** 522–527.
29. JAIN, S. K. & P. HOCHSTEIN. 1980. Polymerization of membrane components in aging red blood cells. Biochem. Biophys. Res. Commun. **92:** 247–254.
30. GHELBERG, N. W., E. BRETTER, L. COSTIN & E. CHITUL. 1966. Investigations on the appearance of Heinz's bodies under the influence of small lead concentrations in the atmosphere. Igiena **15:** 209–219.
31. NATTA, C. & L. MACHLIN. 1979. Plasma levels of tocopherol in sickle cell anemia subjects. Am. J. Clin. Nutr. **32:** 1359–1362.
32. CHIU, D. & B. LUBIN. 1979. Abnormal vitamin E and glutathione peroxidase levels in sickle cell anemia. J. Lab. Clin. Med. **94:** 542–548.
33. OLATUNBOSUN, D., S. MORRIS, F. LICHTE, S. R. KOIRTYOHANN & J. R. VOGT. 1976. Trace element content of hair from Nigerians with sickle cell anemia. *In* Trace Substances in Environmental Health. D. D. Hemphill, Ed. **10:** 383–388. University of Missouri Press. Columbia, Mo.
34. ERENBERG, G., S. S. RINSLER & B. G. FISH. 1974. Lead neuropathy and sickle cell disease. Pediatrics **54:** 438–441.
35. WELSH, S. O. 1979. The protective effect of vitamin E and *N,N'*-diphenyl-*p*-phenylenediamine (DPPD) against methyl mercury toxicity in the rat. J. Nutr. **109:** 1673–1681.
36. NEWMAN, J. G., T. B. NEWMAN, L. J. BOWIE & J. MENDELSOHN. 1979. An examination of the role of vitamin E in glucose-6-phosphate dehydrogenase deficiency. Clin. Biochem. **12:** 149–151.
37. SPIELBERG, S. P., L. A. BOXER, L. M. CORASH & J. G. SHULMAN, 1979. Improved erythrocyte survival with high doses of vitamin E in chronic hemolyzing G6PD and glutathione synthetase deficiencies. Ann. Intern. Med. **90:** 53–54.
38. MCINTIRE, M. S. & C. R. ANGLE. 1972. Air lead: relation to lead in blood of black school children deficient in glucose-6-phosphate dehydrogenase. Science **177:** 520–522.

Discussion

A. L. Tappel (*University of California, Davis, Calif.*): I'd like to ask your viewpoint on the lead catalysis of lipid peroxidation by, for example, decomposition of peroxide. Lead salts were used as accelerators in the early paints based upon lipid peroxidation.

O. A. Levander: Right, that's very true. Of course, lead isn't nearly as potent a catalyst as copper or iron. But we do see these changes in filterability in cases of iron overload or copper excess in animals. Lead is a rather weak catalyst for peroxidation reactions. Instead, lead might be reacting with phosphate groups in the phospholipids and thus disrupting the membrane. As you indicated, structural integrity is a very good antioxidant, and if you could disrupt membrane structure, that might lead to increased lipid peroxidation.

H. H. Sandstead (*Human Nutrition Research Center, U.S. Department of Agriculture, Grand Forks, N. Dak.*): Adult patients with chronic lead poisoning show target cells, spherocytes, and shortened red cell survival. Has anybody ever tried to relate that to vitamin E?

O. A. Levander: The problem is that recently everybody has thought of lead anemia only in terms of the inhibition of heme production. In fact, 40 years ago, workers were thinking mainly in terms of membrane effects, and I think it is time to start thinking about membrane effects again now.

P. Hochstein (*University of Southern California School of Medicine, Los Angeles, Calif.*): You indicated that the cause of spherocytosis is internalization of the membranes. You showed the picture of the dimples in the red cells. What is the evidence of membranes actually being internalized?

O. A. Levander: We haven't done transmission electron microscopy to confirm that. Our evidence is by extrapolation from what other people have shown in some studies with drugs that intercalate in the inner half of the lipid bilayer of the membrane.

P. Hochstein: I would just like to comment that invagination of the membrane is not always followed by internalization and the formation of internal vacuoles. It is not a necessary consequence.

LIPID PEROXIDATION AND THE CYTOTOXICITY OF COPPER*

Paul Hochstein, K. Sree Kumar,† and Stephen J. Forman‡

Department of Pharmacology
University of Southern California School of Medicine
Los Angeles, California 90033

Copper is an essential trace element whose presence in biological systems was first reported over 150 years ago.[1] Early suggestions that the metal might be involved as a catalyst in living cells have been amply confirmed.[2] It is now well established that copper participates in the activity of over a dozen enzyme systems. For example, cytochrome oxidase, superoxide dismutase, and dopamine-β-hydroxylase, to name just a few, all contain copper as an essential constituent.[3-5] Its associations with these enzymes presumably underlie the failure of specific metabolic processes in deficiency states. In humans, a variety of clinical signs accompany inadequacies in either dietary intake of copper or absorption mechanisms.[6,7] Thus, low serum copper levels have been related to disturbances in iron absorption, failures in erythropoiesis, mental deterioration, and death.

Although copper has important therapeutic uses, as is the case with all heavy metals, excessive amounts are highly toxic.[8] Copper toxicosis has been reported after the ingestion of copper salts, after the application of copper compounds to large areas of burned skin, and after the introduction of copper into the circulation during hemodialysis.[9-11]

These instances of copper toxicity presumably result from the presence of copper in amounts in excess of the capacity of specific intracellular and extracellular proteins to adequately sequester the metal. Among the proteins with such a function is ceruloplasmin.[12] It is of special interest that individuals with Wilson's disease exhibit a genetic and lifelong deficiency of this copper-binding plasma protein. In the face of normal ingestion of copper, the livers of these persons may contain up to 50 times the usual amounts of the metal. Ultimately, hepatic copper diffuses into the circulation and may enter tissue compartments with toxic effects on susceptible cells. In these instances, the toxic effects are usually manifested in the liver, the kidney, and the central nervous system. However, in other instances, massive hepatic necrosis may also take place, releasing large amounts of copper to the plasma on an episodic basis and inducing severe hemolysis.[13]

TABLE 1 shows the serum copper, urinary copper, and ceruloplasmin levels in patients with Wilson's disease who have had no hemolysis and from those who have had marked hemolysis. The normal range of values for these parameters is included for comparison. It should be noted that the group of persons with a deficiency of ceruloplasmin and who showed no hemolysis exhibit, as would be expected, lower than normal levels of serum copper. On the other hand, those persons who exhibit hemolysis showed, even with diminished amounts of ceruloplasmin, *elevated* serum copper levels as well as excretion rates in huge excess of the normal range. It is this

* Supported in part by Grant No. AG-00471 from the National Institutes of Health.

† Present affiliation: Department of Chemistry, University of Calicut, Calicut, India.

‡ Present affiliation: Department of Hematology and Bone Marrow Transplantation, City of Hope National Medical Center, Duarte, California 91010.

0077-8923/80/0355-0240 $01.75/0 © 1980, NYAS

TABLE 1

SERUM COPPER, URINARY COPPER, AND CERULOPLASMIN LEVELS IN PATIENTS WITH WILSON'S DISEASE WITH AND WITHOUT HEMOLYSIS

	Normals*	No Hemolysis*	Hemolysis†
Serum Copper (μg/100 ml)	81–147	47	182
Urinary Copper (μg/24 hrs)	11–31	344	3300
Ceruloplasmin (mg/100 ml)	29–36	7	7

* From Strickland and Leu, Reference 36.

† From Reference 36 and including two patients seen at the Los Angeles–University of Southern California Medical Center.

latter group who are seen in medical clinics with extensive red cell damage and jaundice.

Many investigators have attempted to clarify the mechanisms of hemolysis in hypercupremic states, such as those illustrated in TABLE 1. There is general consensus that copper may act to inhibit several key enzymes and metabolic processes.[14–16] The inhibition of glycolytic enzymes, for example, would be expected to result in a depletion of cellular adenosine triphosphate (ATP), a loss of osmotic integrity, and an alteration in surface-to-volume relationships that might produce aberrant rheological behavioral and hemolysis.

We have confirmed the inhibitory effects of copper on glycolytic enzymes, such as hexokinase. In the experiment illustrated in TABLE 2, for example, the incubation of intact erythrocytes with copper sulfate (100 μM) resulted in about 90% inactivation of this enzyme. The enzyme was assayed at the end of the incubation and after the cells had been washed free of medium and hemolysates prepared. In general, the degree of inhibition observed in these experiments was proportional to the concentration of copper (between 5.0 and 100 μM) present during the incubation period. However, it should be noted, in TABLE 2, that if the cells were incubated in the absence of oxygen or if the hemoglobin was first oxidized (with nitrite) to

TABLE 2

THE EFFECTS OF COPPER SULFATE ON THE HEXOKINASE ACTIVITY OF HUMAN ERYTHROCYTES*

	Hexokinase (nmoles NADPH/min/mg Hb)†		
Additions	Aerobic ($HbFe^{+2}$–O_2)	Anaerobic ($HbFe^{+2}$)	Aerobic ($HbFe^{+3}$)
None	0.53 ± 0.02	0.49 ± 0.03	0.41 ± 0.03
$CuSO_4$ (100 μM)	0.04 ± 0.01	0.42 ± 0.02	0.33 ± 0.02
$CuSO_4$ (100 μM) + Glucose (20 mM)	0.39 ± 0.02	0.41 ± 0.03	0.35 ± 0.02
Glucose (20 mM)	0.54 ± 0.03	0.51 ± 0.04	0.44 ± 0.02

* Erythrocytes (5% hematocrit) were incubated for 60 minutes at 37 °C in isotonic NaCl buffered with 20 mM phosphate, pH 7.6. At the conclusion of the incubation, the cells were washed twice with isotonic saline solutions, and hexokinase assay was carried out in aliquots of lysed cells. Cells incubated aerobically were held in an atmosphere of air, while those incubated anaerobically were held, after flushing the incubation flasks, under an atmosphere of argon. $HbFe^{+3}$-containing cells were obtained by treating the erythrocytes with 1% sodium nitrite for 5 minutes and then washing them free of excess nitrite before resuspending them in the incubation medium.

† NADPH is reduced nicotinamide-adenine dinucleotide phosphate.

TABLE 3

COPPER-INDUCED INHIBITION OF YEAST HEXOKINASE

Additions	Hexokinase* (nmoles NADPH/min)
None	0.93 ± 0.04
$CuSO_4$ (20 μM)	0.82 ± 0.03
$CuSO_4$ (20 μM) + Hb (1.0 mg/ml)	0.12 ± 0.02
Hb (1.0 mg/ml)	0.90 ± 0.04

* Cuvettes contained tris-HCl, 50 mM, pH 8.0; $MgCl_2$, 5.0 mM; glucose, 5.0 mM; ATP, 2.0 mM; NADP, 0.2 mM; G-6-PD, 0.5 U.

methemoglobin, the inhibition observed after incubation with copper is markedly diminished. Metz and Sagone have noted that H_2O_2 is formed in erythrocytes exposed to copper;[17] and the effects described above are consistent with the view that copper may enhance the autoxidation of hemoglobin and cause the formation of O_2^-.[18,19] Superoxide would in turn undergo dismutation to form H_2O_2. Although direct effects of copper on hexokinase may be observed at high concentrations (above 100 μM), it seems likely that the inhibitory effects seen at lower concentrations of the metal are a consequence of its interaction with hemoglobin to form oxidant species, such as H_2O_2.

This concept is confirmed by the data illustrated in TABLE 3. It may be seen there that copper at a concentration of 20 μM has only a small direct effect on crystalline yeast hexokinase. However, if hemoglobin is included in the reaction mixture, then a very dramatic inhibition is recorded. One can observe the formation of methemoglobin after the addition of copper to the reaction cuvettes.

It may also be seen in TABLE 2 that when glucose is present in the incubation medium, the oxygen and ferrous hemoglobin-dependent inhibition of hexokinase is not observed. The protection afforded to hexokinase, by glucose, in such experiments may be attributed to the activity of the glutathione peroxidase pathway for peroxide detoxification.[20] Thus, in the presence of glucose, cellular levels of reduced glutathione are maintained (TABLE 4). While glucose metabolism permits the cells to maintain glutathione levels and prevents inhibition of hexokinase, it does not prevent hemolysis of the cells exposed to copper. This is evident in the data in TABLE 4. Also shown in TABLE 4 is that a lipid antioxidant, such as butylated hydroxyanisole (BHA), dramatically suppresses cell damage. This effect suggests that while copper,

TABLE 4

THE EFFECTS OF COPPER ON HEMOLYSIS, REDUCED GLUTATHIONE LEVELS, AND METHEMOGLOBIN FORMATION IN HUMAN ERYTHROCYTES*

	Hemolysis (%)	GSH (nmoles/mg Hb)	$HbFe^{+3}$ (%)
No additions	<1	3.12	<1
$CuSO_4$ (200 μM)	18	0.28	9
$CuSO_4$ (200 μM) + BHA (5.0 μg)	2	0.36	9
$CuSO_4$ (200 μM) + Glucose (20 mM)	16	2.74	3

* Erythrocytes (5% hematocrit) were incubated for 120 minutes in isotonic NaCl buffered with 20 mM phosphate, pH 7.6 The incubation volume was 3.0 ml. BHA was dissolved in ethanol, and equivalent amounts of ethanol (20 μl) were added to control flasks. The values presented are the averages obtained from two experiments each with duplicate tubes.

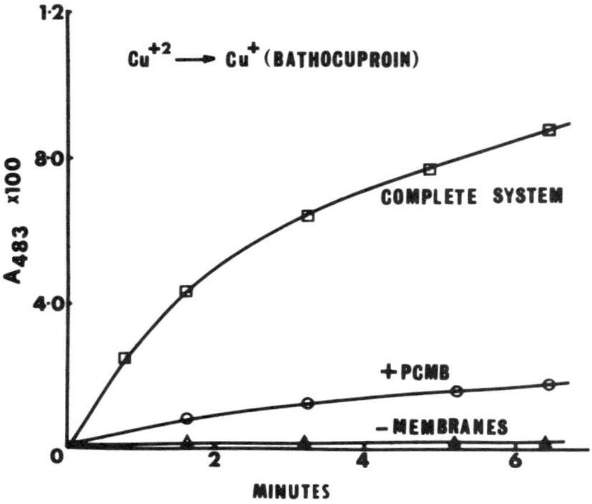

FIGURE 1. The reduction of Cu^{+2} to Cu^{+} as measured by complex formation with bathocuproin. The complete system included tris-HCl, 0.15 M; NaCl, 0.154 M; bathocuproin, 0.25 mM; membrane protein, 3.0 mg; and $CuSO_4$, 100 μM. The concentration of PCMBS was 1.5 mM.

at high concentrations, may have deleterious effects on the internal constituents of the erythrocyte, hemolysis is primarily a consequence of events associated with membrane lipids.

In order to explore the interaction of copper with membrane lipid components, preparations of hemoglobin-free erythrocyte ghosts were first prepared and then exposed to cupric copper in the presence of bathocuproin.[21] FIGURE 1 illustrates the formation of cuprous-bathocuproin complexes, which may be observed in the presence of red cell membranes. In their absence, negligible amounts of chromogen are

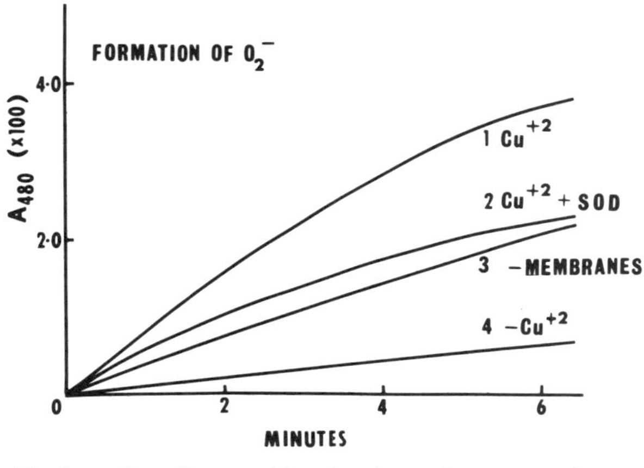

FIGURE 2. The formation of superoxide anions by erythrocyte membranes in the presence of copper. The formation of adrenochrome from epinephrine was measured by the method of McCord and Fridovich.[22] The concentration of copper added to the cuvettes was 25 μM. Other conditions of the reaction system are described in Reference 21.

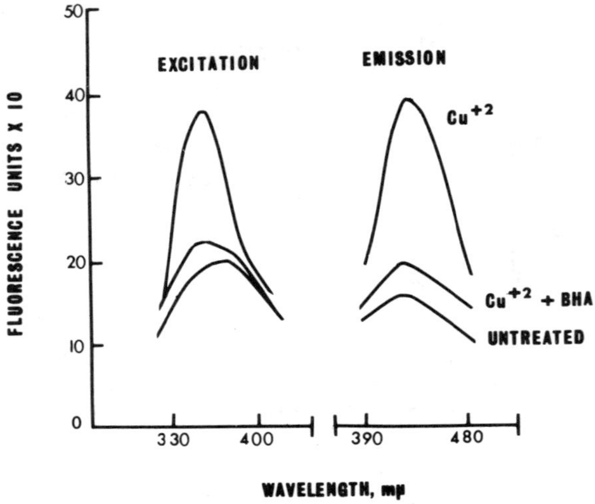

FIGURE 3. The formation of fluorescent chromolipids in human erythrocytes exposed to $CuSO_4$. Cells were incubated for 60 minutes at 37 °C with $CuSO_4$ (200 μM). At the end of the incubation period (little or no lysis was observed in control or treated cells), the erythrocytes were washed three times with isotonic saline solutions and the lipids extracted with isopropanol and chloroform in the cold. The fluorescence of the organic solvent layers was determined in a Farrand spectrofluorimeter standardized with quinine sulfate. Ten fluorescence units are equivalent to 0.01 ng quinine sulfate in 0.1 N HCl.

formed. Also shown in FIGURE 1 is the inhibition of the reduction of copper if the membranes are first treated with *p*-chloromercuriphenylsulfonate (PCMBS) to block their sulfhydryl groups.

The sulfhydryl-dependent formation of cuprous copper, under aerobic conditions, is accompanied by the generation of O_2^-. This is illustrated in FIGURE 2, where the formation of adrenochrome from epinephrine is recorded as an index of superoxide production.[22] The addition of superoxide dismutase (SOD) to the cuvettes (curve 2) reduces adrenochrome formation to the levels observed in the absence of membranes (curve 3). In these experiments, copper itself, in the absence of membranes, caused the formation of material that absorbs light at 480 nm (curve 3). The formation of this material is not sensitive to SOD. In the absence of copper (curve 4), only small increases in absorption are observed.

These experiments illustrate the capacity of cupric copper to react with plasma membrane sulfhydryl groups and to cause the formation of superoxide radicals. Such radicals may either directly or indirectly (after dismutation to form peroxide or after interaction with peroxide to form hydroxy radicals) initiate the peroxidation of unsaturated fatty acids in membrane phospholipids. FIGURE 3 shows that, in fact, fluorescent chromolipids—characteristic of those formed during the peroxidation of phospholipids—are present in the membranes of copper-treated red cells before they undergo hemolysis (after one hour of incubation). If BHA is included in the incubation medium, fluorescent chromolipid formation is reduced almost to the level observed in cells incubated without copper. In the presence of BHA, copper-treated cells do not go on to hemolyze. The fluorescent pigment present in the untreated cells (FIGURE 3) is characteristic of that found in the oldest cells of mixed populations of human erythrocytes.[23]

Although not shown in FIGURE 3, washing of the cells with ethylenediaminetetraacetic acid (EDTA) solutions at the end of the incubations—and before preparing membranes for extraction with organic solvents—did not alter the intensity of the fluorescent peaks. This suggests that the fluorescent material is formed during the incubation of the cells with copper and is not a consequence of the action of the copper on either the isolated membranes or the extracted lipids.

The spectral characteristics of the fluorescent chromolipids are like those of the well-known lipofuscins. Such pigments have been long recognized as the products of the peroxidation of cellular lipids.[24] Their occurrence in certain tissues has been associated with the aging process.[25] The concept that they are derived from peroxidized lipid is substantiated by the observation that their accumulation in the tissues of experimental animals is markedly reduced after the introduction of lipid antioxidants to the diet.[26] The degradation of peroxidized fatty acids may lead to the formation of malonyldialdehyde. This agent has the capacity to cross-link the amino groups of lipids and proteins by the formation of Schiff's bases. Such cross-linked derivatives, when formed with malonyldialdehyde *in vitro,* have characteristics similar to the fluorescent pigments found *in vivo.*[27] Their exact solubility properties and excitation and emission spectra depend on the nature of the lipids and proteins from which they are derived.[28,29] In the red cell, the presence of malonyldialdehyde is associated with the polymerization of specific membrane proteins, such as spectrin, and with the inactivation of membrane-bound enzymes, such as the ATPases.[23,30]

On the basis of these considerations, we visualize that the following reactions may be involved in the sequence of events that leads to hemolysis in the presence of copper. The metal has the capacity to accelerate the autoxidation of ferrous hemoglobin to form methemoglobin and superoxide anions (Reaction 1).§ Superoxide

$$HbFe^{+2}-O_2 \xrightarrow{Cu^{+2}} HbFe^{+3} + O_2^- \quad \textbf{(1)}$$

may serve as a source of hydrogen peroxide through dismutation (Reaction 2). It is

$$2O_2^- + 2H^+ \longrightarrow H_2O_2 + O_2 \quad \textbf{(2)}$$

also possible that copper may enhance the autoxidation of reduced glutathione (Reaction 3). Such a reaction would not only form hydrogen peroxide, but would

$$2GSH + O_2 \xrightarrow{Cu^{+2}} GSSG + H_2O_2 \quad \textbf{(3)}$$

also deplete cells of the reduced glutathione necessary for the detoxification of both hydrogen peroxide and organic hydroperoxides. Reactions such as these—which may involve the autoxidation of other heme proteins and constituents, such as ascorbic acid, phenols, and phenolic amines—may well be the basis for the cytotoxicity of copper in other cells and tissues. However, since we have found that at copper concentrations less than about 100 μM, glucose is able to prevent the loss of reduced glutathione in the red cell and to protect glycolytic enzymes such as hexokinase, but not prevent hemolysis, we assume that peroxide generated by these intracellular mechanisms does not play a major role in the ultimate hemolysis caused by copper. Of course, at higher concentrations of copper, the capacity of the glutathione peroxidase system to detoxify peroxides and of glucose to regenerate reduced glutathione may be overwhelmed and compromised.

We visualize a primary effect of copper to be on the oxidation of membrane (PCMBS-sensitive) sulfhydryl groups to form disulfides. This oxidation is accompanied by the formation of cuprous copper, which may rapidly oxidize with

§ Hb = hemoglobin.

molecular oxygen to form superoxide radicals at membrane sites (Reaction 4). As a

$$Cu^{+} + O_2 \longrightarrow Cu^{+2} + O_2^{-} \qquad (4)$$

result of dismutation, this reaction would serve as a source of hydrogen peroxide. It is also possible that copper participates in the breakdown of peroxide to yield peroxidation-initiating radicals, which may be scavenged by BHA but not by glucose or ethanol (see TABLE 4). The direct participation of copper in an initiating reaction, by electron abstraction from unsaturated fatty acids, is also not excluded by our experiments. In any event, it is not unreasonable to posit that membrane disulfides, formed in the presence of copper, may be in equilibrium with intracellular reduced glutathione and, hence, readily regenerated to their sulfhydryl forms. This would permit a cyclic system for the generation of nonstoichiometric amounts of oxygen radicals through a small pool of membrane sulfhydryl groups (Reaction 5).

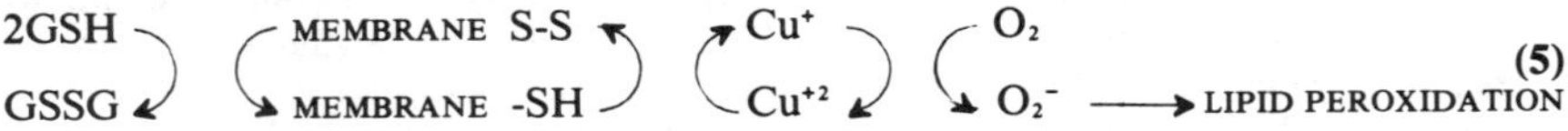

(5)

The formation of lipid peroxides in itself may be sufficient cause for the disruption of membranes and hemolysis merely through the loss of phospholipids.[31] However, the finding of fluorescent pigments in copper-treated erythrocytes suggests that the lipid peroxides may be undergoing extensive degradation. It is of interest that we have previously shown that cuprous salts may accelerate the breakdown of peroxidized lipid in hepatic microsomal systems to form short chain hydrocarbons—which include ethane and ethylene—as well as malonyldialdehyde.[32,33] It is not surprising that copper should have the capacity to generate radicals and peroxides in biological systems.[34] However, it may be the formation of malonyldialdehyde, with its capacity to polymerize essential macromolecules, that terminates the cascade of events leading to hemolysis. These experiments suggest that—in addition to copper-binding drugs, such as penicillamine[35]—there may be some merit in utilizing antioxidants, such as vitamin E, in the treatment of individuals with Wilson's disease who exhibit hemolysis.

REFERENCES

1. SARZEAU, M. 1830. J. Pharm. Chim. **16:** 505.
2. FLEURENT, E. & L. LEVI. 1920. Bull. Soc. Chim. Fr. **27:** 440.
3. KUBOYAMA, M., F. C. YONG & T. E. KING. 1972. J. Biol. Chem. **247:** 6375.
4. KEELE, B. B., J. M. MCCORD & I. FRIDOVICH. 1971. J. Biol. Chem. **246:** 2875.
5. FRIEDMAN, S. & S. KAUFMAN. 1965. J. Biol. Chem. **240:** 4763.
6. GRAHAM, G. G. & A. CORDANO. 1969. Johns Hopkins Med. J. **124:** 139.
7. DANKS, D. M., *et al.* 1972. Pediatrics **50:** 188.
8. OSTER, G. & M. P. SALGO. 1977. Adv. Pharmacol. Chemother. **14:** 327.
9. CHUTTANI, H. K., *et al.* 1965. Am. J. Med. **39:** 849.
10. HOLTZMAN, N. A., D. A. ELLIOTT & R. H. HELLER. 1966. New Engl. J. Med. **275:** 347.
11. BARBOUR, B. H., M. BISCHEL & D. E. ABRAMS. 1971. Nephron **8:** 455.
12. SCHEINBERG, I. H. & D. GITLIN. 1952. Science **116:** 484.
13. ROCH-SICOT, J. & J. P. BENHAMOU. 1977. Ann. Intern. Med. **86:** 301.
14. DEISS, A., G. R. LEE & G. E. CARTWRIGHT. 1970. Ann. Intern. Med. **73:** 413.
15. FAIRBANKS, W. F. 1967. Arch. Intern. Med. **120:** 428.
16. BOULARD, M., K. G. BLUME & E. BEUTLER. 1972. J. Clin. Invest. **51:** 459.
17. METZ, E. N. & A. L. SAGONE. 1972. J. Lab. Clin. Med. **80:** 405.
18. RIFKIND, J. M., *et al.* 1976. Biochemistry **24:** 5337.
19. WINTERBOURNE, C., B. M. MCGRATH & R. W. CARRELL. 1976. Biochem. J. **155:** 493.
20. COHEN, G. & P. HOCHSTEIN. 1961. Science **134:** 1574.

21. Kumar, K. S., C. Rowse & P. Hochstein. 1978. Biochem. Biophys. Res. Commun. **83:** 587.
22. McCord, J. & I. Fridovich. 1969. J. Biol. Chem. **244:** 6049.
23. Jain, S. K. & P. Hochstein. 1980. Biochem. Biophys. Res. Commun. **92:** 247.
24. Ciaccio, C. 1915. Biochem. Z. **69:** 313.
25. Strehler, B. L., *et al.* 1959. J. Gerontol. **14:** 430.
26. Tappel, A., B. Fletcher & D. Deamer. 1973. J. Gerontol. **28:** 415.
27. Chio, K. S. & A. L. Tappel. 1969. Biochemistry **8:** 2821.
28. Dillard, C. J. & A. L. Tappel. 1973. Lipids **8:** 183.
29. Bidlack, W. R. & A. L. Tappel. 1973. Lipids **8:** 203.
30. Jain, S. K. & P. Hochstein. 1980. (In preparation.)
31. Jacob, H. S. & S. E. Lux. 1968. Blood **32:** 549.
32. Hochstein, P. & L. Ernster. 1963. Biochem. Biophys. Res. Commun. **12:** 388.
33. Liberman, M. & P. Hochstein. 1966. Science **152:** 213.
34. Schubert, J. 1964. Copper and Peroxides in Radiobiology and Medicine. Charles C. Thomas, Publishers. Springfield, Ill.
35. Iser, J. H., *et al.* 1974. Gastroenterology **67:** 290.
36. Strickland, G. T. & M. L. Leu. 1975. Medicine **54:** 113.

Discussion

W. G. Hoekstra (*University of Wisconsin, Madison, Wis.*): We have recently examined "whole body" lipid peroxidation by measuring ethane production in animals that were deficient in both vitamin E and selenium. These animals are extremely sensitive to very small amounts of copper, which dramatically increases ethane production. Of course, we do not know the source of the ethane, but it is our impression that it is not from peroxidation of red cell membranes.

Is spectrin a protein specific to the red cell membrane?

P. Hochstein: Yes, it is apparently ubiquitous in mammalian red cells, and it has not been detected in other cell types. However, it occurs in close association with actin (band 5), which has the same molecular weight as muscle actin and which has been shown to form functional actomysin with muscle myosin.

W. G. Hoekstra: Do you suppose that the high degree of specificity of the malonyldialdehyde reaction with spectrin relates to some aspect of the high degree of membrane organization?

P. Hochstein: Yes, in the sense that the close proximity of spectrin monomers on the inner surface of the plasma membrane may permit easy polymerization by either added malonyldialdehyde or by that generated during peroxidation reactions involving phospholipids located in the inner portions of the membrane bilayer.

A. L. Tappel (*University of California, Davis, Calif.*): As you know, there are two possible modes of attack by lipid peroxidation. The first involves malonyldialdehyde formation, and the second, free radical-initiated polymerization reactions. Is it possible that the formation of fluorescent products is only concurrent with a free radical-induced polymerization of protein?

P. Hochstein: That is the case, and from our own experiments, we can only point to the capacity of malonyldialdehyde to form specific polymers with spectrin and not with other membrane proteins. If free radical polymerization were taking place, one would expect other proteins to be involved.

N. F. Suttle (*Moredun Research Institute, Edinburgh, Scotland*): Do you think that these changes are likely to occur *in vivo*? My colleagues Ernest Smith and Harry Rice have found that when albumin is present in the medium *in vitro*, the red cells become very tolerant of copper. It seems likely that copper would be bound to albumin *in vivo.* Did your incubation medium contain protein?

P. HOCHSTEIN: No, we did not include albumin in the experiments that I have described. These experiments were carried out over short periods of time (less than 2 hours). In general, our experience has been that although albumin will protect cells against the effects of copper over these short periods of time, it will not do so during prolonged periods of incubation (up to 20 hours). Presumably, over these longer periods of time, copper that is loosely bound to albumin becomes available for interaction with red cells. I would also presume that this is the situation *in vivo.*

N. F. SUTTLE: I would like to comment that although the red cell is thought to be unresponsive to copper uptake *in vivo,* work in Australia has shown that copper accumulates in superoxide dismutase.

P. HOCHSTEIN: We have been able to demonstrate that copper is taken up by red cells *in vitro,* but since the adult cells have little capacity for new protein synthesis, it would be most surprising if that copper were to be incorporated into any new enzyme molecules.

W. MERTZ (*Beltsville Human Nutrition Research Center, U.S. Department of Agriculture, Beltsville, Md.*): Were your experiments carried out with isolated membranes or with intact cells?

P. HOCHSTEIN: All of the experiments were carried out with intact cells except those that involved the formation of superoxide anions and those in which we measured the reduction of copper.

W. G. HOEKSTRA: There has been some suggestion that the hemolytic crisis in copper toxicity might be related to the release of some hemolytic substance rather than to copper itself. Your experiments suggest that hemolysis is a direct consequence of the action of copper on the cell membrane. Do you have any additional comments to make?

P. HOCHSTEIN: Unfortunately, we have not been able to obtain large quantities of plasma from patients exposed to copper during an active hemolytic episode, so I am not able to make a comment about other substances that might be present in the plasma of these individuals. The presence of such substances would be of considerable interest, although our experiments suggest that there is no need to postulate their presence.

H. H. SANDSTEAD (*Human Nutrition Research Center, U.S. Department of Agriculture, Grand Forks, N. Dak.*): Although patients with Wilson's disease may become overloaded with respect to copper, what level of dietary copper would be necessary to produce these same effects in a normal individual?

W. G. HOEKSTRA: That question is complicated by the extensive storage capacity of the liver for copper.

P. HOCHSTEIN: I am not familiar with the quantitative data; however, under certain circumstances, the margin of safety afforded by storage pools may not be reassuring. I have in mind those individuals who suffer copper toxicity after its acute ingestion, its application to the skin, and during hemodialysis with an apparatus that utilizes copper tubing.

EFFECTS OF VITAMIN C AND IRON ON CADMIUM METABOLISM*

M. R. Spivey Fox, Richard M. Jacobs, A. O. Lee Jones,
B. E. Fry, Jr., and Charles L. Stone

Division of Nutrition
Food and Drug Administration
Department of Health and Human Services
Washington, D.C. 20204

INTRODUCTION

Cadmium is a nonessential element that is present in the United States diet at levels approximating 50 μg per day, which is near the provisional tolerable intakes of 57–71 μg per day of the Food and Agriculture Organization and the World Health Organization.[1,2] Cadmium has a long biological half-time, estimated to be 18 to 33 years in the human kidney, the target organ for damage. At levels near 200 parts per million in the renal cortex (wet weight), proximal tubular damage can be expected, followed by severe bone mineral loss.[3] The latter appears to be secondary to kidney damage; however, the exact etiology is not established. No means are known for removing cadmium from the body without causing kidney damage.

Cadmium-induced toxicosis in immature experimental animals is characterized by depressed growth, anemia, low bone ash, low tissue levels of several essential elements, and pathology of the intestinal mucosa, testis, kidney, and adrenal gland. Some of the same changes have been observed in industrial workers chronically exposed to cadmium-containing dusts or fumes. Adverse effects of cadmium typically occur with 5 ppm or more of dietary cadmium in experimental animals. An exception is an enteropathy that occurred with a two-day exposure of Japanese quail to diets containing 1 ppm of cadmium.[4] Adverse metabolic and physiological effects have been observed with a similar low cadmium exposure when the diet was deficient in copper or iron, apparently due to antagonisms of copper and iron, respectively.[5,6]

An extensive literature now documents the interactions of essential nutrients with dietary cadmium at toxic levels. The nutrients include zinc, iron, manganese, copper, selenium, calcium, ascorbic acid, vitamin D, and proteins. Many of these relationships have been reviewed.[7-10] In general, low levels of the essential nutrients exacerbate the adverse effects of cadmium, whereas high levels of the essential nutrients are protective. These studies have been valuable as a means of quickly identifying nutrients that might affect the absorption and long-term tissue turnover of low levels of dietary cadmium similar to those ingested by humans. Beneficial effects at these low cadmium levels, less than 0.1 ppm, have been reported in experimental animals for a combined supplement of zinc, manganese, and copper, for zinc alone, and in man for iron.[11-14,6]

The purpose of this paper is to review the studies of ascorbic acid and iron interactions with cadmium and to present new data on the effects of these nutrients on tissue retention of very low dietary levels of cadmium, similar to those typically encountered by humans.

* Some of these data were presented at the annual meeting of the Federation of American Societies for Experimental Biology, April 1–10, 1979.

0077-8923/80/0355-0249 $01.75/0 © 1980, NYAS

Interactions between Iron, Ascorbic Acid, and High Levels of Cadmium

Very high levels of dietary cadmium caused anemia in rats, mice, rabbits, chicks, Japanese quail, cattle, and man.[15-23] The iron pigment of rat incisors was also absent.[15] Cadmium exposure during pregnancy produced more severe anemia in newborn mice than in the mothers.[24] Low tissue iron levels associated with cadmium ingestion, which were observed in most of the above studies, also occurred in sheep.[25] Decreased iron in newborn rats occurred when the mothers received 4.3 μg of cadmium/ml of drinking water before and during pregnancy.[26]

Iron absorption was depressed by cadmium.[20,27] Jacobs *et al.* showed that cadmium caused a rapid decline of iron in the duodenum.[28] Under conditions of low iron intake, there was a greater uptake and transport of cadmium from the intestine.[27,29] By 48 hours after dosing, rats with a chronic mild iron deficiency absorbed more of a single dose of cadmium-109 as the citrate (9.9 μg of cadmium) than did controls.[30]

Fox *et al.* showed that feeding iron(II) as the sulfate was effective in preventing the anemia caused by cadmium, whereas supplements of iron(III) as the citrate were essentially ineffective.[31] Oral supplements of Fe(II) as the sulfate were also protective in rats and pigs.[32,33] Injection of iron protected against the anemia produced by cadmium in rats, mice, and pigs.[32,34,24,33]

Dietary supplements of ascorbic acid protected against the growth depression, anemia, and decrease in liver iron concentration produced by dietary cadmium in young Japanese quail.[35] D-Isoascorbic acid was similarly effective, whereas ethoxyquin had no effect.[31] Cadmium at a dietary level of 75 ppm did not reduce liver concentrations of ascorbic acid. Supplements of ascorbic acid had variable effects on tissue concentrations of cadmium in the quail. Maji and Yoshida found that a combined supplement of iron(II) as the sulfate and ascorbic acid reduced cadmium concentrations in the liver and kidneys of rats fed cadmium.[36] Richardson *et al.* showed that supplemental ascorbic acid fed to young Japanese quail alleviated or prevented multiple pathological effects of cadmium, including enteropathy, testicular hypoplasia, decreased granulation of the adrenal medulla, and excessive periodic acid–Schiff reactivity of esophageal mucous glands.[37]

The toxicity of 75 ppm of dietary cadmium, fed to Japanese quail between 7 and 14 days of age, was significantly decreased when the dietary protein was egg white rather than casein plus gelatin or soy isolate.[38] The changes in hematocrit, bone ash, and tissue minerals were indicative of better utilization of iron and zinc in the presence of cadmium with the egg white as compared with the other protein sources.

Interactions between Iron, Ascorbic Acid, and Very Low Levels of Cadmium

Flanagan *et al.* fed cadmium-115m as the chloride to 22 normal human adults in a breakfast of rolled oats and milk (total cadmium, 25 μg).[6] Apparent absorption of the cadmium-115m was 8.9 ± 2.0% [mean ± standard error (SE)] for 10 subjects with low iron stores, as indicated by serum ferritin values less than 20 ng/ml. Twelve subjects with higher serum ferritin absorbed only 2.3 ± 0.3% of the cadmium dose. Although more women than men had low iron stores, both men and women were in each group.

Studies were carried out in our laboratory to assess the effect of mild iron deficiency, an ascorbic acid supplement, and substitution of equal amounts of iron(II) as ferrous sulfate for iron(III) as the citrate on tissue retention of cadmium fed at levels similar to those in human diets.

Experimental Procedures

Day-old Japanese quail (*Coturnix coturnix japonica*) were housed in suspended stainless steel cages with adequate heat, light, demineralized drinking water, and diet at all times. They were wing banded at 7 days of age and were weighed at 7, 9, 14, and 16 days, depending on the experiment. There were 10 birds per group, and in experiments where treatments were begun at 7 days, the birds were redistributed by body weights so that the weights were closely similar for all groups.

The composition and mineral content (by analysis) of the basal purified diet containing casein and gelatin were reported previously.[14] The diet was nutritionally adequate for young quail, and the total levels of zinc, iron (as ferric citrate), manganese, copper, and magnesium met requirements as closely as possible. The total amount of cadmium in the diet was 0.062 ppm. Basal diet was fed to all birds except when they received experimental diets.

In experiment 1, the basal diet and its modifications were fed from 7 to 14 days of age as follows: (1) 50 ppm of iron as ferric citrate; (2) 100 ppm of iron as ferric citrate (basal diet, control); (3) 100 ppm of iron as ferric citrate plus 0.5% ascorbic acid; and (4) 100 ppm of iron as ferrous sulfate. In experiment 2, the same experimental diets were fed from 7 to 16 days except that iron as the citrate was decreased to 25 ppm rather than to 50 ppm (diet modification 1). Each diet was fed to two groups of birds, one of which was killed at 9 days for tissue mineral analysis, and the other dosed at 9 days with cadmium-109 as described below and the birds killed 7 days later at 16 days of age. Experiment 3 was identical to experiment 2 except that the experimental diets were fed from the time of hatching.

In experiment 1, accelerator-produced carrier-free $^{109}CdCl_2$ (New England Nuclear Corp., Boston, Mass.) was mixed with each experimental diet to provide 100 μCi/kg of diet, which was fed during 7–14 days.[14] In experiments 2 and 3, the labeled diets were compressed with a Stokes compacting machine (Pennwalt Corp., Warminster, Penn.) into cylindrical tablets about 5 mm in diameter and 8 mm long weighing 80–100 mg and containing approximately 3.4 μCi of $^{109}CdCl_2$. Powdered stearic acid was mixed in the diet at a level of 0.1% to permit release of the tablet from the dies. The labeled tablets were placed in plastic powder transfer pipets, inserted into the upper esophagus of nonfasted birds midway between the mouth and crop, and the tablet pushed into the esophagus with the pipet plunger. The birds swallowed the tablets and did not appear disturbed by the procedure. Hemoglobin was measured as cyanmethemoglobin at 15 days in experiments 2 and 3 and at 8 days in experiment 3. All birds were killed by decapitation without a prior fast. The duodenum, jejunum-ileum, liver, and kidneys were excised, washed in 0.75% NaCl solution (except the kidney), weighed, solubilized in nitric acid for cadmium-109 measurements, and digested in nitric and perchloric acids before determination of zinc, iron, magnesium, and calcium by atomic absorption spectrophotometry (Model 5000, Perkin-Elmer Corp., Norwalk, Conn.). Details of these procedures have been published.[14]

The labeled diet tablets were placed in small plastic tubes, which were precisely centered and held upright in standard counting vials by a lid adapter with an opening just large enough to accommodate the tube. Radioactivity was measured in an NaI (T1) crystal scintillation detector (Model 5285, Packard Instruments, Des Plaines, Ill.). For each dosing period, radioactivity in 10 labeled tablets was measured after solubilization in nitric acid by procedures used for the diet in experiment 1 and all tissues to adjust for the two types of counting procedures.

Food consumption was not measured in experiment 1 because it was expected to be the same for all groups based on expected and actual body weight similarity. The amount of cadmium-109 in the tissue was expressed as ng/g, based on the specific activity of the diet (100 μCi/62 ng of cadmium) fed from day 7 to day 14; however, cadmium retention could not be calculated. In experiments 2 and 3, the cadmium-109 in the tissue was expressed as percent retention of the dose.

Within experiments, statistically significant differences were based on Student's t test.[39] Correlation and multiple regression analyses were calculated by computer programs of the Statistical Analysis System (SAS Institute, Inc., Cary, N.C.)

RESULTS

All treatments affected cadmium retention, and the trends or significant effects were qualitatively similar in all experiments. In general, cadmium retention was inversely related to tissue iron concentrations.

TABLE 1

EFFECTS OF IRON AND ASCORBIC ACID (AA) TREATMENTS (7–14 DAYS) ON TISSUE MINERAL CONCENTRATIONS, ^{109}Cd FED 7-14 DAYS (EXPERIMENT 1)*

	Dietary Treatment			
Measurement	50 ppm Fe^{3+} 0 AA	100 ppm Fe^{3+} 0 AA	100 ppm Fe^{3+} 0.5% AA	100 ppm Fe^{2+} 0 AA
Body Weight (g)	47 ± 1.1	45 ± 1.1	45 ± 0.9	44 ± 0.9
Duodenum				
Weight (mg)	590 ± 24	628 ± 14	619 ± 20	606 ± 26
Zn (ppm)	38 ± 1.4†	33 ± 1.1	33 ± 0.9	35 ± 0.7
Fe (ppm)	67 ± 14†	115 ± 16	367 ± 39‡	326 ± 33‡
Cd (ppb)	609 ± 78‡	264 ± 29	174 ± 16†	187 ± 11†
Jejunum-Ileum				
Weight (mg)	666 ± 32	675 ± 28	658 ± 20	643 ± 24
Zn (ppm)	32 ± 0.8‡	29 ± 0.6	28 ± 0.6	31 ± 0.6†
Fe (ppm)	38 ± 3‡	64 ± 7	134 ± 15‡	92 ± 9†
Cd (ppb)	122 ± 15	131 ± 17	64 ± 5‡	94 ± 9
Liver				
Weight (g)	1.70 ± 0.074	1.65 ± 0.104	1.75 ± 0.084	1.61 ± 0.056
Zn (ppm)	20 ± 0.5	23 ± 1.2	21 ± 0.7	21 ± 0.6
Fe (ppm)	142 ± 19	140 ± 8.8	251 ± 25.5‡	164 ± 15.2
Cd (ppb)	2.39 ± 0.120†	2.93 ± 0.124	2.59 ± 0.192	3.04 ± 0.183
Kidneys				
Weight (mg)	553 ± 14	548 ± 2	515 ± 17	559 ± 15
Zn (ppm)	20 ± 0.3	20 ± 0.2	20 ± 0.3	19 ± 0.3†
Fe (ppm)	90 ± 4.6	91 ± 3.7	92 ± 4.5	98 ± 5.2
Cd (ppb)	8.38 ± 0.677	9.62 ± 0.410	6.44 ± 0.567‡	8.24 ± 0.506†

* Means ± SE, 10 birds per group, killed at 14 days of age. Control diet wih 0.021 ppm of Cd was fed 0–7 days; experimental diets with 0.062 ppm of Cd with 100 μCi of $^{109}CdCl_2$/kg of diet were fed 7–14 days. Tissue cadmium values were based on specific activity of diet. Iron forms were ferric citrate and $FeSO_4$.

† Significantly different from group fed 100 ppm of Fe^{3+}, $P < 0.05$.

‡ Same comparison, $P < 0.01$.

The results of experiment 1 are presented in TABLE 1. Body weights and tissue or organ weights were not significantly affected by dietary treatment. Cadmium in the duodenum was markedly elevated by low dietary iron and decreased by supplemental ascorbic acid or substitution of iron(II) for iron(III). Iron concentrations were inversely related to those of cadmium. In the jejunum-ileum, only ascorbic acid decreased cadmium. In the liver, low dietary iron caused a decrease in cadmium concentration relative to the control, 100 ppm of iron(III). Both ascorbic acid and iron(II) caused decreased cadmium levels in the kidneys. Tissue zinc changes were relatively small.

In experiment 2 (TABLE 2), changes in the diet for 2 days before dosing with cadmium-109 caused marked changes in tissue iron levels (duodenum, jejunum-ileum, and liver). Hemoglobin was significantly decreased at 16 days by the low iron diet; however, body weight was not affected. Tissue iron concentrations reflected similar treatment effects by 16 days; the effect of iron deficiency on liver iron status was greater at 16 than at 9 days. Cadmium retention in the duodenum was markedly elevated by the low iron diet and decreased by ascorbic acid and iron(II). Similar ef-

TABLE 2

EFFECTS OF IRON AND ASCORBIC ACID (AA) TREATMENTS (7–16 DAYS) ON TISSUE MINERAL CONCENTRATIONS AND RETENTION OF A SINGLE DOSE OF ^{109}Cd GIVEN AT 9 DAYS (EXPERIMENT 2)*

		Dietary Treatment			
Measurement	Age (days)	25 ppm Fe^{3+} 0 AA	100 ppm Fe^{3+} 0 AA	100 ppm Fe^{3+} 0.5% AA	100 ppm Fe^{2+} 0 AA
Body Weight (g)	9	28 ± 0.7	28 ± 0.5	28 ± 0.5	28 ± 0.7
Duodenum					
Weight (mg)	9	418 ± 28	422 ± 20	442 ± 18	480 ± 21
Zn (ppm)		30 ± 1.1	31 ± 1.5	30 ± 1.2	31 ± 1.2
Fe (ppm)		18 ± 2‡	42 ± 5	95 ± 16‡	194 ± 25‡
Mg (ppm)		213 ± 4‡	228 ± 2	220 ± 3	226 ± 2
Ca (ppm)		201 ± 9	194 ± 8	191 ± 11	216 ± 4†
Jejunum-Ileum					
Weight (mg)	9	490 ± 23	478 ± 15	511 ± 21	530 ± 17†
Zn (ppm)		22 ± 0.5	23 ± 0.4	22 ± 0.8	22 ± 0.6
Fe (ppm)		35 ± 5†	53 ± 5	150 ± 19‡	110 ± 10‡
Mg (ppm)		218 ± 3	223 ± 2	219 ± 3	214 ± 4†
Ca (ppm)		271 ± 18	260 ± 14	234 ± 25	255 ± 14
Liver					
Weight (g)	9	1.22 ± 0.08	1.19 ± 0.05	1.20 ± 0.05	1.15 ± 0.04
Zn (ppm)		17 ± 0.9	18 ± 0.5	18 ± 0.4	19 ± 0.7
Fe (ppm)		145 ± 25	161 ± 18	222 ± 23†	354 ± 39‡
Mg (ppm)		216 ± 6†	236 ± 6	237 ± 2	242 ± 2
Ca (ppm)		33 ± 2.4	42 ± 4.2	44 ± 3.1	42 ± 2.5
Kidney					
Weight (mg)	9	358 ± 14	360 ± 13	367 ± 13	366 ± 14
Zn (ppm)		17 ± 0.2	17 ± 0.5	18 ± 0.2	18 ± 0.3
Fe (ppm)		54 ± 3†	71 ± 5	61 ± 5	65 ± 4
Mg (ppm)		197 ± 3	201 ± 3	206 ± 3	206 ± 1
Ca (ppm)		39 ± 2.4†	52 ± 5.3	91 ± 11.4‡	47 ± 5.8
Body Weight (g)	16	49 ± 1.2¶	50 ± 1.1¶	47 ± 1.6¶	49 ± 1.0¶
Hb (g/100 ml)	15	10.9 ± 0.25†	12.1 ± 0.36	11.2 ± 0.34	12.9 ± 0.35

(*cont.*)

TABLE 2 (*cont.*)

Measurement	Age (days)	Dietary Treatment: 25 ppm Fe^{3+} 0 AA	100 ppm Fe^{3+} 0 AA	100 ppm Fe^{3+} 0.5% AA	100 ppm Fe^{2+} 0 AA
Duodenum					
Weight (mg)	16	611 ± 16¶	657 ± 21¶	662 ± 34¶	659 ± 29¶
Zn (ppm)		30 ± 1.6†	36 ± 2.4	32 ± 1.4	32 ± 0.9
Fe (ppm)		26 ± 5‡	125 ± 21¶	350 ± 56‡¶	235 ± 23‡
Mg (ppm)		222 ± 9	225 ± 2	223 ± 5	222 ± 4
Ca (ppm)		210 ± 17	198 ± 12	215 ± 10	205 ± 12
^{109}Cd (%)		9.53 ± 0.938‡	3.18 ± 0.357	0.87 ± 0.166‡	0.50 ± 0.107‡
Jejunum-Ileum					
Weight (mg)	16	743 ± 29¶	733 ± 26¶	695 ± 34¶	715 ± 35¶
Zn (ppm)		28 ± 0.8‡¶	33 ± 1.1¶	29 ± 0.6‡¶	30 ± 0.7†¶
Fe (ppm)		21 ± 3‡§	51 ± 8	162 ± 18‡	184 ± 7‡§
Mg (ppm)		229 ± 7	224 ± 4	224 ± 4	225 ± 3¶
Ca (ppm)		262 ± 20	248 ± 19	320 ± 41	274 ± 32§
^{109}Cd (%)		2.56 ± 0.464	1.60 ± 0.238	0.33 ± 0.039‡	0.53 ± 0.138‡
Liver					
Weight (g)	16	1.73 ± 0.06¶	1.80 ± 0.06¶	1.80 ± 0.07¶	1.83 ± 0.11¶
Zn (ppm)		21 ± 1.4§	22 ± 0.7¶	21 ± 0.8	21 ± 0.4
Fe (ppm)		61 ± 5‡¶	164 ± 19	242 ± 30†	208 ± 23¶
Mg (ppm)		252 ± 11¶	255 ± 4	246 ± 4	243 ± 6¶
Ca (ppm)		39 ± 2§	43 ± 4	38 ± 2	35 ± 2
^{109}Cd (%)		0.40 ± 0.030	0.45 ± 0.021	0.33 ± 0.028‡	0.28 ± 0.040‡
Kidney					
Weight (mg)	16	540 ± 19¶	538 ± 18¶	515 ± 40¶	590 ± 32¶
Zn (ppm)		20 ± 0.9§	20 ± 0.3¶	21 ± 1.1§	19 ± 0.8
Fe (ppm)		66 ± 4§	75 ± 3	81 ± 7§	86 ± 5¶
Mg (ppm)		204 ± 9	213 ± 2	216 ± 10‡	204 ± 8
Ca (ppm)		60 ± 4¶	84 ± 15	80 ± 11	63 ± 6
^{109}Cd (%)		0.59 ± 0.044	0.53 ± 0.038	0.36 ± 0.044†	0.32 ± 0.039‡
Liver & Kidney					
^{109}Cd (%)	16	0.99 ± 0.065	0.98 ± 0.048	0.69 ± 0.071‡	0.60 ± 0.078‡

* Mean ± SE, 10 birds per group, killed at 9 days (no ^{109}Cd dose) and 16 days. Control diet was fed 0–7 days, experimental diets, 7–16 days. A dose of 3.4 μCi of $^{109}CdCl_2$ in about 100 mg of experimental diet was given at 9 days. All diets contained 0.062 ppm of Cd. Values for ^{109}Cd are percent of dose in tissue.

† Significantly different from group fed 100 ppm of Fe^{3+}, killed at same age, $P < 0.05$.

‡ Same comparison, $P < 0.01$.

§ Significantly different from group fed same experimental diet but killed at 9 days, $P < 0.05$.

¶ Same comparison, $P < 0.01$.

fects of these treatments occurred in the jejunum-ileum. Ascorbic acid and iron(II) reduced cadmium concentration in the kidneys. Low dietary iron decreased cadmium retention by the liver; however, the combined cadmium retention of the liver and kidneys was the same as that of the control birds.

The longer duration of feeding the experimental diets before dosing with cadmium-109 (experiment 3, TABLE 3) resulted in more marked effects on tissue iron concentrations by 9 days than occurred in experiment 2. By day 16, the values for experiments 2 and 3 were more similar. In experiment 3, hemoglobin was significantly decreased by iron deficiency at 8 days and was significantly higher with ascorbic acid and iron(II) than in the controls. All hemoglobin values were higher at 16 than at 9 days. The effects of treatments on cadmium retention gave values that were similar for experiments 2 and 3, except that the values were generally higher in the jejunum-ileum in experiment 3. The cadmium in the kidneys of iron-deficient birds was significantly higher than in controls; however, the total in the liver and the kidneys was not different from that of controls. Again, both ascorbic acid and iron(II) caused marked reductions in tissue cadmium retention.

In both experiments 2 and 3, there were some statistically significant changes in tissue concentrations of zinc, magnesium, and calcium with age. Sometimes these were relatively small and were not consistent between experiments 2 and 3. A marked elevation of calcium occurred in the livers of iron-deficient birds in experiment 3.

Discussion

The purpose of these experiments was to determine whether an ascorbic acid supplement and varying iron status, which are known to affect cadmium toxicity,

Table 3

Effects of Iron and Ascorbic Acid (AA) Treatments (0–16 Days) on Tissue Mineral Concentrations and Retention of a Single Dose of ^{109}Cd Given at 9 Days (Experiment 3)*

		Dietary Treatment			
Measurement	Age (days)	25 ppm Fe^{3+} 0 AA	100 ppm Fe^{3+} 0 AA	100 ppm Fe^{3+} 0.5% AA	100 ppm Fe^{2+} 0 AA
Body Weight (g)	9	26 ± 0.4†	28 ± 0.7	28 ± 0.4	28 ± 0.7
Hb (g/100 ml)	8	6.8 ± 0.20‡	9.5 ± 0.38	10.9 ± 0.42†	11.3 ± 0.38‡
Duodenum					
Weight (mg)	9	384 ± 10†	427 ± 17	426 ± 13	475 ± 12†
Zn (ppm)		34 ± 1.3	34 ± 1.6	35 ± 1.2	35 ± 1.2
Fe (ppm)		13 ± 3	20 ± 4	290 ± 31‡	313 ± 25‡
Mg (ppm)		214 ± 2†	227 ± 4	226 ± 2	228 ± 2
Ca (ppm)		208 ± 14	245 ± 28	210 ± 19	259 ± 13
Jejunum-Ileum					
Weight (mg)	9	457 ± 18	501 ± 21	506 ± 27	485 ± 20
Zn (ppm)		23 ± 0.8	22 ± 0.7	23 ± 0.6	23 ± 0.4
Fe (ppm)		17 ± 2‡	67 ± 8	207 ± 8‡	129 ± 10‡
Mg (ppm)		225 ± 9	236 ± 5	227 ± 2	227 ± 3
Ca (ppm)		313 ± 29	275 ± 25	274 ± 26	264 ± 17
Liver					
Weight (g)	9	0.92 ± 0.03‡	1.23 ± 0.08	1.18 ± 0.03	1.15 ± 0.05
Zn (ppm)		18 ± 0.5†	20 ± 1.0	18 ± 0.5	19 ± 0.8
Fe (ppm)		35 ± 3‡	145 ± 18	321 ± 20‡	383 ± 36‡
Mg (ppm)		234 ± 4†	244 ± 3	232 ± 4†	237 ± 5
Ca (ppm)		94 ± 15	65 ± 8	48 ± 8	46 ± 4
Kidney					
Weight (mg)	9	301 ± 12†	344 ± 11	339 ± 8	347 ± 8
Zn (ppm)		17 ± 0.5	17 ± 0.2	18 ± 0.3	17 ± 0.3
Fe (ppm)		27 ± 6‡	52 ± 4	60 ± 4	75 ± 10
Mg (ppm)		204 ± 4	198 ± 2	204 ± 2	201 ± 2
Ca (ppm)		148 ± 30	88 ± 16	64 ± 7	61 ± 6
Body Weight (g)	16	47 ± 1.4¶	50 ± 1.1¶	51 ± 1.4¶	52 ± 1.9¶
Hb (g/100 ml)	15	8.5 ± 0.49‡¶	12.4 ± 0.18¶	12.9 ± 0.22¶	12.6 ± 0.46§

(*cont.*)

TABLE 3 (*cont.*)

Measurement	Age (days)	Dietary Treatment 25 ppm Fe^{3+} 0 AA	100 ppm Fe^{3+} 0 AA	100 ppm Fe^{3+} 0.5% AA	100 ppm Fe^{2+} 0 AA
Duodenum					
Weight (mg)	16	531 ± 23‡¶	634 ± 24¶	677 ± 33¶	680 ± 33¶
Zn (ppm)		33 ± 0.9	36 ± 1.6	33 ± 0.9	38 ± 1.6
Fe (ppm)		15 ± 2‡	102 ± 13¶	341 ± 31‡	305 ± 21‡
Mg (ppm)		220 ± 4†	233 ± 3	233 ± 3§	236 ± 2§
Ca (ppm)		188 ± 21	237 ± 10	242 ± 11	230 ± 20
^{109}Cd (%)		10.23 ± 1.270‡	2.70 ± 0.463	0.70 ± 0.156‡	0.79 ± 0.156
Jejunum-Ileum					
Weight (mg)	16	680 ± 25¶	679 ± 24¶	785 ± 38¶	644 ± 35¶
Zn (ppm)		27 ± 0.7¶	28 ± 0.6¶	26 ± 0.5†¶	30 ± 0.9¶
Fe (ppm)		23 ± 3‡	70 ± 6	121 ± 8‡¶	84 ± 8¶
Mg (ppm)		219 ± 3	223 ± 3§	218 ± 3§	227 ± 3
Ca (ppm)		275 ± 22	279 ± 20	286 ± 13	298 ± 22
^{109}Cd (%)		3.38 ± 0.508	3.43 ± 0.385	0.46 ± 0.104‡	1.84 ± 0.700
Liver					
Weight (g)	16	1.48 ± 0.05†¶	1.65 ± 0.05¶	1.79 ± 0.08¶	1.69 ± 0.10¶
Zn (ppm)		20 ± 0.4†¶	25 ± 1.8†	21 ± 0.6¶	23 ± 0.6¶
Fe (ppm)		30 ± 2‡	154 ± 24	245 ± 32†	294 ± 39‡
Mg (ppm)		240 ± 3	239 ± 2	229 ± 3	238 ± 5
Ca (ppm)		76 ± 13†	43 ± 7	30 ± 1§	31 ± 2§
^{109}Cd (%)		0.32 ± 0.032†	0.42 ± 0.030	0.22 ± 0.015‡	0.35 ± 0.024
Kidney					
Weight (mg)	16	534 ± 11¶	545 ± 14¶	599 ± 23¶	568 ± 38¶
Zn (ppm)		19 ± 0.1¶	19 ± 0.2¶	19 ± 0.4§	19 ± 0.4¶
Fe (ppm)		45 ± 3‡¶	78 ± 5¶	78 ± 4¶	95 ± 7
Mg (ppm)		226 ± 2¶	223 ± 2¶	219 ± 3¶	218 ± 3¶
Ca (ppm)		92 ± 15	58 ± 3	60 ± 2	55 ± 7
^{109}Cd (%)		0.73 ± 0.061†	0.53 ± 0.041	0.26 ± 0.022‡	0.42 ± 0.029
Liver & Kidney					
^{109}Cd (%)	16	1.05 ± 0.084	0.95 ± 0.065	0.48 ± 0.032‡	0.78 ± 0.049†

* Mean ± SE, 10 birds per group, killed at 9 days (no ^{109}Cd dose) and 16 days. All diets were fed 0–16 days. All diets contained 0.062 ppm of Cd. A dose of 3.4 μCi of $^{109}CdCl_2$ in about 100 mg of experimental diet was given at 9 days. Values for ^{109}Cd are percent of dose in tissue.

† Significantly different from group fed 100 ppm of Fe^{3+}, killed at same age, $P < 0.05$.

‡ Same comparison, $P < 0.01$.

§ Significantly different from group fed same experimental diet, but killed at 9 days, $P < 0.05$.

¶ Same comparison, $P < 0.01$.

could modify tissue retention of very low levels of dietary cadmium. The ascorbic acid supplement and sometimes equal weight substitution of iron(II) for iron(III) significantly reduced cadmium retention in all four of the tissues studied. Except for increased duodenal cadmium-109 retention, iron deficiency had a relatively small effect as compared with the control; however, the control level of iron was established at the required level so this group would correspond to the normal adult with no iron stores (i.e., low serum ferritin) reported in the study of Flanagan *et al.*[6]

It appears reasonable to conclude that the major, if not the only, effect of ascorbic acid on cadmium metabolism was due to the effect on improved iron absorption. TABLE 4 summarizes a variety of correlation coefficients; the data from all

TABLE 4

CORRELATION OF TISSUE IRON CONCENTRATIONS AND CADMIUM RETENTIONS—TISSUE VS. TISSUE AND 9 DAYS VS. 16 DAYS (VALUES FOR ALL TREATMENTS COMBINED, EXPERIMENTS 2 AND 3)*

Experiment	Element/Age (days)/ Tissue	r: Tissue Fe, 9 Days D	r: Tissue Fe, 9 Days JI	r: Tissue Fe, 9 Days L	r: Tissue Fe, 9 Days K	r: Tissue Fe, 16 Days D	r: Tissue Fe, 16 Days JI	r: Tissue Fe, 16 Days L	r: Tissue Fe, 16 Days K	r: Tissue Cd, 16 Days D	r: Tissue Cd, 16 Days JI	r: Tissue Cd, 16 Days L
2	**Fe, 9**											
	JI	0.566§	—	—	—	—	—	—	—	—	—	—
	L	0.555§	0.364†	—	—	—	—	—	—	—	—	—
	K	−0.021	−0.076	0.020	—	—	—	—	—	—	—	—
	Fe, 16											
	D	0.437‡	0.688§	0.409‡	0.046	—	—	—	—	—	—	—
	JI	0.359†	0.701§	0.258	0.058	0.919§	—	—	—	—	—	—
	L	0.405†	0.602§	0.367†	0.039	0.695§	0.699§	—	—	—	—	—
	K	0.437‡	0.266	0.550§	−0.067	0.470‡	0.396†	0.432‡	—	—	—	—
	Cd, 16											
	D	−0.544§	−0.601§	−0.554§	−0.187	−0.622§	−0.584§	−0.661§	−0.411‡	—	—	—
	JI	−0.428‡	−0.577§	−0.385†	0.140	−0.575§	−0.553§	−0.603§	−0.407‡	0.751§	—	—
	L	−0.155	−0.372†	−0.303	−0.102	−0.261	−0.302	−0.217	−0.111	0.285	0.359†	—
	K	−0.345†	−0.536§	−0.295	0.086	−0.448‡	−0.408‡	−0.351†	0.191	0.564§	0.597§	0.746§
3	**Fe, 9**											
	JI	0.735§	—	—	—	—	—	—	—	—	—	—
	L	0.819§	0.810§	—	—	—	—	—	—	—	—	—
	K	0.534§	0.484§	0.730§	—	—	—	—	—	—	—	—
	Fe, 16											
	D	0.816§	0.780§	0.827§	0.582§	—	—	—	—	—	—	—
	JI	0.641§	0.714§	0.590§	0.478‡	0.774§	—	—	—	—	—	—
	L	0.629§	0.570§	0.668§	0.342†	0.767§	0.670§	—	—	—	—	—
	K	0.558§	0.474‡	0.695§	0.588§	0.573§	0.502‡	0.666§	—	—	—	—
	Cd, 16											
	D	−0.610§	−0.632§	−0.702§	−0.657§	−0.691§	−0.712§	−0.658§	−0.648§	—	—	—
	JI	−0.480‡	0.505§	−0.455‡	0.328†	−0.480‡	−0.440‡	−0.221	−0.243	0.476‡	—	—
	L	−0.270	−0.302	−0.088	−0.073	−0.315†	−0.358†	0.232	0.090	0.111	0.457‡	—
	K	−0.573§	0.670§	−0.688§	−0.409‡	−0.745§	−0.817§	−0.664§	−0.432‡	0.798§	0.491‡	0.540§

* All correlation coefficients are for four groups of birds, N = 36–40. See first footnotes of TABLES 2 and 3. Abbreviations for tissues: D, duodenum, JI, jejunum-ileum; L, liver; K, kidney. † $P < 0.05$. ‡ $P < 0.01$. § $P < 0.001$.

four treatments were pooled by experiment for experiments 2 and 3. Except for some of the data for the kidneys in experiment 2, there were significant correlations of iron concentrations between tissues at 9 days, at 16 days, and between 9 and 16 days. The kidney responded less sensitively and more slowly than did the liver to changes in iron status (TABLES 2 and 3). In all cases, there was a significant negative correlation between iron concentration in the two small-intestinal segments and their retention of cadmium-109. There were relatively few significant negative correlations of tissue iron concentrations with cadmium retention in liver; however, most corresponding correlations for the kidney were statistically significant.

The virtual absence of changes in tissue zinc and calcium, two elements known to affect cadmium absorption and toxicity, is further evidence of the specificity of the iron effect. Higher calcium levels in livers of iron-deficient birds (experiment 3) have been observed previously in Japanese quail fed 75 ppm of cadmium or a low iron diet.[31] This might be indicative of a change in mitochondrial metabolism; however, there was no change in liver magnesium.

The data show that iron status can influence intestinal uptake and transport of low levels of cadmium to the two organs that typically contain the highest concentrations of this toxic element, the liver and the kidney. Iron deficiency appeared to accelerate movement of cadmium from the liver to the kidney; however, data are needed on the cadmium content of the residual carcass to help establish this mechanism.

Although the absorption and transport of iron appear to influence cadmium absorption and metabolism, further studies are needed to identify intestinal sites and chemical species involved in these processes. One of the highest negative correlations

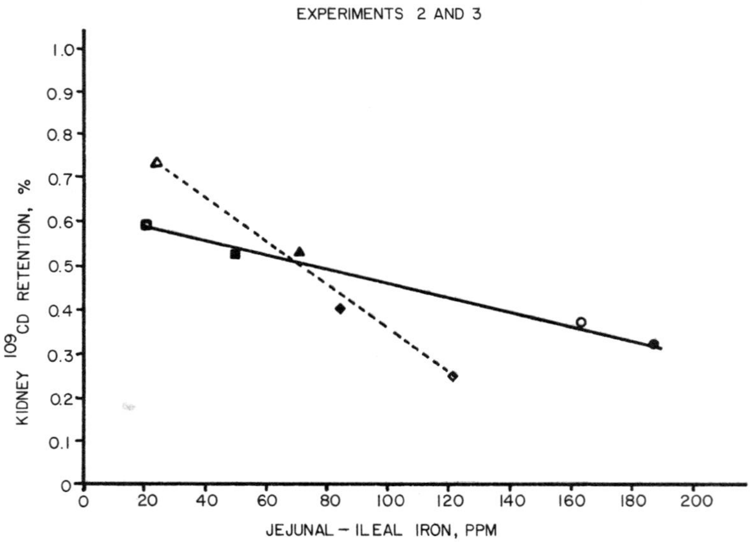

FIGURE 1. The relationship of iron in the jejunum-ileum at 16 days to the retention of cadmium-109 in the kidney by 16 days. For experiment 2 (treatments 7–16 days): ——; □, 25 ppm of Fe^{3+} in the diet; ■, 100 ppm of Fe^{3+} (control); ○, 100 ppm of Fe^{3+} plus 0.5% ascorbic acid; ●, 100 ppm of Fe^{2+}. For experiment 3 (treatments 0–16 days): - - - -; △, 25 ppm of Fe^{3+}; ▲, 100 ppm of Fe^{3+} (control); ◇, 100 ppm of Fe^{3+} plus 0.5% ascorbic acid; ◆, 100 ppm of Fe^{2+}. The equations describing the lines for the means were as follows: experiment 2, $Y = -0.00162X + 0.61904$, $r = 0.999$; experiment 3, $Y = -0.00845X + 0.84653$, $r = 0.996$. Based on individual values, the lines were significantly different, $P < 0.0001$.

was for iron in the jejunum-ileum and cadmium in the kidney (experiment 3). The data for the four treatments from experiments 2 and 3 are shown in FIGURE 1. From these data, it appears that changes of iron status of longer duration (experiment 3) had a more profound effect on kidney cadmium retention (TABLE 4). This effect may have resulted from iron status at the time of cadmium ingestion or may reflect a systemic effect of iron status well after the time of cadmium ingestion. Iron and ascorbic acid may have accelerated cadmium excretion in the urine. The localization of cadmium within the intestinal tissue is not established; however, significant amounts of cadmium remain beyond the period during which epithelial cells would be expected to have been shed. It is not known whether the cadmium from sloughed cells may be taken up by a more distal segment of the intestine.

It has been known for many years that large amounts of cadmium can bind to ferritin *in vitro*. When Stonard and Webb injected 1 mg of cadmium as the chloride/kg of body weight into rats, ferritin isolated from the liver contained 2.5 g atom of cadmium/mole of ferritin, approximately 0.1% of the average iron content.[40] It is not known whether the uptake and absorption of the small amounts of cadmium fed in this study may have involved binding to intestinal ferritin. If the cadmium were bound to ferritin, iron status could be expected to affect cadmium uptake and transport. It is also possible that iron status may influence the level of other cadmium-binding proteins in the intestinal tract.

The ascorbic acid fed in this study represents a level higher than that typically consumed by humans. This level of ascorbic acid produced changes in tissue iron status similar to those elicited by substituting an equivalent amount of iron(II) for iron(III). Iron(II) as the sulfate is utilized about twice as effectively by the young quail as is iron(III) as the citrate (unpublished data). The birds fed the iron(II) might be considered the equivalent of a person with an adequate iron intake who takes a daily supplement of iron(II) equal to the day's requirement.

SUMMARY

Toxic levels of dietary cadmium (5–200 ppm) interfered with iron absorption and produced an iron deficiency. Supplements of iron (particularly the divalent form) and ascorbic acid protected against the cadmium. With very low levels of dietary cadmium (about 0.06–0.08 ppm), typical of those in the diets of humans, supplements of iron(II) and ascorbic acid markedly decreased cadmium concentrations in the liver, kidney, and small intestine. Iron deficiency changed the distribution of cadmium within the body. The effect of ascorbic acid on cadmium metabolism appears to depend primarily, if not entirely, on its influence in improving iron absorption. Maintenance of modest iron stores appears to be very important in minimizing cadmium absorption.

ACKNOWLEDGMENTS

The authors are grateful to Ms. Mildred Johnson for her superior technical assistance and to Mr. James Etherith for care of the animals.

REFERENCES

1. MAHAFFEY, K. R., P. E. CORNELIUSSEN, C. F. JELINEK & J. A. FIORINO. 1975. Environ. Health Perspect. **12:** 63–69.

2. Joint FAO/WHO Expert Committee on Food Additives. 1972. WHO Tech. Rep. Ser. **505:** 20–24, 32.
3. Friberg, L., M. Piscator & G. Nordberg. 1971. Cadmium in the Environment. CRC Press. Cleveland, Ohio.
4. Mason, K. E., M. E. Richardson & M. R. S. Fox. 1977. Fed. Proc. Fed. Am. Soc. Exp. Biol. **36:** 1152.
5. Campbell, J. K. & C. F. Mills. 1974. Proc. Nutr. Soc. **33:** 15A–17A.
6. Flanagan, P. R., J. S. McLellan, J. Haist, M. G. Cherian & M. J. Chamberlain. 1978. Gastroenterology **74:** 841–846.
7. Fox, M. R. S. 1974. J. Food Sci. **39:** 321–324.
8. Fox, M. R. S. 1975. Ann. N.Y. Acad. Sci. **258:** 144–150.
9. Fox, M. R. S. 1979. Environ. Health Perspect. **29:** 95–104.
10. Bremner, I. 1978. World Rev. Nutr. Diet. **32:** 165–197.
11. Jacobs, R. M., A. O. L. Jones, M. R. S. Fox & B. E. Fry, Jr. 1978. J. Nutr. **108:** 22–32.
12. Jacobs, R. M., A. O. L. Jones, B. E. Fry, Jr. & M. R. S. Fox. 1978. J. Nutr. **108:** 901–910.
13. Jacobs, R. M., M. R. S. Fox, A. O. L. Jones, R. P. Hamilton & J. Lener. 1977. Fed. Proc. Fed. Am. Soc. Exp. Biol. **36:** 1152.
14. Fox, M. R. S., R. M. Jacobs, A. O. L. Jones & B. E. Fry, Jr. 1979. Environ. Health Perspect. **28:** 107–114.
15. Wilson, R. H., F. Deeds & W. H. Cox, Jr. 1941. J. Pharmacol. Exp. Ther. **71:** 222–235.
16. Banis, R. J., W. G. Pond, E. F. Walker, Jr. & J. R. O'Connor. 1969. Proc. Soc. Exp. Biol. Med. **103:** 802–806.
17. Bunn, C. R. & G. Matrone. 1966. J. Nutr. **90:** 395–399.
18. Stowe, H. D., M. Wilson & R. A. Goyer. 1972. Arch. Pathol. **94:** 389–405.
19. Hill, C. H., G. Matrone, W. L. Payne & C. W. Barber. 1963. J. Nutr. **80:** 227–235.
20. Freeland, J. H. & R. J. Cousins. 1973. Nutr. Rep. Int. **8:** 337–347.
21. Jacobs, R. M., M. R. S. Fox & M. H. Aldridge. 1969. J. Nutr. **99:** 119–128.
22. Powell, G. W., W. J. Miller, J. D. Morton & C. M. Clifton. 1964. J. Nutr. **84:** 205–214.
23. Friberg, L. 1950. Acta Med. Scand. Suppl. **138** (240).
24. Webster, W. S. 1978. Arch. Environ. Health **33:** 36–42.
25. Doyle, J. J. & W. H. Pfander. 1975. J. Nutr. **105:** 599–606.
26. Petering, H. G., H. Choudhury & K. L. Stemmer. 1979. Environ. Health Perspect. **28:** 97–106.
27. Hamilton, D. L. & L. S. Valberg. 1974. Am. J. Physiol. **227:** 1033–1037.
28. Jacobs, R. M., M. R. S. Fox, B. E. Fry, Jr. & B. F. Harland. 1974. *In* Trace Element Metabolism in Animals. W. G. Hoekstra, J. W. Suttie, H. E. Ganther & W. Mertz, Eds. **2:** 684–685. University Park Press. Baltimore, Md.
29. Valberg, L. S., J. Sorbie & D. L. Hamilton. 1976. Am. J. Physiol. **231:** 462–467.
30. Ragan, H. A. 1977. J. Lab. Clin. Med. **90:** 700–705.
31. Fox, M. R. S., B. E. Fry, Jr., M. E. Schertel & C. E. Weeks. 1971. J. Nutr. **101:** 1295–1306.
32. Pond, W. G. & E. F. Walker, Jr. 1972. Nutr. Rep. Int. **5:** 365–370.
33. Pond, W. G., E. F. Walker, Jr. & D. Kirtland. 1973. J. Anim. Sci. **36:** 1122–1128.
34. Sansi, K. A. O. & W. G. Pond. 1974. Nutr. Rep. Int. **9:** 407–414.
35. Fox, M. R. S. & B. E. Fry, Jr. 1970. Science **169:** 989–991.
36. Maji, T. & A. Yoshida. 1974. Nutr. Rep. Int. **10:** 139–149.
37. Richardson, M. E., M. R. S. Fox & B. E. Fry, Jr. 1974. J. Nutr. **104:** 323–338.
38. Fox, M. R. S., R. M. Jacobs, B. E. Fry, Jr. & B. F. Harland. 1973. Fed. Proc. Fed. Am. Soc. Exp. Biol. **32:** 924.
39. Steel, R. G. D. & J. H. Torrie. 1960. Principles and Procedures of Statistics. McGraw-Hill Book Co. New York, N.Y.
40. Stonard, M. D. & M. Webb. 1976. Chem. Biol. Interact. **15:** 349–363.

Discussion

W. G. Hoekstra (*University of Wisconsin, Madison, Wis.*): Is there any evidence for a direct effect of ascorbate in reducing cadmium uptake into the body?

M. R. S. Fox: Well, I think it's an effect on iron primarily; we don't have any evidence for any other effect.

S. R. Lynch (*University of Kansas Medical Center, Kansas City, Kans.*): Do you have any idea of the form of the cadmium in the duodenum and how long it may remain there?

M. R. S. Fox: No, we don't know the form. From data with soy protein diets, we know that the concentrations in the duodenum and in the jejunum-ileum are maximal by four hours after a single dose of cadmium-109. With respect to tissue concentrations of iron in the two small-intestinal segments, we got the best correlation between iron in the jejunum-ileum and cadmium uptake in the kidney.

W. G. Hoekstra: Would Ian Bremner care to comment on the form of cadmium in the intestine?

I. Bremner (*Rowett Research Institute, Bucksburn, Aberdeen, United Kingdom*): I kind of suspect that the cadmium must be there in metallothioneins. However, I think that it's fair to say that no one has ever characterized the cadmium-binding protein in the gut.

M. R. S. Fox: Also, I don't think anyone has looked at bound forms of cadmium in the intestinal tract with a very low intake of cadmium, which may be different. There is a tremendous difference between the cadmium:iron molar ratio in the intestinal mucosa and that in the kidney.

I. Bremner: I think that's a valid point that is very important. Can I ask your opinion of the work of Flanagan *et al.* that shows the effects of serum ferritin on cadmium retention. How do you think these differences reflect the sex distribution in the two groups?

M. R. S. Fox: Well, there were both men and women in each group, but there were more women in the group with the lower ferritin levels. So sex may be a factor.

H. Sprince (*Veterans Administration Medical Center, Coatesville, Penn.*): I think I ran across a paper wherein cadmium toxicity was prevented by ascorbic acid and the effect was enhanced by zinc.

M. R. S. Fox: I don't remember the paper, but it wouldn't be too surprising. Zinc, copper, iron, and calcium all have been implicated in decreasing the toxicity of cadmium.

J. Parizek (*Czechoslovak Academy of Sciences, Prague, Czechoslovakia*): You have said that iron as well as vitamin C influences both the absorption and the retention of cadmium. Do you have any evidence that points to an effect on half-life?

M. R. S. Fox: No, we don't.

INTERACTIONS OF VITAMIN C WITH LEAD AND MERCURY

C. H. Hill

Department of Poultry Science
North Carolina State University
Raleigh, North Carolina 27607

Ascorbic acid has been found by several investigators to influence mineral metabolism. We found that ascorbic acid increased the severity of the symptoms of copper deficiency, suggesting that the availability of this element was decreased.[1] The results of subsequent studies in which toxic levels of various elements were used indicated that the availability of several elements was decreased by ascorbic acid because ascorbic acid reduced their toxicity.[2] Fox *et al.* have suggested that the reduction in cadmium toxicity by ascorbic acid is indirect and is mediated by the action of the vitamin in reducing ferric to ferrous iron.[3]

In view of the fact that ascorbic acid affects the availability of several elements, it would not be surprising if it were to interact also with lead and mercury either directly or indirectly through an effect on iron metabolism. It has been found by Six and Goyer and Klauder and Petering, for instance, that dietary iron can have an effect on lead metabolism.[4,5] The former workers found that lead retention was increased in the liver, kidney, and bone of rats fed an iron-deficient diet and suggested that this might be the result of increased lead absorption. The latter workers found that both iron deficiency and copper deficiency exacerbated some of the toxic effects of lead in rats.

There has been little experimental evidence until recently on the effect of ascorbic acid on lead toxicity, but some clinical studies have suggested that the vitamin might ameliorate this condition. Holmes *et al.* reported in 1939 that painters who presented a clinical picture of lead poisoning were cured of their symptoms by the daily administration of 100 mg of ascorbic acid.[6] Marchmont-Robinson treated workers exposed to lead with 50 mg of ascorbic acid per day and reported that the workers felt better.[7] Another, more recent report found that treatment with 2 g of ascorbic acid plus 60 mg of zinc per day reduced the blood lead levels of battery workers from toxic values to safe levels.[8] These clinical findings, then, suggested that ascorbic acid might play a role in reducing the availability of lead.

In a direct experimental approach, Suzuki and Yoshida studied the interaction of iron and ascorbic acid with lead in rats.[9] In their studies, they used dietary levels of 500 parts per million lead fed as the acetate, 1% ascorbic acid, and 400 ppm ferrous iron. They found that the combination of ascorbic acid and iron prevented the growth depression and anemia associated with the administration of lead. Furthermore, the lead concentrations in the liver, kidney, and tibia were reduced by this treatment.

In experiments in which iron and ascorbic acid were tested separately, Suzuki and Yoshida found that the beneficial effects as far as lead toxicity was concerned resided entirely with the iron. Iron, alone, increased the growth and prevented the anemia associated with lead feeding. Iron, alone, decreased the amount of lead in the liver and kidney. In further work, these authors found that dietary iron and ascorbic acid had almost no curative effect on established lead toxicity.[10]

In work with chicks conducted in our laboratories, a factorial experiment was

0077-8923/80/0355-0262 $01.75/0

devised to examine the effect of 0.5% ascorbic acid and 1,000 ppm ferrous iron and the combination of the two on the toxicity of 500 ppm lead fed as the chloride. At this level within this time, 500 ppm lead did not result in significantly reduced growth. There was a significant interaction between lead and iron indicative of the fact that growth was increased when iron was added to the lead-containing diet. There was no interaction between ascorbic acid and lead. More important than growth is the finding that iron reduced the lead concentration in the femur and kidney while ascorbic acid had no such effect on the femur and only a moderate effect on the kidney. The experiment with chicks, then, is in accord with those reported by Suzuki and Yoshida[10] in that iron, but not ascorbic acid, reduced the toxic effects of lead.

It would appear from the results presented here that the interaction between lead and ascorbic acid is tenuous indeed. While some clinical reports suggest a possible interaction, experimental studies fail to disclose any in spite of the fact that they do disclose an interaction between lead and iron.

There has been some presumptive evidence of an interrelationship between ascorbic acid and mercury for some time. As long ago as 1840, a London physician noted that scorbutic symptoms were very much aggravated by mercury taken before the scorbutic symptoms made their appearance.[11] The experimental evidence for the interaction between mercury and ascorbic acid rests on very few experiments. In the work of ours referred to previously, ascorbic acid seemed to have a marginal effect in overcoming mercury toxicity in chicks.[2] In subsequent work, a factorial experiment was designed to investigate the effect of both ascorbic acid and iron on mercury toxicity. The growth depression caused by feeding 500 ppm mercury was partially overcome by 0.5% ascorbic acid but not by 1,000 ppm iron. The interaction between mercury and ascorbic acid was statistically significant, as was that between mercury and iron; but in the latter case, added iron resulted in an even greater growth inhibition when mercury was present. The three-way interaction between mercury, iron, and ascorbic acid was also significant, indicating that in the presence of added iron, ascorbic acid was less effective in overcoming mercury toxicity. These findings clearly show that there is an effect of ascorbic acid on mercury metabolism that is evidently not mediated through iron metabolism.

While one might surmise that mercury absorption and/or retention might be decreased under the influence of ascorbic acid, the evidence that exists disputes that supposition. Murray and Hughes reported that ascorbic acid in the drinking water increased the amount of mercury in the liver, brain, and kidneys of guinea pigs given $HgCl_2$ orally but not when the element was injected.[12]

The results of the studies with lead and mercury are in contrast to those reported previously in which both ferrous iron and ascorbic acid were effective in overcoming cadmium toxicity.[3] In the case of lead toxicity, iron but not ascorbic acid is effective, while in the case of mercury, ascorbic acid but not iron is effective in overcoming the toxicity.

In view of these results, it seemed appropriate to examine the interaction of ascorbic acid and iron with cadmium in the chick model. In an experiment in which 400 ppm iron were fed either as the ferric or ferrous form, no difference was found in the degree of cadmium toxicity as measured by growth retardation. Moreover, 0.1% ascorbic acid increased the gain over the cadmium-fed chicks equally with the two forms of iron.[2] On the other hand, the ferrous iron protected against the anemia induced by cadmium, and ascorbic acid added to the ferric iron–containing diet also prevented the cadmium-induced anemia. The results with the hemoglobin changes are in accord with the results reported by Fox *et al.* with Japanese quail, while the results of the growth studies are not.[3]

When the level of iron fed was increased from 400 ppm to 1,000 ppm, it was found that the ferrous iron was much more effective in overcoming the cadmium-induced growth depression than was ferric iron, but ascorbic acid added to the ferric iron-containing diet did not result in an increased growth and actually seemed to result in less growth. While the ferrous iron was effective in preventing cadmium-induced anemia, the addition of ascorbic acid to the ferric-containing diets did not result in a reversal of the anemia. At this level of iron supplementation, then, both the growth and hemoglobin changes are in accord with those reported by Fox *et al.*[3] However, from these results, it seems unlikely that the effect of ascorbic acid in reversing cadmium toxicity in chicks is related to a conversion of ferric to ferrous iron.

Since we had found that the toxicities of selenium, cobalt, vanadium, and copper were reversed by ascorbic acid, it was of interest to determine whether or not they could also be reversed by ferrous iron. In an experiment designed to test this, we found that only copper toxicity was significantly reduced by 400 ppm iron. The effects of greater levels of iron have yet to be tested.

As a result of the studies presented in this report, we would have to conclude that ascorbic acid does counteract the toxic effects of many elements, including mercury, but not of lead. While iron in the ferrous form is effective in counteracting the toxicity of cadmium as well as that of copper or lead, the effect of ascorbic acid appears to be independent of the iron effect.

It is possible that ascorbic acid has a much more direct effect on the elements studied. Lewin has proposed that high dietary levels of ascorbic acid might result in increased urinary excretion of cations to balance the excretion of the ascorbate anion and thus increase the rate of elimination of toxic elements.[13] This proposal was based on physicochemical considerations only and was not tested biologically. Ascorbic acid does form complexes with many biologically important elements, and it is possible that in some instances, the ascorbic acid-metal complex is absorbed and/or excreted differently from the metal alone.

Summary

Ascorbic acid has been found to interact with several elements in such a manner as to render them less available for animals. This property of the vitamin has a negative effect on the animals fed a copper-deficient diet, but a positive effect on those fed toxic levels of copper, selenium, vanadium, and cobalt. The effect of ascorbic acid in alleviating cadmium toxicity has been attributed to the effect of the vitamin on iron metabolism, since ferrous iron will also alleviate cadmium toxicity in the Japanese quail. The results of studies reported here indicate that iron will alleviate lead toxicity but ascorbic acid is ineffective. Ascorbic acid will alleviate mercury toxicity, but iron exacerbates this condition. For these two elements, the effects of iron and ascorbic acid are independent of each other.

References

1. Hill, C. H. & B. Starcher. 1965. Effect of reducing agents on copper deficiency in the chick. J. Nutr. **85**(3): 271–274.
2. Hill, C. H. 1979. Studies on the ameliorating effect of ascorbic acid on mineral toxicities in the chick. J. Nutr. **109**(1): 84–90.
3. Fox, M. R. S., B. E. Fry, Jr., B. F. Harland, M. E. Schertel & C. E. Weeks. 1971.

Effect of ascorbic acid on cadmium toxicity in the young coturnix. J. Nutr. **101**(10): 1295–1305.
4. SIX, K. M. & R. A. GOYER. 1972. The influence of iron deficiency on tissue content and toxicity of ingested lead in the rat. J. Lab. Clin. Med. **79:** 128–136.
5. KLAUDER, D. S. & H. G. PETERING. 1977. Anemia of lead intoxication: a role for copper. J. Nutr. **107**(10): 1779–1785.
6. HOLMES, H. N., K. CAMPBELL & E. J. AMBERG. 1939. The effect of vitamin C on lead poisoning. J. Lab. Clin. Med. **24:** 1119–1127.
7. MARCHMONT-ROBINSON, S. W. 1941. Effect of vitamin C on workers exposed to lead dust. J. Lab. Clin. Med. **26:** 1478–1481.
8. PAPAIDAMNOU, R., A. SOHLER & C. C. PFEIFFER. 1978. Reduction of blood lead levels in battery workers by zinc and vitamin C. J. Orthomed. Psychiatry **7**(2): 94–106.
9. SUZUKI, T. & A. YOSHIDA. 1979. Effectiveness of dietary iron and ascorbic acid in the prevention and cure of moderately long-term lead toxicity. J. Nutr. **109**(11): 1974–1978.
10. SUZUKI, T. & A. YOSHIDA. 1979. Effect of dietary supplementation of iron and ascorbic acid on lead toxicity in rats. J. Nutr. **109**(6): 982–988.
11. HUGHES, R. E. 1974. Nutritional interactions between vitamin C and heavy metals. *In* Vitamin C. G. C. Birch & K. Parker, Eds.: 68–77. John Wiley & Sons, Inc. New York, N.Y.
12. MURRAY, D. R. & R. E. HUGHES. 1976. The influence of dietary ascorbic acid on the concentration of mercury in guinea pig tissues. (abst.) Proc. Nutr. Soc. **35:** 118–119.
13. LEWIN, S. 1973. Evaluation of potential effects of high intake of ascorbic acid. Comp. Biochem. Physiol. B. **46:** 427–441.

DISCUSSION

W. G. HOEKSTRA (*University of Wisconsin, Madison, Wis.*): Have you followed up the effects of ascorbate on selenium toxicity at all? Do you have any idea about at what stage it's affecting selenium toxicity?

C. H. HILL: What I suspect happens is that selenium given as selenite could well be reduced in the diet by high levels of ascorbic acid.

W. G. HOEKSTRA: To elemental selenium.

C. H. HILL: To elemental selenium, and therefore not absorbed. This certainly happens in test tubes.

W. G. HOEKSTRA: You haven't measured selenium?

C. H. HILL: No.

H. SPRINCE (*Veterans Administration Medical Center, Coatesville, Penn.*): Have I heard you correctly, namely, that ascorbic acid can protect against mercury but not against lead?

C. H. HILL: Right.

H. SPRINCE: The question arises whether mercury or lead is more lipophilic with respect to cell membrane. Also, would it be worthwhile considering something like dehydroascorbic acid?

C. H. HILL: I don't know which is more lipophilic, and I can't answer the second question either.

W. G. HOEKSTRA: I think that is certainly an area we should know more about at some time. Dr. Ganther?

H. E. GANTHER (*University of Wisconsin, Madison, Wis.*): Dr. Hill, I wondered if you said selenate or selenite when you were describing the methods used.

C. H. HILL: I was using selenite.

H. E. GANTHER: There is an interesting distinction between the reduction of these two forms of selenium by ascorbic acid. At least we find that if you treat with ascorbic acid, you can reduce selenite quite readily to elemental selenium, whereas selenate stays in solution.

W. G. HOEKSTRA: Have you studied the effects of ascorbate on methylmercury toxicity, or has anyone that you know?

C. H. HILL: I do not know that anyone has.

REACTION OF NITRITE WITH VITAMINS C AND E

Steven R. Tannenbaum

Department of Nutrition and Food Science
Massachusetts Institute of Technology
Cambridge, Massachusetts 02139

William Mergens

Hoffmann-La Roche, Inc.
Nutley, New Jersey 07110

INTRODUCTION

N-Nitroso compounds may be formed whenever a nitrosating agent interacts with a suitable secondary or tertiary nitrogen compound under favorable reaction conditions. The variety of nitrogen compounds susceptible to this process is very large, and nitrosamines have been found in an amazing array of products, including foods, beverages, industrial products, agricultural chemicals, tobacco and tobacco smoke, drugs and pharmaceuticals, and cosmetics.

The same process that leads to the formation of *N*-nitroso compounds in the exogenous environment of man can yield similar products in his endogenous environment, particularly the mouth, gastrointestinal tract, and infected bladder. This process of endogenous nitrosamine formation has recently been discussed in detail.[1]

Why are *N*-nitroso compounds important? Many members of this class (e.g., *N*-nitrosodimethylamine) have been shown to be carcinogens in animals (Reference 2), and they are strongly suspected to be carcinogens in man.

If *N*-nitroso compounds are toxicologically significant, then it is important to prevent their formation through elimination of one or both of the reactants or through prevention of the reactions leading to their formation. Many types of compounds can function in this manner, but two compounds in particular, ascorbic acid and α-tocopherol, have the unique property of being both vitamins and effective blocking agents for nitrosation reactions. As will be seen, their vitamin function is unrelated to their blocking function. It will also be shown how the pair can synergistically inhibit nitrosation in multiphase systems, a desirable characteristic for foods and for the lumen of the gastrointestinal tract.

ASCORBIC ACID AND NITRITE

The chemistry of nitrite is complex and will not be discussed at length in this paper. Some of the key equilibria for conversion of nitrite to a nitrosating agent are shown below (nitrosating agents are italicized):[3]

$$NO_2^- \rightleftharpoons HNO_2 \qquad pKa = 3.4$$
$$HNO_2 + H^+ \rightleftharpoons \mathit{H_2NO_2^+}$$
$$2HNO_2 \rightleftharpoons \mathit{N_2O_3} + H_2O$$
$$HNO_2 + HX \rightleftharpoons \mathit{NOX} + H_2O \qquad (X = \text{halide or pseudohalide})$$
$$2NO_2 \rightleftharpoons \mathit{N_2O_4}$$

0077-8923/80/0355-0267 $01.75/0

Ascorbic acid reacts with all of these nitrosating agents, as first shown by Dahn and coworkers, who studied the reaction under anaerobic conditions.[4] The utility of ascorbic acid as an *in vivo* blocking agent was demonstrated by Mirvish and coworkers, and application to animals and foods was rapidly demonstrated.[5-8] Since then a large number of papers have followed that demonstrate the applicability of ascorbic acid in a variety of systems.

The utility of ascorbic acid is complicated by its chemistry in the presence of oxygen:[9]

$$\text{amine} + N_2O_3 \rightarrow \text{nitrosamine} + NO_2^- + H^+$$
$$\text{ascorbate} + N_2O_3 \rightarrow \text{dehydroascorbate} + 2NO + 2H_2O$$
$$2NO + O_2 \rightarrow 2NO_2 \rightarrow N_2O_4$$
$$\text{ascorbate} + O_2 \rightarrow \text{dehydroascorbate} + H_2O_2$$
$$2H_2O_2 \rightarrow 2H_2O + O_2$$
$$\text{etc.}$$

Because of the complexity of this chemistry, substantially more ascorbic acid is required for complete blocking of nitrosation than is stoichiometrically necessary under anaerobic conditions. This is illustrated in FIGURES 1 and 2. In FIGURE 1, the rate of nitrosation of morpholine is given as a function of the ratio of ascorbate to nitrite for both aerobic and anaerobic conditions. The fact that oxygen controls the stoichiometry is demonstrated by the fact that sparging air or O_2 into the system increased the amount of ascorbate required for complete inhibition of nitrosation to the order of two moles of ascorbate per mole of nitrite.

To explain these findings, we compared the rates of oxidation of ascorbic acid by nitrite in the absence and presence of air. Typical results at pH 4.0 are shown in

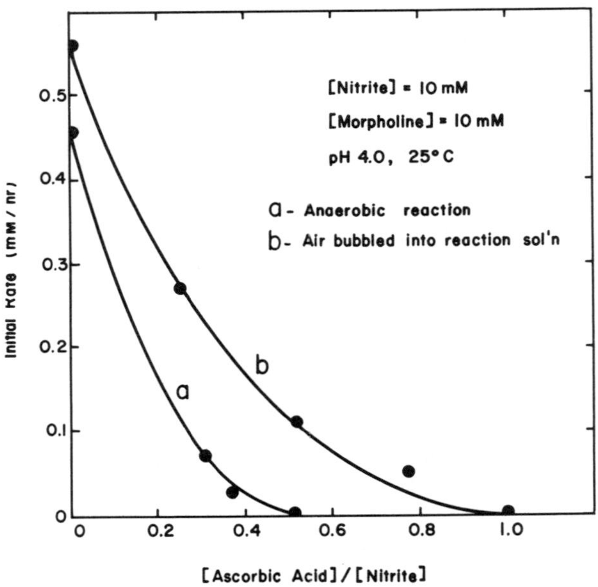

FIGURE 1. Effect of concentration ratio of ascorbic acid to nitrite on the rate of nitrosation of morpholine under aerobic and anaerobic conditions.

FIGURE 2. Under anaerobic conditions, equimolar concentrations of ascorbate and nitrite led to oxidation of only half the ascorbate, as would be expected from the previously established stoichiometry. In the presence of air (bubbled via Pasteur pipette), reaction of 10 mM nitrite with 10 mM ascorbate led to complete oxidation of the ascorbate. This observation may be explained by reaction with oxygen of nitric oxide produced during the oxidation of ascorbate by nitrite, which leads to formation of additional oxidizing equivalents (nitrogen dioxide). The presence of oxygen in the system could also lead to direct oxidation of the ascorbate semiquinone intermediate, which is produced in the initial step of the oxidation by nitrous acid.[10] This would again lead to oxidation of more than half a mole of ascorbic acid by one mole of nitrous acid.

In systems that are above pH 5, nitrite ion and ascorbate can coexist because the reactive species is N_2O_3, and the formation of N_2O_3 is the rate-limiting step in the overall reaction. However, since ascorbate reacts with N_2O_3 far more rapidly than with most amines, no nitrosamines will be formed as long as excess ascorbate is present in the system. Problems may arise when more than one phase is involved, as will be discussed later on in this paper.

α-TOCOPHEROL AS A BLOCKING AGENT

The action of vitamin E as a blocking agent against nitrosamine formation is finding increased use in a number of *in vivo* and *in vitro* applications. In contrast to ascorbic acid, α-tocopherol functions in the lipid phase to scavenge nitrosating agents. However, quite like ascorbic acid, it is presently believed that the role of tocopherol in preventing nitrosamine formation is one of a competitive reaction vs. a susceptible amine for available nitrosating agent. Several studies have demonstrated its utility in bacon and bacon model systems to prevent the formation of nitrosopyr-

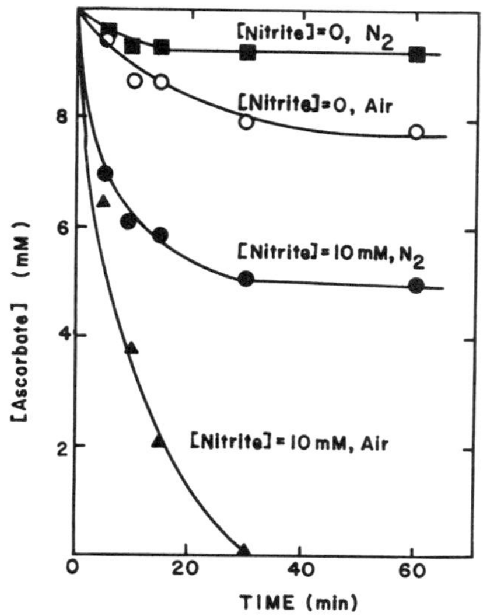

FIGURE 2. Oxidation of 10 mM ascorbic acid under aerobic and anaerobic conditions by 10 mM nitrite at pH 4.0 and 25 °C.

rolidine.[11-14] Fiddler *et al.* have shown that the formation of nitrosopyrrolidine takes place primarily in the adipose tissue of bacon.[15]

Using the rat as a model, Kamm *et al.* evaluated the effect of α-tocopherol and other related compounds on the hepatotoxicity induced by the feeding of aminopyrine and sodium nitrite.[16] The simultaneous incorporation of approximately 1.2 moles of α-tocopherol per mole of nitrite with the feeding regimen was found to totally ameliorate hepatotoxicity. In addition, α-tocopherol was somewhat more effective than was the equivalent amount of γ-tocopherol. α-Tocopherolquinone, the first oxidation product of α-tocopherol, was ineffective in preventing hepatotoxicity.

α-Tocopherol and its related compounds are essentially insoluble in water. In order to facilitate dispersion of these compounds into the stomach contents of the rat, special water-dispersible forms were prepared. The oils were individually emulsified in water, using a food grade "dextrin"-type emulsification agent, and subsequently spray dried to yield a free-flowing solid that contained 33% by weight to test compound.

Reaction of α-Tocopherol with Nitrite

In support of the hypothesis that the mechanism of nitrosamine inhibition by α-tocopherol is one of competition with the amine for the nitrosating agent, Kamm *et al.* reported on an *in vitro* model system in which *dl*-α-tocopherol (8.0 mM) was reacted with sodium nitrite (7.0 mM) at 37 °C in simulated gastric fluid.[16] α-Tocopherol was dispersed in the medium using a sixfold weight excess of polyoxyethylene sorbitan 20, monolaurate (Tween 20), which itself is unreactive toward nitrite. When the results are plotted as mole fraction vs. time (Figure 3), one observes the disappearance of nitrite and the simultaneous formation of α-tocopherolquinone. In this system, tocoquinone was the only observed reaction product. To a first approximation, the results would indicate that one mole of tocopherol consumes one mole of nitrite. This might not be true, since during the ex-

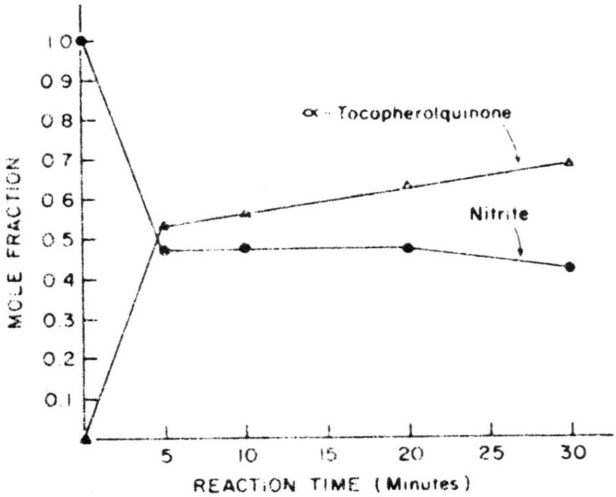

Figure 3. Disappearance of nitrite and formation of α-tocopherolquinone from simulated gastric fluid (pH 1.3) containing nitrite (7.0 mM) and α-tocopherol (8.0 mM). Each point is the mean for duplicate determinations. The results are typical of two separate experiments.

periment, no precautions were taken to eliminate oxygen. If the product of the reaction of tocopherol with nitrite is nitric oxide (NO), as is suspected, then a distinct possibility exists for NO to be reoxidized to NO_2. This regeneration of additional nitrosating capacity would make mole ratio calculations uncertain.

More recently, additional studies have been performed on the α-tocopherol reaction with nitrite.[17] α-Tocopherol dissolved in petroleum ether was allowed to react under a nitrogen atmosphere with an equimolar amount of sodium nitrite dissolved in 0.1 N HCl. After 24 hours at 37 °C, the headspace gas was injected directly into the inlet of a thermal energy analyzer (TEA) (response specific for NO), and a substantial response was measured. Similarly, headspace gases of control samples containing tocopherol alone and nitrite alone were analyzed. No TEA response was observed for the tocopherol control, and only a small response (0.10 of the tocopherol plus nitrite test sample) for the nitrite control. Theoretically, nitrogen dioxide should not respond to the TEA. It does appear, however, that at least some NO_2 or N_2O_3 is pyrolytically converted to NO.[18] The headspace gas from the tocopherol-nitrite mixture remained colorless. Upon transferring 1 ml of headspace gas to a vessel containing oxygen, the gas turned brown. These results strongly suggest that the reaction product of nitrite with tocopherol is nitric oxide. Analysis of the tocopherol reaction products in the petroleum ether phase indicated the presence of tocored and another compound, possibly the paraquinone. No tocoquinone was observed. John and Empte have shown that α-tocopherol is oxidized successively to α-tocopherolquinone, α-tocored, and the yellow paraquinone by nitric acid (FIGURE 4).[19] The presence of tocored has been confirmed in our studies by gas chromatog-

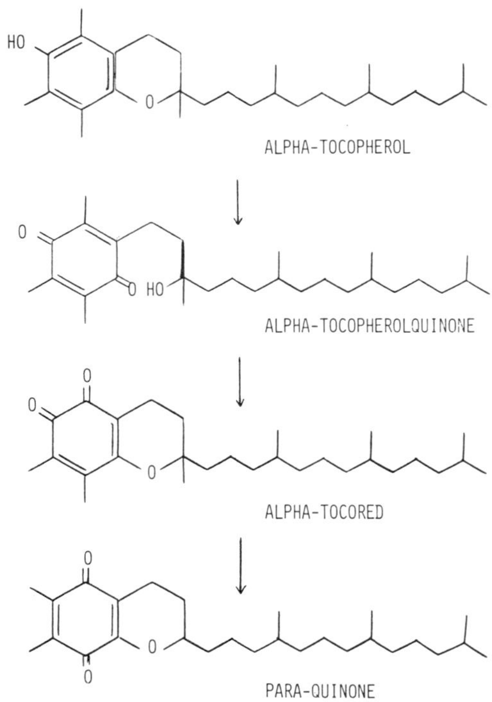

FIGURE 4. Products of α-tocopherol oxidation by nitric acid. (John and Empte, Reference 19.)

raphy–mass spectrometry. The identification of the paraquinone remains to be proven. In view of the sequence of oxidative transformations of the tocopherol molecule reported by John and Empte, the tocopherol-nitrite system was reexamined by sampling at much shorter time intervals under the same conditions described above. Preliminary results indicate that the initial reaction product is tocoquinone, which gradually increases in concentration over a two-hour period, after which evidence appears of further oxidation products. At present, no quantitative information is available.

Pharmaceutical Forms of α-Tocopherol

In addition to the mechanical aspects of properly delivering α-tocopherol to the system under investigation—be it the fat portion of bacon or the lower gastrointestinal tract of man, etc.—there are several other facets of "vitamin E" worth review or at least reiteration. The active form of α-tocopherol is the unesterified or "free alcohol" form of the vitamin, which is the form that exists in nature in plants, seeds, etc. Most of the vitamin E forms of commerce are the esters, particularly the acetate ester and, in some cases, the hemisuccinate. These esters do not naturally appear in food but were developed as a means of stabilizing isolated pure forms of the "natural" *d*-isomer as well as the synthetic *dl* material from oxidation of the phenol groups during processing and storage. This is true particularly in pharmaceutical dosages, such as tablets and capsules. The esters, per se, are inactive as *N*-nitroso blocking agents and, for that matter, as antioxidants as well. Their activity, then, relies upon hydrolysis, which on oral ingestion occurs in the intestinal lumen through the action of pancreatic lipase and the aid of bile salts as part of normal fat digestion. Overall then, *in vitro* applications of tocopherol as an *N*-nitroso compound inhibitor—for example, in bacon, cosmetic formulations, drug products, etc.—would require the use of the unesterified molecule. The same is true for inhibiting nitrosation reactions that could occur in the stomach where lipase activity for hydrolysis is lacking. In the lower gastrointestinal tract, it is conceivable, although not proven, that the esterified forms of vitamin E may be active.

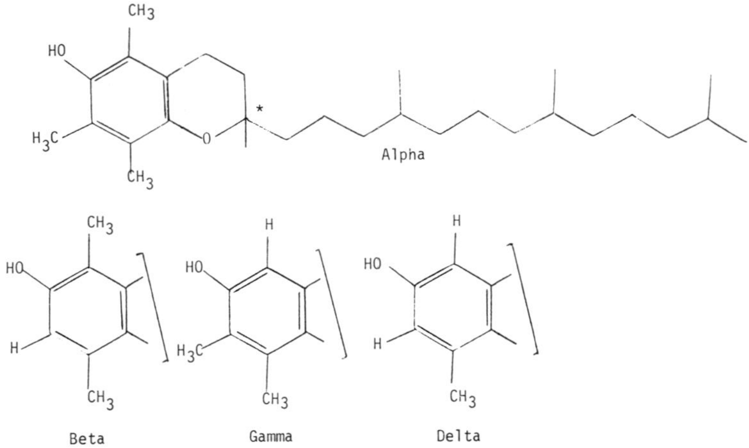

Figure 5. Tocopherols.

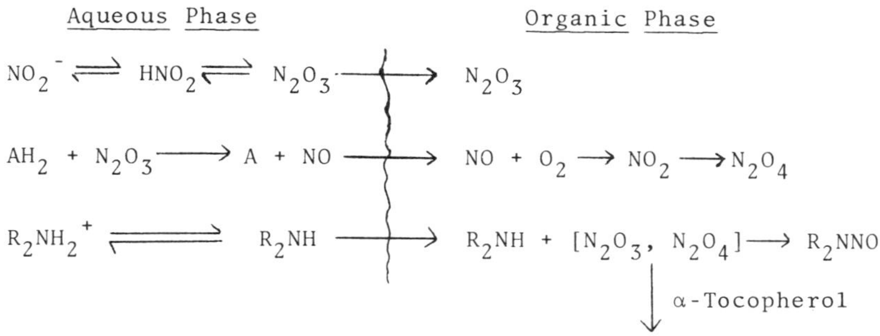

FIGURE 6. Multiphasic inhibition of nitrosamine formation by ascorbic acid and α-tocopherol.

Preliminary studies indicate that after oral administration of 400 mg vitamin E acetate to volunteers, the unabsorbed fraction of the dose (~35%) appearing in feces is essentially all unesterified vitamin E. This study, however, was not coupled with concomitant measurements of fecal nitrosamine determinations.

ISOMERS OF VITAMIN E (FIGURE 5)

Within the family of tocopherols with some vitamin E activity, several distinctions can be made with respect to nitroso compound blocking activity. α-Tocopherol has three asymmetric centers at position 2, 4′, and 8′. The chief distinctions are as follows.

The asymmetric center at position 2, where the side chain joins the chromane ring, is in the optically active "*d*" position in the "natural" form of the vitamin. The racemic "*dl*" form produced by total synthesis is composed of an equal mixture of the *d* form and the *l* form at position 2, the latter having only about one-half the biological activity as a vitamin of the *d* form. The biological activity is determined by biological tests that are at least partly dependent on relative efficiency of absorption and retention into the organism and cellular components, so that the *d* form is considered to have 1.36 times the activity of the synthetic *dl* form.[20] On this basis, the relative biological activities of the α-tocopherol have been assigned in terms of units, not mg, of activity. However, in terms of nitrosation blocking ability, both the *d* and *dl* forms have equal capacity. Thus, they can be considered equivalent on an mg, or weight, basis rather than on a unit of biological activity. The asymmetry at positions 4′ and 8′ appears to have little effect on biological activity.

The other tocopherols, principally beta, gamma, and delta, are biologically less active than is alpha and also appear to be chemically different. In 1948, Quaife described an analytical method of differentiating and estimating α-tocopherol in the presence of its beta, gamma, and delta isomers. This bears directly on the reaction of these compounds with nitrite. The tocopherols contain a phenol group, which is a strong *ortho-para* director. In the presence of a nitrosating agent, β-, γ-, and δ-tocopherol will form a *C*-nitroso derivative. α-Tocopherol, having a fully substituted ring, will not undergo such a reaction; rather, it is simply oxidized to the tocoquinone. It is known that *C*-nitroso and *C*-nitro compounds can act as transnitrosating agents as well as catalysts toward nitrosamine formation.[21,22] The latter effect has been proposed to occur through tautomeric equilibrium of a *C*-nitroso compound with its oxime. Kamm *et al.* have shown that α-tocopherol is somewhat more effective than is gamma as a nitrosamine blocking agent.[16] Whether this relates to the fact that γ-tocopherol can *C*-nitrosate and thus become a nitrosating "donor" to susceptible amines or whether α-tocopherol simply reacts more rapidly with a nitrosating agent than does gamma remains to be demonstrated. A point in favor of the latter argument is that α-tocopherol is oxidized by Fe^{III} much more rapidly than is gamma.[23]

Multiphase Inhibition

Foods and the contents of the digestive tract are not simple monophasic homogeneous systems. They contain aqueous, lipid, micellar, and solid phases. Since nitrosation can potentially take place in at least the first three of these phases, complete blocking would require reactive compounds in each phase.

Ascorbic acid and α-tocopherol can act in concert to effect multiphase inhibition as shown in Figure 6. They are effective in this manner by virtue of the distribution of ascorbate in the aqueous phase and of α-tocopherol in the nonaqueous phase, thus providing synergistic action for the entire system. As stated in the introduction, the desirability of this combined characteristic for foods and for the lumen of the gastrointestinal tract is readily apparent.

References

1. Tannenbaum, S. R. 1979. Endogenous formation of nitrite and *N*-nitroso compounds. *In* Naturally Occurring Carcinogens—Mutagens and Modulators of Carcinogenesis. E. C. Miller *et al.,* Eds.: 211–220. Japan Science Society Press/University Park Press. Tokyo and Baltimore.
2. Walker, E. A., M. Castegnaro, L. Griciute & R. E. Lyle, Eds. 1978. Environmental Aspects of *N*-Nitroso Compounds. IARC Scientific Publication No. 19. International Agency for Research on Cancer. Lyon, France.
3. Mirvish, S. S. 1975. Formation of *N*-nitroso compounds: chemistry, kinetics and *in vivo* occurrence. Toxicol. Appl. Pharmacol. **31:** 325–351.
4. Dahn, H., L. Loewe & C. A. Bunton. 1960. Über die Oxydation von Ascorbinsäure durch salpetrige Säure Teil VI: Ubersicht und Diskussion der Ergebnisse. Helv. Chim. Acta **43:** 320–333.
5. Mirvish, S. S., L. Wallgave, M. Eagen, *et al.* 1972. Ascorbate-nitrate reaction: possible means of blocking the formation of carcinogenic *N*-nitroso compounds. Science **177:** 65–68.
6. Kamm, J. J., T. Dashman, A. H. Conney, *et al.* 1973. Protective effect of ascorbic acid on hepatoxicity caused by sodium nitrite plus aminopyrine. Proc. Nat. Acad. Sci. USA **70:** 747–749.
7. Greenblatt, M. 1973. Ascorbic acid blocking of aminopyrine nitrosation in N20/BI mice. J. Nat. Cancer Inst. **50:** 1055–1056.
8. Fiddler, W., J. W. Pensabene, E. G. Piotrowski, *et al.* 1973. Use of sodium ascorbate or erythorbate to inhibit formation of *N*-nitrosodimethylamine in frankfurters. J. Food Sci. **38:** 1084–1085.
9. Archer, M. C., S. R. Tannenbaum, T. Y. Fan & M. Weisman. 1975. Reaction of nitrite with ascorbate and its relation to nitrosamine formation. J. Nat. Cancer Inst. **54**(5): 1203–1205.
10. Bunton, C. A., H. Dahn & L. Loewe. 1959. Oxidation of ascorbic acid and similar reductones by nitrous acid. Nature London **183:** 163–165.
11. Mergens, W. J., J. J. Kamm, H. L. Newmark, W. Fiddler & J. Pensabene. 1978. Alpha-tocopherol: uses in preventing nitrosamine formation. *In* Environmental Aspects of *N*-Nitroso Compounds. E. A. Walker, M. Castegnaro, L. Griciute & R. E. Lyle,

Eds.: 199–212. IARC Scientific Publication No. 19. International Agency for Research on Cancer. Lyon, France.
12. MERGENS, W. J. & H. L. NEWMARK. 1979. The use of alpha-tocopherol in bacon processing—an update. *In* Proceedings of the Meat Industry Research Conference, March 29–30, 1979: 79–84. American Meat Institute Foundation. Arlington, Va.
13. GRAY, J. I. & L. R. DUGAN. 1975. Inhibition of nitrosamine formation in model food systems. J. Food Sci. **40:** 981.
14. FIDDLER, W., J. W. PENSABENE, E. G. PIOTROWSKI, J. G. PHILLIPS, J. P. KEATING, W. J. MERGENS & H. L. NEWMARK. 1978. Inhibition of formation of volatile nitrosamines in fried bacon by the use of cure-solubilized alpha-tocopherol. J. Agric. Food Chem. **26**(3): 653.
15. FIDDLER, W., J. PENSABENE & A. E. WASSERMAN. 1974. The role of lean and adipose tissue on the formation of nitrosopyrrolidine in fried bacon. J. Food Sci. **39:** 1070.
16. KAMM, J. J., T. DASHMAN, H. L. NEWMARK & W. J. MERGENS. 1977. Inhibition of amine-nitrite hepatotoxicity by alpha-tocopherol. Toxicol. Appl. Pharmacol. **41**(3): 575.
17. MERGENS, W. J. 1980. (Unpublished observations.)
18. HANSEN, T. J., M. C. ARCHER & S. R. TANNENBAUM. 1979. Characterization of pyrolysis conditions and interference by other compounds in the chemiluminescence detection of nitrosamines. Anal. Chem. **51**(9): 1526–1528.
19. JOHN, W. & W. EMPTE. 1940. Uber Einige Neue Oxydationsprodukte der Tokopherole 8. Mitteilung uber Antisterilstatsfaktoren (vitamin E). Hoppe-Seyler's Z. Physiol. Chem. **268:** 85.
20. DRAPER, H. H. 1970. The tocopherols. *In* International Encyclopedia of Food and Nutrition. Fat-Soluble Vitamins. R. A. Morton, Ed. **9** (Chapter V): 333–393. Pergamon Press. Elmsford, N.Y.
21. FAN, T.-Y., R. VITA & D. H. FINE. 1978. *C*-Nitro compounds: a new class of nitrosating agent. Toxicol. Lett. **2:** 5.
22. WALKER, E. A., B. PIGNATELLI & M. CASTEGNARO. 1979. Catalytic effect of *p*-nitrosophenol on the nitrosation of diethylamine. J. Agric. Food Chem. **27**(2): 393.
23. STERN, M. H. & J. G. BAXTER. 1947. Delta-tocopherol. Assay of total tocopherols in mixtures containing delta-tocopherol. Anal. Chem. **19:** 902.

DISCUSSION

H. SPRINCE (*Veterans Administration Medical Center, Coatesville, Penn.*): Nitric oxide has been claimed to be found in cigarette smoke in an amount hazardous to your health, and there have also been claims that vitamin C may be important for heavy smokers. That is, people who are smoking heavily should be taking vitamin C, more than the recommended daily amount. Now I think these two things ought to be considered in the context of smoking. In your system, you've considered ascorbic acid and vitamin E. Have you also considered other redox systems, such as cysteine versus cystine or reduced glutathione and oxidized glutathione?

S. R. TANNENBAUM: It is true that cigarette smoke contains nitric oxide, and in fact, cigarette smoke also contains nitrosamines. In fact, in some types of cigarettes, there are substantial amounts. The interesting thing is that Dr. Mergens first became interested in the application of alpha-tocopherol through the cigarette case, because you can actually build up the levels of vitamin E in lung tissue. The idea was that that might protect against nitric oxide in cigarette smoke.

In answer to the second question, there are a lot of substances that will react with nitrite. Cysteine, as an example, is not a very effective blocking agent because sulfhydryl compounds form *S*-nitroso compounds, which would rapidly oxidize to disulfides and nitric oxide; and for a variety of reasons, these are not particularly effective blocking agents. But again, within a complex system, one would have to take them into consideration.

J. G. BIERI (*National Institutes of Health, Bethesda, Md.*): Do I understand that bacon manufacturers are proposing to add more ascorbic acid and also vitamin E to their product?

S. R. TANNENBAUM: Well, there are already 500 parts per million of vitamin C in the formulation that the government requires. There is further being considered now the addition of alpha-tocopherol to complete the blocking.

J. G. BIERI: How much do they want to put in?

S. R. TANNENBAUM: 500 ppm.

J. G. BIERI: What's known about the possible toxicity or mutagenicity of things like tocored and alpha-tocopherolparaquinone?

S. R. TANNENBAUM: Well, I don't know about the tocored. Tocoquinone is not mutagenic.

J. G. BIERI: Who has ever looked at the mutagenicity of tocored and the paraquinone?; that's what I want to know.

S. R. TANNENBAUM: Dr. Mergens may have a comment on that.

W. MERGENS: In the reaction of tocopherol with oxidizing agents, the reaction can go to tocored and paraquinone. However, the statement was not made that within a system like bacon or within the body, those would be end products. The first product of the reaction is tocopherolquinone, and as far as we know, it is the only product of oxidation in the system.

P. HOCHSTEIN (*University of Southern California School of Medicine, Los Angeles, Calif.*): What are the quantitative aspects of the reaction of nitric oxide with ascorbate and tocopherol? Is there any evidence for recycling of tocopherol or ascorbate?

S. R. TANNENBAUM: In a simple *in vitro* system, clearly not. In an *in vivo* system, it would be the same as what would happen with air oxidation. In other words, if you had a system that had the capacity for recycling dehydroascorbic, then that would be effective.

Once you get out of the gastrointestinal [GI] tract, ascorbic acid appears to have very little to do with nitrites, because at the pH's and the conditions that you encounter, nitrite reacts very rapidly in blood with oxyhemoglobin; so that scrubs it out of the system—stoichiometrically forming nitrate—before it could possibly react with ascorbic acid.

UNIDENTIFIED SPEAKER: What is the residence time for the two vitamins? That is, how long do they actually stay in the intestinal tract? How are they transported through the intestinal wall?

S. R. TANNENBAUM: You've asked a very complex question. The doses of ascorbic acid and alpha-tocopherol that we are talking about are above the RDA [recommended daily allowance]. Absorption is incomplete. A lot of it gets into feces, and the extent isn't known. In addition, alpha-tocopherol is stored to an extent in certain tissues, particularly in lung tissue. I don't know if anyone has studied it along the GI tract, but it would be a very interesting thing to do.

UNIDENTIFIED SPEAKER: I'd like to know what is the idea of adding ascorbic acid to the bacon? Because after you fry it, the ascorbate is gone.

S. R. TANNENBAUM: The original basis for adding ascorbic acid to bacon was because it enhanced color formation. In fact, either isoascorbate or ascorbate is used in all cured meats. It has absolutely nothing to do with increasing the amount of ascorbic acid in the diet. In fact, in the original decision that was made by the Food and Drug Administration, there was some concern about adding too much ascorbic acid to the diet, and this is why they permitted isoascorbate. By the time you fry the bacon, there's very little left in the way of ascorbic acid. But I would say that anyone who consumes bacon for its nutritive value is making a mistake; I think it is a condiment not a food.

UNIDENTIFIED SPEAKER: No, I'm not asking for the nutritive value but to find out how ascorbic acid counteracts nitrosamine formation if you're going to add it to bacon.

S. R. TANNENBAUM: In bacon, the nitrosamine is formed in the frying operation. So the idea of the ascorbate and the alpha-tocopherol is to prevent formation of the *N*-nitroso compounds during cooking. It's not an *in vivo* problem.

H. SPRINCE: Are there any known interactions of aldehyde with nitric oxide?, and can they act synergistically to increase nitrosation?

S. R. TANNENBAUM: You're asking a very complicated question. There are a variety of ways in which interactions can take place. For example, if you condense the aldehyde with the amino compound to form a Schiff base, that will actually enhance nitrosation for reasons that I don't want to go into. It just takes a different reaction pathway. You could have oxidations or reductions taking place. I don't think anyone could give a definitive answer to that question without specifying exactly what the system was.

UNIDENTIFIED SPEAKER: Dr. Tannenbaum, in view of what you said, do you think the RDAs for vitamins C and E are adequate?

S. R. TANNENBAUM: Well, I tried to say very carefully in the beginning of my talk that we are talking about an action here that has nothing to do with the vitamin activity. Clearly the several things that I'm talking about, if correct—in other words, if it were applicable to a certain population—would call for reevaluation of the amounts of vitamins C and E in the diet.

Now I would like to point out that I think what we have here is a classical case of balance of risks. Clearly there could be additional risks from increasing the amounts of vitamins C and E in the diet. In the course of the discussion that I have heard here, I'm impressed by the complexity of interactions of the different trace metals.

We do this every time we make a decision. We have to sit down and say what we think the risk is with regard to the process of carcinogenesis in the population, and is this something that ought to be considered from the point of view of prevention. Is this a good way to do it? And if we do this, then the other risks are brought out.

J. G. BIERI: I'll just make one more comment. We now know that the primary oxidation product when you cook bacon containing vitamin E is going to be tocopherolquinone, at least that was the statement that Dr. Mergens made. Now, unless anyone thinks that tocopherolquinone has no potential toxicity, they might read the old literature of Dr. D. W. Wolley about 30 years ago, who tried tocopherolquinone for biological activity in the rat, and not in very big doses. He ended up with vitamin K deficiency, which was cured by giving vitamin K. Later, Dr. Karl Mason also produced vitamin K deficiency by feeding alpha-tocopherolhydroquinone to rats.

W. MERGENS: The only thing I would like to say at the moment is that during the frying process of bacon, you lose essentially no tocopherol. It is stable through the process of frying. If there is any tocopherolquinone formed, it is in extremely small amounts. The reactions that Dr. Tannenbaum was talking about are reactions that occurred in model systems. I'm not prepared at this time to say to what extent tocored, for example, will be formed under conditions that would mimic the gastrointestinal tract.

VITAMIN C, VITAMIN E, AND THE PREVENTION OF GASTRIC CANCER: DISCUSSION

Discussant: John H. Weisburger

Naylor Dana Institute for Disease Prevention
American Health Foundation
Valhalla, New York 10595

Dr. Tannenbaum has just given us an excellent detailed review of the kinetics of the formation of nitrosamines, and of the rather complex reactions through which nitrite interacts with ascorbic acid and thus becomes unavailable for nitrosation of substrates leading to nitrosamines.

Scientifically, this is an interesting area and has led to major advances in understanding of the reaction mechanisms involving these components. On the basis of a somewhat different line of reasoning, we have been involved in parallel investigations specifically directed toward uncovering the elements responsible for gastric cancer in man. Briefly, epidemiology shows that gastric cancer is one type of neoplastic disease that has exhibited sharply decreased incidence in the United States in the last 50 years.[1] There are areas in the world—such as Japan, western Latin America, northern and eastern Europe, and, within the United Kingdom, Wales—where this disease still has a high incidence, although even there a declining trend has begun.[2,3] Studies of people who have migrated from high to low risk regions, such as Japanese and Scandinavians in the United States, developed the information that one kind of food that such migrants tend to consume more in the low risk country is fresh fruits and vegetables—foods with increased vitamin C and perhaps vitamin E content.[2,3] In high risk regions for gastric cancer, such foods are consumed infrequently, especially so during the late fall through early spring seasons.

We have postulated that the carcinogen responsible for gastric cancer in man might have the structure of an alkylnitrosamide, since Sugimura and Kawachi discovered this type of carcinogen to be capable of inducing gastric cancer in relevant animal models.[4,5] Based on this concept, we have subjected a kind of fish frequently eaten in Japan to nitrosation under conditions prevailing in the stomach. We obtained a powerful, direct-acting mutagen similar in prototype to *N*-methyl-*N'*-nitro-*N*-nitrosoguanidine (MNNG). We have further demonstrated that an extract of nitrite-treated fish can induce glandular stomach cancer in animals. Tatematsu *et al.* have shown that salt has a promoting effect with MNNG in stomach carcinogenesis, and Joossens *et al.* have related the intake of salt in various populations to the occurrence of hypertension and stomach cancer.[6,7] We have further found that not all foods subjected to nitrosation had this mutagen. Of particular importance is the fact that nitrite-treated meats, such as hot dogs and pork, do not produce this mutagen, probably because of the competition of myoglobin in meats.[8]

Simulating the conditions seen in migrants, we have observed that addition of vitamin C prior to treatment of fish with nitrite abolishes the formation of the mutagen.[4] It had been found previously that ascorbate and tocopherol inhibited nitrosation.[9,10]

We are thus in a position to conclude that a regular intake of vitamin C–containing foods from childhood onwards may prevent the development of stomach cancer. It would seem also that a lower intake of salt would be beneficial in reducing the risk of stomach cancer and hypertension.

References

1. Piper, D. W. 1978. UICC Technical Report Series No. 34. Union Internationale Contre le Cancer. Geneva, Switzerland.
2. Haenszel, W., M. Kurihara, F. B. Locke, K. Shimuzu & M. Segi. 1976. J. Nat. Cancer Inst. **56:** 265–274.
3. Hirayama, T. 1979. Nutr. Cancer **1:** 67–81.
4. Weisburger, J. H., H. Marquardt, H. F. Mower, N. Hirota, H. Mori & G. Williams. 1980. Prev. Med. **9:** 352–361.
5. Sugimura, T. & T. Kawachi. 1978. *In* Gastrointestinal Tract Cancer. M. Lipkin & R. Good, Eds: 327–342. Plenum Press. New York, N.Y.
6. Tatematsu, M., M. Takahashi, S. Fukashima, M. Hananouchi & T. Shirai. 1975. J. Nat. Cancer Inst. **55:** 101–104.
7. Joossens, J. V., H. Kesteloot & A. Amery. 1979. N. Engl. J. Med. **300:** 1396.
8. Marquardt, H., R. Rufino & J. H. Weisburger. 1977. Food Cosmet. Toxicol. **15:** 97–100.
9. Mirvish, S. S. 1977. J. Toxicol. Environ. Health **2:** 1267–1277.
10. Mergens, W. J., J. J. Kamm, H. L. Newmark, W. Fiddler & J. Pensabene. 1978. *In* Environmental Aspects of *N*-Nitroso Compounds. IARC Scientific Publication No. 19: 199–212. International Agency for Research on Cancer. Lyon, France.

INTERACTIONS OF VITAMINS WITH TOXIC MINERALS: GENERAL DISCUSSION

Moderator: W. G. Hoekstra

Department of Biochemistry
University of Wisconsin
Madison, Wisconsin 53706

A. L. Tappel (*University of California, Davis, Calif.*): As you know from Dr. Hochstein's discussion, fluorescent products can be used as a measure of damage to membranes. I believe that you were measuring both lipid-soluble and aqueous fluorescent products, and so I would like to have your comment as to how useful this is in measuring damaged membranes. You have very high sensitivity with fluorescent measurements.

P. Hochstein (*University of Southern California School of Medicine, Los Angeles, Calif.*): Yes, we measured the fluorescence excitation and emission spectra of chloroform-isopropanol extracts of membranes. That material is composed primarily of lipids. The polymerized protein is usually present in the aqueous extracts. They were not fluorescent.

With regard to the fluorescent material extracted with organic solvents, this seems to us to be a most sensitive way of looking at lipid peroxidation, certainly much more sensitive than the TBA [thiobarbituric acid] reaction, although less sensitive than pentane production.

W. G. Hoekstra: My understanding is that extractable fluorescent pigments don't correlate very well with other indices of peroxidative damage. It is a very complicated situation in terms of the fluorescence products that are present and whether they are extractable or unextractable with solvents.

J. G. Bieri (*National Institutes of Health, Bethesda, Md.*): We have a recent paper in *Lipids* where we looked at the lipofuscin or ceroid pigment in the vitamin E-deficient rat uterus. Most of it is insoluble, but if you extract it, you get a little bit of something that gives characteristic fluorescence spectra. But the correlation between gross pigmentation and extractable fluorescence isn't particularly good in our hands when we use some of the established techniques trying to purify this particular mixture of pigments.

On the other hand, I have a collaborator in the eye institute who's looking at the retina. He finds that the lipofuscin granules in the pigment epithelium of the retina, formed in the absence of vitamin E, form more in the presence of vitamin A than in the absence of vitamin A. Thus, in contrast to our conclusion that vitamin A is not involved in the uterine pigmentation, it now appears that vitamin A may play some role in the pigment epithelium granules.

W. G. Hoekstra: I believe Dr. Csallany at the University of Minnesota has studied this quite extensively and has a number of soluble fluorescent pigments, some of which seem to correlate and some of which don't. There is a differential distribution of these things or extractabilities at least in different organs. It is a very complicated situation according to the way I understand it.

P. Hochstein: I wonder if there isn't a difference between the fluorescent pigments that are obtained from storage granules and those that are acutely formed by initiating reactions in the preparations that I described. It seems reasonable that after storage, higher degrees of polymerization may result in altered patterns of extraction. The question really should be one that relates to the properties of newly formed fluorescent polymers in membranes and those that are accumulated. Making these distinctions may be helpful over the long run.

H. BHAGAVAN (*Hoffmann-La Roche, Inc., Nutley, N.J.*): I'd like to ask Dr. Hochstein if he isolated the polymers from patients with Wilson's disease?

P. HOCHSTEIN: No, we have not isolated these polymers from red cells in patients with Wilson's disease. The polymers that I showed were formed after *in vitro* incubation of human red cells with copper. That is obviously the thing we would like to do next.

INTERACTIONS OF TOXIC ELEMENTS WITH ESSENTIAL ELEMENTS: INTRODUCTION

Harold H. Sandstead

Human Nutrition Research Center
U.S. Department of Agriculture
Science and Education Administration
Grand Forks, North Dakota 58202

Papers in this session are concerned with interactions of toxic elements with essential elements. Such interactions are important because they illustrate the ways in which toxic elements can impair metabolic processes that depend upon essential elements. The occurrence of these impairments under controlled experimental conditions suggests that similar abnormalities might occur in free-living man and animals under circumstances of increased exposure to toxic elements. Conversely, the finding that certain elements can prevent some of the adverse effects of some toxic elements suggests that the presence of those essential elements in the diet might contribute to the protection of man and animals from effects of low levels of toxic elements.

The complexity of the possible interactions is inferred by FIGURE 1. Some of the interactions involve competition for ligands; others are noncompetitive. The occurrence of an interaction probably has implications for the metabolism of elements other than those primarily involved. Under usual circumstances, a variety of responses occur that are responsible for the maintenance of homeostasis. Toxicity occurs when the levels of toxic elements exceed homeostatic capabilities.

Some of the effects of toxic elements and the protective effects of essential elements might be attributed to competition for binding sites on ligands that have important roles in homeostasis. Possibly the binding of copper, cadmium, and zinc

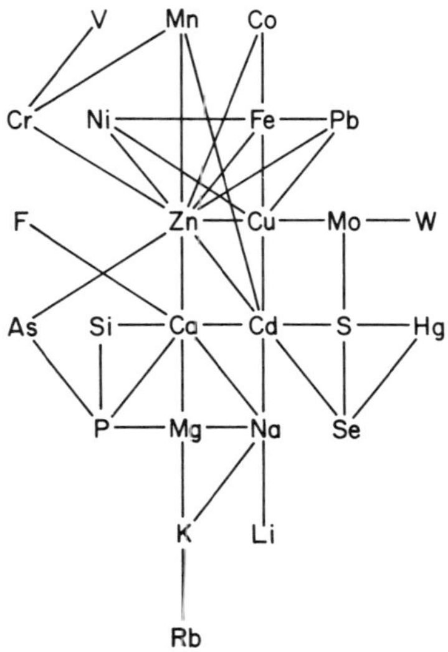

FIGURE 1. Interactions among essential and toxic elements.

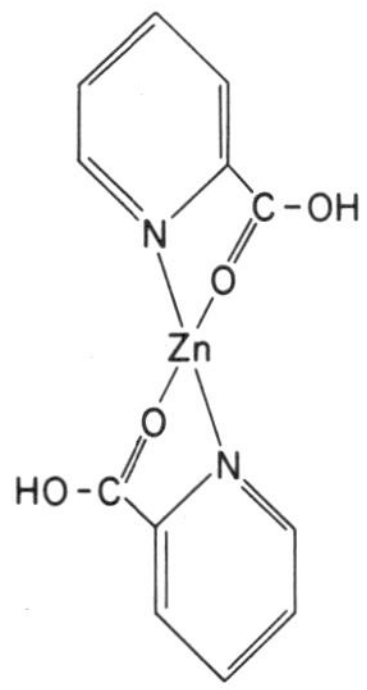

FIGURE 2. Formula of zinc picolinate.[4]

to metallothionein is an example of such a competition. *In vitro* measurements of the binding of these metals to metallothionein suggest that copper displaces cadmium and zinc and that cadmium displaces zinc.[1,2] *In vivo* studies have generally been consistent with these *in vitro* observations.[3]

Another example is suggested from studies of the mechanisms of zinc absorption. A metabolite of tryptophan, picolinic acid, that forms bidentate complexes with zinc (FIGURE 2) facilitates zinc absorption and retention in rats.[5-8] Presumably, this phenomenon also occurs in man. The stability constants of picolinic acid with toxic and essential elements (TABLE 1)[9] suggest that picolinic acid may have a role in the intestinal absorption of other essential elements and that toxic elements may interfere with absorption of essential elements by formation of complexes with picolinic acid. Possibly the adverse effects of toxic elements on absorption increase in situations that limit the level of picolinic acid, such as deficiencies in dietary tryptophan and/or vitamin B_6.

The discovery that picolinic acid facilitates the intestinal absorption of zinc is so new that its implications have not yet been appreciated. As far as I know, interactions between picolinic acid and toxic elements have not been studied in biological systems. I hope my comments will stimulate research in this area because some of the puzzling relationships between dietary toxic and essential elements might be resolved by such studies.

TABLE 1

SOME STABILITY CONSTANTS OF METAL COMPLEXES OF PICOLINIC ACID (PYRIDINE-2-CARBOXYLIC ACID)[9]

Ca^{+2}	3.79
Mg^{+2}	3.95
Mn^{+2}	4.60
Sr^{+2}	4.71
Cd^{+2}	8.25
Pb^{+2}	8.57
Zn^{+2}	10.01
Co^{+2}	10.53
Cu^{+2}	12.20
Fe^{+2}	12.30
Ni^{+2}	12.45
Fe^{+3}	12.80
Hg^{+2}	15.40

The numerous interactions of cadmium, lead, and mercury with essential elements have been reviewed in the past. Persons interested in this literature should begin by reading two reports by the Permanent Subcommittee on the Toxicology of Metals, reports of the National Research Council's Subcommittee on Geochemical Environment in Relation to Health and Disease, Underwood's text on *Trace Elements in Human and Animal Nutrition,* and portions of a Nutrition Foundation symposium on *Trace Elements in Human Health and Disease.*[10-16] These references and the publications of the participants in today's session give perspective to the research we are about to hear described.

References

1. Kagi, J. H. R. & B. L. Vallee. 1961. Metallothionein: a cadmium and zinc-containing protein from equine renal cortex. J. Biol. Chem. **236:** 2435.
2. Hartmann, H. J. & V. Weser. 1977. Copper-thionein from fetal bovine liver. Biochim. Biophys. Acta **491:** 211.
3. Sandstead, H. H. 1977. Nutrient interactions with toxic elements. Adv. Mod. Toxicol. **2:** 241–256.
4. Paul, R. C., R. S. Chopra, R. K. Shambri & G. Singh. 1974. Metal complexes of ethyl picolinate. J. Inorg. Nucl. Chem. **36:** 3703.
5. Evans, G. W. & P. E. Johnson. 1980. Characterization and quantitation of a zinc binding ligand in human milk. Pediatr. Res. **14:** 876.
6. Evans, G. W. & E. C. Johnson. 1980. Zinc absorption in rats fed a low protein diet and a low protein diet supplemented with tryptophan or picolinic acid. J. Nutr. **110:** 1076.
7. Evans, G. W. & E. C. Johnson. 1979. Zinc absorption in rats fed varying levels of vitamin B_6 and a vitamin B_6 antagonist. (abst.) Clin. Res. **27:** 682.
8. Evans, G. W. 1980. Normal and abnormal zinc absorption in man and animals: the tryptophan connection. Nutr. Rev. **38:** 137.
9. Sillen, L. G. & A. E. Martell. 1964. Stability Constants of Metal-Ion Complexes: 496. Chemical Society, Burlington House. London, England.
10. Nordberg, G. F., Ed. 1976. Effects and Dose Response Relationships of Toxic Metals. Elsevier. Amsterdam, The Netherlands.
11. Nordberg, G. F., Ed. 1978. Factors influencing metabolism and toxicity of metals. Environ. Health Perspect. **25:** 1.
12. Subcommittee on the Geochemical Environment in Relation to Health and Disease. 1974. Geochemistry and the Environment **1.** National Academy of Sciences. Washington, D.C.
13. Subcommittee on the Geochemical Environment in Relation to Health and Disease. 1977. Geochemistry and the Environment **2.** National Academy of Sciences. Washington, D.C.
14. Subcommittee on the Geochemical Environment in Relation to Health and Disease. 1978. Geochemistry and the Environment **3.** National Academy of Sciences. Washington, D.C.
15. Underwood, E. J. 1976. Trace Elements in Human and Animal Nutrition. Academic Press, Inc. New York, N.Y.
16. Prasad, A. S., Ed. 1976. Trace Elements in Human Health and Disease **1** & **2**. Academic Press, Inc. New York, N.Y.

METABOLIC INTERACTIONS: LEAD, CALCIUM, AND IRON

Kathryn R. Mahaffey and Jeanne I. Rader

Division of Nutrition
Food and Drug Administration
Cincinnati, Ohio 45226

Introduction

The metabolism of lead and susceptibility to the toxicity of lead are influenced by the nutritionally required metals calcium and iron. A number of similarities exist between the metabolism of calcium, lead, strontium, and barium. Awareness of metabolic relationships between calcium and lead has existed for many years. In 1926, Aub stated that the "lead stream" follows the "calcium stream."[1] Certain of the physiologic mechanisms that control calcium metabolism have also been shown experimentally to alter absorption and tissue distribution of lead in experimental animals. Interactions between lead and iron are far less well understood. Much of what we do know was learned from studies of low-income urban children, in whom iron deficiency and lead toxicity are both prevalent. Iron deficiency results in increased absorption and tissue retention of lead, but the metabolic mechanisms involved are not nearly as well understood as those for calcium. Conversely lead can produce marked alterations in iron metabolism.

Within the available literature, possibly conflicting reports have appeared. In part, these potential differences are a reflection of the type of study performed. Chronic feeding studies have been used to determine the overall lead/nutrient interactions in the whole animal. Observation of changes is usually followed by an interest in determining the mechanism or mechanisms producing these effects. Subsequent research—frequently involving an isolated organ system, e.g., the gastrointestinal tract—may show lead-induced changes in that organ system or nutrient-induced changes in the manner in which the organ system metabolizes lead. However, in the intact animal or person, numerous physiologic mechanisms and the effects of other organ systems may minimize the importance of the observed changes in the isolated organ system studied. Other reasons for possibly conflicting reports are differences in route of lead exposure and dosage of lead. Some experimental studies have utilized routes of exposure, e.g., intravenous injection, and extremely high doses of lead that are of limited value in predicting those changes occurring under more physiologic conditions. However, this type of study has the advantage of providing direction to future experimental work using chronic exposure and doses of lead that produce body burdens of lead comparable to those commonly prevalent in humans.

Calcium and Lead

General Effects

Early investigation indicated that vitamin D, calcium, and phosphorus influence deposition of lead in soft tissue and bone.[2] Shields and Mitchell reported that lowering the calcium and/or phosphorus intake at low levels of lead intake [32 parts per million (ppm)] could increase bone or soft tissue lead.[3] These workers also observed

0077-8923/80/0355-0285 $01.75/0

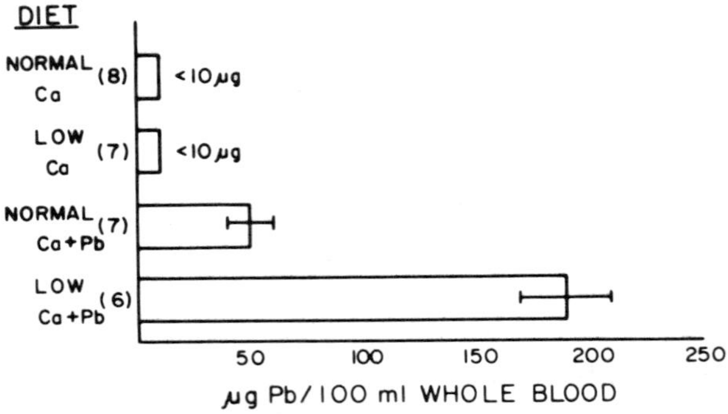

FIGURE 1. Influence of dietary calcium on blood lead levels. (Reprinted from Reference 32 with permission of the C. V. Mosby Company.)

that the influence of calcium intake on lead metabolism was seen primarily at low levels of calcium intake; increasing dietary calcium to high levels, 1.1% of the diet, did not decrease tissue stores of lead below those found on a normal calcium diet. Many of the early studies were carried out with the hope that manipulation of dietary calcium would be preventive or useful in treatment of occupational lead poisoning. In fact, it was customary at that time in Great Britain, and to a lesser extent in the United States, to provide workmen in lead industries with free milk while they were working.[4] One difficulty in interpreting many of the older papers arises from the emphasis on the dietary calcium/phosphorus ratio, which resulted in the investigators changing more than one nutrient in the same experiment, e.g., calcium, phosphorus, and vitamin D.

Several decades later, the effect of lowered dietary calcium in increasing tissue lead content and the biochemical and morphological changes associated with lead toxicity were reported, providing a new awareness that low dietary calcium greatly enhanced susceptibility to the pathological effects of lead.[5] Ingesting a low calcium diet and a given quantity of lead resulted in approximately a fourfold increase in blood lead concentration in rats (FIGURE 1). Tissue lead concentrations were greatly elevated with low calcium diets (TABLES 1 and 2); however, the increase of lead in

TABLE 1

EFFECT OF DIETARY CALCIUM DEFICIENCY ON KIDNEY AND FEMUR Pb CONCENTRATION IN RATS*

	Kidney Pb (µg/g)†	Femur Pb (µg/g)†
Normal Ca‡	2.6 ± 1.2§	2.2 ± 1.0
Low Ca¶	4.4 ± 0.6	9.7 ± 2.2
Normal Ca + Pb‖	29.6 ± 7.0	202.0 ± 22.2
Low Ca + Pb	691.0 ± 203.0	225.0 ± 15.2

* Reference 32.
† Wet weight.
‡ 0.7% of diet.
§ Mean ± standard error of the mean (SEM).
¶ 0.1% of diet.
‖ Pb in drinking water; 200 ppm Pb added as lead acetate.

TABLE 2

RENAL AND FEMUR LEAD CONTENT OF RATS FED NORMAL (0.7%) AND LOW (0.1%) CALCIUM DIETS*

	Renal Pb (μg/g)		Femur Pb (μg/g)	
Pb in Drinking Water (ppm)	Normal Ca Diet	Low Ca Diet	Normal Ca Diet	Low Ca Diet
ND†	1.0 ± 0.1‡	3.6 ± 0.5	4.8 ± 1.1	50 ± 13
12	1.9 ± 0.1	19.6 ± 2.0	16.8 ± 2.8	240 ± 14
200	21.3 ± 3.8	942 ± 362	236.5 ± 5.4	922 ± 188

* Reference 5.
† ND = not detectable, <0.1 ppm Pb.
‡ Mean ± SEM.

soft tissue was much greater than for bone. Urinary excretion of delta-aminolevulinic acid (dALA) was markedly increased by low calcium diets in lead-treated animals, as were morphological changes in the proximal tubules of the kidney. The magnitude of the calcium effect was illustrated by the observation that rats ingesting water containing 12 ppm lead on a low calcium (0.1%) diet had similar concentrations of tissue lead to those of rats receiving water containing 200 ppm lead but a normal calcium (0.7%) diet.[5] Reduction of dietary calcium to approximately 40–50% of the dietary recommendation, approximating the physiologic requirement for calcium in the rat, was necessary before increases in tissue lead content occurred.[6] Possibly, part of the interaction between low calcium diet and lead occurs only when physiologic mechanisms adapting the body to a low calcium diet are activated.

Similar effects of low calcium diet on susceptibility to lead toxicity in the rat were reported by Quarterman and Morrison.[7] Confirmation of the role of calcium in increasing toxicity of a particular dose of lead has been reported for the dog, pig, horse, and lamb.[8-11]

Absorption

Lederer and Bing observed that lowered dietary calcium increased deposition of lead in the femur when lead acetate was fed in the diet, but did not affect femur lead content when lead acetate was administered by daily intraperitoneal injection, suggesting that the changes brought about by low dietary calcium were due to increased gastrointestinal absorption of lead.[12] Specific studies of the gastrointestinal absorption of lead subsequently have shown a more complex situation than was first envisioned. The most complete work published to date on this subject is the study by Barton *et al.*[13] Using ligated intestinal loop techniques to measure lead absorption, these workers observed that when the concentration of calcium in the intubation media was varied within physiologic ranges, lead absorption decreased with increasing calcium concentration (FIGURE 2). However, prior conditioning by low or high calcium diets did not significantly alter the rat's lead absorption *in vivo*. Similar results, indicating that decreasing concentrations of calcium in the intubation media, but not calcium deficiency per se, increased lead absorption in rats and chicks, have been observed by Mahaffey and coworkers during studies on the role of vitamin D in lead absorption.[14] Reduced lead uptake from ligated gut loops following levels of calcium in intubation media have been reported by Barltrop and Khoo.[15] Meredith *et*

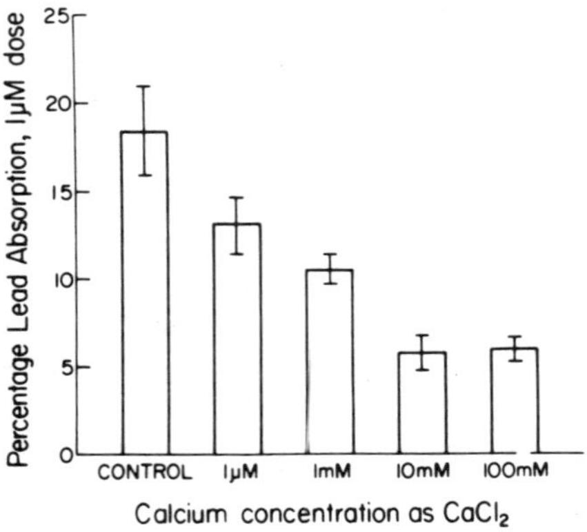

FIGURE 2. Effect of variation of calcium chloride in the intubation media on the absorption of a single dose of radiolabeled lead chloride. (Reprinted from Reference 13 with permission of the C. V. Mosby Company.)

al. have shown that oral calcium administered immediately before lead was highly effective in decreasing lead absorption in rats.[16] Results of these animal studies suggest that simultaneous ingestion of lead with a low calcium diet enhances the absorption of lead.

Similar effects resulting from decreasing dietary calcium have been demonstrated in human infants and toddlers, using balance study techniques.[17] Ziegler *et al.* observed that not only did young children absorb a greater percentage of ingested lead than did adults but that lead absorption and retention were inversely correlated with the calcium content of the diet.[17] When dietary calcium level was higher, lead absorption decreased. Interestingly, the various calcium levels used in this study were all greater than those recommended by the National Research Council as adequate for human infants and toddlers.

Both lead and calcium absorption are stimulated by 1,25-dihydroxycholecalciferol, but these enhancements occur primarily in the distal small intestine for lead and in the duodenum for calcium.[14,18] Recent evidence suggests that calcium and lead compete for similar sites on intestinal mucosal proteins but that lead is bound to a higher molecular weight protein while calcium is bound to a lower molecular weight protein. The higher molecular weight protein is probably not vitamin D-dependent.

Excretion

Barton *et al.* observed that excretion of injected lead by rats on calcium-deficient diets was slower than by rats receiving normal calcium diets.[3] Rats receiving the diets containing higher than normal calcium showed lead retention similar to those rats on normal calcium diets. The pattern of these changes again illustrates that the major calcium effects on lead metabolism occur when dietary calcium is deficient. Little influence of calcium on lead metabolism is observed if elevated levels of calcium are compared with normal dietary calcium intake.

Tissue and Organ Distribution of Lead

Ingestion of low calcium diets increases the lead by far greater percentages in tissues such as kidney and blood than in bone. However, the much higher absolute concentration of lead in bone allows the sequestering of much more lead in this tissue than could be possible in kidney or blood without development of severe symptoms of lead toxicity. It is not clear at this time whether the great increases in renal lead content observed with a low calcium diet are due to (1) a reduced deposition of lead in bone; (2) a decreased rate of bone formation; or (3) a mobilization of lead from bone arising as a result of the stimulatory effect on bone resorption of a low calcium diet. Using *in vitro* bone organ culture techniques, Rosen and Wexler demonstrated that low media levels of calcium with or without parathyroid hormone or 1,25-dihydroxycholecalciferol enhanced the release of radioactive lead from bone explants.[19] Under these conditions, lead may be mobilized from osseous tissue to critical organ sites in soft tissue, such as kidney or brain. In recent *in vivo* studies, Norimatsu and Talmage observed that pretreatment of rats with calcitonin reduced the initial uptake of intravenously injected lead by trabecular and compact bone by as much as 50%.[20] This effect was observed at 30 minutes after lead injection but was not observed at 12 hours after lead injection.

Lead and calcium also interact in neural tissue. Lead appears to block presynaptic neural transmission by reducing the release of acetylcholine. Using *in vitro* techniques, this lead effect was reversed by adding calcium to the incubation medium.[21,22]

Using rat heart mitochondria, Parr and Harris have demonstrated that very low concentrations of Pb^{2+} decreased the capacity of heart mitochondria to remove Ca^{2+} from the incubation medium.[23] Below 0.5 nmol Pb^{2+}/mg protein, this effect had the characteristics of competitive inhibition. Addition of 1 nmol Pb^{2+}/mg protein resulted in almost complete inhibition of Ca^{2+} sequestering. Although these results were based almost entirely on *in vitro* work, the authors calculated that 0.5 nmol of Pb^{2+}/mg protein is equivalent to between 3 and 9 ppm Pb^{2+} in whole tissue. Persons without unusual exposure to lead have much lower concentrations of cardiac lead; however, in persons with unusually high lead exposure, the aorta showed the highest lead concentrations of any soft tissue, in the region of 2 ppm wet weight basis.[24] Cardiac complications are considered an unusual sequela of lead exposure in humans, although a few cases have been reported. For example, Freeman reported myocarditis in a three-year-old child with severe lead poisoning; cardiac status returned to normal within four days of chelation therapy with ethylenediaminetetraacetic acid (EDTA) for reduction of body burden of lead.[25] Others have reported cardiac changes accompanying lead intoxication.[26-28]

Effects of Lead on Calcium Metabolism

Lead-induced changes in calcium metabolism also have been observed. Varying effects of lead on calcium absorption have been reported. Doses of lead acetate greater than 20 μg/day decreased the transfer of calcium across the duodenal wall in rats, as determined by everted gut sac methods.[29] Doses of lead up to 200 μg/day continued to reduce calcium transfer; however, above 200 μg/day, no further decreases occurred. Similar results were seen for whole body retention of ^{47}Ca when measured three days after oral dosing with ^{47}Ca. Animals used in these experiments were not on chronic lead administration, but received lead for only seven days before measurement of ^{47}Ca retention. In contrast to these *in vitro* results, *in vivo* experiments demonstrated increased gastrointestinal absorption of calcium only at high orally administered doses of lead (20 mg Pb/day or greater) and only when the lead and calcium were given simultaneously.[30] In discussing reasons for differences in their *in vitro* and *in vivo* results, these authors note that *in vitro* everted gut sac techniques provided information primarily about transfer of substances through the intestinal wall, whereas their *in vivo* techniques permitted evaluation of lead-induced effects on the entire gastrointestinal tract; only the duodenum was studied in their *in vitro* studies.[31] Another difference between their *in vivo* and *in vitro* techniques was that *in vivo* transport takes place mainly through the mucosa and submucosa to blood vessels, whereas *in vitro* transfer was measured through all layers of the intestinal walls, including the lamina muscularis and serosa.

Contrasting results also have been reported for the effects of lead on serum calcium level. Total serum calcium was reduced ($P = 0.01$) in rats fed 200 ppm lead for 70 days.[32] This dose of lead for this time period produces blood lead concentrations of approximately 50 μg/dl in rats fed nutritionally adequate diets.

Increased serum calcium concentration in rats in response to acute administration of high doses of lead has been reported by several authors.[33-35] Yamaguchi and Yamamoto observed increases in serum calcium beginning 6 hours after a single intraperitoneal injection of 20 mg lead acetate/100 g body weight and lasting for about 60 hours.[33] The source of serum calcium in these studies was thought to be bone, although effects of lead on calcium homeostatic mechanisms in kidney or intestine cannot be excluded. Administration of thyrocalcitonin 23 hours after the lead injection caused a marked reduction in serum calcium levels.[33] Prolonged hypercalcemia induced by the administration of lead might be expected to stimulate the secretion of calcitonin to maintain calcium homeostasis. However, Peng *et al.* observed severe hypercalcemia in rats (serum calcium 20 mg/dl) within 90 minutes after an intravenous dose of 2.25 mg lead/100 g body weight.[35] The hypercalcemic response was due entirely to an increase in the nondialyzable fraction of serum calcium and was unaccompanied by increased secretion of calcitonin.[35] This could be due to the absence of change in the level of ionic calcium, which is known to regulate secretion of calcitonin, or to the direct effects of lead.[36,37] Chronic exposure of rats to lead has been reported to cause hyperplasia of the C-cells of the thyroid as well as hypersecretion of calcitonin.[35] The mechanisms responsible for these apparent differences in acute and chronic responses to lead have not been defined.

Lead administration can affect soft tissue calcium concentration. For example, kidney calcium concentration was dramatically increased ($P = 0.002$) when lead was fed with a low calcium diet. Because renal lead content and the percentage of rats with renal intranuclear inclusion bodies were both increased, the elevation in renal calcium content simply may be secondary to generalized renal damage and pathological tissue calcification.

Lead-induced changes also can be observed in bone metabolism of calcium. Some years ago, the lead line resulting at the metaphysis of lead-exposed children was described by Park *et al.* as due to an abnormal calcification of cartilage.[38] Hsu *et al.* observed inclusion bodies in multinucleated giant cells in bone and indicated that the osteoclasts became poisoned during osteolysis of bone containing high concentrations of lead.[9] Eisenstein and Kawanoue demonstrated that the histological lesion was due to impaired resorption of cartilage, depressed bone deposition on cartilaginous surfaces, and the accumulation of numerous multinucleated giant cells, some containing lead inclusions.[39] These investigators, using electron microscopy, identified these cells as osteoclasts and chondroclasts containing large amounts of mineralized cartilage matrix.

Parathyroid hormone, calcitonin, and vitamin D are highly important in phys-

TABLE 3

DIETARY CALCIUM INTAKE IN CONTROL AND LEAD-BURDENED CHILDREN*

	Control Children	Lead-Burdened Children
Mahaffey *et al.*, 1976[40]	570 ± 23†	457 ± 18†
Sorrell *et al.*, 1977[41]	800 ± 30†	580 ± 15†
Johnson & Tenuta, 1979[42]	615 ± 245‡	463 ± 152‡

* Mg Ca/day.
† Mean ± SEM.
‡ Mean ± standard deviation (SD).

iologic regulation of calcium metabolism. The release of calcitonin and formation of 1,25-dihydroxycholecalciferol are altered in lead-burdened animals and humans.

Clinical Associations

Dietary intake of calcium by lead-burdened children (blood Pb > 30 μg/dl) has been shown to be lower than the level of calcium ingested by matched controls in three cross-sectional studies conducted in Washington, D.C., New York City, and Milwaukee, Wisconsin.[40-42] Results of these studies are shown in TABLE 3. In these studies, control children were selected from similar neighborhoods and socioeconomic groups as the lead-burdened children, in some cases being siblings of the children with elevated blood lead concentrations. Such studies demonstrate only association and do not prove that the children had higher lead burdens because of ingesting a low calcium diet. However, if such dietary patterns persist in the presence of continued lead exposure, body burdens of lead could rise to a greater extent than would occur if the children were ingesting a nutritionally adequate diet.

Children with high body burdens of lead (blood Pb > 60 μg/dl) in the New York City study reported by Sorrell *et al.* had reduced dietary vitamin D intake by dietary history, which was confirmed by a lower concentration of 25-hydroxycholecalciferol than was observed in controls.[41] In these lead-poisoned children, serum levels of 1,25-dihydroxycholecalciferol were reduced to levels observed in hypoparathyroidism, uremia, and metabolic bone disease.[43] In lead-poisoned children, 1,25-dihydroxycholecalciferol levels returned to normal after chelation therapy with

TABLE 4

INFLUENCE OF DIETARY IRON ON SUSCEPTIBILITY TO LEAD TOXICITY IN RATS*

	Low Pb Exposure†		High Pb Exposure‡	
Dietary Fe	Blood Pb (μg/dl)	Kidney Pb (ppm)	Blood Pb (μg/dl)	Kidney Pb (ppm)
Deficient (10 ppm)	5.9 ± 0.05§	1.3 ± 0.18	159 ± 8	311 (254,382)¶
Adequate (40 ppm)	9.7 ± 1.8	1.05 ± 0.14	113 ± 11	44 (33,61)
High (120 ppm)	5.8 ± 1.0	0.85 ± 0.10	76 ± 7	26 (19,36)

* Reference 46.
† Deionized water, diet <0.01 ppm Pb.
‡ 200 ppm Pb in water, diet <0.01 ppm Pb.
§ Mean ± SEM.
¶ Data log transformed, error estimates not symmetrical about the mean.

TABLE 5

INFLUENCE OF DIETARY IRON ON SUSCEPTIBILITY TO LEAD TOXICITY IN RATS*

	Femur Pb (ppm)	
Dietary Fe	Low Pb Exposure†	High Pb Exposure‡
Deficient (10 ppm)	3.11 ± 0.26§	339 ± 14
Adequate (40 ppm)	1.04 ± 0.14	209 ± 22
High (120 ppm)	5.8 ± 1.0	187 ± 23

* Reference 46.
† Deionized water, diet <0.01 ppm Pb.
‡ 200 ppm Pb in water, diet <0.01 ppm Pb.
§ Mean ± SEM.

$CaNa_2EDTA$, whereas the serum 25-hydroxycholecalciferol concentration did not change with chelation therapy. These data provide evidence that the biosynthesis of 1,25-dihydroxycholecalciferol is inhibited in lead-burdened children.

IRON AND LEAD

General Effects

Overall, substantially less is known about the effects of iron on lead metabolism than on the interactions of calcium and lead. Iron deficiency increased susceptibility of rats to lead intoxication.[44] Iron-deficient rats have increased concentrations of lead in kidney and bone (TABLES 4 and 5) compared with rats ingesting equivalent quantities of water containing 200 ppm lead and an iron-adequate diet.

The degree of iron deficiency associated with increased body burden of lead need not be severe. Experimental animals with increased lead burden showed only a slight decrease in hematocrit; however, liver iron stores were greatly reduced. Although lead toxicity and iron deficiency act at different steps in the heme biosynthetic pathway, the degree of anemia produced by the combination of iron-deficient diet and lead intoxication is greater than that resulting from either alone. Measurement of various intermediate compounds in heme synthesis illustrates both independent and combined effects of iron and lead. For example, erythrocyte protoporphyrins are increased moderately in iron deficiency but are greatly increased by lead

TABLE 6

URINARY DELTA-AMINOLEVULINIC ACID (dALA) EXCRETION BY RATS FED NORMAL AND LOW Fe DIETS WITH AND WITHOUT Pb*

Dietary Group	*N*	Urinary dALA, (μg/24 hr)
Normal Fe	9	20 ± 5†
Low Fe	8	22 ± 5
Normal Fe + Pb‡	8	180 ± 25
Low Fe + Pb‡	8	355 ± 50

* Reference 44.
† Mean ± SEM.
‡ 200 μg Pb/ml drinking water.

intoxication. Generally, lead intoxication results in far greater increases in free erythrocyte protoporphyrins than does iron deficiency.[45] Urinary excretion of dALA is not increased by iron deficiency alone but is elevated by lead toxicity (TABLE 6). Simultaneous occurrence of these conditions results in higher dALA excretions than those produced by lead alone; however, this may be due to an increased body burden of lead in iron deficiency. High levels of iron appear to decrease susceptibility to lead toxicity. Mahaffey *et al.* observed that increasing dietary iron concentrations to levels three times those recommended for nutritional purposes decreased kidney, femur, and blood lead levels in rats fed varying concentrations of iron for 10 weeks (TABLES 4 and 5).[46]

Absorption

Using retention of ^{210}Pb as an estimate of gastrointestinal absorption, Ragan demonstrated sixfold increases in tissue lead in rats when body iron stores were reduced but before frank iron deficiency developed.[47] Based on results obtained by *in situ* ligated gut loop techniques, Barton *et al.* have demonstrated that iron deficiency secondary to bleeding and iron-deficient diets increased lead absorption and that iron loading decreased lead absorption (FIGURE 3).[48] Ferritin has been shown to bind lead both *in vivo* and *in vitro*.[49] In rats fed an iron-deficient diet, the ferritin concentration would be low, permitting increased transfer of lead to blood rather than retention in the small intestine, bound to ferritin.[50] Transferrin is increased in iron deficiency anemia due to increased transferrin synthesis.[51] Although it binds iron preferentially, transferrin will also transport a number of trivalent and divalent cations, such as plutonium, americium, chromium, cobalt, manganese, and copper.[52,53]

Excretion

Barton *et al.* also determined whole body retention of a single intravenous injection of ^{210}Pb over a period of four weeks and found that rats retained similar quan-

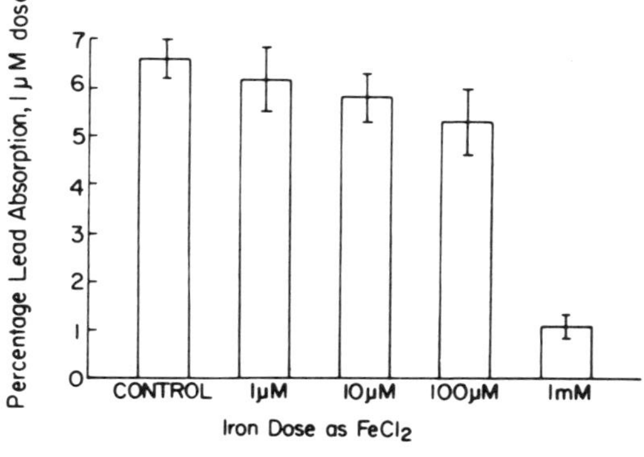

FIGURE 3. Effect of variation of iron chloride in the intubation media on the absorption of radiolabeled lead chloride. (Reprinted from Reference 48 with permission of the C. V. Mosby Company.)

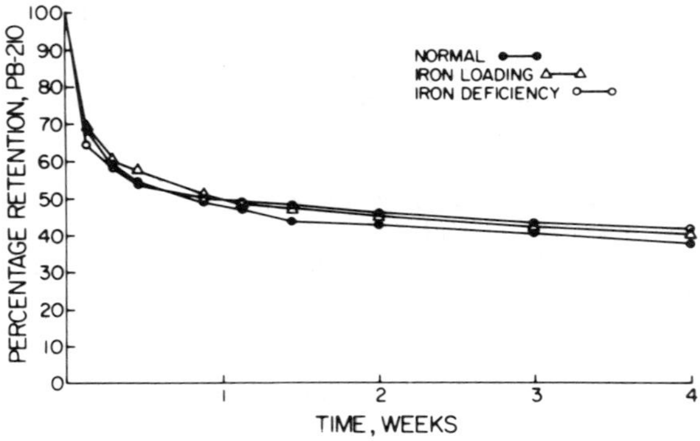

FIGURE 4. Comparison of the retention of ^{210}Pb by normal, iron-loaded, and iron-deficient rats. (Reprinted from Reference 48 with permission of the C. V. Mosby Company.)

tities of lead whether or not they were iron-deficient, normal, or iron loaded (FIGURE 4), demonstrating that body iron status does not alter lead excretion.[48]

Tissue and Organ Distribution of Lead

Unlike the changes occurring in calcium deficiency, iron-deficient animals do not show a more marked deposition of lead in nonosseous than in osseous tissues (TABLE 7).

Cellular Effects

Lowered tissue iron levels in iron-deficient animals can alter effects of lead on enzyme systems. Waxman and Rabinowitz, using incubation of reticulocytes, reported that lead inhibited hemoglobin synthesis as a specific antagonist of heme synthesis and as a general heavy metal inhibitor of cell metabolism.[54] Addition of ferrous iron protected both functions against the action of lead. An interaction exists between the effects of lead and iron on general cellular synthetic reactions. Borsook *et al.* reported that incorporation of C^{14}-labeled amino acids into rabbit reticulocytes was increased by iron and inhibited by lead.[55] Based on these observations, decreasing tissue iron content in iron deficiency may account for increased biochemical effects produced by a specific dose of lead on an iron-deficient diet.

Administration of lead to animals inhibits the activity and level of some iron-containing enzymes. Goldberg *et al.* demonstrated that pretreatment of rats by intraperitoneal injection of lead resulted in a decrease in hepatic microsomal P-450 and b_5 content, with a more marked effect on P-450 than on b_5.[56] Rhyne and Goyer found that rats receiving 1% lead acetate in the diet had a reduced concentration of cytochrome a_3.[57]

Effects of Lead on Iron Metabolism

Liver iron concentration is usually considered a reliable general index of nutritional status for iron. Total liver iron was unaffected, but kidney iron was

TABLE 7

COMPARISON OF TISSUE CONCENTRATIONS OF LEAD IN RATS FED DIETS DEFICIENT IN CALCIUM (LCa) AND IRON (LFe) AND NUTRITIONALLY ADEQUATE DIETS (NCa, NFe)*

Diet	Pb (μg/g wet tissue) Bone	Kidney
No Pb		
NCa, NFe	2.2 ± 1.0†	2.6 ± 1.2
LFe	10.6 ± 3.0	1.9 ± 0.4
LCa	9.7 ± 2.2	4.4 ± 0.6
200 μg Pb/ml H_2O		
NCa, NFe	74 ± 12	22 ± 4.3
LFe	225 ± 15	28.7 ± 4.8
LCa	202 ± 202	691 ± 203

* Reference 44.
† Mean ± SEM.

significantly lowered by the addition of 200 ppm lead to both iron-deficient and iron-adequate diets.[44] The parameter measured was the quantity of iron present in the total organ. However, total organ iron content does not adequately reflect the iron/lead interaction. Lead exposure produces substantial changes in iron metabolism and distribution of iron at the cellular level.

Decreases in heme synthesis reduce the utilization of iron, whereas the hemolytic component of lead-induced anemia could be associated with increases in iron entering the reticuloendothelial system. Wibowo *et al.* found a negative correlation between serum ferritin and whole blood lead concentration in male, but not female, adults.[58] Kochen and Greener reported binding of lead by serum transferrin, while Kochen and Greener and Rüssell observed binding of lead by ferritin in liver, kidney, and spleen.[59,60,49] Lead has a variety of effects on metabolism of iron or on enzymes related to iron metabolism. Saturation of total iron-binding capacity markedly suppressed uptake of plasma lead by red blood cells and increased uptake of lead by liver.[59] Lead does not interfere with incorporation of iron into red cell precursors; however, transfer of nonheme iron into hemoglobin was nearly completely blocked.[61] These authors suggested that the actual blockage of iron transport by lead occurred between the ferritin fraction and iron compounds in the mitochondria. Lead toxicity causes a sideroblastic anemia. Jensen *et al.* using electron microscopy have shown that in lead intoxication, red cell precursors contain many grossly swollen mitchondria, with ferritin particles and ferruginous micelles accumulating in the mitochondria as well as scattered in the cytoplasm.[62] Jensen *et al.* also demonstrated that nonheme iron is associated with cellular basophilic stippling induced by lead.[62] Sassa, in a review of effects of lead on heme metabolism, noted that lead interferes with utilization of iron for heme formation in the mitochondria, producing excessive accumulation of iron and destruction of the mitochondria.[63] Borová *et al.* and Pǒnka and Neuwirt indicate that accumulation of iron in the mitochondria is due to increased uptake of iron from the cytoplasm as well as to decreased iron utilization.[64,65]

Clinical Association

Iron deficiency is potentially of greater clinical significance than is calcium deficiency in altering susceptibility of children to lead toxicity because of the relative prevalence of iron and calcium deficiencies. Some of the types of data that are available for effects of dietary calcium level on lead metabolism do not exist yet for iron. For example, balance study data on lead absorption by iron-deficient children are not yet available. Further, dietary surveys have not shown a clear reduction in dietary iron intake among lead-burdened children. Clinically, the role of iron is in prevention of accumulation of body burden of lead rather than in stimulating excretion of lead. Angle *et al.* have reported that administration of oral iron therapy did not influence blood lead concentrations among children exposed to lead.[66] However, the subjects had elevated blood lead concentrations at the start of their therapeutic programs. When this study is viewed in light of the knowledge that iron status does not alter lead excretion, the negative findings are understandable.

References

1. Aub, J. C., L. T. Fairhall, A. S. Minot & P. Reznikoff. 1926. Lead Poisoning. Medical Monographs **7**. Williams & Wilkins Company. Baltimore, Md.
2. Sobel, A. E., H. Yusha, D. D. Peters & B. Kramer. 1940. J. Biol. Chem. **132:** 239–265.
3. Shields, J. B. & H. H. Mitchell. 1941. J. Nutr. **21:** 541.
4. Hunter, D. 1975. The Diseases of Occupations. 5th edit.: 275. The English Universities Press, Ltd. London, Great Britain.
5. Mahaffey, K. R., R. A. Goyer & J. Haseman. 1973. J. Lab. Clin. Med. **82:** 92–100.
6. Mahaffey, K. R., T. A. Banks, C. L. Stone, S. G. Capar, J. F. Compton & M. H. Gubkin. 1975. Effect of varying dietary calcium on susceptibility to lead toxicity in the rat. *In* International Conference on Heavy Metals in the Environment. T. C. Hutchinson, Ed. **3:** 155–164. Institute for Environmental Studies. Toronto, Canada.
7. Quarterman, J. & J. N. Morrison. 1975. Br. J. Nutr. **34:** 351–362.
8. Calvery, H. O., E. P. Laug & H. J. Morris. 1938. J. Pharmacol. Exp. Ther. **64:** 365–367.
9. Hsu, F. S., L. Krook, J. N. Shively & J. R. Duncan. 1973. Science **181:** 447–448.
10. Willoughby, R. A., T. Thirapatsakun & B. J. McSherry. 1972. Am. J. Vet. Res. **33:** 1165–1173.
11. Morrison, J. N., J. Quarterman & W. R. Humphries. 1977. J. Comp. Pathol. **87:** 417–429.
12. Lederer. L. B. & F. C. Bing. 1940. J. Am. Med. Assoc. **114:** 2457–2461.
13. Barton, J. C., M. E. Conrad, L. Harrison & S. Nuby. 1978. J. Lab. Clin. Med. **91:** 367–376.
14. Mahaffey, K. R., C. Smith, Y. Tanaka & H. F. DeLuca. 1979. Fed. Proc. Fed. Am. Soc. Exp. Biol. **38:** 384.
15. Barltrop, D. & H. E. Khoo. 1975. Postgrad. Med. J. **57:** 795–800.
16. Meredith, P. A., M. R. Moore & A. Goldberg. 1977. Biochem. J. **166:** 531–537.
17. Ziegler, E. E., B. B. Edwards, R. L. Jensen, K. R. Mahaffey & S. J. Fomon. 1978. Pediatr. Res. **12:** 29–34.
18. Frolik, C. A. & H. F. DeLuca. 1971. Arch. Biochem. Biophys. **147:** 143–147.
19. Rosen, J. G. & E. G. Wexler. 1977. Biochem. Pharmacol. **26:** 650–653.
20. Norimatsu, H. & R. V. Talmage. 1979. Proc. Soc. Exp. Biol. Med. **161:** 94–98.
21. Kostial, J. & V. B. Vouk. 1957. Br. J. Pharmacol. Chemother. **12:** 219–222.
22. Silbergeld, E. 1973. Fed. Proc. Fed. Am. Soc. Exp. Biol. **32:** 275.
23. Parr, D. R. & E. J. Harris. 1976. Biochem. J. **158:** 289–294.
24. Barry, P. S. I. 1978. Distribution and storage of lead in human tissues. *In* Biogeochemistry of Lead. J. Nriagu, Ed.: 124. Elsevier/North Holland Biomedical Press. Amsterdam, The Netherlands.
25. Freeman, R. 1973. Clin. Toxicol. Bull. **3:** 75–89.
26. Kline, T. S. 1960. Am. J. Dis. Child. **99:** 48–54.
27. Read, J. L. & J. P. Williams. 1952. Am. Heart J. **44:** 797–802.
28. Myerson, R. M. & J. H. Eisenhauer. 1963. Am. J. Cardiol. **11:** 409–412.

29. Gruden, N. 1975. Toxicology **5:** 163–166.
30. Gruden, N. & M. Buben. 1977. Bull. Environ. Contam. Toxicol. **18:** 303–307.
31. Gruden, N. & M. Buben. 1979. Environ. Res. **18:** 270–275.
32. Mahaffey-Six, K. & R. A. Goyer. 1970. J. Lab. Clin. Med. **76:** 933–942.
33. Yamaguchi, N. & F. Yamamoto. 1974. Toxicol. Appl. Pharmacol. **29:** 233.
34. Kato, Y., S. Takimoto & H. Ogura. 1977. Calcif. Tissue Res. **24:** 41.
35. Peng, T. C., N. J. Gitelman & S. C. Garner. 1979. Proc. Soc. Exp. Biol. Med. **160:** 114–117.
36. Munson, P. L. 1976. Physiology and pharmacology of thyrocalcitonin. *In* Handbook of Physiology. G. D. Auerbach, Ed. **7**(Section 7): 443-464. American Physiological Society. Washington, D.C.
37. Peng, T. C., S. C. Garner, H. J. Gitelman & P. Petrusz. 1978. Abstract No. 388. Seventh International Congress of Pharmacology, Paris, France.
38. Park, E. A., D. Jackson, T. C. Goodwin & L. Kadji. 1933. J. Pediatr. **3:** 265–298.
39. Eisenstein, R. & S. Kawanoue. 1975. Am. J. Pathol. **80:** 309–316.
40. Mahaffey, K. R., S. Treloar, T. A. Banks, B. J. Peacock & L. E. Parekh. 1976. (abst.) J. Nutr. **107**(7): xxx.
41. Sorrell, M., J. F. Rosen & M. R. Roginsky. 1977. Arch. Environ. Health **32:** 160–164.
42. Johnson, N. E. & K. Tenuta. 1979. Environ. Res. **18:** 369–376.
43. Rosen, J. R., R. W. Chesney, A. Hamstra, H. F. DeLuca & K. R. Mahaffey. 1980. N. Engl. J. Med. **302:** 1128–1131.
44. Mahaffey-Six, K. & R. A. Goyer. 1972. J. Lab. Clin. Med. **79:** 128–136.
45. Piomelli, S. 1977. Clin. Chem. **23:** 264–269.
46. Mahaffey, K. R., C. L. Stone, T. A. Banks & C. Reed. 1978. Reduction in tissue storage of lead in the rat by feeding diets with elevated iron concentration. *In* Proceedings of the Third International Symposium on Trace Element Metabolism in Man and Animals. M. Kirchgessner, Ed.: 584–588. Arbeitskreis fur Tierernahung-Storschung. Freising-Weihenstephan, Federal Republic of Germany.
47. Ragan, H. A. 1977. J. Lab. Clin. Med. **90:** 700–706.
48. Barton, J. C., M. E. Conrad, S. Nuby & L. Harrison. 1978. J. Lab. Clin. Med. **92:** 536–547.
49. Rüssell, H. A. 1970. Bull. Environ. Contam. Toxicol. **5**(2): 115–124.
50. Worwood, M. 1974. Iron and the trace metals. *In* Iron in Biochemjstry and Medicine. A Jacobs & M. Worwood, Eds.: 335–367. Academic Press, Inc. New York, N.Y.
51. Awai, M. & E. B. Brown. 1963. J. Lab. Clin. Med. **61:** 369–396.
52. Taylor, D. M. 1972. Health Phys. **22:** 575–581.
53. Aisen, P. & E. B. Brown. 1977. The iron-binding function of transferrin in iron metabolism. *In* Iron Excess. Aberrations of Iron and Porphyrin Metabolism. U. Muller-Eberhard, P. A. Miescher & E. R. Jaffé, Eds.: 31–53. Grune & Stratton, Inc. New York, N.Y.
54. Waxman, H. S. & M. Rabinovitz. 1966. Biochim. Biophys. Acta **129:** 369–379.
55. Borsook, H., E. H. Fischer & G. Keighley. 1957. J. Biol. Chem. **229:** 1059.
56. Goldberg, A., P. A. Meredith, S. Miller, M. R. Moore & G. C. Thompson. 1978. Br. J. Pharmacol. **62:** 529–536.
57. Rhyne, B. C. & R. A. Goyer. 1971. Exp. Mol. Pathol. **14:** 386.
58. Wibowo, A. A. E., P. Delcastilho, R. F. M. Herber & R. L. Zielhuis. 1977. Int. Arch. Occup. Environ. Health **39:** 113–120.
59. Kochen, J. & Y. Greener. 1975. (abst. no. 400). Pediatr. Res. **9:** 323.
60. Kochen, J. & Y. Greener. 1975. (abst. no. 399). Pediatr. Res. **9:** 323.
61. Lothe, K. & I. Falbe-Hansen. 1963. Clin. Sci. **24:** 47–54.
62. Jensen, W. N., G. D. Moreno & M. Bessis. 1965. Blood **25:** 933–943.
63. Sassa, S. 1978. Toxic effects of lead with particular reference to porphyrin and heme metabolism. *In* Handbook of Experimental Pharmacology. Heme and Hemoproteins. F. DeMatters & W. N. Aldridge, Eds. **44:** 333–371. Springer-Verlag. New York, N.Y.
64. Borová, J., P. Pŏnka & G. Neuwirt. 1973. Biochim. Biophys. Acta **320:** 143–156.
65. Pŏnka, P. & G. Neuwirt. 1975. N. Engl. J. Med. **293:** 406.
66. Angle, C. R., K. L. Stelmark & M. S. McIntire. 1976. Lead and iron deficiency. *In* Trace Substances in Environmental Health. D. D. Hemphill, Ed. **9:** 377. University of Missouri Press. Columbia, Mo.

THE INFLUENCE OF DIETARY ZINC AND COPPER ON THE BIOLOGIC EFFECTS OF ORALLY INGESTED LEAD IN THE RAT

Harold G. Petering

Kettering Laboratory
University of Cincinnati
Medical Center
Cincinnati, Ohio 45219

Lead is a biologically nonessential metal to which human beings and domestic animals are widely and variably exposed because of its many industrial uses and, therefore, its wide dissemination. At the levels to which human beings are exposed in the workplace as well as in the general environment, lead has been shown to be a toxic element in most of its chemical forms, whether it is inhaled or ingested in water or food. It has now become a ubiquitous contaminant of the human environment and as such is a cause for great and increasing concern to the medical community.

This paper will deal with some of the biologic effects of inorganic lead compounds that are ingested via the oral route. These effects may or may not result in overt toxicity of lead as usually defined, but, as our work and that of other investigators imply, such biologic effects may contribute to ill health in general and to the incidence and severity of some chronic diseases that afflict modern society. We are concerned, therefore, with definable effects of lead on biochemical and cellular processes that in themselves may not be accepted as symptoms of lead toxicity. As an introduction to the discussion of the interaction of zinc and copper nutriture with the effects of oral lead, it may be of value to list the recognized manifestations of lead toxicity that occur when biochemical and cellular processes become severely impaired. The symptoms of lead toxicity, as given in TABLE 1, are not always fully reversible when exposure to lead is stopped.

Among the best recognized and most studied manifestations of lead toxicity are depression of hematopoiesis and inhibition of heme synthesis, which ultimately result in anemia of the microcytic hypochromic type. This anemia, as we shall show, is a result of copper and iron metabolic impairment. Some of the early signs of the inhibition of heme synthesis—such as increased urinary δ-aminolevulinic acid (ALA), decreased erythrocyte δ-aminolevulinic acid dehydratase (ALA-D), or increased free erythrocyte porphyrin (FEP)—are used to monitor the level of lead ingestion.

Another well-defined indication of lead toxicity is that of peripheral neuropathy in adults and central nervous system (CNS) damage in children. Gastrointestinal disturbances and distress as well as renal damage are also a result of chronic exposure to relatively high doses of lead.

Epidemiologic and clinical as well as experimental evidence exists to indicate that ingestion of inorganic lead causes reproductive failure and thyroid disturbances. Recently, experimental and clinical reports have indicated that lead exposure can result in elevated blood pressure and cardiomyopathy.[1,2]

As we critically evaluate the toxic symptoms, the biochemical effects, and the pathologic lesions of lead ingestion as listed in TABLE 1, we find that a number of these suggest an alteration in the nutritional and biochemical roles of the essential micronutrients zinc and copper. In addition to their separate biologic functions, zinc and copper must be kept in balance in the diet if they are to play their metabolic roles

0077-8923/80/0355-0298 $01.75/0 © 1980, NYAS

TABLE 1

MAJOR TOXIC EFFECTS OF LEAD

1. Depression of Hematopoiesis—leading to anemia
2. Depression of Iron Metabolism
3. Depressive Effects on Nervous System
a. Peripheral neuropathy of adults
b. CNS lesions of children—lead encephalopathy
4. Renal Damage
a. Fanconi syndrome—aminoaciduria, glycosuria, and phosphaturia
b. Nephropathy
c. Atrophy of convoluted tubules
5. Effects on Other Organs
a. Impaired I uptake by thyroid
b. Hypertension—vascular system
c. Cardiomyopathy—abnormal electrocardiograph—heart

effectively, as was early shown by Cox and Harris and Magee and Matrone, and as has recently been confirmed by others.[3-5]

ZINC-LEAD INTERACTION

Interactions of zinc with lead have been demonstrated in several areas of biologic and toxic reactions. These involve the inhibition of heme synthesis by lead, the effect of lead on the brain and central nervous system, and the absorption of lead from the gastrointestinal tract.

The history of the effect of lead ingestion on the hematopoietic system has been reviewed by Waldron and Stöfen.[6] It has been recognized for many years that lead poisoning in humans results in the appearance of excess porphyrin in the urine, and the effects of lead on the hematopoietic system have been studied by many clinical and experimental scientists.[6] The heme synthetic pathway is shown in FIGURE 1, in which the steps inhibited by lead are indicated. The steps that are inhibited, as clearly indicated by a great deal of research, are those involving the enzyme ALA-D and ferrochelatase or heme-synthetase. The former enzyme catalyzes the dehydration of δ-aminolevulinic acid to form porphobilinogen, and the latter one catalyzes the insertion of iron into protoporphyrin IX, which also requires the presence of glutathione and ascorbic acid. The enzymes are reasonably sensitive to lead inhibition, while some work has shown that δ-aminolevulinate synthetase and coprogenase may possibly be affected by very large concentrations of lead that are not of physiologic significance.

δ-Aminolevulinate dehytratase (ALA-D) has been found to be activated *in vitro* by zinc ions and, by Finelli *et al.*, to be a zinc-dependent enzyme *in vivo*.[7-10] The consequence of the inhibition of ALA-D is an increase in the amount of plasma and urinary ALA. Thus, the inhibition of ALA-D by lead can be detected either by increased excretion of urinary ALA or by a decrease in blood or red blood cell (RBC) enzyme activity. Not only is the inhibition of ALA-D contributory to a reduction in heme synthesis, but it has become a very sensitive measure of the exposure of an individual to lead, and one that many investigators regard as more sensitive or more reliable than the blood lead level or the urinary excretion of lead.[11] The biological

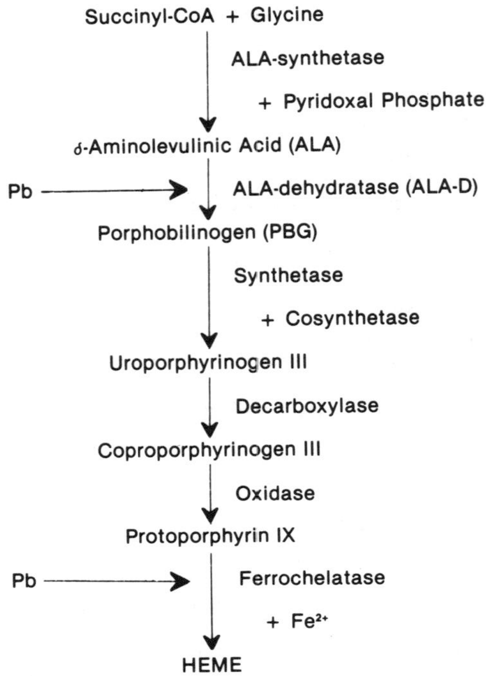

FIGURE 1. Heme synthetic pathway with inhibitory effects of lead shown.

importance of ALA-D is still in question, since it is not considered to be a rate-limiting enzyme in the heme synthetic pathway; but it still represents a useful system for the study of zinc-lead interactions.

The fact that zinc is required for ALA-D activity has been shown by a number of investigators, beginning with the observations of Komai and Neilands.[7] In 1971, Abdulla and Haeger-Aronsen found that the activity of ALA-D in erythrocytes and liver of young rats was directly related to the amount of zinc in the diet and that Zn^{2+} added in concentrations of 10^{-7} to 10^{-3} M to erythrocyte enzyme preparations markedly increased the enzyme activity.[8] In 1975, Finelli and associates reported that lead-inhibited blood ALA-D of rats *in vivo* was not restored to normal levels after lead administration was stopped if the dietary intake of zinc was low.[12] Their results are shown in FIGURE 2. In the same report, these investigators showed that the reduced blood ALA-D activity could be restored *in vitro* by the addition of Zn^{2+} to the enzyme preparation. These results are shown in FIGURE 3. In this figure, one can also see that there was a higher enzyme activity realized in the high dietary zinc controls than in the controls getting only 5 ppm dietary Zn. It was also found in this experiment that *in vitro* concentrations of Zn^{2+} greater than 10^{-4} or 10^{-3} resulted in enzyme inhibition.

Following the direction of the work of Finelli *et al.*, Thomasino *et al.* found that these same relationships of lead to zinc could be demonstrated in a patient with lead poisoning.[12,13] Their work showed that chelation therapy with ethylenediaminetetra-acetate to remove lead from soft tissues of the patient caused a great increase in urinary excretion of zinc with a concomitant decrease in serum zinc and a reduction

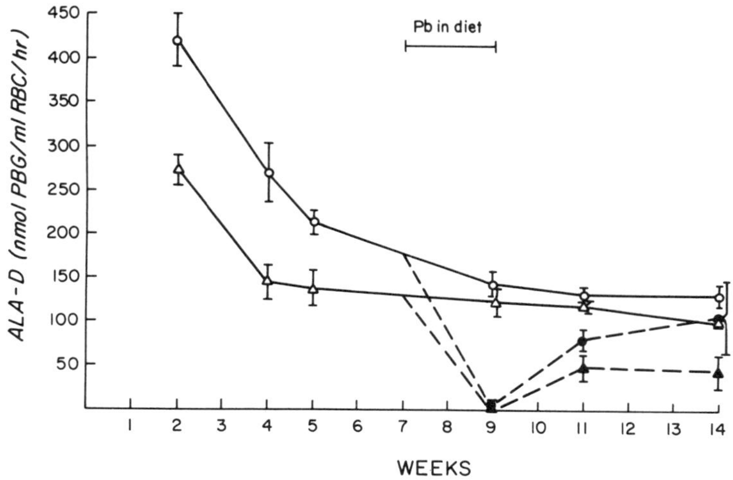

FIGURE 2. Erythrocyte ALA-D activity of rats fed a semipurified diet low in zinc and supplemented in the drinking water as follows: 40 μg Zn/ml (○——○); 40 μg Zn/ml + 200 μg Pb/ml (● ---- ●); 2.5 μg Zn/ml (△——△); 2.5 μg Zn/ml + 200 μg Pb/ml (▲ ---- ▲). Lead given as acetate as indicated. (Reprinted from Reference 12 with permission of Academic Press, Inc.)

of RBC ALA-D activity. Giving the patient extra zinc restored the RBC ALA-D levels promptly.

In a recent article, Dutkiewicz *et al.* reported that mixed exposure of workers to lead and zinc rather than to lead alone resulted in a reduced excretion of ALA and had a tendency to result in lower blood lead levels.[14] This finding confirms what

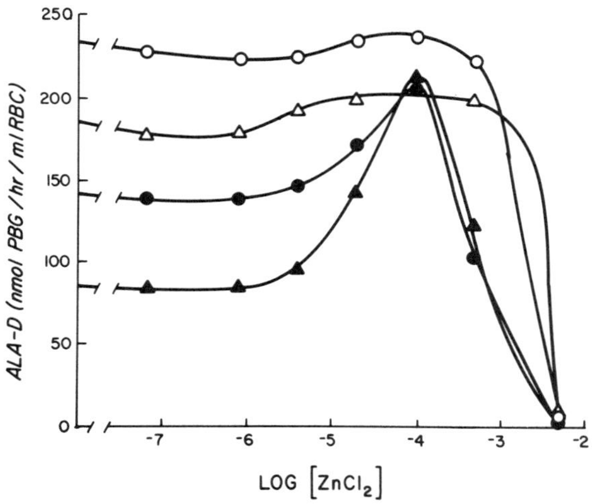

FIGURE 3. ALA-D activation *in vitro* by addition of $ZnCl_2$ to blood preparation of rats exposed to conditions given in FIGURE 2. (Reprinted from Reference 12 with permission of Academic Press, Inc.)

TABLE 2

SOME EFFECTS OF DIETARY ZINC ON LEAD TOXICITY IN THE RAT*

Zn in Diet† (ppm)	8	35	200
Blood Pb (μg/100 g)	86.0 ± 9.0	66.0 ± 5.0	36.0 ± 5.0
Tibia Pb (μg/g ash)	191.0 ± 11.0	204.0 ± 29.0	91.0 ± 12.0
U-ALA (μg/mg creatinine) (% of control)	361.0 ± 24.0	318.0 ± 30.0	183.0 ± 12.0
% Pb Absorbed (based on food intake and fecal analysis)	25.0 ± 4.2	16.1 ± 4.0	10.0 ± 2.2

* Data taken from Cerklewski and Forbes, Reference 15.

† The basal diet was a semipurified one deficient in Zn to which 200 ppm Pb (as acetate) and the indicated amounts of Zn (as carbonate) were added. Values are given as means ± standard error of the mean (SEM). U-ALA is urinary ALA.

would be expected from the studies described here on the experimental protection of extra zinc on lead absorption and toxicity. Thus, epidemiologic and clinical studies cannot be based solely on lead exposure but must also take into consideration other concomitant exposures—in this case, that of a protective agent, namely, zinc.

There are other manifestations of the interaction between zinc and lead. Cerklewski and Forbes found that lead absorption was markedly reduced when dietary zinc of rats was increased to very high levels.[15] This was shown by blood and tibia lead, ALA urinary excretion, and fecal lead, as indicated in TABLE 2. High dietary zinc was definitely related to decreased absorption of lead and to reduced retention of lead as indicated by low tibia lead.

In several recent publications, Finelli and El-Gazzar have shown that lead caused an increase in prothrombin time of the clotting of rat blood when the dietary zinc was 5 ppm, whereas it had no effect when dietary zinc was 50 ppm after the rats received 100 ppm Pb in the diet for 90 days.[16] After 140 days of lead ingestion by the rats, the level of dietary zinc made no difference in the prothrombin time, a fact that suggests a time-dose effect of dietary Zn in inhibiting this biologic effect of lead. In the same experiment, El-Gazzar *et al.* showed that 100 ppm lead in the diet caused a significant reduction in plasma, tibia, and liver zinc levels and that high dietary Zn

TABLE 3

EFFECT OF LEAD ON ZINC METABOLISM*

Dietary Supplements† (μg/ml)		Zinc Concentrations‡		
Zn	Pb	Plasma (μg/ml ± SEM)	Liver (μg/g ± SEM)	Tibia (μg/g ± SEM)
5	0	1.70 ± 0.12^{c}	36.0 ± 2.5^{b}	136.6 ± 15.9^{a,c}
5	100	1.34 ± 0.07^{c}	23.5 ± 1.0^{b}	94.6 ± 6.0$^{a',c}$
50	0	1.81 ± 0.24$^{c'}$	30.5 ± 1.7	325.2 ± 12.8$^{a,c'}$
50	100	1.46 ± 0.07$^{c'}$	27.5 ± 1.6	286.6 ± 7.9$^{a',c'}$

* Data taken from El-Gazzar *et al.*, Reference 17.

† Basal semipurified diet with <1 ppm Zn was fed to all male rats for 140 days. Supplements were given in the drinking water.

‡ Statistical differences in each set of values are given by identical superscripts in vertical columns (a, a′ = $P < 0.001$; b = $P < 0.01$; c, c′ = $P < 0.05$).

(50 ppm) reduced this effect in liver and tibia.[17] These results are summarized in TABLE 3.

Michaelson and Sauerhoff reported in 1973 that chronically ingested inorganic lead by rat neonates through the dam's milk caused a marked reduction of Zn in the cerebral cortex, cerebellum, and caudate nucleus portions of their brains.[18] These reductions cannot be explained by the increased edema, with its resultant increased retention of blood, since increased blood in the tissue would have produced an increase in tissue Zn because of the high Zn content of the RBC. Furthermore, there was an increase of Fe only in the cerebellum and not in the other portions mentioned above. These findings, which are given in TABLE 4, are associated with paraplegia in the neonates and may relate to the mental retardation found in lead-poisoned children. They should be viewed in light of the reports of Warkany and Petering, who found that Zn deficiency during the gestation period of rats even for as short a time as six days caused extensive brain damage to occur.[19,20] Thus it might be well to explore further the relationship of dietary Zn intake to CNS damage due to lead in children and animal models using neonatal ingestion of lead.

COPPER-LEAD INTERACTIONS

The role of copper nutrition in lead intoxication is less well established than is that of zinc nutrition, but recent work by Klauder has definitely shown that there are important copper-lead interactions.[21] In fact, Klauder found that the lead-induced reduction of kidney zinc was greatly minimized by increasing the dietary intake of copper in the rats under experimentation, a fact that suggests a definite Zn-Cu-Pb interaction.

In 1972, Klauder *et al.* presented data that indicated that copper nutrition markedly altered the effect of 2.5% lead acetate trihydrate (1.37% Pb) in the diet of rats.[22] This level of lead intake also affected copper metabolism, including several indications of copper deficiency symptoms. Thus, there was reduced growth and lowered serum copper and ceruloplasmin in lead-treated rats as well as increased ab-

TABLE 4

ZINC, COPPER, AND LEAD CONCENTRATIONS OF BRAIN TISSUES OF RAT NEONATES*†

		Metal Concentrations of Tissues‡ [μg/g (wet wt) ± SEM]		
		Pb	Zn	Cu
Cerebral Cortex	−Pb	0.07 ± 0.02[a]	16.0 ± 3.0[b]	3.2 ± 1.0
	+Pb	6.0 ± 0.8[a]	7.0 ± 2.0[b]	3.0 ± 1.0
Cerebellum	−Pb	0.15 ± 0.03[a′]	11.0 ± 0.7[a]	2.5 ± 0.4[b]
	+Pb	12.5 ± 3.5[a′]	6.0 ± 1.0[a]	1.2 ± 0.26[b]
Caudate Nucleus	−Pb	0.08 ± 0.02[a″]	15.0 ± 2.0[a′]	4.8 ± 1.6
	+Pb	6.2 ± 0.4[a″]	8.0 ± 0.5[a′]	2.9 ± 0.4

* Stock diet with or without 2.5% Pb (as acetate) was fed to dams of suckling neonates as indicated. Data were taken on 25th day after birth.

† Data taken from Michaelson and Sauerhoff, Reference 18.

‡ Statistically significant differences are shown by matching superscripts of each column (a, a′, a″ = $P < 0.01$; b = $P < 0.02$).

TABLE 5

EFFECT OF DIETARY COPPER ON LEAD TOXICITY IN THE RAT*

	Dietary Concentration of Copper†‡ (μg/g)		
	0.5	4.5	8.5
RBC Pb (μg/100 g)	169_a	148	131_a
Kidney Pb (μg/g dry wt)	340_a	275	155_a
Liver Pb (μg/g dry wt)	25^{AB}	12^{A}	9^{B}
Brain Pb (μg/g dry wt)	12.3^{A}_{a}	6.5_a	3.8^{A}

* Data taken from Klauder, Reference 21.
† Semipurified diet containing 0.5% Pb was fed to growing rats for 17 weeks.
‡ Statistical differences at $P < 0.01$ are indicated by identical superscripts; and at $P < 0.05$, by identical subscripts.

sorption of lead if the dietary copper was low. Increasing the dietary copper restored normal copper metabolism.

Giving a high dietary intake of lead to lactating female rats was shown by Michaelson and Saurhoff to cause paraplegia in suckling neonates.[18] The cerebella of the neonates also showed a marked reduction in the normal concentration of copper (cf., TABLE 4). Since one of the metabolic roles of copper is as an active component of metalloenzymes involved in the synthesis of catecholamine neurotransmitters, it is possible that an interference of brain copper metabolism may be involved in the development of the paraplegia found in lead-exposed neonates.

In 1975, Klauder and Petering reported that dietary copper deficiency in rats receiving a relatively low level of lead (500 ppm) in the diet resulted in an elevation of erythrocyte and kidney lead and a marked depression of hematopoiesis as shown by low hematocrit and hemoglobin values.[23] In another experiment in which 0.5% lead was given to growing male rats, Klauder found that as the dietary copper was raised, the concentrations of lead in RBC, kidney, and liver were reduced in a dose-related

TABLE 6

EFFECT OF LEAD AND COPPER ON HEMATOPOIESIS AND COPPER METABOLISM IN THE RAT*†

		Copper Concentrations of Diets‡ (μg/g)	
		0.5	8.5
Hematocrit (% volume)	−Pb	44.3^{A}_{a}	47.7_a
	+Pb	41.1^{A}_{b}	46.2_b
Hemoglobin (g/100 ml blood)	−Pb	13.4^{A}	14.2
	+Pb	11.7^{A}_{a}	13.6_a
Plasma Copper (μg/100 ml)	−Pb	38.0^{A}_{a}	106.5_a
	+Pb	25.6^{A}_{b}	113.0_b
Kidney Copper (μg/g)	−Pb	14.4_a	41.1^{A}_{a}
	+Pb	10.4_b	24.4^{A}_{b}

* Experimental conditions same as those given in TABLE 5.
† Data taken from Klauder, Reference 21.
‡ Statistical differences ($P < 0.01$) are indicated by matching superscripts in columns and subscripts in rows.

fashion.[21] In the same experiment, he found that specific liver and heart weights (g/100 g body weight) were increased significantly by lead and that increased dietary copper diminished these effects. Some of his data are given in TABLES 5 and 6.

In a more recent report on the effects of lead and copper on iron metabolism, Klauder and Petering concluded that iron metabolism is impaired by 500 ppm of dietary lead when dietary iron is sufficient and copper is low.[24] Their work, as indicated in TABLE 7, extended the earlier observations of Goodman and Dallman, who showed that lead severely interfered with iron metabolism of erythroblasts and reticulocytes only when dietary copper was low.[25] These studies show that both copper and iron are necessary to prevent the effects of lead on the hematopoietic system and on both iron and copper metabolism. Williams *et al.* found that rats that had been subjected to lead only during the suckling period exhibited norepinephrine-induced arrhythmias in adult life.[26]

In a recent report by Stemmer *et al.,* it was found that the administration of 0.5% lead to rats receiving only 0.5 ppm Cu in the diet caused cardiomyopathy characterized by focal atrophy with mild lymphocytic infiltration.[2] When the dietary copper was elevated to 8.5 ppm, there were no lesions of the heart muscle caused by lead. These indications of heart pathology induced by lead may be related to a coexisting heart enlargement that had been found by Klauder.[21]

These findings clearly show that there are copper-lead interactions and suggest that increased intake of dietary copper can protect against a number of the biochemical effects of lead as well as against its toxicity. Finally, it should be pointed out that a recent publication of Murthy *et al.* shows that there is severe growth restriction and depression of hematopoiesis when lead is administered to rats receiving a diet low in both zinc and copper.[27]

TABLE 7

EFFECT OF LEAD ON COPPER AND IRON METABOLISM*†

	Dietary Copper Intake‡	
	0.5 ppm	8.5 ppm
Body Weight (12 weeks) (g)		
− Pb	369^{A}	371
+ Pb	269^{A}_{a}	327_{a}
Hemoglobin (μg/ml RBC)		
− Pb	285^{A}	291
+ Pb	251^{A}_{a}	282_{a}
Plasma Fe (μg/100 ml)		
− Pb	108^{A}_{a}	154_{a}
+ Pb	86^{A}_{b}	150_{b}
TIBC§ (μg/100 ml)		
− Pb	527	495
+ Pb	593_{a}	473_{a}

* A 55% milk powder diet containing starch, corn oil, and added vitamins and minerals was fed to weanling rats for 12 weeks. The basal diet contained 0.5 μg Cu/g and was supplemented in the drinking water for the groups indicated above with 8 μg Cu/ml and 500 μg Pb/ml.

† Data taken from Klauder, Reference 21, and Klauder and Petering, Reference 24.

‡ Statistical differences (P < 0.01) are indicated by matching superscripts in columns and subscripts in rows.

§ TIBC = total iron-binding capacity of serum.

Discussion

From this discussion, we may learn that there are two ways in which lead toxicity may be expressed, namely, by direct action on biochemical and cellular processes and by the indirect action of interfering with the availability and function of such essential nutrients as zinc and copper. It seems obvious that this same statement can be made of many toxic elements or chemicals. The direct action of lead may arise in one instance by virtue of its capacity to react with sulfhydryl groups or ligands, as Ulmer and Vallee have shown.[28] As we know, there are many other chemicals and even drugs that also can inactivate essential sulfhydryl groups and thus produce toxic reactions. Lead ingestion, on the other hand, can reduce the nutritional efficacy of zinc and copper by causing a decease in absorption of these nutrients. It also can reduce the biochemical and cellular function of zinc and copper and thus reduce the metabolic actions vital to hematopoiesis, cellular respiration, and other vital functions. We have shown that the interactions among lead, zinc, and copper may manifest themselves also by reducing body growth, depressing the central nervous system, producing cardiomyopathy and hypertension, and interfering with iron metabolism.

As this conference has revealed, there are a number of other effects of lead on the nutritional or physiologic effects of essential elements or vitamins other than zinc and copper. When these are considered as a whole, a message comes through that optimal nutritional status of human beings is a first line of defense against the toxicity of widespread dissemination of lead in our environment. Indeed, it seems that pediatricians and those interested in occupational medicine should now begin to realize this and to take steps to utilize the kind of information that has been developed in experimental studies linking poor nutrition with the toxicity of lead and many other materials. This aspect is of importance, since there is evidence that a substantial portion of our population may not receive adequate amounts of such basic nutrients as zinc and copper.

Since there are many chelating chemicals and drugs that impinge on man's physiologic processes—all of which in one way or another may also reduce the efficacy of many essential elements, especially zinc, copper, and iron—it would seem appropriate to interject a word of encouragement for research into the effects of such logical combinations of agents. One of the most important risk factors in cancer and heart disease, namely, tobacco smoke, is a potent source of such chelating agents as well as the toxic element cadmium.

Acknowledgments

The author wishes to express his thanks to Drs. V. N. Finelli and K. L. Stemmer for helpful discussions during the preparation of this paper.

References

1. Perry, H. M., Jr. & M. W. Erlanger. 1977. Effect of a second metal on cadmium-induced hypertension. *In* Trace Substances in Environmental Health. D. D. Hemphill, Ed. **11:** 280. University of Missouri Press. Columbia, Mo.
2. Stemmer, K. L., H. G. Petering, L. Murthy, D. S. Klauder & V. N. Finelli. 1980. The cardiotoxicity of lead and cadmium. Environ. Health Perspect. (In press.)
3. Cox, D. H. & D. L. Harris. 1960. Effects of excess zinc on iron and copper in the rat. J. Nutr. **70:** 514–520.

4. MAGEE, A. C. & G. MATRONE. 1960. Studies on growth, copper metabolism, and iron metabolism of rats fed high levels of zinc. J. Nutr. **72:** 233–242.
5. MURTHY, L. & H. G. PETERING. 1976. Effect of dietary zinc and copper interrelationships on blood parameters of the rat. Agric. Food Chem. **24:** 808–811.
6. WALDRON, H. A. & D. STÖFEN. 1974. Pathological effects of lead. *In* Sub-Clinical Lead Poisoning (Chapter 3): 77–112. Academic Press. London, England.
7. KOMAI, H. & J. B. NEILANDS. 1968. Effect of zinc ions on δ-aminolevulinate dehydratase in *ustilago sphaerogena*. Arch. Biochem. Biophys. **124:** 456.
8. ABDULLA, M. & B. HAEGER-ARONSEN. 1971. ALA-dehydratase activation by zinc. Enzyme **12:** 708–710.
9. GURBA, P. E., R. E. SENNETT & R. D. KOBES. 1972. Studies on the mechanism of action of δ-aminolevulinate dehydratase from bovine and rat liver. Arch. Biochem. Biophys. **150:** 130.
10. FINELLI, V. N., L. MURTHY, W. B. PEIRANO & H. G. PETERING. 1974. δ-Aminolevulinate dehydratase, a zinc-dependent enzyme. Biochem. Biophys. Res. Commun. **60:** 1418–1421.
11. HERNBERG, S. & J. NIKKAMEN. 1970. Enzyme inhibition by lead under normal urban conditions. Lancet **1:** 63–64.
12. FINELLI, V. N., D. S. KLAUDER, M. A. KARAFFA & H. G. PETERING. 1975. Interaction of zinc and lead on δ-aminolevulinate dehydratase. Biochem. Biophys. Res. Commun. **65:** 303–311.
13. THOMASINO, J. A., E. ZUROWESTE, S. M. BROOKS, H. G. PETERING, S. I. LERNER & V. N. FINELLI. 1977. Lead, zinc, and erythrocyte δ-aminolevulinic acid dehydratase: relationships in lead toxicity. Arch. Environ. Health **32:** 244–247.
14. DUTKIEWICZ, B., T. DUTKIEWICZ & G. MILKOWSKA. 1979. The effect of mixed exposure to lead and zinc on ALA levels in urine. Int. Arch. Occup. Environ. Health **42:** 341–348.
15. CERKLEWSKI, F. L. & R. M. FORBES. 1976. Influence of dietary zinc on lead toxicity in the rat. J. Nutr. **106:** 689–696.
16. FINELLI, V. N. & R. M. EL-GAZZAR. 1977. Interaction of lead and zinc on the prothrombin activity in rats. Toxicol. Lett. **1:** 33–39.
17. EL-GAZZAR, R. M., V. N. FINELLI, J. BOIANO & H. G. PETERING. 1978. Influence of dietary zinc on lead toxicity in rats. Toxicol. Lett. **1:** 227–234.
18. MICHAELSON, I. A. & M. W. SAUERHOFF. 1973. The effect of chronically ingested inorganic lead on brain levels of Fe, Zn, Cu, and Mn of 25-day-old rats. Life Sci. **13:** 417–428.
19. WARKANY, J. & H. G. PETERING. 1972. Malformations of the central nervous system in rats produced by maternal zinc deficiency. Teratology **5:** 319–334.
20. WARKANY, J. & H. G. PETERING. 1973. Congenital malformations of the brain produced by short zinc deficiencies in rats. Am. J. Ment. Defic. **77:** 645–653.
21. KLAUDER, D. S. 1975. The effects of dietary copper, iron, and zinc on the toxicity of lead in male rats. Ph.D. Dissertation: 115–119 and 171–186. University of Cincinnati. Cincinnati, Ohio.
22. KLAUDER, D. S., L. MURTHY & H. G. PETERING. 1972. Effect of dietary intake of lead acetate on copper metabolism in male rats. *In* Trace Substances in Environmental Health. D. D. Hemphill, Ed. **11:** 131. University of Missouri Press. Columbia, Mo.
23. KLAUDER, D. S. & H. G. PETERING. 1975. Protective value of dietary copper and iron against some toxic effects of lead in rats. Environ. Health Perspect. **12:** 77–80.
24. KLAUDER, D. S. & H. G. PETERING. 1977. Anemia of lead intoxication: a role for copper. J. Nutr. **107:** 1779–1785.
25. GOODMAN, J. R. & P. R. DALLMAN. 1969. Role of copper in iron localization in developing erythrocytes. Blood **34:** 747–753.
26. WILLIAMS, B. J., W. H. GRIFFEN, C. M. ALBRECHT, J. H. PIRCH, M. R. HEJTMANCIK, JR. & B. R. NECHAY. 1977. Cardiac effects of chronic lead poisoning. *In* Clinical Chemistry and Chemical Toxicology of Metals. S. S. Brown, Ed.: 127–130. Elsevier/North-Holland Biomedical Press. Amsterdam, The Netherlands.
27. MURTHY, L., S. HIGHHOUSE, L. LEVIN, E. E. MENDEN & H. G. PETERING. 1975. A study of the combined toxic effects of oral cadmium and lead in rats. *In* Trace Substances in

Environmental Health. D. D. Hemphill, Ed. **9:** 395–401. University of Missouri Press. Columbia, Mo.
28. ULMER, D. D. & B. L. VALLEE. 1968. Effects of lead on biochemical systems. *In* Trace Substances in Environmental Health. D. D. Hemphill, Ed. **2:** 7–27. University of Missouri Press. Columbia, Mo.

DISCUSSION

O. A. LEVANDER (*Beltsville Human Nutrition Research Center, U.S. Department of Agriculture, Beltsville, Md.*): Dr. Petering, I wonder if you have any comment about the use of ALA-D inhibition as a diagnostic tool now that you see the effects of dietary zinc.

H. G. PETERING: Severe inhibition of erythrocyte ALA-D in persons suspected of having been exposed to lead is still accepted as a good biologic indicator of such exposure, but there is increasing concern by Dr. Finelli and others in our group about the quantitative relationships of ALA-D concentrations in erythrocytes and blood lead. Dr. Finelli believes that the degree of reactivation of erythrocyte ALA-D by zinc ions in the bioassay will indicate the potential enzyme concentration and the degree of lead inhibition and thus may give a more accurate picture of lead exposure.

H. H. SANDSTEAD (*Human Nutrition Research Center, U.S. Department of Agriculture, Grand Forks, N. Dak.*): Would you comment on the possible implications of the lead-copper interactions as they relate to atherosclerosis.

H. G. PETERING: In work with rats, we find that the cardiomyopathy produced by low copper levels is severely exacerbated by feeding lead and even more so by cadmium.

R. H. WASSERMAN (*New York State College of Veterinary Medicine, Cornell University, Ithaca, N.Y.*): I wonder if you have any thoughts from your work on the relationship of lead to zinc and metallothionein.

H. G. PETERING: We have no evidence that lead is involved in the zinc-metallothionein relationships, and I know of no other group that has reported any effect of lead in this regard.

N. F. SUTTLE (*Moredun Research Institute, Edinburgh, Scotland*): I would like to ask about the dose used to demonstrate your lead-copper interaction. The levels of lead used seemed to be macronutrient, rather than micronutrient, quantities.

H. G. PETERING: We have lowered the dietary concentrations of lead used in our experiments from about 25,000 ppm (2.5% Pb) to amounts in the range of 50–500 ppm.

Our experiments used weanling rats, which are more susceptible to lead intoxication than are adult rats. Therefore, any extrapolation to human beings must be made first of all to infants and growing children, who have also been found to be much more susceptible to lead intoxication than are adults. Dr. Chisholm of Johns Hopkins University Medical Center has recently reported that the iron-lead interactions found in animal studies seem to be prevalent in undernourished children exposed to lead.

BIOLOGICAL INTERACTIONS OF CADMIUM WITH CALCIUM

Helena S. Jones* and Bruce A. Fowler

Laboratory of Organ Function and Toxicology
National Institute of Environmental Health Sciences
Research Triangle Park, North Carolina 27709

INTRODUCTION

Alteration of human calcium metabolism by chronic cadmium exposure has been shown to be associated with development of an osteomalacia syndrome in Japan known as Itai-itai disease.[1-3] This disorder is clinically characterized by reduced calcification of the skeleton, leading to severe pain in the vertebral column and legs because of bone weakness and to development of fractures from mild trauma. The etiology of the disease appears to involve cadmium-mediated perturbation of normal calcium metabolism operating in concert with low dietary intakes of calcium, vitamin D, and protein. Studies by workers in several countries using experimental animals have shown that low dietary intakes of calcium and/or protein enhance the deleterious effects of chronic cadmium exposure on bone thickness and calcium content.[4,5] The exact *in vivo* biochemical/physiological mechanisms responsible for the effects of cadmium on calcium metabolism are presently unknown due to the fact that calcium homeostasis is regulated by a number of factors (FIGURE 1). Dietary calcium level, vitamin D intake and metabolism, function of the parathyroid glands (PTGs), calcitonin secretion and metabolism, gastrointestinal absorption of calcium, and bone synthesis/degradation patterns as well as kidney function form an integrated network of factors that must be considered both individually and as a whole in assessing the impact of cadmium on calcium metabolism *in vivo*. The present study was designed to investigate the effects of chronic cadmium exposure in conjunction with low dietary calcium status on the relationship between serum calcium and phosphorus levels and the morphology of the PTGs in rats, since the effects of cadmium on organs that regulate calcium metabolism *in vivo* have not been well studied.

MATERIALS AND METHODS

Male Charles River CD rats (150–200 grams) were placed on a casein-based semipurified diet containing low (0.1%) or normal (0.7%) levels of calcium and were given access to deionized drinking water containing 0, 0.2, 2.0, 20, or 200 parts per million (ppm) cadmium as $CdCl_2$ for 6 or 12 weeks.[6] The animals were sacrificed under anesthesia, and one PTG was dissected out under a dissecting microscope, fixed in buffered formalin, and stained with hematoxylin and eosin for light microscopy. Morphometric determinations of PTG nuclear density were performed on five adjacent high-power fields for each gland from four rats per treatment group. The remaining parathyroid gland from each animal was fixed in a glutaraldehyde-

* Present affiliation: Department of Biology, University of Wisconsin, Eau Claire, Wisconsin 54701.

0077-8923/80/0355-0309 $01.75/0 1980, NYAS

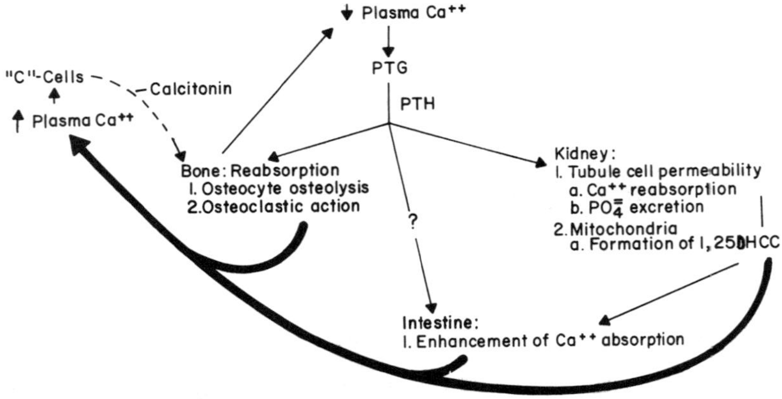

FIGURE 1. Factors that regulate plasma calcium levels, showing the regulatory effects of the parathyroid gland (PTG) and parathyroid hormone (PTH) on *in vivo* calcium metabolism.

formaldehyde fixative and processed for electron microscopy as previously described.[7]

Serum concentrations of calcium, phosphorus, total protein, and alkaline phosphatase were obtained using a clinical chemistry analyzer on blood samples drawn by cardiac puncture at the time of sacrifice. Statistical comparisons for the above parameters between the various groups were made using standard analysis of variance procedures.[8]

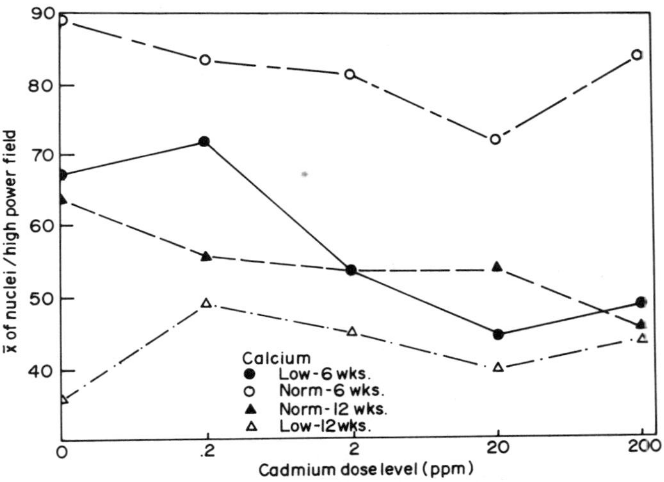

FIGURE 2. Mean parathyroid nuclei counts per high-power field from rats on low and normal calcium diets at 6 and 12 weeks. Note that counts are lowest for rats on the low calcium diet at both time points and most decreased by concomitant cadmium exposure in rats on the low calcium diet at 6 weeks and normal calcium diet at 12 weeks.

RESULTS

The effect of chronic cadmium exposure in conjunction with low or normal dietary calcium status on numbers of PTG nuclei per high-power field is given in FIGURE 2. The observed decrease in numbers of nuclei per field in animals on low calcium diets in comparison with those on normal calcium diets at both 6 and 12 weeks is readily apparent. Decreased numbers of PTG nuclei per high-power field are interpreted as being indicative of cellular hypertrophy associated with increased metabolic activity, since no mitotic figures were observed in any of the PTG slides examined. Concomitant cadmium exposure caused further reductions in numbers of nuclei per field. This effect was found to result in up to a 30% reduction in the PTG nuclei count for rats on the 20 and 200 ppm Cd dose levels, relative to controls. Rats on the low calcium diet at 6 weeks and the normal calcium diet at 12 weeks were most markedly affected by cadmium exposure. The lack of change in numbers of nuclei per field in cadmium-treated rats on the low calcium diet at 12 weeks could suggest that a maximum response by the PTGs had occurred from low dietary calcium intake and that no further response was possible.

Ultrastructural examination of PTG cells from control and cadmium-treated rats on the low calcium diet at 6 weeks is given in FIGURES 3, 4, and 5. Increased amounts of rough endoplasmic reticulum (RER), Golgi, prosecretory vesicles, and

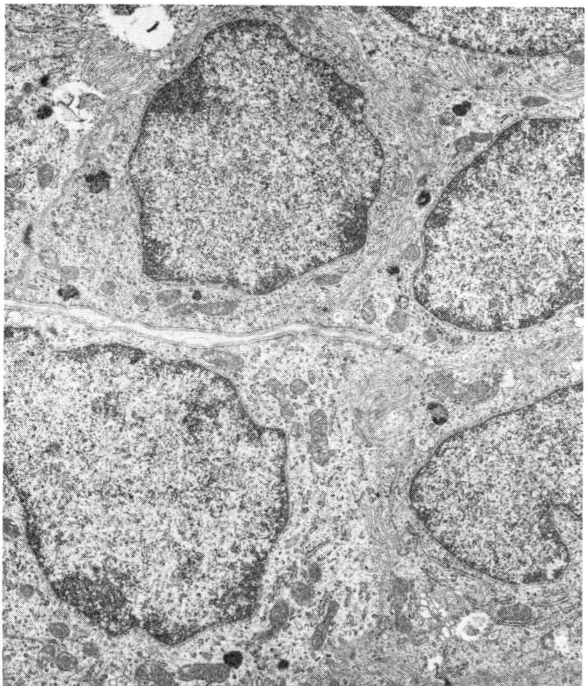

FIGURE 3. Electron micrograph of PTG cells from a control rat on the normal calcium diet at six weeks. ×6,703.

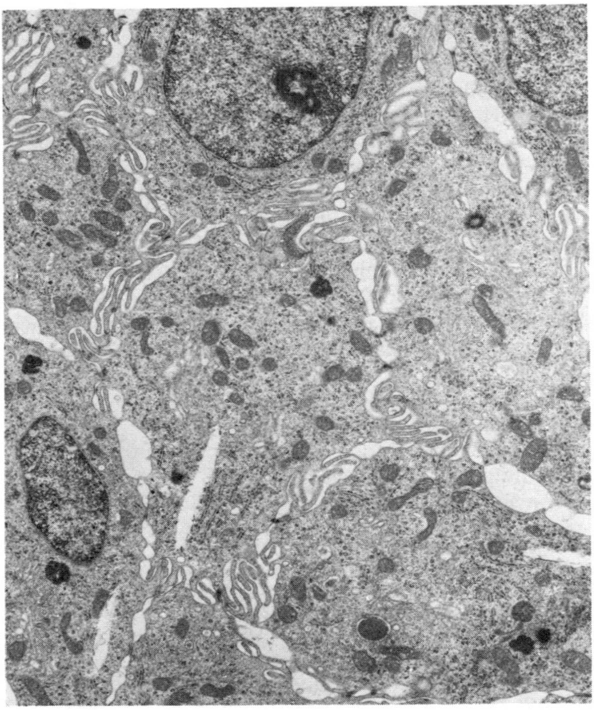

FIGURE 4. Electron micrograph of PTG cells from a rat on the low calcium diet at six weeks, showing essentially normal architecture but fewer nuclei per field. × 6,703.

dense cytosomes were observed in cells from cadmium-treated rats. This morphological appearance is similar to that extensively described in PTGs of animals actively secreting PTG hormone.[9]

Serum calcium and phosphorus values for the various treatment groups are presented in FIGURES 6 and 7 respectively. There are dose-related changes in serum calcium values in the cadmium-treated animals, with an apparent increase at low doses of cadmium and a progress towards decreased calcium values at the higher cadmium doses. The observed decreases are most marked for rats on the low calcium diet after 12 weeks. Perhaps this is due to a failure of the PTGs to compensate further for low calcium intake. Serum phosphate values show a somewhat opposite trend, with mildly decreased values at low doses and increased values at the 200 ppm cadmium dose levels. The exception to this trend is the 12-week normal dietary calcium group.

Total serum protein values (FIGURE 8) for all treatment groups except those on the low calcium diet at 12 weeks remained fairly constant. Animals on the low calcium diet showed a total serum protein pattern similar to that of serum calcium, with elevated values at low dose levels and decreased values at the 20 and 200 ppm cadmium dose levels. Total serum alkaline phosphatase activity showed a pattern characterized by an overall increase in activity in rats exposed to cadmium. Dietary calcium level was not found to alter this parameter.

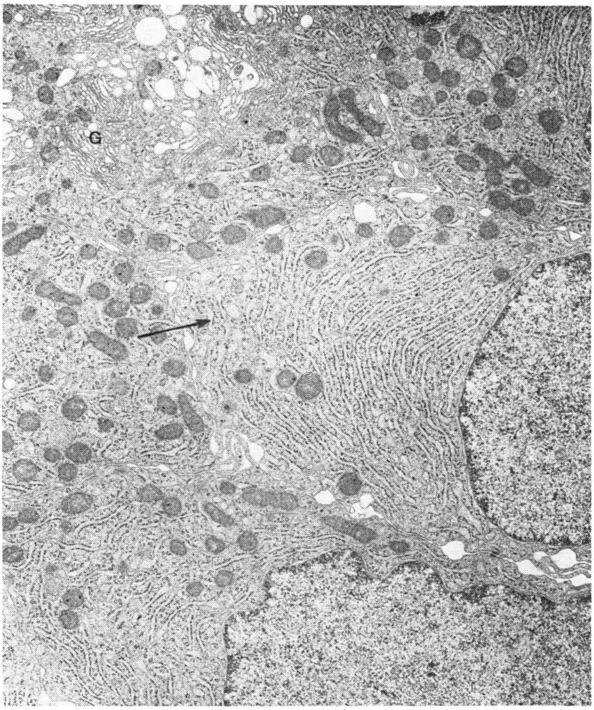

FIGURE 5. PTG cells from a rat on the low calcium diet at six weeks that also received 20 ppm cadmium in the drinking water. Note the marked proliferation of rough endoplasmic reticulum (arrow) and extensive Golgi (G). ×6,703.

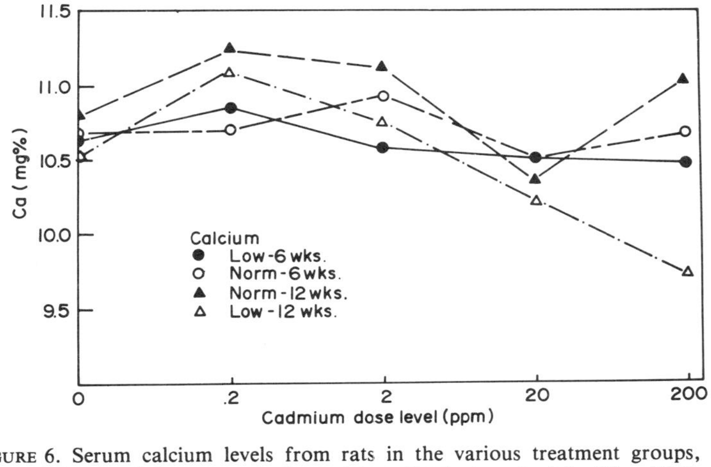

FIGURE 6. Serum calcium levels from rats in the various treatment groups, showing decreased calcium levels in rats on the low calcium diet that received the 20 and 200 ppm cadmium dose levels for 12 weeks.

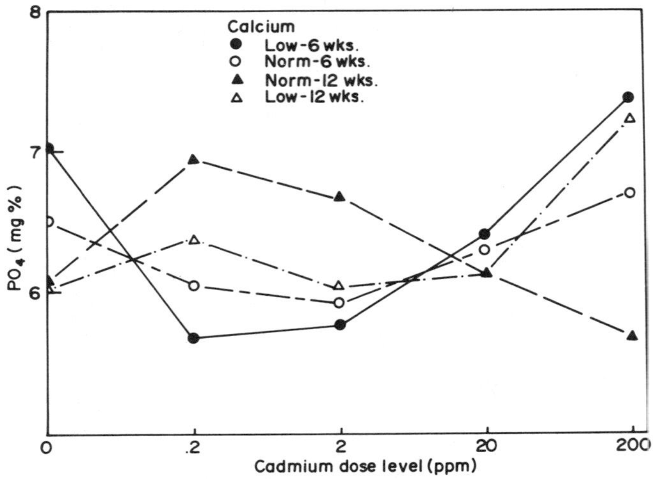

FIGURE 7. Serum phosphate levels for the various treatment groups, showing essentially opposite pattern to that observed for calcium, with mild increases in concentrations at the higher cadmium dose levels in rats receiving low dietary calcium.

Results of analysis of variance for the various clinical serum parameters measured in this study as a function of dietary calcium level, weeks, and cadmium dose level are presented in TABLE 1. These analyses indicate statistically significant differences for serum calcium levels and alkaline phosphatase activity as a function of cadmium dose level. Total serum protein and serum calcium were found to be statistically altered as a function of dietary calcium level. Total serum protein and alkaline phosphatase were also found to show alterations as a function of duration of exposure.

DISCUSSION

The results of this study indicate that dietary calcium level does influence the deleterious effects of chronic cadmium exposure on *in vivo* calcium metabolism and at least one of the organ systems involved in its regulation. The combination of low dietary calcium intake and high cadmium dose levels was found to significantly decrease serum calcium levels in a synergistic fashion. These findings are consistent with those of others, which have shown that low dietary calcium levels enhance cadmium effects on bone calcium content and shaft thickness.[4,5] The role of the PTGs in modulating the magnitude of cadmium and dietary calcium effects on *in vivo* calcium metabolism has received little attention to date, but results of the present study suggest that this organ does respond to both dietary calcium level and cadmium exposure, with more pronounced effects being observed when the effects of low calcium are combined with those of cadmium. It is hence clear that any explanation for the *in vivo* effects of cadmium on calcium metabolism must take the response of the PTGs into account. This is particularly true with respect to effects of cadmium on bone, since administration of excess parathyroid hormone (PTH) has been shown to produce bone demineralization due to increased osteoclast activity.[10]

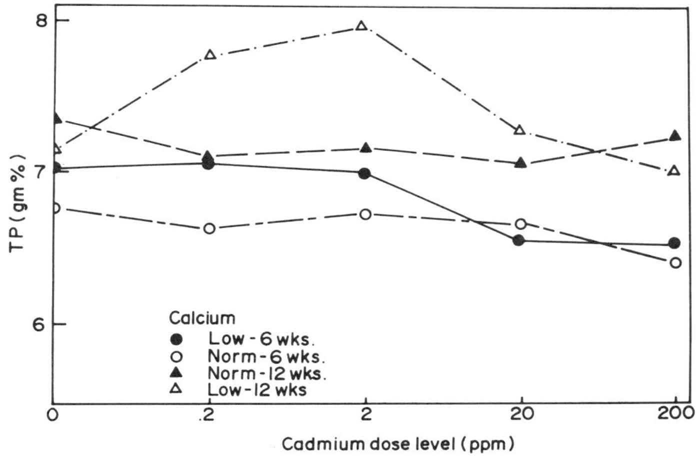

FIGURE 8. Total serum protein (TP) concentrations, showing essentially constant values for all groups except those on the low calcium diet at 12 weeks, where an increase is observed at the two lowest cadmium dose levels and values near those of controls for the two highest cadmium treatment groups.

In terms of the overall mechanism of cadmium alteration of *in vivo* calcium metabolism, there are several possibilities. Cadmium has been shown to inhibit the 1-hydroxylation of vitamin D *in vitro;*[11,12] but this effect has also been shown to be readily prevented by the presence of cadmium-thionein, suggesting that cadmium interference with renal formation of 1,25-dihydrocholecalciferol *in vivo* is not likely to occur.

Another possibility is that cadmium deposition in bone interferes with normal calcification, with subsequent decalcification and resorption.[5,13] The observed statistical increases in serum alkaline phosphatase as a function of cadmium dose level but not of dietary calcium level in the present study are consistent with such a hypothesis and suggest that cadmium may cause bone demineralization either directly or indirectly. Further research is needed to clarify this observation.

TABLE 1

RESULTS OF ANALYSIS OF VARIANCE TESTS FOR BLOOD CHEMISTRIES OF CADMIUM-TREATED ANIMALS ON NORMAL OR LOW CALCIUM DIETS

	Total Protein	Alkaline Phosphatase	Ca	PO_4
Doses	NS*	$P < 0.05$	$P < 0.05$	NS
Diets	$P < 0.05$	NS	$P < 0.05$	NS
Weeks	$P < 0.01$	$P < 0.01$	NS	NS
Doses × Diets	NS	NS	NS	NS
Doses × Weeks	NS	NS	NS	NS
Diets × Weeks	NS	NS	NS	NS
Doses × Diets × Weeks	NS	NS	NS	NS

* NS means not significant.

Cadmium interference with calcium absorption at the level of the gastrointestinal tract has also been suggested by the work of several investigators.[14–16] Richardson and Fox have shown morphological damage to the intestinal villi of quail exposed to dietary cadmium for prolonged periods.[14] More recently, Tsuruki and coworkers, using the everted gut sac technique in rats, have demonstrated cadmium-induced inhibition of vitamin D-stimulated calcium transport *in vitro*.[15] The major point is that cadmium may interfere with intestinal calcium absorption by physical damage to cells of the gut epithelium and/or by functional damage involving a hormone-receptor relationship. It is clear that further work in this area is needed to elucidate these effects more clearly as well as those alterations in functional responses of target tissues, such as the gut and kidney, to PTH or calcitonin.

Finally, the possibility exists that cadmium may interfere with calcium metabolism *in vivo* by a combination of the above mechanisms, and in order to completely understand the effects of cadmium on calcium metabolism, some comprehensive and detailed studies that take all of the above systems into account are necessary.

References

1. Friberg, L., M. Piscator, G. F. Nordberg & T. Kjellström. 1974. *In* Cadmium in the Environment. 2nd edit.: 192–195. CRC Press. Cleveland, Ohio.
2. Emerson, B. T. 1970. "Ouch ouch" disease: the osteomalacia of cadmium nephropathy. Ann. Intern. Med. **73:** 854.
3. Friberg, L., T. Kjellström, G. F. Nordberg & M. Piscator. 1979. Cadmium. *In* Handbook on the Toxicology of Metals. L. Friberg, G. F. Nordberg & V. Vouk, Eds.: 355–381. Elsevier/North Holland Biomedical Press. Amsterdam, The Netherlands.
4. Larsson, S.-E. & M. Piscator. 1971. Effects of cadmium on skeletal tissue in normal and calcium deficient rats. Isr. J. Med. Sci. **7:** 495–498.
5. Itokawa, Y., T. Abe & S. Tanaka. 1973. Bone changes in experimental chronic cadmium poisoning. Radiological and biological approaches. Arch. Environ. Health **26:** 241–244.
6. Mahaffey-Six, K. R. & R. A. Goyer. 1970. Experimental enhancement of lead toxicity by low dietary calcium. J. Lab. Clin. Med. **16:** 933–942.
7. Fowler, B. A., H. S. Jones, H. W. Brown & J. K. Haseman. 1975. The morphologic effects of chronic cadmium administration on the renal vasculature of rats given low and normal calcium diets. Toxicol. Appl. Pharmacol. **34:** 233–252.
8. Snedecor, G. W. & W. G. Cochran. 1967. Statistical Methods: 339–381. Iowa State University Press. Ames, Iowa.
9. Shannon, W. A. & S. I. Roth. 1974. An ultrastructural study of acid phosphatase activity in normal, adenomatous and hyperplastic (Chief cell type) human parathyroid gland. Am. J. Pathol. **77:** 493–505.
10. Weisbrode, S. E., C. C. Capen & L. A. Nagode. 1974. Effects of parathyroid hormone on bone of thyroparathyroidectomized rats. Am. J. Pathol. **75:** 529–542.
11. Suda, T., N. Horiuchi, E. Ogata, I. Ezawa, N. Otaki & M. Kimura. 1974. Prevention by metallothionein of cadmium-induced inhibition of vitamin D activation reaction in kidney. FEBS Lett. **42:** 23–26.
12. Kimura, M., N. Otaki, S. Yoshiki, M. Suzuki, N. Horiuchi & T. Suda. 1974. The isolation of metallothionein and its protective role in cadmium poisoning. Arch. Biochem. Biophys. **165:** 340–348.
13. Furuta, H. 1978. Cadmium effects on bone and dental tissues of rats in acute and subacute poisoning. Experientia **34:** 1317–1318.
14. Richardson, M. E. & M. R. S. Fox. 1974. Dietary cadmium and enteropathy in Japanese quail. Lab. Invest. **31:** 722–731.
15. Tsuruki, F., Y. Otawara, H. L. Wang, S. Moriuchi & N. Hosoya. 1978. Inhibitory effect of cadmium on vitamin D-stimulated calcium transport in rat duodenum *in vitro*. J. Nutr. Sci. Vitaminol. **24:** 237–242.

16. HAMILTON, D. L. & M. W. SMITH. 1978. Inhibition of intestinal calcium uptake by cadmium and the effect of a low calcium diet on cadmium retention. Environ. Res. **15:** 175–184.

DISCUSSION

H. H. SANDSTEAD (*Human Nutrition Research Center, U.S. Department of Agriculture, Grand Forks, N. Dak.*): Would you comment about the levels of cadmium intake that women with Itai-itai disease have and maybe tell how the disease occurs and whether this sort of phenomenon is known to occur in man anyplace else in the world.

B. A. FOWLER: Yes, the situation most frequently occurred in those areas of Japan where water effluent containing cadmium was used to irrigate rice fields and the cadmium was picked up by the rice and ingested by humans. The population group that seems to be at greatest risk for this particular phenomenon are individuals whose nutritional status is not all that it might be. In particular, multiparous women who have experienced birth of several children seem to be at greatest risk. The disease itself is characterized by an osteomalacia with almost spontaneous fracturing of the bones that is extremely painful. The term itai-itai, for those of you who aren't familiar with Japanese, means ouch-ouch because the individuals involved with this disease are in a great deal of pain.

Now in terms of the second part of your question about other areas of the world. I think there are some preliminary studies that have been conducted on individuals who are in much better dietary status, and there are also suggestions of bone lesions similar to this, but the full syndrome that's observed in the Japanese has not been reported.

R. H. WASSERMAN (*New York State College of Veterinary Medicine, Cornell University, Ithaca, N.Y.*): We have done some studies in the chick in terms of cadmium toxicity using dietary levels of about 20 ppm, and what we find is quite supportive of what you say. We measured directly the one vitamin D-hydroxylase in these chicks and could find either no difference due to cadmium intake or a slight increase, which goes along with the parathyroid studies. But in the chick, what we find is a hypercalcemia not a hypocalcemia. We tried to explain whether this is an effect on bone or the kidney.

B. A. FOWLER: I think one thing that we learned from our study is the real need for running a wide dose-response curve. One could conclude one thing about the effects of cadmium exposure on serum calcium levels by picking one or two of the doses and get a curve that looked one way, or if you picked a higher dose level, for instance, you would get a curve that looked another way.

So probably from this point of view—until these things get sorted out a little more clearly for different species—the need for running pretty wide dose curves is there.

N. F. SUTTLE: (*Moredun Research Institute, Edinburgh, Scotland*): Are tissue cadmiums higher on the low calcium diet?

B. A. FOWLER: They are statistically higher, but it isn't a twofold difference, more like a 20% increase. Statistically, we showed that they are elevated relative to the normal calcium animals.

N. F. SUTTLE: It seemed that you were interpreting your results primarily in terms of an effect of cadmium on calcium metabolism. I wasn't quite sure whether you might not really be looking at effects of calcium on cadmium metabolism.

B. A. FOWLER: That's right; your point is well taken, and we certainly are aware that if one changes dietary calcium status, this can certainly affect the absorption of metals like cadmium.

H. SPENCER (*Veterans Administration Hospital, Hines, Ill.*): I believe that the phosphorus depletion plays the greatest role, because when cadmium is deposited in the renal tubules, you get what is called a Fanconi syndrome with phosphaturia. Serum phosphorus levels are very low, and secondary to the phosphorus depletion, there is calcium loss. I believe this is one of the important mechanisms for bone dissolution.

T. BERGLUND (*Institute of Theoretical Physics, University of Stockholm, Stockholm, Sweden*): Is there an interaction between cadmium and calcium in the intestinal mucus?

B. A. FOWLER: That's a fairly anionic kind of material, and it's entirely possible; but I'm not aware that anyone has studied it.

J. PARIZEK (*Czechoslovak Academy of Sciences, Prague, Czechoslovakia*): In connection with the discussion on the effects of cadmium on bones and cadmium-calcium interactions, I should like to mention that these problems—including the reports on bone changes (and renal stones) observed in workers exposed to cadmium and the studies on Itai-itai disease—have been reviewed in detail in previous monographs by Professor Friberg [see Reference 1 and Friberg, L., T. Kjellström, G. F. Nordberg & M. Piscator. 1975. *Cadmium in the Environment* **3.** Publication No. EPA-650/2-75-049. U.S. Environmental Protection Agency. Research Triangle Park, N.C.] as well as in the recently issued World Health Organization document EHE/EHC/79.20 [*Environmental Health Criteria for Cadmium—Interim Report*]. Evaluation of factors possibly involved in the etiopathogenesis of Itai-itai disease can be found also in a recent monograph *Cadmium Studies in Japan: A Review,* edited by K. Tsuchiya in 1978 [Kodanshi Ltd., Tokyo and Elsevier/North-Holland Biomedical Press, Amsterdam, New York, Oxford].

THE INFLUENCE OF DIETARY COPPER INTAKE ON THE TOXICITY OF CADMIUM*

Ian Bremner and James K. Campbell†

The Rowett Research Institute
Bucksburn, Aberdeen AB2 9SB
United Kingdom

Introduction

There has been an increased awareness in recent years that the toxicity of metals can be influenced by a range of nutritional and physiological factors. Cadmium is no exception in this regard, and it has been shown that its accumulation in tissues and the development of pathological lesions attributable to its presence are determined not only by the intake of this metal but also by that of several essential elements, including calcium, iron, zinc, and copper.[1]

In this paper, particular attention will be given to the effects of copper on the toxicity of cadmium and to the effect of cadmium on copper metabolism in animals. However, it would be a mistake to restrict this discussion solely to the simple two-way interaction between these metals. A close interrelationship exists between the metabolism of both cadmium and copper and that of zinc. Since environmental contamination with cadmium is frequently associated with increased exposure to zinc, it is of some practical interest to consider also the influence of zinc on the cadmium-copper interaction.

Historical Aspects

The complexity of the interactions between cadmium, zinc, iron, and copper was evident in some of the earliest studies of this topic.[2-5] It was shown that when rats, mice, and chicks were maintained on diets with >75 mg cadmium/kg, mortality increased, growth was impaired, and anemia developed. In addition, there was degeneration of aortic elastin and a significant reduction in tissue concentrations of copper. These changes were indicative of copper deficiency, and many of them could be overcome by increasing the dietary copper intake of the animals. It appeared therefore that under these particular experimental conditions, at least some of the toxic effects of cadmium could be related to its antagonistic effect on copper metabolism.

These early studies did not provide any biological explanation for this apparent interaction between cadmium and copper, but it was suggested that it was a consequence of the similar physicochemical properties of the two metals, which enabled cadmium to substitute for copper in certain essential, but unspecified, biological sites.[2]

* Supported in part by Rio Tinto Zinc Services Limited, United Kingdom, and by the International Lead Zinc Research Organization.

† Present affiliation: Boots Company Limited, Thurgerton, Nottingham NG14 7GX, United Kingdom.

0077-8923/80/0355-0319 $01.75/0 © 1980, NYAS

Environmental Considerations

These and other related investigations clearly demonstrated that when experimental animals receive diets containing relatively large amounts of cadmium, pathological lesions related to disturbances in the metabolism of essential metals can rapidly develop, prior to any significant accumulation of cadmium in target organs. Unfortunately, the experimental conditions used in many of these studies were such that the findings could not be extrapolated readily to situations where environmental pollution with cadmium represents a problem for man or farm animals. For example, the amounts of cadmium used in the experimental diets were often two to three orders of magnitude greater than those found in most foodstuffs. In addition, the diets used were on occasion extremely low in copper, and also in zinc and iron, with the result that the susceptibility of the animals to the toxic effects of cadmium would have been greatly enhanced.

However, recent reports from East Germany indicate that the adverse effects of cadmium on copper metabolism indeed can be of major significance in sheep grazing in areas contaminated with cadmium from industrial plants.[6] Tissue copper levels were abnormally low in these animals, and the incidence of the demyelinating disease enzootic ataxia, or swayback, in their offspring was greatly increased, even though pasture copper contents were normal. Renal cadmium concentrations in adult sheep in the most polluted area were 40 mg/kg dry matter (DM), which is only 20% of the level at which renal dysfunction is thought to occur in other species. Because kidney cadmium concentrations in most species increase with age, concentrations in the lambs with swayback would undoubtedly have been much less than this. In these circumstances, therefore, disturbances in copper metabolism presented a more important practical problem in animal husbandry than did other lesions commonly associated with cadmium poisoning.

Similar problems may exist throughout the industrial world. Certainly in the United Kingdom there has been concern about the poor growth and reproductive performance of cattle grazing near some industrial plants, where appreciable emission of cadmium- and zinc-containing dusts has occurred. The symptoms in these animals again suggested that they might be suffering from copper deficiency. A detailed study therefore has been carried out at the Rowett Institute on the influence of cadmium and zinc, individually and in combination, on copper metabolism with a view to assessing the likely biological significance of these effects for farm animals grazing contaminated pastures.

In setting up these studies, care was taken to use levels of cadmium, and of zinc, that reflected those that have been found near smelting plants in the United Kingdom. Mills and Dalgarno reported that cadmium concentrations in herbage a few miles downwind from industrial plants ranged from 1–40 mg/kg, depending on the season of the year and the distance from the probable source of emission.[7] Zinc concentrations in the same pastures ranged from 200–3,000 mg/kg.

In addition, the copper content of the experimental diets was adjusted so that it was in most cases only just sufficient to satisfy the animal's normal requirement for this element. Moreover, attention was concentrated on pregnant and on young, growing animals, as it was considered that they constituted the population groups most at risk from any decrease in the availability of a limited supply of dietary copper.

Effect of Cadmium on Copper Status of Sheep

Decreases in liver and spleen copper concentrations of between 30 and 70% have been reported in sheep maintained on diets containing from 5 to 15 mg cadmium/kg.[7,8] Similar effects were found in growing male lambs and in ewes that received cadmium-containing diets during the later stages of pregnancy and lactation.[8,7] Even greater reductions in liver copper concentration occurred in the eight-week-old offspring of the ewes, which had also been allowed access to the cadmium-containing diets during the weaning period. Indeed, liver copper reserves in those lambs were so depleted that plasma copper and ceruloplasmin concentrations also were reduced. There were no comparable changes in plasma copper in their parent ewes or the older lambs, but this is not surprising as liver copper concentrations in these animals were in the range 60 to 360 mg/kg DM, which is far in excess of the level at which hypocupremia usually develops in sheep.[7,8] In accord with these findings, there were no clinical signs of copper deficiency in these animals, other than a change in wool quality and a nonsignificant trend towards reduced weight gain.[7,8]

There also appeared to be important effects of cadmium on the developing fetuses, as liver copper concentrations in the newborn lambs were reduced by up to 60% when the ewes received the cadmium-containing diets for the last six weeks of pregnancy.[7] This is consistent with other studies where pregnant goats have received diets with 75 mg cadmium/kg and sheep have grazed cadmium-contaminated pastures.[9,6] In the former case, the birth weight and viability of the goat kids were also reduced, despite the lack of any significant transfer of cadmium to the newborn animal. It would appear, therefore, that cadmium can exert an inhibitory effect on the placental transfer of copper and that this can contribute to the poor condition of the neonatal animal.

In view of these findings, it seemed to Mills and Campbell that even lower intakes of cadmium might seriously disturb copper metabolism in pregnant ewes and their offspring provided that:[10,11]

1. The copper intake was further reduced to a level that was only marginally adequate under most circumstances to permit normal growth and reproductive performance but that would not necessarily maintain copper reserves;
2. The period during which cadmium was given was extended to include most of gestation and also the postweaning growth phase of the lambs;
3. The dietary zinc concentration was also increased, since, under conditions of industrial pollution, cadmium and zinc are frequently cocontaminants and it is known that high dietary intakes of zinc can also affect copper metabolism in animals.

An experiment was therefore carried out in which six groups of ewes, up to six weeks pregnant, were maintained throughout the remainder of pregnancy and lactation on a semipurified diet that contained only 2.5 mg copper/kg.[10,11] The diet was supplemented with cadmium and zinc so that it contained 0 or 3 mg cadmium and 30, 150, or 750 mg zinc/kg. Contrary to expectations, no significant disturbances in reproductive performance or in copper metabolism occurred in the ewes receiving the cadmium-containing diets with either 30 or 150 mg zinc/kg. Plasma copper concentrations prior to parturition were normal in all animals, and liver copper concentrations at the end of lactation were unaffected by cadmium intake (TABLE 1). Although the copper status of the ewes and the viability of the newborn lambs were severely affected when the zinc content was increased to 750 mg/kg, these effects were quite independent of dietary cadmium intake.[10,11]

The inclusion of as little as 3 mg cadmium/kg diet, however, did have an effect on the neonatal lambs. Thus their birth weights tended to be less than those of lambs from ewes receiving no cadmium, and in addition their growth rate after weaning was reduced (TABLE 2). Although plasma copper concentrations in the lambs at 12 days of age were not affected by dietary treatment, the subsequent rate of change of plasma copper up to and immediately after weaning depended on both cadmium and zinc (TABLE 3). Thus, cadmium tended to increase the rate of decline in plasma cop-

TABLE 1

EFFECT OF CADMIUM ON LIVER METAL CONCENTRATIONS IN EWES AT END OF LACTATION

Dietary Concentration (mg/kg)		Liver Metal Concentration (mg/kg DM)		
Cadmium	Zinc	Copper	Zinc	Cadmium
<0.1	30	15.2	107.8	<0.1
<0.1	150	39.3	135.1	<0.1
3.0	30	12.3	115.7	6.61
3.0	150	31.5	143.9	8.51

per, whereas zinc had the opposite effect. Since there appeared to be a significant relationship between the decline in growth rate and the rate of change in plasma copper concentration, it appeared that this disturbance in copper metabolism could be responsible for the growth impairment. However, subsequent results did not always support this view, as normal growth rates were not restored when the dietary copper content was increased to 4.5 mg/kg in the animals receiving 30 mg zinc/kg, even though plasma and liver copper concentrations in the control and cadmium-supplemented lambs were increased to the same level (TABLE 4). It is of interest that cytochrome oxidase activity in the duodenal mucosa of the cadmium-treated lambs was reduced by about 50%. This could have arisen from a localized deficit in copper supply and could have contributed to the low growth rate in the lambs.

It was found that the effects of cadmium on growth were abolished when the zinc content of the diet was increased to 150 mg/kg. The reason for this is not clear, but it was associated in both control and cadmium-treated lambs with an increase in liver copper concentrations and in the proportion of hepatic copper present as metallothionein. While the latter change is consistent with earlier observations on hepatic copper distribution in sheep, previous experiments in which sheep received similar zinc supplements resulted in a decrease in liver copper concentrations.[12,13]

When the dietary copper concentration was increased in the last phase of the experiment to 15 mg/kg, which is far in excess of the sheep's normal requirement for copper, the effects of cadmium on growth disappeared (TABLE 4), again indicating

TABLE 2

EFFECT OF CADMIUM SUPPLEMENTATION DURING PREGNANCY ON BIRTH WEIGHT AND GROWTH RATE OF LAMBS*

Dietary Concentration (mg/kg)		Birth Weight (kg)	Growth Rate for Period 3 Weeks after Weaning (g/day)
Cadmium	Zinc		
<0.1	30	5.29	165
<0.1	150	5.03	224
3.0	30	3.95	38
3.0	150	4.33	97
Residual Standard Deviation		1.25	123

* Ewes were maintained on the experimental diets for about 14 weeks, and lambs were weaned at 7–8 weeks of age. The dietary copper concentration was 2.5 mg/kg.

TABLE 3

EFFECT OF CADMIUM ON PLASMA COPPER CONCENTRATIONS IN LAMBS

Dietary Concentration (mg/kg)		Plasma Cu (mg/l) at 12 Days	Rate of Change in Plasma Cu* (mg/l/100 days)
Cadmium	Zinc		
<0.1	30	1.09	−0.46
<0.1	150	1.07	0.22
3.0	30	1.23	−1.18
3.0	150	0.91	−0.12
Residual Standard Deviation		0.18	0.65

* The rate of change in plasma copper was measured from birth to weaning at about eight weeks of age.

the existence of some cadmium-copper interaction. The beneficial effect of copper was still less than that obtained by increasing the zinc intake from 30 to 150 mg/kg.

These results are therefore difficult to interpret in terms of direct antagonist effects of zinc and cadmium on copper metabolism. However, they do support the view that the young, growing animal is particularly at risk from increased exposure to cadmium and show that particular attention must be paid to the dietary intakes of copper and zinc in assessing an animal's susceptibility to cadmium poisoning. They also indicate that marked species differences may exist in the response to cadmium and zinc ingestion, as it has been found that these metals can have an additive effect in inducing copper deficiency in the rat.[11,14]

EFFECT OF CADMIUM ON COPPER STATUS OF THE RAT

The young, growing rat was shown in these studies to be very susceptible to relatively small increases in dietary cadmium content when the dietary copper intake was only marginally adequate for maintenance of growth and normal tissue copper levels.[11,14] Thus, when weanling male rats received a semisynthetic diet containing 2.6 mg copper, 30 mg zinc, and 1.5, 6.1, or 18 mg cadmium/kg, significant decreases rapidly occurred in plasma and tissue copper concentrations (TABLE 5). As little as

TABLE 4

GROWTH RATES AND DUODENAL CYTOCHROME OXIDASE ACTIVITIES IN LAMBS*

Dietary Concentration (mg/kg)		Growth Rate (g/day)		Cytochrome Oxidase at 35 Weeks (U/g)
Cadmium	Zinc	15–35 Weeks	35–46 Weeks	
<0.1	30	168	140	11.0
<0.1	150	166	113	9.8
3.0	30	18	70	—
3.0	150	146	129	5.6
Residual Standard Deviation		35	54	1.1

* The dietary concentration of copper was 4.5 mg/kg from 15–35 weeks and 15.0 from 35–46 weeks.

1.5 mg cadmium/kg diet was sufficient to reduce plasma copper and ceruloplasmin concentrations by about half.

Kidney copper concentrations also were reduced at this low intake of cadmium, and there was a trend for liver copper concentrations to decline also. Increasing the cadmium intake to 6.1 and 18 mg/kg generally increased the magnitude of these effects. The skeletal development of the rats was impaired by cadmium ingestion, as is illustrated by the reduced cortical bone index in the femurs. This decrease is typical of that found in copper-deficient rats. The achromotrichia that developed in the rats receiving 18 mg cadmium/kg is also indicative of the development of copper deficiency.

Unlike the findings in lambs described above, where zinc tended to alleviate the toxicity of cadmium, the severity of the copper deficiency induced in the rats by cadmium was increased by zinc supplementation. Thus, increasing the zinc content of the cadmium-containing diets to 300 and 1,000 mg zinc/kg further reduced tissue and plasma copper concentrations. In addition, the growth of the rats was impaired. The final live weights of the control rats and those receiving 18 mg cadmium and 1,000 mg zinc/kg diet were 363 and 305 g respectively. It should be pointed out, however, that direct interactions also appeared to occur between cadmium and zinc, with zinc decreasing the tissue accumulation of cadmium. For example, final kidney cadmium concentrations in the rats receiving 18 mg cadmium and 30, 300, or 1,000 mg zinc/kg diet were 12.7, 7.4, and 6.1 μg/g respectively.

Many of the findings in this experiment are consistent with a direct antagonist effect of cadmium, and zinc, on copper metabolism. One would therefore expect an increase in copper supply to overcome these effects, and this indeed has been shown to occur.[11] As can be seen from TABLE 6, increasing the dietary copper content from 2.6 to 7.8 mg/kg prevented the decreases in plasma and liver copper concentrations that occurred at cadmium intakes of 1.5 and 6.1 mg/kg diet. In addition, copper supplementation tended to overcome the effects of cadmium on cortical bone index.

Petering and his colleagues have made similar findings on rats receiving semi-synthetic diets with low copper and zinc contents.[15] Moderate increases in cadmium intake reduced plasma copper and ceruloplasmin concentrations, and these changes were prevented by copper supplementation. In contrast, no changes occurred in plasma and liver copper concentrations in several other investigations where rats were fed on stock colony diets, even at dietary cadmium contents as great as 100 mg/kg.[16,17] It is probable that the relatively high copper content of these diets was responsible for the absence of any significant changes in copper status. An unexpected feature of these experiments was the increase that occurred in renal copper concentrations, which is at variance with the decrease that was found when the dietary intakes of both cadmium and copper were much lower (TABLE 5).

TABLE 5

EFFECT OF DIETARY CADMIUM ON COPPER STATUS OF RATS*

Dietary Cadmium Content (mg/kg)	0.2	1.5	6.1	18.0
Plasma Cu concentration (mg/l)	0.71	0.44	0.18	0.03
Plasma ceruloplasmin (U/l)	44.3	18.6	8.9	6.5
Liver Cu concentration (mg/kg)	4.5	3.8	3.5	2.3
Kidney Cu concentration (mg/kg)	6.8	5.3	4.5	4.3
Cortical bone index in femur	0.44	0.40	0.39	0.38

* Male weanling rats received the experimental diets for nine weeks. Tissue concentrations refer to fresh weight.

TABLE 6

EFFECTS OF INCREASED DIETARY INTAKES OF COPPER AND CADMIUM IN THE RAT*

Dietary Copper Concentration (mg/kg)	2.6			7.8		
Dietary Cadmium Concentration (mg/kg)	0.16	1.5	6.1	0.16	1.5	6.1
Plasma Cu concentration (mg/l)	1.0	0.80	0.51	1.31	0.97	1.12
Liver Cu concentration (mg/kg)	4.9	4.2	4.0	5.1	4.8	5.4
Kidney Cd concentration (mg/kg)	<0.1	0.43	4.63	0.1	0.43	3.11
Cortical bone index in femur (%)	40.7	38.3	38.8	40.3	40.6	39.1

* Male weanling rats received the experimental diets for nine weeks. Tissue concentrations refer to the fresh weight.

In addition to preventing the development of cadmium-induced copper deficiency in rats, an increase in dietary copper intake was found to be of benefit in reducing the accumulation of cadmium in the kidneys. For example, there was a 33% reduction in kidney cadmium when the dietary copper content was increased from 2.6 to 7.8 mg/kg (TABLE 6). Similarly, kidney cadmium concentrations in rats receiving diets with 5 mg cadmium and 1, 2.5, or 5 mg copper/kg for nine weeks were 6.2, 5.5, and 5.0 mg/kg respectively.[18] Since the development of renal dysfunction in cadmium-poisoned animals including man is a direct consequence of renal accumulation of this metal, it would appear that in some circumstances, copper supplementation could be used to lessen the risk of kidney damage in subjects exposed to cadmium.

EFFECT OF CADMIUM ON COPPER ABSORPTION

While the above results have clearly confirmed that a mutual antagonism exists between copper and cadmium, they have not cast much light on the mechanism whereby this occurs. Van Campen and Starcher identified the intestine as the likely site of interaction between the metals.[5,19] Thus, Van Campen found that the addition of cadmium to a ligated segment of small intestine in the rat inhibited the subsequent transfer of ^{64}Cu from the gut loop into the carcass by about half. The validity of these results is perhaps questionable, however, since cadmium is known to have enteropathic properties and the addition of up to 0.7 mg cadmium into a duodenal loop could well have had nonspecific effects on nutrient absorption.[20] Moreover, the molar ratios of cadmium to copper used by these workers were 150:1 and 20:1 and were therefore much greater than those required in other experiments to induce disturbances in copper metabolism.[5,19] For example, significant reductions in plasma copper occurred in rats when the molar ratio of cadmium:copper in the diet ranged from only 1:1 to 4:1 (TABLE 5).

Davies and Campbell therefore examined the effects of feeding low levels of dietary cadmium for one week on the absorption of a single dose of ^{64}Cu given in the feed.[21] Copper absorption was reduced by about half when the diet contained 2.6 mg copper and 17.6 mg cadmium/kg (i.e., a molar ratio of cadmium:copper of 4:1) (TABLE 7). However, copper absorption was not affected at lower cadmium intakes, even though such treatment had been found to decrease liver and plasma copper concentrations in an earlier experiment (TABLE 5). It may be that the difference in apparent response in the two experiments merely reflects their different durations.

Cadmium had no effect on the internal organ distribution of the absorbed ^{64}Cu,

TABLE 7

EFFECTS OF CADMIUM AND ZINC ON COPPER ABSORPTION AND ON METALLOTHIONEIN (MT) CONCENTRATIONS IN THE INTESTINAL MUCOSA OF THE RAT*

Dietary Concentration (mg/kg)			^{64}Cu MT	Total Concentration of Metal on
		^{64}Cu Absorption	Concentration (% of control	MT (μmoles/
Cadmium	Zinc	(% of dose)	level)	g mucosa)
<0.1	30	38.7	100	0.032
4.4	30	40.3	455	0.042
8.8	30	33.1	272	0.043
17.6	30	21.6	182	0.056
—	30	43.4	100	0.018
—	150	38.6	113	0.035
—	450	43.2	168	0.056
—	900	26.7	627	0.410

* Data are taken from Davies and Campbell and Hall *et al.*[21,23]

but it did increase the amount of isotope retained by the intestinal tissue at all levels of cadmium intake, perhaps by blocking the exit of ^{64}Cu from the mucosal cells. Fractionation of the cytosolic fraction of the intestinal mucosa on Sephadex G-75 revealed that some of the increased mucosal ^{64}Cu was associated with a protein with an apparent molecular weight of about 10,000. This protein was not identified, but there are strong grounds for believing that it is metallothionein, synthesis of which is induced by cadmium (see Reference 1 for review). Evans has suggested that this protein plays an important role in the homeostatic regulation of copper absorption,[22] and it is possible that the increased incorporation of ^{64}Cu into this protein in the cadmium-treated animals is at least partly responsible for the decrease in ^{64}Cu absorption. However, it remains to be explained why the binding of ^{64}Cu to this protein was inversely proportional to the cadmium intake (TABLE 7) and why there was no decrease in ^{64}Cu absorption in the rats that had the highest levels of mucosal ^{64}Cu-metallothionein, i.e., those receiving diets with equimolar cadmium and copper concentrations. The possibility must therefore remain that cadmium inhibits copper absorption by some other unidentified mechanism.

As was discussed earlier, zinc can also function as a potent copper antagonist in the rat and induce a copper-deficient state. It is of interest, therefore, that the decrease in ^{64}Cu absorption caused in rats by increasing the dietary zinc content to 900 mg/kg was associated with a sixfold increase in the incorporation of ^{64}Cu into intestinal metallothionein.[23] Lower levels of zinc neither affected copper absorption nor increased the amount of ^{64}Cu bound to metallothionein in the intestine by more than 70% (TABLE 7). Thus, there are stronger grounds for suggesting that in zinc-treated rats, the binding of ^{64}Cu to mucosal metallothionein may result in decreased uptake of the ^{64}Cu into the carcass. It is also noteworthy in this regard that the differences between cadmium and zinc in their potency as inhibitors of copper absorption are mirrored by the differences in their ability to increase concentrations of intestinal metallothionein (TABLE 7).

These findings of increased incorporation of ^{64}Cu into intestinal metallothionein in response to cadmium or zinc administration are at variance with earlier observations by Starcher and Evans *et al.,* since these authors suggested that both these metals caused displacement of ^{64}Cu from metallothionein.[19,24] While the reason for this lack of agreement in results has not been unequivocally established, it is probably associated with the different experimental conditions used in the different investigations. In particular, the short time course of the early experiments would have precluded any significant induction of further metallothionein synthesis.[19,24] If this is so, then the procedure adopted by Davies and Campbell and Hall *et al.* may give a more appropriate indication of the response of animals to long-term exposure to both cadmium and zinc.[21,23]

Interaction between Cadmium and Copper in Kidneys

There is reason to believe that metallothionein is also involved in the interaction that occurs between cadmium and copper in the kidneys of certain species. Ingestion of relatively large amounts of cadmium by rats and also by lambs can lead to substantial increases in kidney copper concentrations.[16,17,8] These increases in renal copper, and cadmium, have been found to be greater in female than in male rats, suggesting some possible hormonal influence on this response.[25] Fractionation of these kidneys has indicated that both metals are bound principally by metallothionein, although the copper protein has yet to be fully characterized. It is of interest therefore that similar, but smaller, increases in renal copper-metallothionein concentrations occur in growing female and to a lesser extent in male rats without any exposure to cadmium.[26] It may be that cadmium—and perhaps other metals, such as mercury, gold, and bismuth—can potentiate this tendency for copper-metallothionein to accumulate in kidneys. This could arise from stabilization of the renal copper protein by cadmium. The biological stability of copper-metallothionein in liver and kidneys is normally much less than that of the cadmium protein;[27] and it is perhaps significant that Cain and Holt have demonstrated recently that the half-life of hepatic and renal metallothionein in the rat increases as the cadmium:copper ratio increases.[28]

Interaction between Cadmium and Copper in Liver

Several reports have been published indicating that interactions may also occur between cadmium and copper in the liver, but few of these have been based on experiments where cadmium was included in the diet at low concentrations similar to those found in contaminated foodstuffs.

For example, it has been reported that the incorporation of hepatic copper into ceruloplasmin is inhibited in rats receiving diets with 100 mg cadmium/kg.[31] The biliary excretion of copper by rats is also decreased when the animals are repeatedly injected with large amounts of cadmium, and it was suggested that this response could have been related to the increased concentrations of hepatic metallothionein in these animals.[30]

Irons and Smith have also implicated hepatic metallothionein in the adverse effects of copper injection on the response of rats to repeated subcutaneous injections of large amounts of cadmium.[29] The increased mortality in the copper-treated animals was associated with a lack of any significant binding of hepatic cadmium to metallothionein, whereas in most other situations where hepatic cadmium concentrations are increased, the metal is bound almost exclusively by this protein. It is of interest in this regard that the binding of hepatic cadmium to metallothionein in sheep receiving diets with up to 12 mg cadmium/kg was inversely related to the copper content of the liver.[1] In some samples with liver copper concentrations greater than 50 μg/g fresh weight, less than 5% of the hepatic cadmium was present as metallothionein. These results were consistent with a displacement of cadmium from metallothionein by copper, which is known to have a greater affinity for the protein. However, it has not been established whether this displacement occurs *in vivo* or *in vitro* during processing of the liver.

CONCLUSION

There are clearly complex interactions between the chemically similar metals cadmium, copper, and zinc that can significantly affect the metabolism of each of the metals. Variations in copper and zinc intake may modify the accumulation of cadmium in the body and the ultimate development of any lesions, such as renal dysfunction, that result from high tissue concentrations of cadmium. In other circumstances, the effects of cadmium on copper metabolism and on the development of copper deficiency may be of greater consequence. This will generally be of most importance when cadmium intakes are high and when dietary copper intakes are relatively low, as is sometimes the case with farm animals. The effects of zinc on cadmium toxicity may vary between species and will depend to some extent on whether zinc interacts directly with cadmium, when it may have a protective role, or whether it is acting as an antagonist of copper, in which case it will exacerbate the effects of cadmium.

Considerable interest has been shown in the binding of these three metals to metallothionein in liver, kidneys, and the intestinal mucosa. Although some evidence has been produced that is consistent with an involvement of this protein in the complex interactions between cadmium, copper, and zinc, it would be unrealistic at present to claim that this has been unequivocally proven. Further investigations on the role of this protein are clearly merited.

Finally, in considering the mechanisms of interaction between these metals, attention should perhaps also be directed to the modifying effect of iron on cadmium metabolism and the enhanced susceptibility of iron-deficient animals to cadmium toxicosis. Both copper deficiency and high zinc intakes result in changes in tissue iron concentrations and ultimately in the development of anemia. It is possible therefore that these disturbances in iron metabolism could also contribute to the relatively low tolerance of copper-deficient animals to cadmium and to the exacerbating effect of zinc on cadmium toxicity in some animals.

ACKNOWLEDGMENT

The authors thank Dr. C. F. Mills for his advice and encouragement.

REFERENCES

1. BREMNER, I. 1978. World Rev. Nutr. Diet. **32:** 165–197.
2. HILL, C. H. & G. MATRONE. 1970. Fed. Proc. Fed. Am. Soc. Exp. Biol. **29**: 1474–1481.
3. BUNN, C. R. & G. MATRONE. 1966. J. Nutr. **90:** 395–399.
4. HILL, C. H., G. MATRONE, W. L. PAYNE & C. W. BARBER. 1963. J. Nutr. **80:** 227–235.
5. VAN CAMPEN, D. R. 1966. J. Nutr. **88:** 125–130.
6. GRUN, M., M. ANKE & M. PARTSCHEFELD. 1977. *In* Kadmium-Symposium: 253–257. Friedrich-Schiller-Universitat. Jena, German Democratic Republic.
7. MILLS, C. F. & A. C. DALGARNO. 1972. Nature London **239:** 171–173.
8. DOYLE, J. J. & W. H. PFANDER. 1975. J. Nutr. **105:** 599–606.

9. ANKE, M., A. HENNIG, H.-J. SCHNEIDER, H. LUDKE, W. VON GAGERN & H. SCHLEGEL. 1969. *In* Trace Element Metabolism in Animals. C. F. Mills, Ed.: 317–320. Livingstone. Edinburgh, United Kingdom.
10. CAMPBELL, J. K. & C. F. MILLS. 1979. Environ. Res. **20:** 1–13.
11. CAMPBELL, J. K. 1979. Ph.D. Thesis. University of Aberdeen. Aberdeen, United Kingdom.
12. BREMNER, I. & R. B. MARSHALL. 1974. Br. J. Nutr. **32:** 293–300.
13. BREMNER, I., B. W. YOUNG & C. F. MILLS. 1976. Br. J. Nutr. **36:** 551–561.
14. CAMPBELL, J. K. & C. F. MILLS. 1974. (abst.). Proc. Nutr. Soc. **33:** 15A–17A.
15. RICE, D. P., L. MURTHY, E. MENDEN & H. G. PETERING. 1973. *In* Trace Substances in Environmental Health. D. D. Hemphill, Ed. **7:** 305–311. University of Missouri Press. Columbia, Mo.
16. STONARD, M. D. & M. WEBB. 1976. Chem. Biol. Interact. **15:** 349–363.
17. WASHKO, P. W. & R. J. COUSINS. 1977. J. Nutr. **107:** 920–928.
18. GALLAGHER, J. A. 1977. M.Sc. Thesis. University of Aberdeen. Aberdeen, United Kingdom.
19. STARCHER, B. W. 1969. J. Nutr. **97:** 321–326.
20. RICHARDSON, M. E. & M. R. S. FOX. 1975. Lab. Invest. **31:** 722–731.
21. DAVIES, N. T. & J. K. CAMPBELL. 1977. Life Sci. **20:** 955–960.
22. EVANS, G. W. 1979. *In* Metallothionein. J. H. R. Kagi & M. Nordberg, Eds.: 321–329. Birkhauser Verlag. Basel, Boston, Stuttgart.
23. HALL, A. C., B. W. YOUNG & I. BREMNER. 1979. J. Inorg. Biochem. **11:** 57–66.
24. EVANS, G. W., P. F. MAJORS & W. E. CORNATZER. 1970. Biochem. Biophys. Res. Commun. **40:** 1142–1148.
25. MURTHY, L., D. P. RICE & H. G. PETERING. 1978. *In* Trace Element Metabolism in Man and Animals. M. Kirchgessner, Ed. **3:** 557–561. Arbeitskreis fur Tierernahrungsforschung. Weihenstephan, Federal Republic of Germany.
26. BREMNER, I., W. G. HOEKSTRA, N. T. DAVIES & R. B. WILLIAMS. 1978. *In* Trace Element Metabolism in Man and Animals. M. Kirchgessner, Ed. **3:** 44–51. Arbeitskreis fur Tierernahrungsforschung. Weihenstephan, Federal Republic of Germany.
27. BREMNER, I., W. G. HOEKSTRA, N. T. DAVIES & B. W. YOUNG. 1978. Biochem. J. **174:** 883–892.
28. CAIN, K. & D. E. HOLT. 1979. Chem. Biol. Interact. **28:** 91–106.
29. IRONS, R. D. & J. C. SMITH. 1976. Chem. Biol. Interact. **15:** 289–294.
30. KLAASSEN, C. D. 1978. Am. J. Physiol. **234:** E47–E53.
31. WHANGER, P. D. & P. H. WESWIG. 1970. J. Nutr. **100:** 341–348.

DISCUSSION

J. C. SMITH, JR. (*Beltsville Human Nutrition Research Center, U.S. Department of Agriculture, Beltsville, Md.*): I appreciate your comments regarding the need for care in giving supplementary zinc to pregnant women. I wonder if you could give some indication of how far the zinc supply in the ruminant animals exceeded their normal requirements. How much zinc do you think pregnant women would have to ingest before comparable effects occurred? Would it be 5 or 10 times the recommended daily allowance [RDA] of 20 mg?

I. BREMNER: The zinc intake of the pregnant sheep was certainly much greater than normal. However, I cannot really say what the minimum level of zinc required to produce these effects would be. Reproduction was impaired at a dietary zinc content of 750 mg/kg but not at 150 mg/kg. Intermediate levels of zinc were not studied, but it is possible that they also could have had adverse effects on the fetus.

I cannot really speculate at what level of zinc problems might arise in pregnant women. However, it is significant that in one limited study in India where pregnant women were given zinc supplements, there was an increased incidence of abortion.

J. C. SMITH, JR.: The recommended level of zinc in sheep is around 50 mg/kg, isn't it?

I. BREMNER: Yes, about that level. I acknowledge that the amounts of zinc used in this experiment were considerably greater than this. All I am suggesting is that pregnant women may be particularly at risk from excessive zinc supplementation and that care should be taken in prescribing zinc for such patients.

J. C. SMITH, JR.: I think it is a good point. However, I think it would be difficult for a pregnant women to normally ingest sufficient zinc to be at risk. I agree that supplementing the daily intake with 200 or 100 mg zinc might be a problem, but hopefully the levels derived for the RDA are quite safe.

H. H. SANDSTEAD (*Human Nutrition Research Center, U.S. Department of Agriculture, Grand Forks, N. Dak.*): I believe zinc supplementation at high levels is clearly hazardous. There's a paper in the *Journal of the American Medical Association*—Volume 240, 1978, by Prasad *et al.*—reporting supplementation of patients with sickle-cell anemia with 150 milligrams of zinc daily. Some of the patients developed copper deficiency. In the past, supplementation with this amount of zinc was believed safe. I believe people should be very cautious about supplementing themselves with zinc because I have a feeling that an intake greater than three to four times the recommended allowance may result in inhibition of the intestinal absorption of other essential trace elements, such as copper. Caution may be particularly appropriate in pregnant women.

C. H. HILL (*North Carolina State University, Raleigh, N.C.*): Dr. Bremner, do you think that metallothionein plays any role in the normal absorptive processes of zinc, copper, and cadmium? Do you find metallothionein in any tissues of animals fed normal nutritional intakes of these metals?

I. BREMNER: You can find metallothionein in quite appreciable amounts in tissues from normal animals. For example, up to 30 micrograms of copper and zinc may be bound as metallothionein in the kidneys of female rats, although only trace amounts of the protein may be present in the liver of these animals.

We should appreciate that there are quite marked differences between species in the amount of metallothionein present in tissues. I think the rat is perhaps abnormal in this regard, since it has evolved over the generations an efficient homeostatic control mechanism that often prevents any buildup of metal concentrations in the liver and other tissues. If the metal concentration does not increase, then you won't find any metallothionein.

In other species, including man, where liver zinc concentrations are greater than in the rat, then more metallothionein is present. Indeed, you almost invariably find that as liver zinc concentrations increase, then about 75% of the additional zinc will be present as metallothionein.

Regarding your other question about the role of metallothionein in the absorption of metals, I do not think it functions in any way as a transport protein. It seems more likely that it acts in the control of absorption, perhaps as a type of blocking agent. Professor Cousins has been investigating the involvement of metallothionein in the regulation of zinc absorption, and his evidence certainly supports this view.

H. G. PETERING (*University of Cincinnati Medical Center, Cincinnati, Ohio*): I would like to comment about the possibility of agents other than metals inducing metallothionein. We've been working with the alpha-mercapto-beta-arylacrylic acid drugs, which can elevate serum zinc by as much as 10 to 15 times. These compounds considerably disturb the metabolism of cadmium and zinc, and you find metallothionein induction of very high order in the liver and kidneys. I think that we might keep our eyes open for other agents, drugs, or chemicals that can increase metallothionein concentrations as effectively as higher zinc or cadmium intakes. We may find that these compounds may then alter some other things as well.

I. BREMNER: I think the problem when you work with these mercapto-aryl-acrylic acids is that it is never very clear whether you are observing a direct effect on metallothionein synthesis or whether you are dealing with secondary effects of major changes in metal concentrations.

H. G. PETERING: I think that's right. In my view—and I think Dr. Giroux is of the same opinion—the principal effect is really one of zinc mobilization. Once this happens, then the animal's response is the same as if you gave a massive dose of zinc, and you get increased induction of metallothionein.

I. BREMNER: But how do you explain the increase in copper concentrations, presumably as copper-metallothionein, in the kidneys of the animals receiving these drugs? This occurs without any increase in serum or liver copper concentrations.

I. S. JAMALL (*University of Cincinnati Medical Center, Cincinnati, Ohio*): I'd like to make a comment on possible side effects after zinc supplementation therapy. I've been treating a patient with acrodermatitis enteropathica with zinc since 1975. He has been given between 400 and 600 milligrams of zinc a day, and we monitored plasma alkaline phosphatase, which is an indirect way of measuring zinc, and also hair levels of zinc, copper, and iron. We have found that both the zinc and copper levels have been within a normal range.

I accept that these are not very sensitive indications of disease and that there may be other effects. However, we have found no gross lesions so far, after five years of experiments in which all the symptoms of acrodermatitis have been repaired.

H. H. SANDSTEAD: I might comment that a supplementation at that level of zinc is perhaps more than others have found necessary to eliminate the symptoms of acrodermatitis. I believe that in Detroit, they find that as little as 60 mg zinc daily can control the disease.

For those who do not know what acrodermatitis is, acrodermatitis enteropathica [AE] is a genetic disease that arises from a malabsorption of zinc. It is a human analog of lethal trait A46, which occurs in Friesian cattle, and has been studied here in the United States, in Denmark, and also in Aberdeen.

The human disease results in severe dermatitis, alopecia, diarrhea, increased susceptibility to infection, and death if not treated appropriately. In 1974, it was discovered that AE is responsive to zinc. Prior to that time, AE was treated with diiodohydroxyquin. Recent studies with experimental animals have shown that picolinic acid, a metabolite of tryptophan, facilitates the intestinal absorption of zinc. Research is under way in Detroit to assess the effects of zinc picolinate on infants with AE.

I. S. JAMALL: I would just like to make one further comment. We tried reducing the zinc intake to 200 mg/day and found that the symptoms of acrodermatitis reappeared.

H. H. SANDSTEAD: Okay, but there may be quite a difference in response between individual patients with acrodermatitis. Some may require more zinc than do others, conceivably because there is a difference in the degree to which zinc absorption is blocked.

P. D. WHANGER (*Oregon State University, Corvallis, Oreg.*): We find that metallothionein levels were very high in neonatal fetal tissues.

I. BREMNER: We certainly find very high levels of zinc metallothionein in fetal tissue from lambs. In fact, when we looked at the distribution of zinc in the fetuses at around midterm, we found that about 50% of the total zinc in the body was present in the liver as metallothionein.

L. SASSER (*University of Tennessee, Knoxville, Tenn.*): We have also found very high levels of metallothionein in fetal tissue. However, I would like to raise another question regarding the disposal of sewage, especially in urban or industrial areas. There has been some concern in this country about the use of sewage as a fertilizer, since it frequently contains quite high levels of cadmium and other heavy metals. Do you think the type of interaction that you described between cadmium and other metals could be of some relevance in this regard?

I. BREMNER: I think the practice of using sewage containing large concentrations of heavy metals could, in some circumstances, be quite hazardous. Unfortunately, few detailed studies have been carried out as yet on the topic, and it is impossible to describe how serious a problem it really is. I believe the European Economic Community is currently drafting some legislation that will limit the amounts of sludge and of heavy metals that can be disposed of as fertilizer. However, one major problem is that a distinction is not always made between the rates of application that will affect plant production and those that will lead to accumulation of heavy metals in the plants, with subsequent effects on animals, including man, eating those foodstuffs.

INTERACTIONS OF ZINC AND SELENIUM ON THE BINDING OF CADMIUM TO RAT TISSUE PROTEINS*

P. D. Whanger, J. W. Ridlington, and C. L. Holcomb

Department of Agricultural Chemistry
Oregon State University
Corvallis, Oregon 97331

Based on similar chemical parameters for zinc and cadmium,[1] a biological interaction between these two elements would be expected to occur. Several workers have shown that cadmium will influence the metabolism of zinc.[2-4] As would be predicted from the chemical parameter hypothesis,[1] cadmium should cause a decrease in the tissue zinc content. Instead, the opposite trend is obtained. Cadmium causes zinc to accumulate in tissues, and the reason for this is not entirely clear. The investigation of the interaction of cadmium and zinc on metallothionein (MT) synthesis, however, has provided some insights on this relationship.

Cadmium is known to cause selective injury to the testes following injection of a single subacute dose to animals with scrotal testes.[5-7] The ability of zinc to prevent cadmium injury to testes is apparently due to competitive mechanisms.[5,6] Cysteine and other thiols also protect the testes from cadmium, but the most efficient protector known is selenium.[6,7] In a study to investigate the mechanism of selenium and cadmium interaction, selenium was shown to divert the binding of cadmium from low molecular weight (MW) proteins to higher MW ones in the testes of rats.[8] Thus, in light of these results, the interaction of selenium and zinc on cadmium binding to tissue proteins was investigated.

Cadmium-Zinc Interaction

In our initial studies on the turnover of MT, the injection of cadmium also was found to cause an accumulation of zinc in the MT fraction.[9] The accumulated zinc was found to disappear at a parallel rate with the degradation of the MT protein moiety, but in contrast, cadmium remained constant in this fraction. The cadmium even was found to be at the same level 19 days after injection. This failure of cadmium to disappear with the degradation of the MT protein moiety has been confirmed by work of other investigators.[10] The reasons cadmium does not disappear from the MT fraction are not entirely clear, but apparently the released cadmium from degradation of the protein moiety is available for further binding to newly synthesized MT, resulting in a continuous cycle. Alternately, the released cadmium could stimulate the synthesis of new MT.

In a long-term experiment, the effect of dietary cadmium on zinc accumulation in liver and kidney MT was investigated (Figure 1). Cadmium accumulated at a linear rate in kidney MT during the entire 300-day experiment, whereas the accumulation of cadmium in liver MT started to plateau after 80 days. The accumulation of cadmium in MT was accompanied by an increase of zinc in both liver and kidney, with zinc reaching a higher concentration in liver MT than in kidneys. In both tissues, the zinc levels in MT declined after day 80 even though the rats were still con-

* Supported by National Institutes of Health Grants No. AM19285 and DE04615.

0077-8923/80/0355-0333 $01.75/0

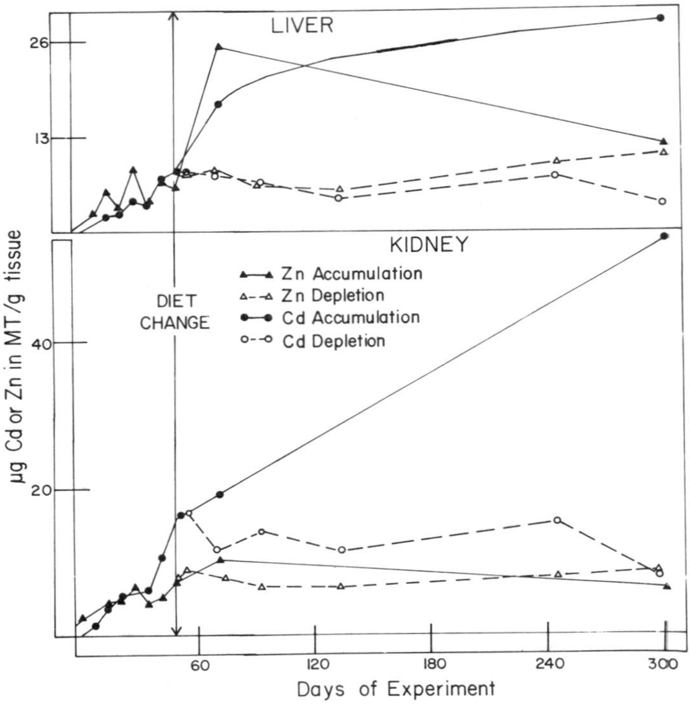

FIGURE 1. Accumulation and depletion of cadmium in liver and kidney MT of rats. The treatment of rats, the gel filtration procedures, and the calculation of the amount of cadmium and zinc in MT are indicated by Deagen *et al.* (Reference 13). The solid lines indicate those rats that were continued on the cadmium-containing diet; and the dashed lines, those that were changed to the diet without cadmium. These animals are indicated as zinc or cadmium "depletion."

suming the diet containing cadmium. This influence of dietary cadmium on zinc accumulation in MT is consistent with work by others and with work where cadmium was injected.[4,11,12] Cadmium administration even has been shown to increase the zinc content of MT in zinc-deficient rats.[12,13] The origin of this zinc, however, has not been definitely established. The inability of the tissues to eliminate cadmium has been suggested to lead to a tissue zinc trap, and this "trapping" ability depends upon the tissue concentration.[12] The data of FIGURE 1 indicate that the accumulation of zinc in MT reached a saturation point with time and then decreased. Thus, the "zinc-trapping" ability of cadmium is not a permanent effect.

In contrast to cadmium, zinc accumulates and depletes from MT very rapidly.[14,15] Excess zinc has been shown to accumulate almost exclusively in tissue MT, but this accumulated zinc depletes to presupplementation levels after only three days of feeding a low zinc diet to rats and chicks.[15,16] Thus, the zinc that accumulates in tissue MT as the result of feeding high levels of zinc is very labile, but the zinc that accumulates as the result of cadmium administration is not very labile.

The half-life of MT is dependent upon the metals used to stimulate its synthesis (TABLE 1). When cadmium was used to stimulate MT synthesis, half-life values of 2.8 to 5.8 days were found for the hepatic protein and 3.7 to 6.3 days for the renal pro-

TABLE 1

EFFECT OF VARIOUS METALS ON THE TURNOVER OF MT IN RATS AS REPORTED BY DIFFERENT INVESTIGATORS*

Metals and Method of Administration	Liver	Kidney	Reference
Cadmium injection	4.2 days	—	Chen *et al.*[9]
Cadmium injection	3.5 days	3.7 days	Feldman *et al.*[10]
Cadmium injection	2.8 days	5.0 days	Shaikh and Smith[17]
Cadmium injection	3.8 days	3.3 days	Cain & Holt[19]
High cadmium injection	6.3 days	5.8 days	Cain & Holt[19]
Basal diet	4.3 days	3.6 days	Cain & Holt[19]
Basal diet	3.4 days	2.0 days	Oh *et al.*[18]
Dietary cadmium	3.3 days	3.6 days	Oh *et al.*[18]
Zinc injection	18.0 hours	—	Feldman & Cousins[22]
Zinc injection	26.0 hours	—	Andersen *et al.*[21]
Copper injection (−Zn rats)	12.3 hours	—	Bremner *et al.*[20]
Copper injection (+Zn rats)	16.9 hours	—	Bremner *et al.*[20]
High dietary zinc then basal	31 hours	31 hours	Oh *et al.*[18]
High dietary zinc	65 hours	53 hours	Oh *et al.*[18]
Dietary zinc (young rats)	29 hours	53 hours	Oh & Whanger[23]
Dietary zinc (adult rats)	48 hours	163 hours	Oh & Whanger[23]

* [**Note added in proof:** After this manuscript was in press, it was discovered that a paper by Day *et al.* (1978. *Bioinorg. Chem.* **8:** 93) had been overlooked and should have been cited in TABLE 1. These workers reported that the half-lives were 10 hours for zinc thionein, 4.53 days for zinc thionein in rats injected with cadmium, and 6.80 days for cadmium thionein.]

tein.[9,10,17-19] Significantly shorter half-life values, however, have been obtained when zinc was used to stimulate MT synthesis. A range in values of 12 to 32 hours have been reported for hepatic MT and 19 to 34 hours for the renal protein.[18,20-22] The range in values obtained by the various investigators could be due to several factors, among which could be zinc status of the animal, degree of metal saturation of MT, and age of animals. The half-life of MT was found to be 16.9 hours in liver of zinc-adequate rats but only 12.3 hours in zinc-deficient rats.[20] Low doses of cadmium resulted in half-life values of 3.3 and 3.8 days respectively in liver and kidney MT, whereas high doses resulted in half-life values of 5.8 and 6.3 days respectively for liver and kidney MT.[19] These authors concluded that the cadmium:zinc ratios in the liver and the cadmium:zinc:copper ratios in the kidney determine the respective rates of degradation of MT. In addition to zinc accumulation, cadmium treatments also cause significant accumulations of copper in kidney MT. The half-life of MT was found to be significantly longer in old rats than in young ones.[23] The *in vivo* work on MT degradation is consistent with *in vitro* work on its degradation. Lysosomal enzymes were found to degrade the metal-free proteins most rapidly, followed by MT containing zinc, and most slowly for MT containing cadmium.[24] This provides further evidence that the degradation of MT is regulated *in vivo* by the species of metal bound to it.

The available evidence indicates that zinc disappears at a parallel rate with the degradation of liver MT in adult rats, suggesting that the release of zinc occurs simultaneously with the degradation of the protein moiety.[20,22] However, this is not true for renal MT or for liver MT in young rats. The disappearance of zinc from the renal MT fraction is slower than the degradation of the protein moiety, and the half-life of zinc in MT fraction from liver and kidney of young rats is about twice as long as that of the protein moiety.[18,23] Thus, the half-life of the metal in the MT fraction cannot be used to accurately estimate the turnover of MT under all conditions and in all tissues.

It has been well documented that zinc will stimulate the synthesis of MT.[18,22] Therefore, if the accumulation of zinc in MT as the result of cadmium exposure is due exclusively to the stimulation of MT synthesis, then zinc would also be expected to cause cadmium to accumulate in MT. However, zinc was not found to cause an accumulation of cadmium in MT,[13] suggesting that other factors beside stimulated synthesis of MT are involved in the accumulation of zinc due to cadmium exposure. Thus, these results appear to be due to the "trapping" ability of cadmium,[12] and zinc does not possess the capacity to "trap" cadmium.

Even though dietary cadmium causes zinc to accumulate in MT of liver and kidney, this metal does not cause such accumulation in the low MW testis protein (FIGURE 2). The lack of influence of cadmium on zinc accumulation in testis MT is similar to reported results for oysters.[25] This may be because the amino acid analysis of the cadmium-binding protein in oysters indicates that it is not MT.[26] This similarity prompted us to investigate the properties of this low MW protein in the testis. Our preliminary amino acid analysis indicates a cysteine content of about 3% in this protein from rat testis,[27] suggesting that it is also not MT. Thus, this could be one of the reasons cadmium does not cause zinc to accumulate in the low MW cadmium-binding protein in testis. Thus, similar elution volumes of metals from gel filtration columns cannot be taken as evidence of the metals bound to MT. The present work suggests that not even cadmium in all kinds of tissue preparations can be assumed to be bound to MT.

SELENIUM-CADMIUM INTERACTION

Chen *et al.* showed that the injection of selenium as selenite diverted the binding of cadmium in rat testes.[8] We extended these studies to determine whether this diversion also occurred in other tissues. Selenium was found to divert the binding of only a small amount of cadmium in the liver, about 50% of the cadmium binding in kidneys, but nearly all of the cadmium binding in plasma from low MW proteins to high MW ones.[28] Thus, the extent of this diversion in cadmium binding is tissue dependent.

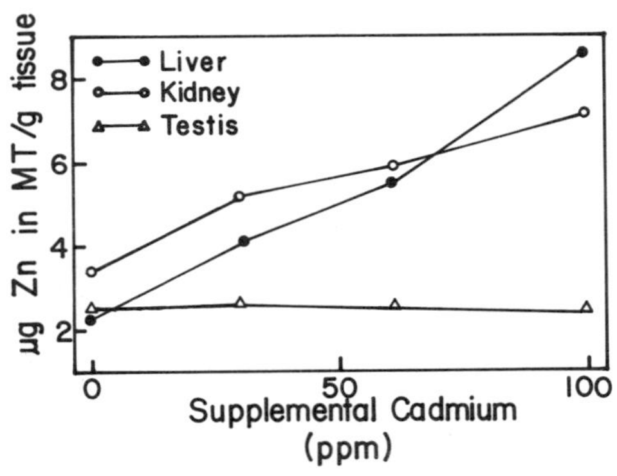

FIGURE 2. Effect of dietary cadmium on the accumulation of zinc in MT of liver, kidney, and testes. Rats were fed a basal casein diet containing 18 ppm zinc or this diet plus additions of either 30, 60, or 100 ppm cadmium for six weeks. The amount of zinc in MT was determined by gel filtration as described by Deagen *et al.* (Reference 13).

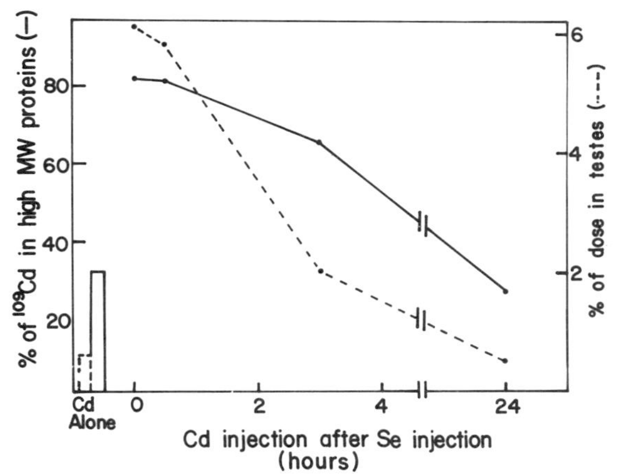

FIGURE 3. Effect of time of cadmium injection after the injection of selenium on the percentage of cadmium binding to higher molecular weight proteins in rat testes. Male rats (350 g) were injected with 0.01 mmole selenium as selenite per kg body weight and with 0.01 mmole cadmium chloride plus 280 μCi ^{109}Cd per kg body weight either simultaneously or 30 minutes, 3 hours, or 24 hours after selenium injection. The testis cytosol was subjected to gel filtration (G-75 Sephadex) as indicated in FIGURE 4. The percentage of cadmium in the high MW proteins was determined by dividing the sum of the three peaks into that found in the high MW peak.

Since the testis was one of the organs in which the greatest amount of cadmium diversion occurred, this tissue was used for further investigations. It was of interest to determine the time differential of selenium injection and the influence of different chemical forms of selenium on the binding of cadmium to tissue proteins. As shown in FIGURE 3, the greatest amount of cadmium in the high MW proteins occurred when selenium was injected simultaneously with cadmium, but the injection of cadmium 30 minutes after the injection of selenium was very similar. There was significantly less cadmium in the high MW proteins when cadmium was injected 3 hours after the injection of selenium, and the injection of cadmium 24 hours after selenium injection was essentially the same as when cadmium was injected alone. Thus, this indicates that the greatest diversion occurs when these two elements are injected fairly close together. It is also apparent that the greatest percentage of the cadmium dose in the testis is present at the same time that the greatest amount of cadmium is present in the high MW proteins.

The injection of selenite and selenate caused a diversion in the binding of cadmium to the cytosolic proteins in testis of rat (FIGURE 4). In contrast, very little diversion in the binding of cadmium occurred when selenomethionine was the form of selenium injected. In other work (not shown), we found that selenite diverted the binding of a portion of the cadmium in the kidneys but that selenomethionine had no influence on cadmium binding in this organ. Thus, the chemical form of selenium is important in diverting the binding of cadmium in tissues.

The administration of selenide as well as selenite by this method also caused the diversion in the binding of cadmium in the testis of rats (FIGURE 5). However, the administration of selenocystine did not cause significant diversion in the binding of cadmium in the testis, but the amount of cadmium in the high MW proteins appeared to be slightly greater than that of controls. This small amount of diversion by selenocystine could be due to its conversion to chemical forms that cause the diver-

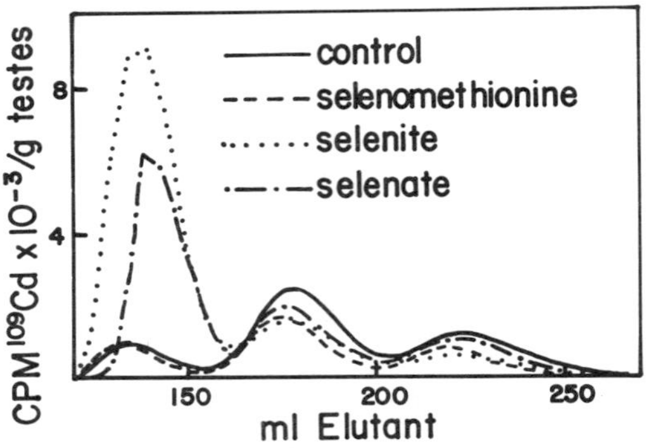

FIGURE 4. Effect of selenate, selenite, and selenomethionine on the binding of cadmium to cytosolic proteins in rat testes. Male rats (330 g) were injected simultaneously at different sites with 0.01 mmole selenium as either selenate, selenite, or selenomethionine and 0.01 mmole cadmium chloride plus 280 μCi ^{109}Cd per kg body weight. The controls were rats that were injected with only cadmium in saline. The rats were killed one hour later, and the testes cytosol chromatographed on Sephadex columns (2 × 100 cm) with 0.05 M Tris buffer, pH 7.4, at a flow rate of 20 ml per hour at 4 °C. About 4 ml were collected per fraction.

sion of cadmium. Evidence has been presented to indicate that selenocystine is metabolized similarly to inorganic selenium whereas selenomethionine is not.[29] Other time periods between the injection of the organic selenium compounds and cadmium injections were not tested.

As indicated in TABLE 2, in general the greatest amount of protection of the testis was obtained when the concentration of cadmium was the highest. Selenate and selenide offered complete protection, whereas selenite and selenocystine offered almost complete protection against cadmium-induced testicular damage. However,

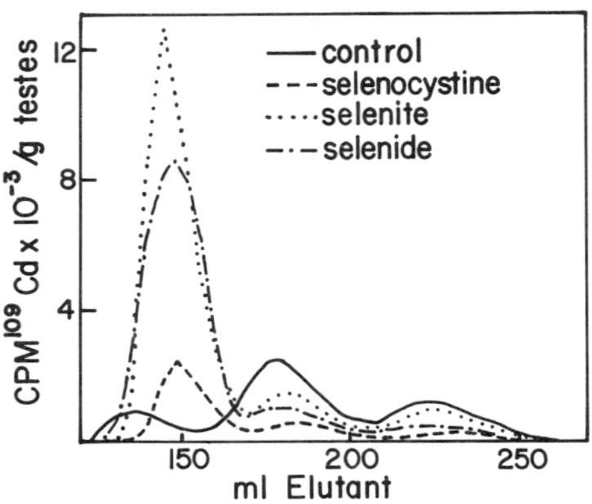

FIGURE 5. The influence of selenocystine, selenide, and selenite on the binding of cadmium to cytosolic proteins in rat testes. Male rats (350 g) were given 0.01 mmole selenium per kg body weight as either selenocystine, selenide, or selenite in a small slit in the body cavity while the rats were anesthetized. At the same time, 0.01 mmol cadmium chloride plus 280 μCi ^{109}Cd per kg body weight was injected intraperitoneally. The rats were killed 90 minutes later, and the testes cytosolic proteins chromatographed as indicated in FIGURE 4.

TABLE 2

EFFECT OF SELENATE, SELENITE, SELENIDE, SELENOMETHIONINE, AND SELENOCYSTINE ON TESTICULAR DAMAGE DUE TO CADMIUM AND ON THE CADMIUM CONTENT OF RAT TESTES*

Selenium Compound Injected	Degree of Testicular Damage	Cadmium Content of Testes (μg/g)
None	4.0	0.08
Selenate	0.0	0.37
Selenite	0.5	0.42
Selenide	0.0	1.10
Selenomethionine	3.0	0.13
Selenocystine	0.5	0.47

* Mature male rats (350 g) were given the selenium compounds and stable cadmium as indicated in FIGURES 4 and 5. The rats were killed 48 hours later, and the degree of testicular damage assessed using a score of 0–4, with 4 representing the most severe damage. The testes were then analyzed for cadmium content.

the cadmium content in the testes was the highest for those given selenide, followed by those given selenocystine, selenite, and selenate in decreasing order. Selenomethionine offered very little protection against cadmium damage, and the cadmium content of the testis was similar to that in rats given only cadmium. These results are consistent with those showing that selenocystine is metabolized similarly to inorganic selenium compounds whereas selenomethionine is not.[29] It appears that the selenium compounds that offer the greatest protection also cause cadmium to accumulate in testis in greater concentrations, presumably in a less toxic form; this suggests that cadmium levels alone, without a knowledge of other factors, cannot be used under all circumstances to assess possible cadmium toxicity.

The differences between these results of the testicular damage study and those obtained on the diversion of cadmium binding may be due to the different times the animals were killed after cadmium and selenium injections. The rats were killed 60 to 90 minutes after injection in the diversion studies, whereas those in the testicular damage study were killed 48 hours after injection with these compounds. This longer time period may have been sufficient to allow some of the selenium compounds, such as selenocystine, to be converted to forms that would protect against cadmium damage. The times used in the present study were chosen because 48 hours are needed to assess testicular damage due to cadmium,[8] whereas the greatest diversion in the binding of cadmium occurs when selenium as selenite is given near the same time as cadmium (FIGURE 3). Obviously, other time differentials need to be investigated.

Other workers have shown that the injection of selenium in rats did not prevent the increased production of MT due to cadmium injection in liver and kidney.[30] However, the injection of selenium did prevent the increased production of MT as the result of mercury injection in liver and kidney. These observations may be explained by some of the results from our laboratory. Selenium was found to divert the binding of only a small amount of cadmium from low MW proteins (MT) to high MW ones in the liver and about 50% of binding in the kidney, whereas essentially all of the mercury binding was diverted in liver and kidney by selenium.[28,31] Thus, if selenium diverts the binding of the major portion of a metal from MT to other proteins, this will apparently counteract the metal's ability to increase the tissue MT levels.

Based on the present results and those of other workers, we conclude that selenium must be in the selenide form to cause diversion of cadmium binding. It is known that animal tissues can reduce selenate and selenite to the selenide level.[32] Other workers found that a cadmium-selenium complex was formed either after incubation of selenite, cadmium, erythrocytes, and plasma or after incubation of selenide, cadmium, and plasma *in vitro*.[33] No interaction occurred, however, with the incubation of cadmium, selenite, and plasma *in vitro*, indicating the requirement for erythrocytes when selenite is the form of selenium used. These authors concluded that their results indicate that hydrogen selenide or a similarly reduced selenide is the product of selenite metabolism by erythrocytes and that this form of selenium is responsible for the diversion of cadmium binding in plasma. Since erythrocytes are known to possess glutathione (GSH) reductase,[32] this appears to be a logical possibility. Some preliminary evidence from our laboratory indicates that the injection of chromate, an inhibitor of GSH reductase, will prevent the diversion of cadmium binding by selenite in rats. This is consistent with the hypothesis indicating that selenide is the form of selenium responsible for the diversion of cadmium binding.

Since cysteine and BAL (2,3-dimercaptopropanol, or British antilewisite) have been shown to protect the testes against cadmium damage,[34] it was of interest to determine the influence of these compounds on cadmium binding. Cysteine and BAL were found to give maximum protection when injected respectively 30 minutes and 6 hours before cadmium,[34] and these time periods were used in the present study. As shown in FIGURE 6, cysteine and BAL do not appear to counteract cadmium by the same mechanisms as does selenium. Cysteine appeared to reduce the uptake of cadmium by the testis, which is reflected by a lower amount in each of the cadmium binding peaks. In contrast, BAL increased the uptake of cadmium, but this increase was in both the high and low MW peaks. Therefore, these results indicate that BAL, cysteine, and selenium counteract cadmium-induced testicular damage by different mechanisms.

SELENIUM-ZINC INTERACTION

Since zinc and cadmium possess similar chemical parameters,[1] it would be logical to conclude that if selenium diverted the binding of cadmium, this element

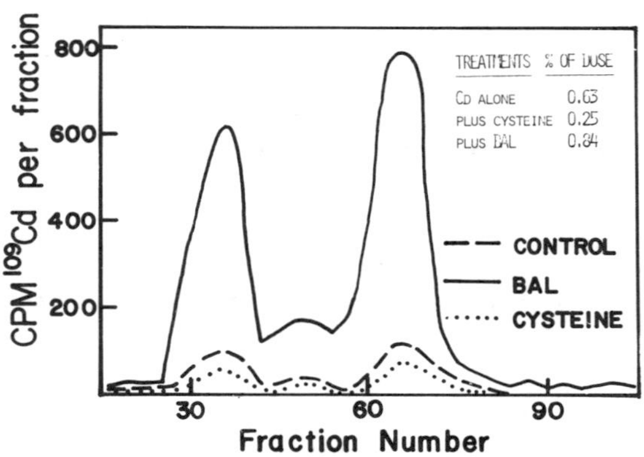

FIGURE 6. The influence of cysteine and BAL on the binding of cadmium to the cytosolic proteins in rat testes. Male rats (350 g) were injected (intraperitoneally) with 400 times (4 mmoles/kg) cysteine 30 minutes before or with 30 times (0.3 mmoles/kg) BAL as cadmium (0.01 mmoles/kg) six hours before the injection of cadmium. The rats were killed one hour after cadmium injection. Stable and radioactive cadmium levels injected and gel filtration procedures are the same as indicated for FIGURE 4.

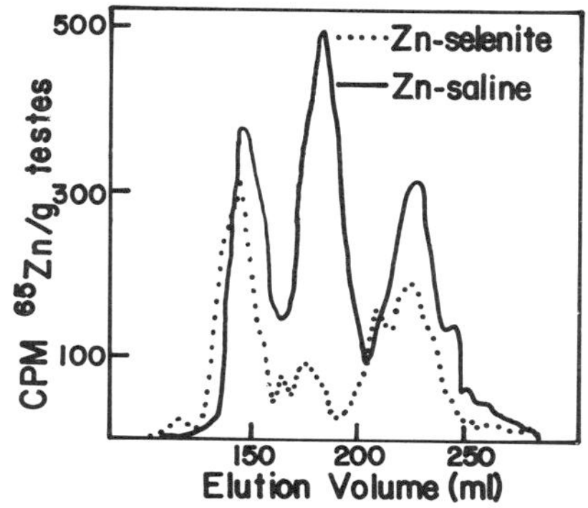

FIGURE 7. Effect of selenium as selenite on the binding of zinc to the cytosolic proteins in rat testes. Male rats (350 g) were injected simultaneously (intraperitoneally) with 0.01 mmole $ZnCl_2$ (280 μCi ^{65}Zn) and 0.01 mmole selenium as selenite per kg body weight, and the rats killed 90 minutes later. The testis cytosolic proteins were chromatographed on gel filtration as indicated in FIGURE 4.

might also divert the binding of zinc in tissues. As indicated in FIGURE 7, selenium did not influence the binding of zinc to testis cytosolic proteins similarly to cadmium. Selenium reduced the amount of zinc in the second peak (160 ml to 200 ml) but had no influence on the zinc content of the other peaks. Similar to the patterns for cadmium, however, three zinc peaks were obtained upon gel filtration with G-75 Sephadex, which is consistent with other work from our laboratory.[13] Even though selenium did not have any major effect on the binding of zinc to proteins in the testis, other work has shown that zinc will influence the metabolism of selenium. Precipitation of selenium deficiency in chicks by high dietary levels of zinc has been observed.[35] High dietary levels of zinc have been shown to promote liver necrosis in vitamin E- and selenium-deficient rats.[36] Thus, there appears to be a metabolic relationship between selenium and zinc even though zinc binding to proteins is not significantly affected by selenium, as judged by the testis.

SELENIUM-ZINC-CADMIUM INTERACTIONS

In an experiment to evaluate the influence of selenium on the binding of cadmium and zinc to testes proteins, rats were fed a basal diet or this diet plus 3 parts per million (ppm) selenium as selenite. Radioactive cadmium was injected, and the radioactivity and stable zinc levels evaluated in the cytosolic proteins of testes. As shown in FIGURE 8, there was a small amount of diversion in the binding of cadmium from the two lower MW peaks (volumes 155 to 170, and 195 to 200 ml) to the higher MW one (volumes 125 to 145 ml). However, this was not as marked as when the selenium was injected. Thus, we conclude that the major part of the dietary selenium had been converted to other chemical forms that could not divert the binding of cadmium. These changes could have occurred in the digestive tract or during absorption from the intestine. The small amount of diversion that did occur was probably due to the presence of selenide in tissues that was derived primarily from the reduction of selenite.[32] The insert of FIGURE 8 indicates that dietary selenium had no influence on the deposition of zinc in the testes cytosolic proteins. Thus, the binding of cadmium is diverted by selenium if it is in the proper chemical form, but selenium has very little influence on the binding of zinc to tissue proteins.

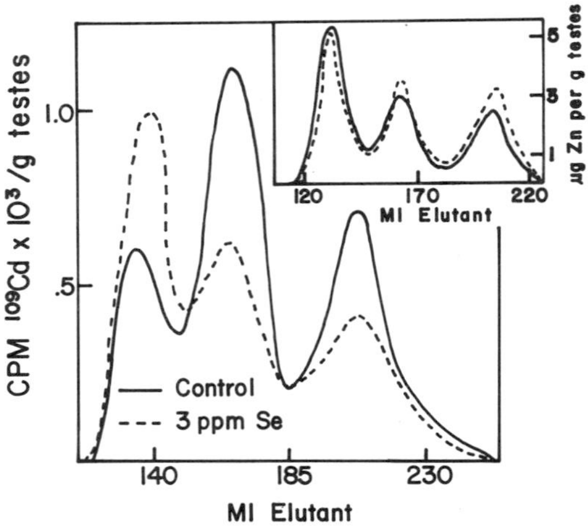

FIGURE 8. Influence of dietary selenium on cadmium binding and on zinc levels in cytosolic proteins of the rat testes. Weanling rats were fed a basal casein diet or this diet plus 3 ppm selenium as selenite for six weeks. They were injected with 0.01 mmole cadmium plus 280 μCi ^{109}Cd per kg body weight. The rats were killed one hour later, and the testes cytosolic protein chromatographed on gel filtration as indicated for FIGURE 4.

In order to present a unified concept, a schematic representation of the metabolic interrelationships of selenium, zinc, and cadmium is offered in FIGURE 9. This scheme was composed to illustrate the different effects of zinc and cadmium in relation to MT synthesis and degradation and is not presented to imply that zinc and cadmium stimulate the production of different MTs. All the available evidence indicates that these two metals stimulate the production of identical MTs by the same mechanisms.[37,38] The exposure of animals to zinc results in an increase of polyribosomal thionein mRNA.[37] This increase is maximal five hours after the administration of zinc, indicating a short-lived polyribosomal mRNA. By use of inhibitors of protein synthesis, evidence has been obtained to indicate a requirement for transcription of MT mRNA *de novo* after zinc administration. During synthesis of MT (zinc thionein), zinc becomes bound to this protein. In the liver of adult animals, the zinc disappears from the MT fraction as it is degraded.[9,22,23] Most of the degraded MT and released zinc is then apparently excreted. In the kidney and in liver of the young animal, some of the zinc is apparently reincorporated into MT, since the half-life of the zinc in the MT fraction is longer than that of the protein moiety.[23] Only a small percentage of the amino acids from the degradation of MT is reincorporated into this protein.[18]

Likewise, cadmium appears to result in increased synthesis of MT by similar mechanisms to zinc.[38] Cadmium stimulates the production of polyribosomal thionein mRNA, which is transcribed to produce thionein. The cadmium then binds to this protein to produce cadmium-thionein. During this process, zinc from either the diet or endogenous sources also becomes bound to the thionein protein. In contrast to zinc in zinc-thionein, the cadmium and zinc in MT as the result of cadmium exposure do not disappear from the MT fraction with degradation of the protein moiety.[9,10,13] The released cadmium then either stimulates the production of new mRNA or becomes attached to newly synthesized thionein, thus creating a continuous cycle. This creates a zinc "trap,"[12] and the zinc that accumulates as the result of cadmium exposure is apparently also recycled. The degree of "trapping" of zinc, however, is

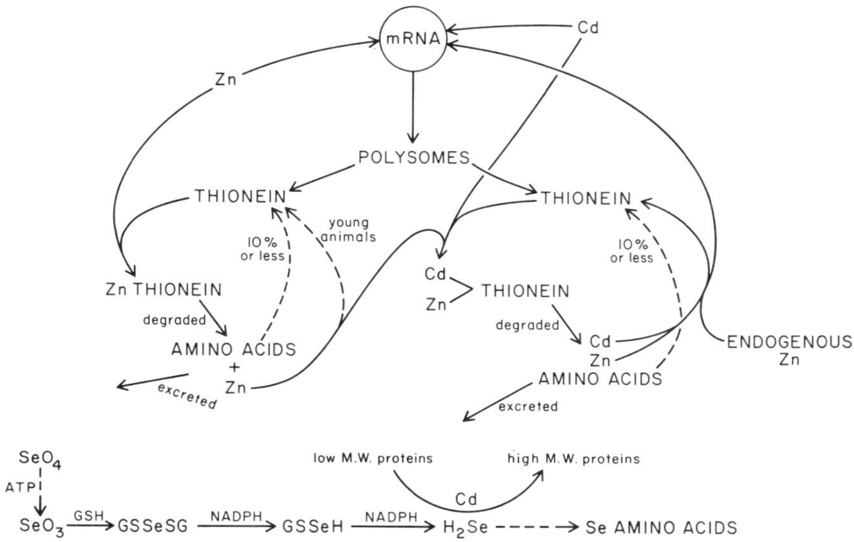

FIGURE 9. Proposed metabolic relationship between selenium, cadmium, and zinc.

dependent upon the extent of cadmium saturation of the tissues.[19] Only a small amount (up to 10%) of the amino acids derived from the degradation of cadmium-thionein is reutilized for synthesis of new MT.[18]

The available evidence indicates that it is the selenide form of selenium that diverts the binding of cadmium and that the diversion of cadmium by more oxidized forms of selenium is the result of their reduction to the selenide level.[32,33] We propose that any interaction between zinc and selenium is also at the selenide level. Although not clearly established, the reduction of selenate to selenite probably involves adenosine triphosphate (ATP) and ATP sulfurylase. The reduction of selenite to selenide occurs by a series of reactions involving a nonenzymatic reaction with GSH to form a selenotrisulfide intermediate, followed by nicotinamide-adenine dinucleotide phosphate (NADPH)-linked reduction of this intermediate by GSH-reductase to hydrogen selenide.[32] This form of selenium is then converted to selenoamino acids by pathways yet to be established. A highly probable pathway for synthesis of selenocysteine could be the substitution of selenide for sulfide in the reaction with serine, which is catalyzed by cysteine synthase.[39] We propose that the incorporation of selenium from selenite into protein is the reason why very little cadmium is diverted when inorganic selenium is given orally. The inorganic selenium is reduced to the selenide level and converted to selenoamino acids during metabolism, and only transient amounts of selenide are available for cadmium diversion. Much higher levels of selenide are available for diversion when inorganic selenium is injected either simultaneously with or shortly after the injection of cadmium.

SUMMARY

The administration of cadmium to rats by either oral or injection routes causes zinc to accumulate in the low molecular weight (MW) protein metallothionein (MT) of liver and kidney, but not in a low MW protein in the testis. Preliminary evidence indicates that the low MW cadmium-binding protein in testes is not MT. Feeding high levels of zinc to rats results in its accumulation with tissue MT, and the zinc is very labile. In contrast, the zinc that accumulates in MT as the result of cadmium exposure is not very labile. In the reverse situation, zinc does not cause cadmium to accumulate in MT. The turnover of MT is shorter when saturated with zinc than when cadmium is the predominant metal bound to it. Even though selenium will counteract testicular damage due to cadmium, it causes cadmium to accumulate in this organ at higher levels than in animals exposed to cadmium without selenium. Injection of selenate, selenite, and selenide—but not selenomethionine or selenocystine—diverts the binding of injected cadmium from low MW proteins to higher MW ones in the testes. Selenium injections had only minor influences on the binding of zinc to testicular proteins. In contrast, very little diversion occurred in the binding of either cadmium or zinc in tissues of rats fed high levels of selenium. The data suggest that it is the selenide form of selenium that causes the diversion of cadmium binding in tissues, thus providing protection of testes against cadmium exposure.

References

1. Hill, C. H. & G. Matrone. 1970. Chemical parameters in the study of *in vivo* and *in vitro* interactions of transition elements. Fed. Proc. Fed. Am. Soc. Exp. Biol. **29:** 1474.
2. Hill, C. H., G. Matrone, W. L. Payne & C. W. Barber. 1963. *In vivo* interactions of cadmium with copper, zinc and iron. J. Nutr. **80:** 227.
3. Banis, R. S., W. G. Pond, E. F. Walker & J. R. O'Connor. 1969. Dietary cadmium, iron and zinc interactions in the growing rat. Proc. Soc. Exp. Biol. Med. **130:** 802.
4. Stonard, M. D. & M. Webb. 1976. Influence of dietary cadmium on the distribution of the essential metals copper, zinc and iron in tissue of the rat. Chem. Biol. Interact. **15:** 349.
5. Parizek, J. 1957. The destructive effect of cadmium ion on testicular tissue and its prevention by zinc. J. Endocrinol. **15:** 56.
6. Mason, K. E. & J. O. Young. 1967. Effectiveness of selenium and zinc in protecting against cadmium-induced injury of the rat testis. *In* Selenium in Biomedicine. O. H. Muth, J. E. Oldfield & P. H. Weswig, Eds.: 383. Avi Publishing Co. Westport, Conn.
7. Kar, A. B. & R. P. Das. 1963. The nature of protective action of selenium on cadmium-induced degeneration of rat testis. Proc. Nat. Inst. Sci. India Part B. **29:** 297.
8. Chen, R. W., P. A. Wagner, W. G. Hoekstra & H. E. Ganther. 1974. Affinity labelling studies with ^{109}cadmium in cadmium-induced testicular injury in rats. J. Reprod. Fertil. **38:** 293.
9. Chen, R. W., P. D. Whanger & P. H. Weswig. 1975. Biological function of metallothionein. I. Synthesis and degradation of rat liver metallothionein. Biochem. Med. **12:** 95.
10. Feldman, S. L., K. S. Squibb & R. J. Cousins. 1978. Degradation of cadmium-thionein in rat liver and kidney. J. Toxicol. Environ. Health **4:** 805.
11. Sugawara, N. 1977. Influence of cadmium on zinc distribution in the mouse liver and kidney: role of metallothionein. Toxicol. Appl. Pharmacol. **42:** 377.
12. Winge, D. R., R. Premakumar & K. V. Rajagopalan. 1978. Studies on the zinc content of Cd-induced thionein. Arch. Biochem. Biophys. **188:** 466.
13. Deagen, J. T., S. H. Oh & P. D. Whanger. 1980. Biological function of metallothionein. VI. Metabolic interaction of cadmium and zinc in rats. Biol. Trace Element Res. **2:** 65.
14. Richards, M. P. & R. J. Cousins. 1976. Metallothionein and its relationship to the metabolism of dietary zinc in rats. J. Nutr. **106:** 1591.
15. Chen, R. W., E. J. Vasey & P. D. Whanger. 1977. Accumulation and depletion of zinc in rat liver and kidney metallothioneins. J. Nutr. **107:** 805.
16. Oh, S. H., H. Nakaue, J. T. Deagen, P. D. Whanger & G. H. Arscott. 1979. Accumulation and depletion of zinc in chick tissue metallothioneins. J. Nutr. **109:** 1720.
17. Shaikh, Z. A. & J. C. Smith. 1976. The biosynthesis of metallothionein in rat liver and kidney after administration of cadmium. Chem. Biol. Interact. **15:** 327.

18. Oh, S. H., J. T. Deagen, P. D. Whanger & P. H. Weswig. 1978. Biosynthesis and degradation of liver and kidney metallothionein in rats fed diets containing zinc or cadmium. Bioinorg. Chem. **8:** 245.
19. Cain, K. & D. E. Holt. 1979. Metallothionein degradation: metal composition as a controlling factor. Chem. Biol. Interact. **28:** 91.
20. Bremner, I., W. G. Hoekstra, N. T. Davies & B. W. Young. 1978. Effect of zinc status of rats on the synthesis and degradation of copper-induced metallothioneins. Biochem. J. **174:** 838.
21. Andersen, R. D., W. P. Winter, J. J. Maher & I. A. Bernstein. 1978. Turnover of metallothioneins in rat liver. Biochem. J. **174:** 327.
22. Feldman, S. L. & R. J. Cousins. 1976. Degradation of hepatic zinc-thionein after parenteral zinc administration. Biochem. J. **160:** 583.
23. Oh, S. H. & P. D. Whanger. 1979. Biological function of metallothionein. VII. Effect of age on its metabolism in rats. Am. J. Physiol. **237:** 318.
24. Feldman, S. L., M. L. Failla & R. J. Cousins. 1978. Degradation of rat liver metallothioneins *in vitro*. Biochim. Biophys. Acta **544:** 638.
25. Frazier, J. M. 1979. Bioaccumulation of cadmium in marine organisms. Environ. Health Perspect. **28:** 75.
26. Ridlington, J. W. & B. A. Fowler. 1979. Isolation and partial characterization of a cadmium-binding protein from the American oyster (C.Virginica). Chem. Biol. Interact. **25:** 127.
27. Deagen, J. T., C. L. Holcomb & S. H. Oh. 1980. Interaction of selenium and cadmium in rat testes. Fed. Am. Soc. Exp. Biol. **39:** 622.
28. Chen, R. W., P. D. Whanger & P. H. Weswig. 1975. Selenium-induced redistribution of cadmium-binding to tissue proteins: a possible mechanism of protection against cadmium toxicity. Bioinorg. Chem. **4:** 125.
29. Latshaw, J. D. & M. Osman. 1975. Distribution of selenium in egg white and yolk after feeding natural and synthetic selenium compounds. Poultry Sci. **54:** 1244.
30. Piotrowski, J. K., E. M. Bem & A. Werner. 1977. Cadmium and mercury binding to metallothionein as influenced by selenium. Biochem. Pharmacol. **26:** 2191.
31. Chen, R. W., P. D. Whanger & S. C. Fang. 1975. Diversion of mercury binding in rat tissues by selenium: a possible mechanism of protection. Pharmacol. Res. Commun. **6:** 571.
32. Ganther, H. E. 1979. Metabolism of hydrogen selenide and methylated selenides. Nutr. Res. **2:** 107.
33. Gasiewicz, T. A. & J. C. Smith. 1978. Properties of the cadmium and selenium complex formed in rat plasma *in vivo* and *in vitro*. Chem. Biol. Interact. **23:** 171.
34. Gunn, S. A., T. C. Gould & W. A. D. Anderson. 1966. Protective effect of thiol compounds against cadmium-induced vascular damage to testis. Proc. Soc. Exp. Biol. Med. **122:** 1036.
35. Jensen, L. S. 1975. Precipitation of a selenium deficiency by high dietary levels of copper and zinc. Proc. Soc. Exp. Biol. Med. **149:** 113.
36. Whanger, P. D. & P. H. Weswig. 1978. Influence of 19 elements on development of liver necrosis in selenium and vitamin E deficient rats. Nutr. Rep. Int. **18:** 421.
37. Shapiro, S. G., K. S. Squibb, L. A. Markowitz & R. J. Cousins. 1978. Cell-free synthesis of metallothionein directed by rat liver polyadenylated messenger ribonucleic acid. Biochem. J. **175:** 833.
38. Cousins, R. J. 1979. Metallothionein synthesis and degradation: relationship to cadmium metabolism. Environ. Health Perspect. **28:** 131.
39. Olson, O. E. & I. S. Palmer. 1976. Selenoamino acids in tissues of rats administered inorganic selenium. Metabolism **25:** 299.

DISCUSSION

J. PARIZEK (*Czechoslovak Academy of Sciences, Prague, Czechoslovakia*): First of all, I should like to do justice to an old paper by Tobias *et al.* [Tobias, J. M., C. C. Lushbaugh, H. M. Pratt, S. Postel, M. N. Swift & R. W. Gerard. 1946. *J. Pharmacol. Exp. Ther.* Suppl. **87**(4): 102–118]. These authors, reporting on their research on BAL [2,3-dimercaptopropanol], noted that selenite had a protective effect when injected in mice exposed to an otherwise lethal dose of cadmium chloride mist via inhalation. This, to my knowledge, was the first observation on the protective effect of selenium compounds against the toxicity of cadmium salts, a protective effect that was overlooked for a long time before it was rediscovered by Kar *et al.* [Kar, A. B., R. P. Das & B. Mukerji. 1960. *Proc. Nat. Inst. Sci. India Part B* Suppl. **26:** 40] in connection with the effects of cadmium on testes.

My second comment is related to the experiments in which you used selenomethionine. You may recall that in one of our papers on selenium-mercury and selenium-cadmium interactions [Parizek, J., I. Benes, I. Ostadalova, A. Babicky, J. Benes & J. Lener. 1969. *Physiol. Bohemoslov.* **18:** 95–103], we studied the effect of selenite and DL-selenomethionine administration on the blood level of injected cadmium and concluded that the remarkable increase in the blood level of cadmium in the selenium-treated rats resulted from increased binding of cadmium with selenium in macromolecular fractions of blood plasma. Both selenite and selenomethionine were effective in increasing blood cadmium levels in our *in vivo* experiments; however, with selenomethionine, a higher dose and longer time interval were needed to observe a comparable effect. This indicated that for conversion into an active form, selenomethionine took longer than did selenite. Our preliminary experiments, mentioned in the same paper, indicated that hepatectomy would interfere with some steps in the selenomethionine conversion. More recently, in a very important piece of work, Gasiewicz and Smith [Gasiewicz, T. A. & J. C. Smith. 1978. *Environ. Health Perspect.* **24:** 133–136] have demonstrated the role of erythrocytes in the conversion of selenite into the active form reacting with cadmium in the blood plasma.

My last comment relates to the proteins that you have discussed as not being identical with metallothionein. May I say that this conclusion is certainly well supported, not only by your results on cysteine, but also—if I recollect correctly your relevant table—by your data on the content of aromatic amino acids and histidine.

INTERACTIONS OF SELENIUM-MERCURY AND SELENIUM-SELENIUM COMPOUNDS

J. Parizek* and J. Kalouskova

Institute of Physiology
Czechoslovak Academy of Sciences

J. Benes and L. Pavlik

Radioisotope Laboratories of the
Institutes for Biological Research
Czechoslovak Academy of Sciences
Prague, Czechoslovakia

As reported previously, administration of selenite proved to be highly effective in preventing the toxicity of mercuric compounds.[1,2] Reviews of the research on this protective effect and its mechanisms—as well as the results of other studies dealing with the similar protective effect of selenite against the toxicity of certain other metals, including cadmium—have been presented elsewhere.[2-9] In the present paper, another aspect of mercury-selenium interactions will be discussed—reviewing research instigated by observation of the unexpected death of one rat, which was recorded in one of our first experiments revealing the protective effect of selenite against the toxicity of mercuric compounds.[1] In a group of 40 rats given mercuric chloride in a subcutaneous dose of 20 μmole/kg body weight, followed within one hour by a subcutaneous injection of sodium selenite in a dose of 30 μmole/kg body weight, 1 rat died within a few hours of the injection; at autopsy, pulmonary edema and pleural and pericardial effusions were the dominant signs. No signs typical of intoxication by mercuric compounds were found in this rat or in the other 39 animals of this group, which survived without any apparent harm up to the end of the experiment (one week), in contrast to rats given this (in controls, lethal) dose of mercuric chloride without selenite. Further research showed that the frequency of the peculiar lethal reaction—which was connected with convulsions and tended to occur suddenly about six hours after treatment (with the above-mentioned characteristic changes at autopsy)—varied with the dose of mercury and selenium but, in particular, could be substantially increased by two factors: first, by administering selenite a few hours before, instead of after, the mercuric compounds; and second, by using adult males instead of females in the experiment.

The combination of these two factors resulted in a remarkable increase in the lethal reaction, which occurred in 95% of 20 adult male rats given 20 μmole/kg body weight of sodium selenite intraperitoneally followed two hours later by a subcutaneous injection of mercuric chloride in a dose of 30 μmole/kg body weight. Of an analogous group given the same doses of selenite and mercury, but in the reverse order, only 20% of the males died.

The unexpected risk of this lethal reaction was, of course, scientifically intriguing, but it was particularly important in view of any potential use of selenite in the therapy or prevention of intoxications by mercuric compounds.

The nature of the signs observed—which were similar to those described after the administration of a very high dose of dimethylselenide by McConnell and Port-

* Present affiliation of all authors: Institute of Nuclear Biology and Radiochemistry, Czechoslovak Academy of Sciences, Prague.

0077-8923/80/0355-0347 $01.75/0 1980, NYAS

man[10]—and the dependence of the frequency of the lethal reaction on the sequence and timing of administration of the mercury and selenium compounds have made us suspect that methylated selenium metabolites could be involved in the lethal reaction observed. However, the amount of dimethylselenide (and related methylated selenium metabolites) that could be produced in the organism from selenite given in a dose of 20 μmole/kg body weight (resulting, in the above-mentioned experiment, in 95% lethality in the males given selenite and mercuric chloride) is more than 1,000 times less than the amount of dimethylselenide corresponding to the LD_{50} established by McConnell and Portman in 1952.[10]

We realized that the hypothesis of the involvement of dimethylselenide (or related compounds) in the observed lethality could be acceptable under two conditions; we decided to test them in further experiments, posing two questions:

1. Does simultaneous exposure to mercuric compounds increase the toxicity of dimethylselenide and trimethylselenonium ions?
2. Are these methylated selenium metabolites more toxic to males than to females?

The results of our experiments, reviewed elsewhere, have made it possible to answer both questions affirmatively.[2,3]

Sex-Linked Difference in the Toxicity and Body Retention of Methylated Selenium Metabolites

A single parenteral dose of dimethylselenide or trimethylselenonium salts was substantially more toxic in adult male rats in comparison with females.[2,3] This remarkably increased sensitivity of the adult males was, however, not yet fully apparent in males 1 month old. As shown in further experiments, the LD_{50} values established after a single parenteral dose of dimethylselenide in 1-month-old rats of both sexes and in 3½-month-old females agreed well with the extremely low toxicity of dimethylselenide reported by McConnell and Portman with LD_{50} values exceeding a dose of 20 mmole dimethylselenide/kg body weight.[10,11] In contrast, dimethylselenide was much more toxic in adult male rats, both when given undiluted and when the sex-linked difference was studied with dimethylselenide diluted in pharmaceutical *Oleum Olivae* or *Ol. helianthis.*[2,3]

Another sex-linked difference was observed in our experiments when animals were given, parenterally, ^{75}Se-dimethylselenide or ^{75}Se-trimethylselenonium salts (iodide or citrate).[2,3,13] (For methods of preparation of the methylated selenium compounds used and their characteristics, see Reference 14.) Slower urinary excretion of trimethylselenonium ions was found to be responsible for a higher whole body retention of ^{75}Se in males when compared with females given ^{75}Se-dimethylselenide or ^{75}Se-trimethylselenonium salts.[12] A highly significant sex-linked difference in ^{75}Se retention was found with these rats, particularly in the kidneys, but also in other organs or tissues.[12]

Further experiments brought out several results indicating that this substantially slower elimination of methylated selenium metabolites in males cannot per se explain the sex-linked difference in their toxicity:

1. The sex-linked difference in the renal excretion of ^{75}Se-trimethylselenonium ions developed during the third decade of postnatal life and was highly significant in one-month-old rats, that is, at the age where male rats did not yet manifest substantially increased sensitivity to the toxicity of dimethylselenide or trimethylselenonium ions characteristic in our experiments for adult males.

2. The sex-linked difference in the retention of ^{75}Se-trimethylselenonium ions was stictly androgen dependent, being abolished by the castration of the males; administration of androgens (or anabolic steroids) to castrated males or to females increased the ^{75}Se retention in animals given ^{75}Se-dimethylselenide or ^{75}Se-trimethylselenonium salts.[12] On the other hand, as shown in FIGURE 1, previous castration of the animals of both sexes, performed at the age of two months, decreased to some extent the toxicity of dimethylselenide given two months later, that is, at four months. However, the difference in toxicity between males and females remained significant even after castration.

3. Sex-linked difference in the whole body ^{75}Se retention entirely disappeared when selenium dimethylselenide was given to adult males and females after bilateral nephrectomy. On the other hand, nephrectomy did not abolish the sex-linked difference in the toxicity of methylated selenium compounds.[11,15]

These results indicate that the increased retention and increased toxicity of methylated selenium metabolites observed in adult males, in comparison with females, are parallel phenomena; nor can the increased toxicity be explained by increased retention, but must result from increased sensitivity of the male organism to

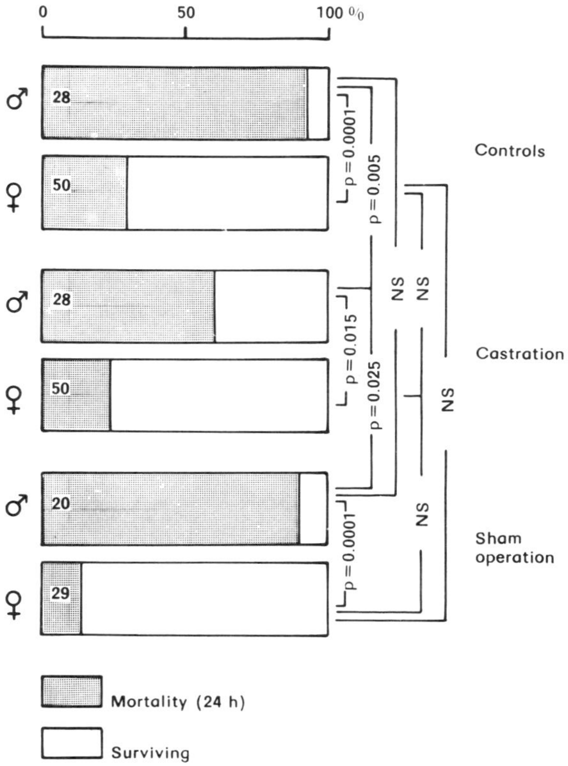

FIGURE 1. Sex-linked difference in the toxicity of dimethylselenide: gonad independent. Rat males or females four months old that were castrated or sham operated at the age of two months. Dimethylselenide was given at 200 μmole/kg body weight intraperitoneally (ip). Exact Fisher's test.

a toxic effect not directly dependent on the presence of gonads in the organism and the actual secretion of gonadal steroids.

Potentiating Effect of Mercuric Compounds on the Toxicity of Methylated Selenium Metabolites

As reported previously, simultaneous exposure to mercuric compounds and to dimethylselenide or trimethylselenonium salts results in a remarkable potentiation of the toxicity of the methylated selenium metabolites.[2] An equimolar dose of zinc or cadmium salts does not result in a similar potentiation.[2] However, an analogous phenomenon was described with arsenite.[16]

In our experiments the potentiating effect of mercuric compounds was observed with parenteral administration of dimethylselenide as well as with respiratory exposure to dimethylselenide vapor.[2] The frequency of the characteristic lethal syndrome was dependent on both the dose of mercuric compounds and the dose of dimethylselenide.[2,3]

In male rats given mercuric chloride subcutaneously in a dose of 1 μmole/kg body weight, 60% mortality was observed in the animals given, simultaneously, an intraperitoneal dose of 1 μmole dimethylselenide/kg body weight (corresponding to 79 μg selenium/kg body weight).[3] This means that in adult male rats exposed to mercuric compounds, dimethylselenide was more than 10,000 times more toxic than in adult females or one-month-old females and males in the experiments performed in our laboratory, or in the rats in the experiments of McConnell and Portman.[10] In view of this, it was possible to accept the hypothesis mentioned above, namely, that the toxicity of methylated selenium metabolites was causally involved in the lethal syndrome observed in rats, particularly in males given small amounts of selenite and of mercuric compounds.

As regards the mechanism responsible for the potentiating effect of mercury and the metabolic changes involved, at least two other results seem to be important. First, it should be noted that exposure to small amounts of mercuric chloride did not increase the whole body ^{75}Se retention after ^{75}Se-dimethylselenide administration.

$HgCl_2$ - μmole/kg b. w.	h before DMSe	DMSe - μmole/kg b. w.	Number of rats	Mortality (24h), %
–	–	5	20	10
1	1	5	10	70
5	1	5	10	90
1	24	5	10	0
5	24	5	10	0

p = 0.002
NS
p = 0.0001

FIGURE 2. Lethal toxic syndrome dependent on time interval (hours, h) between injection of $HgCl_2$ and dimethylselenide. Female rats two months old. $HgCl_2$ was injected subcutaneously (sc). Dimethylselenide (DMSe) was injected ip. Exact Fisher's test.

Second, the period of increased toxicity of dimethylselenide was limited to the first few hours after mercuric chloride injection (FIGURE 2). In further experiments, the increased toxicity of dimethylselenide was clearly manifest when it had been given as a single dose, one, three, or six hours after administering mercuric chloride (in a dose of 1 μmole/kg body weight). Groups consisting of 10 adult females were used; 24-hour mortality was 70%, 80%, and 60% respectively. However, when the same dose of dimethylselenide (20 μmole/kg body weight) was administered nine hours after the above-mentioned dose of mercuric chloride, no difference was observed between these rats (10% mortality) and the controls given dimethylselenide without mercuric chloride exposure (20% mortality). This rapid disappearance of the potentiating effects of mercury seems to indicate that this potentiation is more a function of actual exposure to mercury than of body burden, and this conclusion is, of course, of importance when evaluating the risk of a similar reaction under conditions of long-term low-level exposure to mercury. More experiments are needed, including those involving repeated or long-term exposure, to confirm the validity of this important conclusion.

The Toxicity of Dimethylselenide in Lactating Animals

In the experiments in which the toxicity of dimethylselenide was investigated when administered at different stages of ontogenic development, we were struck by the incidental observation of death of lactating mothers nourishing sucklings that had received a dimethylselenide injection. These untreated mothers, which were exposed to methylated selenium compounds that had passed through the bodies of dimethylselenide-injected pups, died with the signs of dimethylselenide intoxication, although the treated sucklings survived without apparent harm.

This seemed to indicate that lactation could be another situation connected with increased sensitivity to the toxic effects of methylated selenium metabolites. Further experiments in which dimethylselenide was given parenterally to lactating rats confirmed this suspicion.[13,17] Sensitivity to the toxic effect of dimethylselenide increased gradually during the first two weeks after delivery (that is, during the period of complete nutritional dependence of the sucklings on the mother), gradually decreasing during the second half of lactation (FIGURE 3).

This suggested an association with the intensity of lactation, even though further experiments revealed that variation in the number of animals nourished by the mother (3 or 14 sucklings) did not affect the frequency of the lethal reaction in mothers given dimethylselenide. On the other hand, artificial removal of sucklings from the mothers resulted in decreased dimethylselenide toxicity to levels observed in nonlactating females (FIGURE 3). Further experiments revealed that the toxicity remained high during the first 12 hours after removal of the sucklings, decreasing gradually within the following 12 hours. In preliminary experiments, this decrease in sensitivity was observed also in the animals that, after removal of the sucklings, had no access to food.

No increase in the whole body ^{75}Se retention was observed in lactating compared with nonlactating females.[17] It seems, therefore, that endocrine and/or metabolic changes connected with lactation are responsible for the increased toxicity of dimethylselenide in the lactating animals. Although access to food did not apparently influence the decrease in dimethylselenide toxicity after artificial removal of the sucklings, and though a reduced number of sucklings nourished did not affect the toxicity, the association of increased toxicity with the period of maximum lactation indicated a possible association with the nutritional status of the lactating animals.

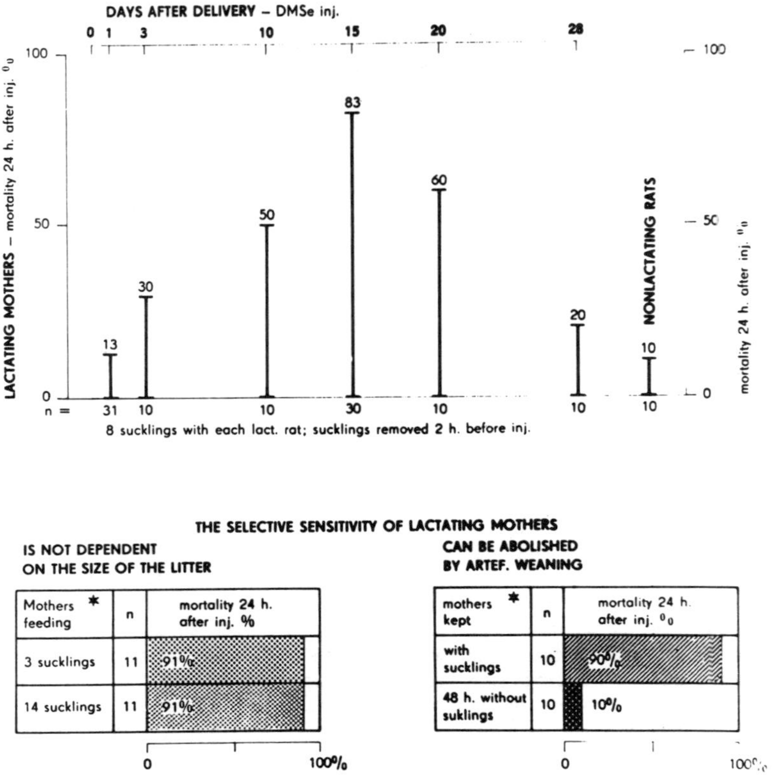

FIGURE 3. Lactation and the toxicity of dimethylselenide (200 μmole/kg body weight ip). * = injected DMSe 15th day after delivery. n = number of lactating mothers or controls in each group.

Effect of the Level of Previous Selenium Exposure on the Toxicity of Dimethylselenide

Two previous, independent studies demonstrated the role of adaptation to a high level of selenium intake in chronic selenium toxicity.[18-20] In this connection, it is of interest that Shtutman *et al.* observed increased synthesis of glutathione and increased glutathione levels as well as other changes, particularly in methionine metabolism, in the liver of rats a few hours after a single dose of selenite, suggesting the importance of this metabolic effect for detoxication reactions involving selenium and its toxicity.[21,22]

Occasionally, increased toxicity of selenite has been reported when given in the usual prophylactic doses to sheep in low-selenium areas.[23,24] The nature of the lethal reaction observed in these sheep and the lethal reaction occurring in rats in the experiments descibed in this paper are strikingly similar.

In all the experiments referred to so far in this paper, the Wistar rats used were kept on a standard, commercially available laboratory diet. This so-called Larsen diet (for composition, see e.g. Reference 25) has been used for more than two dec-

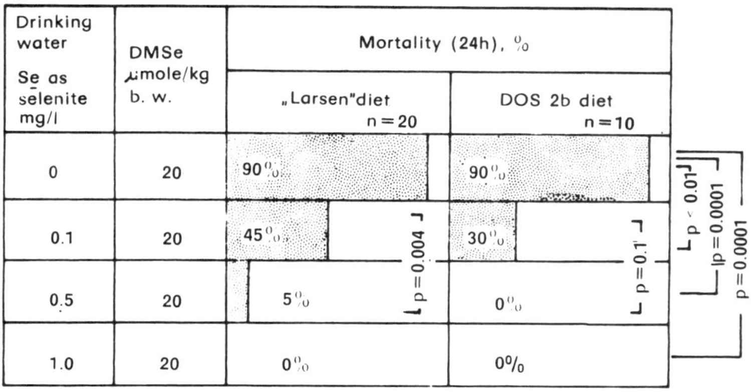

FIGURE 4. The protective effect of increased peroral selenium intake on the toxicity of dimethylselenide. Male rats two months old were given drinking water with the specified selenium content for three days before dimethylselenide injection. DMSe: dimethylselenide 20 µmole/kg body weight ip. Se content in the diet used: "Larsen" diet, 0.052 ± 0.005 mg/kg; DOS 2b diet, 0.044 ± 0.001 mg/kg. Exact Fisher's test.

ades. Generations of rats kept on this diet have not shown any signs of selenium deficiency at regular health status checks of the stock colony (checks that cover body growth and reproduction surveillance, external—including hair—inspection, hematology, and examination of internal organs), despite the relatively low selenium content in the diet. In different batches analyzed, selenium levels varied from 0.045 to 0.07 mg/kg of the diet.[26] Two independent analytical procedures (neutron activation analysis and atomic absorption spectrophotometry) used in parallel showed very good agreement. A description of the methods used for selenium determination and an evaluation of their specificity, detection limits, precision, and accuracy have been presented elsewhere.[26,27]

In further experiments, we decided to test how far the level of previous selenium exposure could influence the toxicity of dimethylselenide. One possibility was that suboptimal selenium intake, still sufficient to maintain the good health of the animals, was responsible for their decreased resistance to dimethylselenide toxicity, particularly under the conditions of increased demand for selenium. The experiments revealed that increased oral exposure to selenite dramatically decreased the toxicity of dimethylselenide in adult rats.[28] This protective effect of previous exposure to small amounts of selenite was dose dependent and was quite clear, whether selenite was added to the drinking water or whether it was added to the diet.

FIGURE 4 compares the results of three days of exposure to drinking water with increased levels of selenite in adult male rats kept on two different laboratory diets, both low in selenium. The semisynthetic diet DOS 2b contained tocopherol acetate at a level of 100 mg/kg diet.

Further experiments showed that the fortification of this diet with selenite one day before the injection of dimethylselenide was sufficient to protect the animals against toxicity. Male rats (two months old) used in this experiment were given a dose of dimethylselenide of 200 µg/kg body weight intraperitoneally, and the mortality was registered for 24 hours afterwards. Four groups of 10 rats each were used; they received the DOS 2b diet without or with selenite fortification to selenium levels of 0.1, 0.5, and 1.0 mg/kg diet (dry weight). When left on the basal diet without the addition of selenite (dietary selenium level of about 0.05 mg/kg), 90% of the rats died within 24 hours of dimethylselenide administration, with the typical signs of toxicity caused by methylated selenium compounds. Dimethylselenide given after one day on the diet with the 0.1 mg/kg selenium level resulted in 60% mortality, and with the 0.5 mg/kg selenium level, in 30% mortality; while all rats in the group given, one day before the dimethylselenide injection, the diet containing 1.0 mg selenium/kg diet survived without any sign of intoxication. In another experiment in which four similar groups of male rats were given the same diets for seven days, all the animals receiving 0.1 mg selenium (or more)/kg diet survived, in comparison with 60% mortality in the group kept on the basal diet, i.e., at a selenium dietary level of about 0.05 mg/kg. Dimethylselenide in this experiment was given intraperitoneally in a dose of 20 μmole/kg.

As already mentioned, no signs of selenium deficiency were ever observed in the rats kept for generations on either of the experimental diets used. However, both were relatively low in selenium, and this could well represent a common denominator explaining why such different factors as male sex, lactation, or acute exposure to mercuric compounds (or even exposure to arsenic compounds) are connected with remarkably increased toxicity of methylated selenium compounds.

Several papers indicate that males, as opposed to females, demand more selenium, being prone to selenium deficiency and retaining less ^{75}Se-selenium from the administered trace dose of ^{75}Se-selenite.[29,30] In our laboratory, lower renal selenium levels were found in adult male than in adult female rats fed the "Larsen" diet.[26] This difference was not present in 20-day-old rats (analogous work to determine the blood levels of selenium and of glutathione peroxidase is in progress). As already mentioned, lactation in the rat, particularly during the second and third postnatal weeks, could well represent another situation connected with an increased demand for selenium. Finally, it should be noted that both mercuric compounds and arsenic compounds interfere with selenium metabolism, mercuric compounds and arsenic compounds being more potent on an equimolar basis than are the salts of cadmium.[31,32]

In view of this, it seems that the following working hypothesis could be proposed. The fact that the precursor (selenite) protects against the toxicity of its metabolic products (methylated selenium compounds) could explain why the toxicity of these methylated selenium metabolites, rapidly excreted from the organism, can be very low and why biosynthesis of these compounds has been considered as detoxication. It is well established that the excretion and thus production of methylated selenium metabolites are proportional to the level of selenium intake, and it may be expected that methylated selenium metabolites and their precursors are, under normal conditions, in a long-term balance in the organism. However, under conditions of suboptimal selenium intake close to borderline deficiency, sudden exposure to larger amounts of selenium compounds and/or changes in selenium metabolism or effects caused by exposure to chemical factors, such as mercuric or arsenic compounds, could change this balance and unmask the toxicity of methylated selenium metabolites.

A final understanding of these interrelations will depend, of course, on the identification of the molecular mechanisms responsible for the toxicity of methylated selenium metabolites and for the protective effect of selenite and possibly other selenium compounds.

Further research is in progress to identify the sex-linked metabolic differences and the metabolic changes induced by lactation or exposure to mercury that could modify probable conversion of dimethylselenide and trimethylselenonium ions to the form acting at tissue level, and/or modify the sensitivity of the target tissues to the deleterious action of these metabolites.

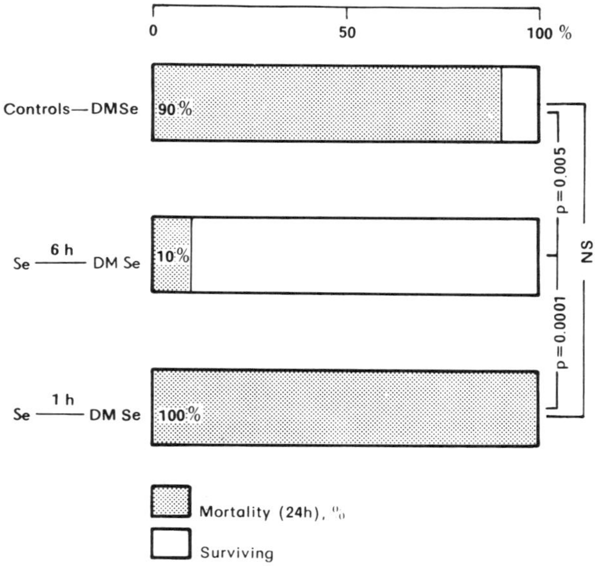

FIGURE 5. The effect of selenite pretreatment on the toxicity of dimethylselenide. DMSe: dimethylselenide 20 μmole/kg body weight ip. Se: Na_2SeO_3 1 μmole/kg body weight sc one hour or six hours before dimethylselenide injection. Controls: saline injected six hours before dimethylselenide, n = 10. Exact Fisher's test.

An important step in identifying these molecular mechanisms seems to be recognition of the relatively short time needed for the induction and disappearance of increased sensitivity to the toxic effects of methylated selenium metabolites. As already mentioned, remarkably increased sensitivity to dimethylselenide appears and disappears within a few hours of the administration of mercuric salts. The sensitivity of lactating rats remains high for 12 hours after artificial removal of sucklings from the mother; it then drops rapidly down to control levels within the next 12 hours. Further experiments revealed that the metabolic changes responsible for the protective effects of selenite developed within a few hours of the injection of a very small amount of selenite.[28]

Animals in these experiments were kept on the "Larsen" diet used in the previous work. A small dose of selenite, 1 μmole/kg body weight, was given subcutaneously one hour or six hours before intraperitoneal injection of dimethylselenide. This small dose of selenite, when given six hours (but not one hour) before dimethylselenide, significantly decreased dimethylselenide toxicity in males (FIGURE 5), in lactating females (FIGURE 6), and, in a similar way, in the animals exposed simultaneously to mercuric chloride and dimethylselenide.

Several studies indicate that a period of a few hours after selenite injection is sufficient for induction of significant biochemical effects. As already mentioned, increased synthesis and a higher level of glutathione, as well as other biochemical changes involving methionine metabolism, were found by Shtutman *et al.* in the liver of rats after parenteral administration of selenite in a dose of 4 μmole/kg body weight or higher.[21,22] A significant increase in the activity of hepatic mitochondrial δ-aminolevulinate synthetase and microsomal heme oxygenase was observed in rats given subcutaneously a high dose of selenite (50 μmole/kg body weight), the max-

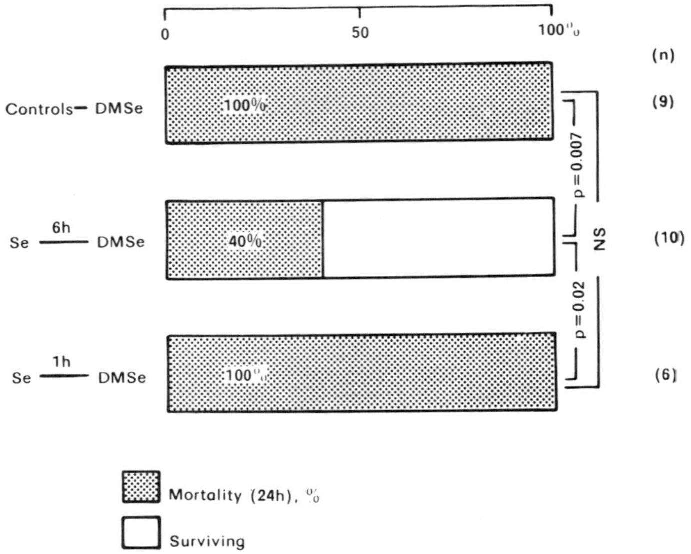

FIGURE 6. The effect of selenite pretreatment on the toxicity of dimethylselenide in lactating rats. Lactating rats 14–16 days after delivery. Six hours after removal of sucklings, dimethylselenide (DMSe) was injected at 200 μmole/kg body weight ip. Controls: saline injected sc six hours before dimethylselenide injection. Se: Na_2SeO_3 1 μmole/kg body weight sc one hour or six hours before dimethylselenide injection. Exact Fisher's test.

imum being reached within two hours of the injection.[33] The doses of selenite used in these experiments were higher than the dose (1 μmole/kg body weight) that, in the aforementioned experiments, ensured protection against the toxicity of dimethylselenide.[28] However, more recent work by Correia and Burk revealed that a single injection of a similar low dose (0.6 μmole per rat of 250–300 g body weight), given to selenium-deficient animals one to six hours before phenobarbital, significantly lowered and finally abolished the phenobarbital-mediated stimulation of microsomal heme oxygenase activity observed in the selenium-deficient, but not in the control, rats.[34]

It is evident that an increased glutathione level could be of crucial importance for the detoxication of methylated selenium metabolites. The biochemical effects of selenite administration described by Shtutman *et al.* could, of course, play a more general role in the protective effect of selenium against various toxicants.[21,22]

In this connection, it should be mentioned that selenium protects against the toxic effects of methylmercury[35] (for more recent reviews, see e.g. References 4, 5, 7, 9, 36, and 37), and, as previously discussed elsewhere, a similarity in the protective mechanisms against the toxicity of methylated selenium compounds and methylmercury cannot be excluded.[8] Although the toxic effects and the biokinetics (rate of elimination and organ distribution) of methylated selenium compounds and methylmercury are, of course, very dissimilar, some of the basic mechanisms of their metabolic activation into the form responsible for their toxicity and/or action at tissue level could be similar. In this respect, the mechanism suggested recently by Ganther as being responsible for the selenium-methylmercury interaction and involving free radicals seems to deserve attention also in the case of selenite-induced protection against the toxicity of methylated selenium compounds.[36] The possible toxi-

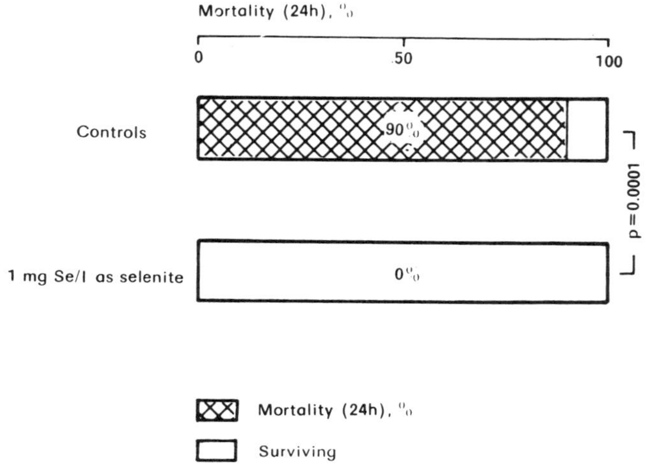

FIGURE 7. The protective effect of increased peroral intake of selenite on the incidence of the lethal reaction in rats given mercuric chloride and selenite. Male rats two months old were injected with Na_2SeO_3 at 10 μmole/kg body weight sc two hours before $HgCl_2$ at 10 μmole/kg body weight sc. Two groups of 20 animals each were kept for three days on deionized water or on water containing 1 mg Se/l as selenite. Exact Fisher's test.

cological significance of the formation of dimethyldiselenide, found in small amounts in the air exhaled by the rats in our experiments, may be of interest in this respect.[2,38]

The above-mentioned effect of selenite administration on the enzymes connected with heme metabolism opens, perhaps, another interesting possibility, and further experiments should elucidate whether methylated selenium metabolites are involved in the induction of microsomal heme oxygenase observed by Maines and Kappas in rats given selenite in a high dose of 50 μmole/kg body weight;[33] whether this effect depends on the dietary level of selenium; and whether pretreatment by small amounts of selenite could abolish the stimulation of this enzyme activity in selenium-deficient animals, as it did with phenobarbital induction in the experiment of Correia and Burk.[34]

Present knowledge does not allow us to confirm or reject any of these possibilities. However, even though the corresponding molecular mechanism cannot be identified yet, it now seems that it is at least possible to understand why some rats occasionally die when given selenite and mercuric compounds.

It may be concluded that a remarkable increase in the toxicity of methylated selenium metabolites is responsible for this lethal reaction and that this increased toxicity can be prevented by previous exposure to a small amount of selenite. In full accordance with these conclusions, the high incidence of lethal reactions observed in rats given selenite and mercuric compounds can be prevented by pretreatment with a small parenteral dose of selenite or by increasing the level of previous oral selenium intake (FIGURE 7).

As previously discussed elsewhere, the risk of a fatal reaction could represent a serious obstacle for practical exploitation of the protective effect of selenium against mercury toxicity.[39] The results presented indicate that this risk is a function of previous selenium intake, which opens up means for its effective control.

However, to close this paper—which is the last in the section dealing with micronutrient interactions and hazardous elements—it seems pertinent to mention one problem of a more general character. Remarkable progress in the science of nutrition has made it possible to devise modern laboratory diets containing optimum, and sometimes even superoptimum, levels of micronutrients recognized as essential. This is, of course, highly important and beneficial for nutrition research, particularly the research oriented towards optimization of human or farm-animal nutrition. However, high dietary levels of these micronutrients could, through interaction, mask some of the toxic effects of chemicals investigated in toxicological studies. A similar problem was discussed by Fox and also by Petering—in the latter case, particularly in connection with some of the effects of long-term exposure to cadmium and the well-known cadmium-zinc interaction.[40-42] The results reviewed in the present paper have brought up another example: the toxic effect of methylated selenium metabolites would not have been manifest at high levels of dietary selenium intake. This masking of toxicity would be highly misleading if it occurred when testing important new chemicals for toxicity, in particular, in long-term experiments entailing exposure to low levels of the chemicals in question. Given the growing demand for such testing, including the long-term low-exposure experiments, the question of possible interference of interaction—and of optimal levels of micronutrients in the diets used in toxicological research—seems very important and demands joint effort from nutritionists and toxicologists.

References

1. Parizek, J. & I. Ostadalova. 1967. Experientia **23:** 142–145.
2. Parizek, J., I. Ostadalova, J. Kalouskova, A. Babicky & J. Benes. 1971. The detoxifying effects of selenium. Interrelations between compounds of selenium and certain metals. *In* Newer Trace Elements in Nutrition. W. Mertz & W. E. Cornatzer, Eds.: 85–122. Marcel Dekker, Inc. New York, N.Y.
3. Parizek, J., J. Kalouskova, A. Babicky, J. Benes & L. Pavlik. 1974. Interaction of selenium with mercury, cadmium, and other toxic metals. *In* Trace Element Metabolism in Animals. W. G. Hoekstra, J. W. Suttie, H. E. Ganther & W. M. Mertz, Eds. **2:** 119–131. University Park Press. Baltimore, Md.
4. Diplock, A. T. 1976. CRC Crit. Rev. Toxicol. **4:** 271–329.
5. Parizek, J. 1976. Interrelationships among trace elements. *In* Effects and Dose-Response Relationships of Toxic Metals. G. F. Nordberg, Ed.: 489–510. Elsevier Scientific Publishing Company. Amsterdam, Oxford, New York.
6. Berlin, M. 1978. Environ. Health Perspect. **25:** 67–69.
7. Levander, O. A. 1978. Environ. Health Perspect. **25:** 77–80.
8. Parizek, J. 1978. Environ. Health Perspect. **25:** 53–55.
9. The Task Group on Metal Interaction. (G. F. Nordberg, Ed.) 1978. Environ. Health Perspect. **25:** 3–41.
10. McConnell, K. P. & O. W. Portman. 1952. Proc. Soc. Exp. Biol. Med. **79:** 230–231.
11. Kalouskova, J. 1975. A study on sex-linked differences in the excretion and toxicity of methylated selenium metabolites. Ph.D. Thesis. Institute of Physiology, Czechoslovak Academy of Sciences. Prague, Czechoslovakia. (In Czech.)
12. Parizek, J., J. Kalouskova, J. Benes, L. Pavlik, A. Babicky & J. Kopoldova. 1972. Physiol. Bohemoslov. **21:** 424–425.
13. Parizek, J., J. Kalouskova, J. Benes, A. Babicky, L. Pavlik & J. Kopoldova. 1975. Some hormonal and environmental factors influencing selenium metabolism and action. *In* Proceedings, Ninth International Congress of Nutrition, Mexico, 1972. S. Basta & A. Chavez, Eds. **1:** 110–114. Karger. Basel, Switzerland.
14. Parizek, J. & J. Benes. 1973. Methylated radioselenium compounds: their synthesis, metabolism and practical use. *In* Radiopharmaceuticals and Labelled Compounds **2:** 141–144. International Atomic Energy Agency. Vienna, Austria.

15. Kalouskova, J., J. Parizek, L. Pavlik & J. Benes. 1978. Studies on the mechanism of sex-linked difference in the toxicity and retention of methylated selenium compounds. *In* Trace Element Metabolism in Man and Animals. M. Kirchgessner, Ed. **3:** 611-613. Institut für Ernährungsphysiologie, Technische Universität München. Freising-Weihenstephan, Federal Republic of Germany.
16. Obermeyer, B. D., I. S. Palmer, O. E. Olson & A. W. Halverson. 1971. Toxicol. Appl. Pharmacol. **20:** 135-146.
17. Parizek, J., J. Kalouskova, L. Pavlik, A. Babicky & J. Benes. 1973. Physiol. Bohemoslov. **22:** 422.
18. Ermakov, V. V. & V. V. Kovalskij. 1969. Geochimicheskaya ekologiya organismov pri povyschennom soderzhanii selena v srede. (Geochemical ecology of organisms at increased environmental levels of selenium.) Tr. Biogeokhim. Lab. Akad. Nauk SSSR. **12:** 204-237. (In Russian.)
19. Jaffe, W. G. & M. C. Mondragon. 1969. J. Nutr. **97:** 431-436.
20. Jaffe, W. G. & M. C. Mondragon. 1975. Br. J. Nutr. **33:** 387-397.
21. Shtutman, C. M., R. V. Chagovets, A. M. Sukharevskaya & T. I. Kashleva. 1968. Vopr. Pitan. **27**(2): 3-7. (In Russian.)
22. Shtutman, C. M., V. P. Artyuhk, A. A. Biber & R. V. Chagovets. 1972. Vopr. Pitan. **31**(3): 12-17. (In Russian.)
23. Caravaggi, C., F. L. Clark & A. R. B. Jackson. 1970. Res. Vet. Sci. **11:** 146-149.
24. Gabbedy, B. J. 1970. Aust. Vet. J. **46:** 223-226.
25. Ostadalova, I. & J. Parizek. 1968. Physiol. Bohemoslov. **17:** 217-228.
26. Pavlik, L., J. Kalouskova, M. Vobecky, J. Dedina, J. Benes & J. Parizek. 1979. Selenium levels in the kidneys of male and female rats. *In* Nuclear Activation Techniques in the Life Sciences 1978: 213-223. International Atomic Energy Agency. Vienna, Austria.
27. Vobecky, M., L. Pavlik & J. Benes. 1977. Radiochem. Radioanal. Lett. **29:** 159-164.
28. Parizek, J., J. Kalouskova, V. Korunova, J. Benes & L. Pavlik. 1976. Physiol. Bohemoslov. **25:** 573-576.
29. Siami, G., A. R. Schulert & R. A. Neal. 1972. J. Nutr. **102:** 857-862.
30. Brown, D. G. & R. F. Burk. 1973. J. Nutr. **103:** 102-108.
31. Levander, O. A. & L. C. Argrett. 1969. Toxicol. Appl. Pharmacol. **14:** 308-314.
32. Parizek, J., I. Benes, A. Babicky, J. Benes, V. Prochazkova & V. Lener. 1969. Physiol. Bohemoslov. **18:** 105-111.
33. Maines, M. D. & A. Kappas. 1976. Proc. Nat. Acad. Sci. USA **73:** 4428-4431.
34. Correia, M. A. & R. F. Burk. 1978. J. Biol. Chem. **253:** 6203-6210.
35. Ganther, H. E., C. Goudie, M. L. Sunde, M. J. Kopecky, P. Wagner, S. OH & W. G. Hoekstra. 1972. Science **175:** 1122-1124.
36. Ganther, H. E. 1978. Environ. Health Perspect. **25:** 71-76.
37. Skerfving, S. 1978. Environ. Health Perspect. **25:** 57-65.
38. Vlasakova, V., J. Benes & J. Parizek. 1972. Radiochem. Radioanal. Lett. **10:** 251-258.
39. Parizek, J. 1972. Toxicological studies involving trace elements. *In* Nuclear Activation Techniques in the Life Sciences 1972: 177-194. International Atomic Energy Agency. Vienna, Austria.
40. Fox, M. R. S. 1978. Environ. Health Perspect. **25:** 137-140.
41. Petering, H. G. 1974. The effect of cadmium and lead on copper and zinc metabolism. *In* Trace Element Metabolism in Animals. W. G. Hoekstra, J. W. Suttie, H. E. Ganther & W. M. Mertz, Eds. **2:** 311-325. University Park Press. Baltimore, Md.
42. Petering, H. E. 1978. Environ. Health Perspect. **25:** 141-145.

Discussion

H. E. Ganther (*University of Wisconsin, Madison, Wis.*): I would like to ask two questions. First, does vitamin E duplicate the protective effect of treatment with selenium? And second, does starvation of animals, which decreases liver glutathione content considerably, have any effect on the interaction?

J. PARIZEK: As regards your first question, I can only say that, as explained in our paper, two laboratory diets were used in our experiments. The semisynthetic diet DOS 2b contained tocopherol acetate at a level of 100 mg/kg diet. The content of vitamin E in the other laboratory diet ("Larsen" diet) has been monitored for many years of its use by Dr. Hruba at the Institute of Nutrition [now the Institute of Experimental and Clinical Medicine] in Prague. The level of vitamin E in this diet varied, it was lower than that in the DOS 2b diet, but even the "Larsen" diet cannot be considered as vitamin E deficient. As shown in FIGURE 4 of our paper, no significant difference was found in the toxicity of dimethylselenide in rats kept on these two diets. Of course, the possibility cannot be excluded that vitamin E deficiency or the use of diets overfortified with vitamin E could modify the toxicity of methylated selenium compounds, and such experiments certainly deserve further consideration. On the other hand, with the administration of vitamin E by injection, we could not expect any protective effect to appear as rapidly as with selenite, where the protective effect becomes manifest within a few hours of injection. For that reason I would be cautious in making any final statement as regards vitamin E.

Concerning your second question, we are just now in the middle of experiments in which we are trying two different ways, including food deprivation or administration of different chemicals, to modify the level of glutathione and to test dimethylselenide toxicity under these conditions. However, the only experiment with food deprivation to which I can refer today is the experiment in which we removed sucklings from lactating mothers and in which simultaneous food deprivation apparently did not influence the decline in the sensitivity of these mothers to the lethal effects of dimethylselenide.

H. SPRINCE (*Veterans Administration Medical Center, Coatesville, Penn.*): I'd like to ask about pulmonary edema.

We've been interested in protecting against aldehyde toxicity and find we can do this particularly with doses of ascorbic acid. Pulmonary edema is associated with lethal doses of acetaldehyde. There's also a loss of ascorbic acid that occurs in pulmonary edema. Have you considered the possible prevention of pulmonary edema by large doses of ascorbic acid?

J. PARIZEK: We have tried to do some work with large doses of ascorbic acid, not for the reason mentioned, but in connection with some older reports on ascorbic acid and the toxicity of selenium compounds. [See Rosenfeld, I. & O. A. Beath. 1964. *Selenium.* Academic Press, Inc. New York and London.] Our first results were not very encouraging, but a definite answer would certainly need more experiments.

May I take this opportunity to repeat that what is of particular interest in our situation is not only the lung edema but the massive accumulation of fluid in the pleural cavity and in the pericardium, which develops rapidly after a lag time of a few hours and which is followed by the death of the animals.

INTERACTIONS OF ESSENTIAL MINERALS WITH TOXIC MINERALS: GENERAL DISCUSSION

Moderator: Harold H. Sandstead

Human Nutrition Research Center
U.S. Department of Agriculture
Science and Education Administration
Grand Forks, North Dakota 58202

P. D. WHANGER (*Oregon State University, Corvallis, Oreg.*): I'd like to make some comments bearing on the results of Dr. Bremner. Although I told him yesterday that I have a gut-level feeling he may be right, I guess I'm looking for data to convince me of this.

We fed high levels of copper in the diet to rats, and copper accumulated to the greatest extent in the liver in a protein of about 30,000 molecular weight [MW], and very little of the copper is present where metallothionein elutes from the column. Cadmium does cause copper to accumulate in the metallothionein fractions.

In contrast to the pattern in the liver, copper accumulates in a lower MW protein, presumably metallothionein, in the kidney. So we have this difference between the liver and the kidney when copper is given orally. It doesn't make any difference whether we inject copper or include it in the diet, the copper presumably is bound to metallothionein in the kidney, but I still have some questions about the liver; the next slide will point this difference out by dietary exposures to copper.

Here one sees that the accumulation of copper in peak 3, which is metallothionein, in the kidney goes up with increased copper content in the diet; whereas in the liver, there is very little increase in the copper content in the metallothionein fractions, with the greatest increase in peak 2 [30,000 MW protein].

Now if you inject the copper in rats fed the basal diet and elute the liver cytosol through a gel filtration column, the greatest amount of copper elutes where metallothionein elutes. If we take the metallothionein [MT] fraction and elute through DEAE cellulose columns, we do not get discrete separation of the MT peaks. If we take the peak fraction and elute that through a column of hydroxyapatite, we lose the copper.

In contrast, if you inject copper in rats fed 100 ppm cadmium in the diet, copper also elutes from this gel filtration column in the same areas as does MT. If each of the MT species is eluted through the DEAE cellulose columns, you get two metallothionein species separated as it should be if it is metallothionein. If you take either one of these peaks here and elute it through hydroxyapatite, you do not lose the copper, but it comes through the column with the protein. This suggests either that cadmium stabilizes the protein so that you do not lose the copper when you elute it from hydroxyapatite or that copper is bound to a different protein other than metallothionein. Is it possible that your diets or your strain of animals would be causing analogous effects to that of dietary cadmium?

I. BREMNER (*Rowett Research Institute, Bucksburn, Aberdeen, United Kingdom*): I agree with you that there are marked differences in the binding of metals, and particularly of copper to metallothionein in the liver and kidneys. Although only trace amounts of metallothionein are usually present in rat liver, we find that when our weanling rats are maintained on either stock colony diets or on semisynthetic diets, there is gradual increase with age in the concentration of copper in the kidneys.

0077-8923/80/0355-0361 $01.75/0 © 1980, NYAS

Most of this copper is bound to a protein that we think is metallothionein. This increase with age in copper-metallothionein concentrations is most evident in female rats, and, as I said in my own talk, up to 20 μg of copper may be bound in this form per gram of tissue.

As regards the identity of the protein, we have carried out the usual isolation procedures for metallothionein, using gel filtration on Sephadex and ion exchange chromatography on DEAE-Sephadex, taking care to use anaerobic conditions and to work in the cold room as far as possible. The separation pattern we observed was identical to that reported for copper-metallothionein from the livers of copper-injected rats and of pigs on high copper rations. That is, we found that one copper fraction did not bind to the DEAE-Sephadex and that two fractions were eluted with dilute Tris-acetate buffer.

I must admit, however, that we have not been able to isolate copper proteins from rat kidneys with 30% cysteine residues, which is what is generally found in metallothionein. In most of our preparations, we find only about 20% cysteine. This probably reflects incomplete purification, but a slight possibility remains that the kidney protein is not identical to the liver protein. Nevertheless I would stress that the amino acid composition of our kidney proteins is far removed from what other research groups have reported for nonmetallothionein copper proteins.

Perhaps I should point out to members of the audience who are not familiar with this topic that there has been considerable controversy as to the nature of the copper protein that is induced in the liver of copper-injected rats. We have successfully isolated copper-metallothionein from these animals, but four or five other research groups have reported that other proteins are synthesized instead. These have a much lower cysteine content. Different groups have reported cysteine contents of from 2 to 14%.

H. H. Sandstead: I might say that some of the differences may be due to techniques and how people do their column work. Isn't that right, Dr. Bremner?

I. Bremner: Yes. The copper proteins are not very stable, and that's why I stress the fact that we use anaerobic conditions for the isolation of protein.

P. D. Whanger: Would you speculate on the reasons for the differences in the behavior on DEAE cellulose with and without cadmium in the diet.

I. Bremner: I don't really know. I know that in the original papers on chelatin from the Duke University group, they found a similar difference. Thus the pure copper-induced protein was apparently bound irreversibly to DEAE cellulose, whereas a preparation that contained a combination of cadmium and copper behaved quite conventionally on DEAE columns.

P. D. Whanger: We found that if you let the copper solution stand in a cold room for two or three days and then elute through DEAE cellulose, the copper becomes bound to the resin and does not elute from the column. I think probably that's the reason the Duke group obtained their results. However, if you take the fraction directly from the gel filtration column and then elute through DEAE cellulose, it does not stick to the resin. Therefore, probably some of it is related to storage techniques. But in our studies, the conditions were the same. It's obviously different, and I was interested in knowing your reaction: Are we dealing with a stability problem or are we dealing with different types of protein here?

I. Bremner: I certainly think it is the same protein. I think perhaps the nature of the metal bound may have an effect on the chemical stability of the protein.

P. Marfey (*State University of New York, Albany, N.Y.*): I'd like to ask Dr. Whanger an additional question. Do I understand correctly that perhaps you have multiple forms of metallothionein due to disulfide interchange because there's a number of sulfhydryl groups available for this type of binding? You have shown by

DEAE cellulose and Sephadex chromatography that you can resolve several components. Can the situation be reversed if you add a reducing agent, like mercaptoethanol or some other compound? Are metallothioneins only found in cytosol?

P. D. WHANGER: There's a possibility of polymerization by forming disulfide bonds between MT molecules. Certainly the copper protein seems to be very much more subject to oxidation, and there appears to be a need for reducing agents, such as glutathione, in the buffer. With MT containing zinc or cadmium, however, the need for reducing agents in the buffer is not as critical.

Regarding your second question, metallothionein is present in other organelles and is not solely in the cytosol. About 60 to 70% is present in cytosol, and most of the remainder is present in the mitochondrial fraction. So it is not exclusively in the cytosolic fraction.

H. G. PETERING (*University of Cincinnati Medical Center, Cincinnati, Ohio*): A few years ago we published a paper on the metallothioneinlike proteins found in the liver cytosol fraction obtained from rats receiving different dietary levels of cadmium, finding that at high levels of cadmium intake, a substantial amount of cytosolic cadmium was bound to high molecular weight fractions.

This finding has recently been examined by a group of biochemists at the University of Wisconsin, Milwaukee, under the direction of Dr. David Petering, who found that the high molecular weight protein fractions containing cadmium appear to be polymerized metallothionein. So, in addition to the techniques of handling metallothionein fractions and storing them, we also may find that there is a need to relate metallothionein metabolism to dosage and perhaps to body burden of cadmium.

There is one other comment that I would like to make regarding your suggestion that there may be differences in the accumulation or handling of cadmium by males and females. We have found that this appears to be the case in the rat, and in a recent publication, we have indicated that our data suggest that female rats ingested much more of the water in which we were administering the cadmium than did males. Thus, there was actually a greater intake of cadmium with respect to body size in females than in males.

W. MERTZ (*Beltsville Human Nutrition Research Center, U.S. Department of Agriculture, Beltsville, Md.*): Excuse me for coming back to a different subject. Several people during the past few days have asked me whether I knew anything about interactions of chromium. Well, we certainly don't know enough about it to talk here at the meeting in a paper.

I would like to mention, however, one finding that I think is important. One of the first steps of chromium metabolism is its attachment to transferrin during or after the absorption process and then its subsequent transport to the organs. This is one step at which chromium is subject to many interferences. Theoretically, we know of at least half-a-dozen elements that interact with transferrin, but we also know one element that has been shown to have practical importance, namely, iron.

The one well-documented interaction of chromium is with iron, and this was shown by the group at the radiation lab at Berkeley. Hemochromatotics, that is, people suffering from iron overload, have significantly different metabolic compartments for chromium than do normals. In other words, they have turnover times and pool sizes that are significantly different from those of normals.

This might explain the frequent observation of impaired glucose tolerance in hemochromatotics. As a matter of fact, there is such a thing as diabetes in hemochromatosis. I might also mention the beneficial effects of chromium that have been observed in a few patients with hemochromatotic diabetes: an increased chromium supplementation under these conditions of iron overload seems to help.

J. C. Smith, Jr. (*Beltsville Human Nutrition Research Center, U.S. Department of Agriculture, Beltsville, Md.*): I'm responding to previous comments concerning the composition of experimental animal diets.

The American Institute of Nutrition [AIN] has published recommended vitamin and mineral mixtures for experimental animal diets. Last year we found that some rats fed the AIN vitamin mix over a long-term experiment exhibited hemorrhaging, which was overcome by giving extra vitamin K.

The AIN-suggested mineral and vitamin mix is an attempt to improve our experimental diets. However, many of us are using experimental diets that we have used for many years, and we are loath to change the composition even though it could be improved.

I would also point out that we're concerned that we are feeding 70% glucose or sucrose to get zinc-deficient animals. We are getting some fatty livers and perhaps some dental caries. It is like feeding candy. I think we should look more closely at our experimental diets. Many of the mineral mixtures still in use do not contain zinc, and in some cases, copper has not been added.

H. H. Sandstead: Jim Smith's comments are strongly supported by the work that Forrest Nielsen presented yesterday. Many investigators do experimental studies with so-called purified diets, but almost nobody in this room—with the exception of Nielsen and maybe a couple of other people—has ever attempted to study nickel, arsenic, and vanadium. These people will be in trouble unless they begin to understand the interactions of those elements and what's in their experimental diets, and that opens up a whole new group of things for us to do research on.

J. Parizek (*Czechoslovak Academy of Sciences, Prague, Czechoslovakia*): I should like to make it quite clear that, in my opinion, we are facing two problems. One is that which was taken up by Dr. Smith, dealing with the need to use defined diets—not only in nutritional, but also in toxicological, research. All of us would probably agree that knowledge on the composition of the diets used in experiments is essential and that relevant information, in as much detail as possible, should be given when describing the experimental conditions.

The other problem is, in my opinion, more complicated. What dietary composition should be used in animal experiments aimed at the toxicological evaluation of chemicals, particularly in experiments with long-term exposure to low levels of the chemicals being tested? Should such a diet contain, for instance, optimal or even superoptimal levels of micronutrients?; or would this approach entail the risk of interactions that will mask some of the toxic effects? I should like to make it clear that this does not mean working with clearly deficient diets and on unhealthy animals. To clarify this point, let me use an example—returning to selenium. I apologize for referring back to our own paper instead of using other possible examples, but for the sake of brevity, this is probably the most feasible approach. In the paper we presented to this meeting, we were able to show that different levels of dietary selenium—within the range of intake levels not connected per se with signs of deficiency on the one hand or of toxicity on the other—can very profoundly modify the toxicity of methylated selenium compounds. Assuming that selenium intake could modify the dose-response relationship with some other chemicals in an analogous way, what level of dietary selenium intake should be used when testing those chemicals, the adverse effects of which are known or suspected to be prevented by selenium? Of course, under ideal conditions, more than one dietary level of selenium should be used; but in view of the number of chemicals to be tested, this would add to the already existing burden of long-term toxicological experiments.

The demands on the actual quantitative composition of the diets used in nutritional research and in long-term toxicological experiments might not be identical.

However, I feel that this conference has again shown that the diets used in toxicological experiments should be well defined and acceptable from the viewpoint of present knowledge on nutrition, taking into account also our knowledge of interactions. The problem—so pertinent at present in view of the growing demands for toxicity testing—can be attacked only by joint efforts and through further fruitful, much needed "interactions" of nutritionists and toxicologists.

N. F. SUTTLE (*Moredun Research Institute, Edinburgh, Scotland*): First of all, access to the mike gives me a chance to thank the organizers for inviting me over here and for giving me the opportunity to participate in what for me has been a most stimulating symposium. One thing that strikes me is that looking back over the animal models that we've used, we have been confining ourselves largely to the young, rapidly growing or pregnant animal. Looking around at the audience here, we are all adults and mostly nonpregnant. In Ian Bremner's study, we saw some examples of the different courses that an interaction can take. With the weanling rat, the effects of cadmium and zinc on copper status were additive, whereas in the ewe, they were not additive, and different things were happening in the fetus and the ewe. I think we have to be careful in extrapolating from the very responsive young, rapidly growing animal, which gives us our results and our papers. Somewhere, sometime, somebody should be looking at the chronic effects of trace element exposure and trace element interactions in the adult, nonpregnant animal.

The second general point that I would like to make is that in many of the interactions described, we are dealing with nonspecific effects. Walter Mertz gave us the example of transferrin, which seems to be involved in chromium transport, zinc transport, and iron transport. High zinc intakes depress the absorption of elements as diverse as cadmium, lead, and copper; and when a low calcium diet is fed, we find it enhances the absorption of calcium, lead, and cadmium. This has led to the exasperated response that "everything is interacting with everything" and that in terms of experimentation, we need to put more factors into our experiments. I would like to suggest that if we do this, we will be looking merely at the same basic mechanism of interaction in a number of different ways. It might be better if some of us got down to looking at the common mechanisms of interactions more intensely.

H. H. SANDSTEAD: Thank you, Dr. Suttle. Are there other comments that people would like to make? Dr. Davis, would you like to say something, being the senior member of the group?

G. K. DAVIS (*University of Florida, Gainesville, Fla.*): Thank you for the opportunity. I too would like to thank the organizers for putting together this rather stimulating symposium.

I tried in my paper the second day to indicate that there are at least 6 different situations in which interactions can occur and about 10 different circumstances under which these may be influenced. I agree with Dr. Suttle that we need to look at the common mechanism whereby some of these interactions may occur.

I think that not only the senior citizens are involved but also the, shall I say, adults who are most active; because here again, we find that there are differences in maturity, and we have to look at what has happened in the years past. We do accumulate, but we also excrete; and so we have an opportune situation, especially when we look at human mechanisms.

NUTRITION INTERACTIONS OF GOVERNMENT, ACADEMIA, AND THE PRIVATE SECTOR: CLOSING REMARKS*

D. Mark Hegsted

Human Nutrition Center
U.S. Department of Agriculture
Science and Education Administration
Washington, D.C. 20251

A review of papers presented in this symposium suggests that practically everything has interactions with almost everything. This is probably true, or almost true. The body is a pretty finely tuned machine, and it seems likely that any change in one metabolic process will require adjustments in many others. The topics discussed here have dealt primarily with rather simple interactions of one nutrient with another. There are some 40 essential nutrients now known, and of course, we are not only dealing with essential nutrients. Even at the dietary level, we are concerned with other dietary constituents—fat, fiber, toxic materials, drugs, etc.—and their interactions with essential nutrients and with each other. The number of permutations and combinations of researchable topics is staggering, and it is clear that the significance of interactions depends on the amounts of materials provided. It seems quite certain that these kinds of effects will also depend on the species of animals studied, or that strains of animals and individuals within such strains will demonstrate substantial differences in the way they respond. We have only scratched the surface in this general area of research, but we will probably never have the scientific capability, money, manpower, or facilities to carry it to its logical conclusions.

Obviously, we are not going to throw up our hands and forget about it, but it does have some important implications. Someone has said that if you want to do important research, you have to select an important problem. I would just point out that in a complex area like this, someone has to decide what the important questions are. Many of us were raised in the rather halcyon days when research in the United States, and particularly biological research supported by the National Institutes of Health (NIH), was expanding at a very rapid rate. If I remember correctly, when I was on the nutrition study section, we were funding about 85% of all applications. Almost anyone with a reasonably good idea and with reasonable capabilities could expect his research to be supported. It is not likely that we are going to see those days again.

I would simply emphasize that this means that everyone in the system—the individual researcher, the review panels, whoever makes the ultimate judgment—must keep this in mind. We are all in favor of basic research and argue that the payoff from basic research cannot be predicted. This must be correct, yet judgments about the most useful expenditure of funds must be made. We all understand the weaknesses in the system. The system undoubtedly favors the status quo. That genius out there somewhere may never be discovered or have the opportunity he deserves. The only point I would make is that none of us can defend the position that just because we are scientists, we should be supported and left alone to do our thing. We all have some responsibility to make the system work better, both individually and collec-

* These remarks were presented as a dinner speech at the symposium banquet.

0077-8923/80/0355-0366 $01.75/0 © 1980, NYAS

tively, and we must arrive at a conclusion—a judgment—as to what is or is not important or worthy of further work. Which of the interactions described in this symposium are the important ones?

It is worth pointing out that the judgment on this will change. Research in nutrition has not been well supported for the past 15 or 20 years or so, and there is evidence that this is changing. The public and congressional interest in nutrition is high. If we are smart enough to handle this situation correctly and with some finesse, the opportunities in nutrition research should be greater than they have been for many years. The system does change.

Judgments have to be made not only about what research we should do but about what the research means. When we look at these complex fields and recognize how much we do not know, we are likely to argue ourselves into an intellectual paralysis that prevents us from drawing conclusions. The easiest position for us to take is that we don't know enough, that we need more money and more time, and then we will have the answer. It becomes increasingly clear that that argument won't fly anymore. The congress and the public, who support research, want to know and deserve to know what we have learned and what it means. This is particularly true in nutrition at the moment. The public is smart enough to know that the reason we do research is to change our opinions and conclusions. Otherwise we would not be doing research. They don't expect the final and definitive answer, but they do expect us to interpret our findings so that they can be utilized.

Practically all important decisions are made without an adequate data base. If we knew enough, the decision would be almost automatic. We accept the most far-reaching decisions from the Supreme Court on a five to four vote—not even a statistically significant majority—not because we think they always arrive at the correct decision, but because we recognize that a decision must be reached. Nutrition happens to be "up front" today, and our knowledge must be interpreted for the public. If we are unwilling to make those interpretations, there are plenty of others who are willing to make them.

The complexities of biological interactions are reminiscent of interactions within and between government agencies. Nutrition has to do with what people eat. There are innumerable activities that directly or indirectly affect what people eat. It has been said that there are something like 19 house and senate committees that deal with nutritional topics. It is difficult to decide even what we mean by "nutrition," or by human nutrition research. One interpretation would be that practically all research in the U.S. Department of Agriculture (USDA) deals with food production and delivery, which affects the nutritional status of the public, and thus that practically all research in the USDA is nutritional. At the other extreme, some would conclude that only research dealing with human subjects could be classified as human nutrition research. Neither is acceptable, but some decision has to be made about what we mean by human nutrition research.

However it is defined, one can identify legitimate research efforts in human nutrition at Health, Education, and Welfare, primarily but not solely at NIH and the Food and Drug Administration, in the USDA, the Department of Defense, the Veterans Administration, the National Science Foundation, the National Oceanic and Atmospheric Administration, the National Aeronautics and Space Administration, the Federal Trade Commission, and the Agency for International Development. There may be others. Everyone agrees that there should be some coordination of activities in various agencies to assure effective programs. The issue, of course, is how to do it. The arrangement we have is based partly on historical precedence and partly on the needs and opportunities in the individual agencies. With limited budgets and concerns over the extent of the bureaucracy, there is considerable interest in coordination or simplification of the system, primarily in the interests of efficiency and avoidance of duplication.

In all of this, my major concern is that while we need some coordination of efforts, it is very easy to devote so much effort to coordination that the job the agency should do becomes secondary. Furthermore, much of the coordination is paper thin. One can set up elaborate organizational charts with arrows running all over the place that have very little effect below the people who do the so-called coordination. There is also a tendency to think that consolidation of effort into a single agency will necessarily produce an effective and efficient program. I prefer to argue that the total American system has presumably been based on competition, and the value of competition between individual researchers and agencies also has advantages. We know that if there is any activity where duplication of effort is necessary—indeed, absolutely required—it is in research. We simply can't accept findings of one person or group as valid until they have been repeated. We know that two or more individuals working on exactly the same problem with similar methods do not necessarily produce the same result or conclusion. If there is any place within the government where duplication must be preserved, it is in research.

It would also seem quite clear that nutrition is the legitimate concern of various agencies. They have different needs, different perspectives, and different clienteles. Assigning responsibility to one agency does not guarantee that these perspectives and needs will be adequately covered.

Several government agencies have issued reports upon the state of nutrition research in recent years, including the Office of Science Technology and Policy, the General Accounting Office, and the Office of Technology Assessment. It is noteworthy that although there is broad agreement upon several aspects, there is also disagreement upon priorities among these groups. This further emphasizes the inherent dangers in limiting participation in the research effort.

One of the things that all of these groups did agree on was that given the current interest and emphasis in nutrition, we are not training enough first-class researchers to fill the anticipated needs. It should be clearly emphasized that this need must be filled by the universities and that researchers are trained by doing research. It would seem quite clear to me that although the competitive grants system—pioneered by NIH and the National Science Foundation, and now being incorporated into the USDA—has done an excellent job, it also has weaknesses as the primary mechanism for support of graduate education. Many of us know that when it takes four or five years to train a Ph.D., it is not easy to provide the continuity of support required from a series of two- or three-year grants that may or may not be renewed. Competitive grants are most effective when they supplement a more permanent base of support. I believe that the next major objective we should try to sell to the administration and to congress as we expand the nutrition research effort is some longer range support in the universities. I believe this should be competitive. I would not, for example, favor the provision of x thousands of dollars for every medical school to support nutrition, as some have recommended. But nutrition research, and particularly research using human subjects, which requires a substantial investment in facilities and a varied faculty, cannot be expected to thrive with typical two- or three-year grants. Who, for example, can afford to get into lifetime studies with animals for the study of nutrition and aging, or nutrition and cancer, unless there is some reasonable guarantee of continued support?

So, while I believe that the machinery now in place needs additional support and expansion, the major new interaction that should be developed between government and academia is a system that recognizes the nature of the problems we must attack and the kinds of facilities and support required for this research. One can see some movement in this direction, but it will require additional effort.

Now I have more difficulty dealing with interactions in nutrition between the private sector—industry—and government and academia. Some years ago—for a paper that was never written—I reviewed the papers in several nutrition journals for the past five years. To say the least, the input from industry was discouraging. Although I recognize that much of the research conducted in industry does not get published in such places, I believe it is fair to say that relatively little fundamental nutrition research is conducted by the food industry. What does one make of this in light of the facts that the food industries have responsibility for the nutritional health of the American public, since they provide the food, and that their total sales are over $200 billion per year—in the aggregate, the largest industry in the United States—and some of the larger companies have advertising budgets that exceed the total budget of the Institute of Arthritis, Metabolism, and Digestive Diseases, which has been one of the primary sources of support for nutritional research.

I can find at least two fairly obvious explanations. One is that most nutrition research does not lead to patents. Why should a company spend a lot of money, time, and effort on developing a product that can be duplicated by almost anyone once the work is done? Another reason, I think, is that although research appears to be good public relations for government and academia, it tends to backfire in the food industries. Research done by industry is often labeled as self-serving, whatever the results, so why should they do it? The skepticism about the results is probably justified. Not many of us expect industry to publish data that are, or appear to be, contrary to the best interest of the industry. Academia comes in for similar criticism when it is supported by industry. This must discourage the support of research in universities by industry.

If I understand the administration's position during the immediate past, it has been that the government should not support the kind of research that industry should do, that is, research that will yield a profit to industry. While I don't believe this has had much influence on nutrition research, it has had a substantial influence on the so-called postharvest technology research into food harvesting, processing, and distribution, which is nutrition-related research. While I think this position is understandable, the question that appears unanswered is: What will happen if industry does not perform the research that someone has decided it should perform? Do we simply forget about it? It is not entirely logical for the USDA, for example, to devote a great deal of research to the production of food and other products and then either ignore or leave to others the entire field by which the products are made available to the public.

Dr. Press, the president's science advisor, emphasized recently that there will be a new initiative to emphasize cooperative arrangements between government and industry. He pointed to a joint effort by government and the automobile industry to undertake a long-range research effort to improve the design and efficiency of automobiles. There should be substantial opportunities in food and nutrition for industry, government, and academia in arrangements of this kind to encourage greater expenditure and participation by industry (which I feel they can afford and owe the public), especially in long-range projects of uncertain payoff that the industry cannot be expected to tackle alone.

Whether we look at the biological systems or the organizational systems with which we have to deal, it is obvious that they are complex. No one, I think, will deny that governmental, academic, and industrial activities are appropriate and that each has peculiar responsibilities, although the dividing lines are not clear-cut and will undoubtedly change with time. Research is inevitably inefficient as compared to many other activities because we often do not know what we will find or, in many instances, what we want to find. If we did know, the research would not be required. The current "proposition 13 attitude" in many places endangers research, but it is comforting to see that the president's 1981 budget does provide for substantial increases in research dollars.

There are special opportunities for nutrition research because of widespread public and congressional interest in nutrition. If this support is to be maintained, however, the meaning of our efforts must be interpreted for the public. This is a two-edged sword. On one hand, the broadcast of unconfirmed results or conclusions undermines confidence in the scientific establishment; on the other, there are many who expect to stay in their ivory tower forever, and this undermines confidence in the utility of research. We can only plead for responsibility at all levels to those who ultimately support the research effort—the public.

The ultimate source of all expertise in research is the academic community. This does not mean that they should do all the research, but to my mind, the most urgent problem in nutrition is to establish more efficient and effective academic programs that recognize the nature of the problems we must deal with in human nutrition research.

Another urgent problem, particularly at this time, is to recognize the diversity of the enterprise in which we are engaged. A great many governmental agencies, university departments, and different types of industry have legitimate interests in nutrition and nutrition research. While a reasonable degree of coordination and cooperation is required, it is neither effective nor desirable to avoid apparent duplication in research, nor will the efficiency of the enterprise necessarily be improved by overly ambitious attempts to organize everything sensibly. This does not, of course, deny that the organization should be studied and changes made.

And, finally, I believe there must be serious and continuing efforts to involve the food industries. Although I may stand to be corrected, I believe that much of the talent in these industries is poorly utilized, often in the development of products that have relatively little social merit. The food industries have the ultimate responsibility for the nutritional health of the American public. It is an extremely large, although diversified, industry. The problem is how to improve the interactions of government, academia, and industry and produce a more efficient and effective research system with maximal benefit for the public to which we are all ultimately responsible.

INDEX OF CONTRIBUTORS

(Italicized page numbers refer to comments made in discussion.)